A TEXTBOOK OF ADVANCED ORAL AND MAXILLOFACIAL SURGERY VOLUME 2

Edited by **Mohammad Hosein Kalantar Motamedi**

A Textbook of Advanced Oral and Maxillofacial Surgery Volume 2
http://dx.doi.org/10.5772/58687
Edited by Mohammad Hosein Kalantar Motamedi

Contributors

Mehmet Cemal Akay, Mazen Almasri, Payam Varedi, Shiva Solahaye Kahnamouii, Gholamreza Shirani, Mohammad Hosein Kalantar Motamedi, Roozbeh Kahali, Alireza Tootoonchian, Reza Tabrizi, Barbad Zamiri, Sertac Aktop, Onur Gonul, Hasan Garip, Kamil Göker, Farzin Sarkarat, Mohammadali Ghavimi, Hamid Mahmood Hashemi, Abdolreza Jamilian, Alireza Darnahal, Letizia Perillo, Dragana Gabrić Pandurić, Goran Batinjan, Marko Blašković, Vanja Vucicevic Boras, Anja Baraba, Irina Filipović Zore, Elizabeta Gjorgijevska, Shahram Nazerani, Petr Schütz, Bashar Rajab, Hussein Hassan Hamed Ibrahim, Seied Omid Keyhan, Arash Khojasteh, Peyman Mehriar, Seifollah Hemmat, Jan Rustemeyer, Ata Garajei, Fina Navi, Hossein Behnia, Flaviana Soares Rocha, Rodrigo Paschoal Carneiro, Aparecido Magalhães, Darceny Zanetta-Barbosa, Lair Mambrini Furtado, Marcelo Caetano Parreira Da Silva, Jonas Dantas Batista, Cláudia Jordão Silva, Roberto Bernardino-Júnior, Luis Henrique Araújo Raposo, Koroush Taheri Talesh, Shahram Mehrzad, Mohammad Ghasem Shams, Javad Yazdani, Mohammad Esmaeelinejad, Farzad Aghdashi, Massoud Seifi, Farid Bourzgui, Hakima Aghoutan, Sana Alami, Samir Diouny, Anuja Antony, Katherine Rodby, Ryan Jacobs, Eric Zielinski, Eric Barker, Fereydoun Pourdanesh, Dina Ameen, Mehdi Sezavar, Taghi Azizi

CBS, Edition **2017**

Published by InTech

Janeza Trdine 9, 51000 Rijeka, Croatia

Publishing Process Manager Danijela Duric

Technical Editor InTech DTP team

Cover InTech Design team

Additional hard copies can be obtained from orders@intechopen.com

A Textbook of Advanced Oral and Maxillofacial Surgery Volume 2, Edited by Mohammad Hosein Kalantar Motamedi

p. cm.

ISBN 978-953-51-2035-3

INTECH

open science | open minds

Contents

Preface

I was astonished to find that the first volume of "A Textbook of Advanced Oral and Maxillofacial Surgery" had been extremely well received in the international medical community. I was also surprised to note the numerous testimonials and positive feedback sent to me by distinguished international authors and world renown peers via email; some of which I have listed below:

"Many thanks. Great job!! "

Daniel M. Laskin, DDS, MS, Professor and Chairman Emeritus

VCU Oral and Maxillofacial Surgery, USA

"Thank you for sharing your lovely textbook. "

Edward Ellis III, DDS, MS

Professor and Chair, Oral and Maxillofacial Surgery

University of Texas Health Science Center at San Antonio, USA

" Congratulations for your new book. It looks very interesting. Is there any possibility to send me a hard copy as a gift for my library?"

Georgios E. Romanos, DDS, PhD

Prof. Dr. med. dent. Professor and Associate Dean for Clinical Affairs

Stony Brook University, School of Dental Medicine, NY, USA

"Thank you very much for the opportunity to have a closer look at this great book and congratulations for this successful, tremendous work."

Christoph Kunz MD, DDS, PD

Associate Professor, Oral and Craniomaxillofacial Surgery University Hospital Basel

"I just dowloaded your valuable book. Thank you very much for your contribution and efforts to our speciality of OMFS."

Dr. Zekai Yaman

American Hospital OMFS Specialits Istanbul, Turkey

"I had the chance to quickly review its different chapters which are written in a new format which is different from any other maxillofacial surgery book and I like it very much. Congratulations for this valuable addition to the maxillofacial surgery books."

Professor Ibrahim El-Hakim

Oral and Maxillofacial Surgeon Riyadh Colleges of Dentistry and Pharmacy, KSA

"This interesting book of advanced oral & maxillofacial surgery reflects the effort you spent for this outstanding book."

Dr. Raja Kummoona

Emeritus Professor of Maxillofacial Surgery, Iraq

Having received these emails, I found the incentive and motivation to prepare the second volume. Once again, national and international experts have been invited to submit chapters. I was fortunate in that they accepted the invitation and devoted their valuable time and efforts to contribute to this second volume. Undoubtedly, this text could not have taken shape without the contributions of these specialists. I am indebted to all of them and am obligated hereby to express my sincere gratitude for their support. As all academicians may know, preparing an academic text of this scale is an extremely arduous and painstaking task; it involves working in tandem with an assembly of highly-creative, well-educated, up-to-date and talented individuals. This book is the fruition of those whom, despite their busy schedule and academic obligations, generously spared time to share their knowledge on a global scale.

Volume 2 is the work of over 100 contributors from 9 countries culminating in 14 sections and 35 chapters. The contents of this second volume essentially complement volume one and cover both basic and advanced concepts on complex topics in the field of oral and maxillofacial surgery namely: Advanced Local Anesthesia Techniques and Modifications, Advanced Surgical Orthodontics, Surgical Treatment of Periapical Lesions, Management of Cysts of the Maxillary Sinus, Treatment of Benign Tumors of the Jaws in Children, Immunohistochemistry in Maxillofacial Lesions, Complex Oral and Maxillofacial Infections, Diagnosis and Treatment of Sleep Apnea, Diagnosis and Management of Ankylosis of the Temporomandibular Joint, Diagnosis and Management of Frontal Sinus Fractures, Basics of Endoscopic Oral and Maxillofacial Surgery, Bone grafting and Regenerative Techniques for Implant Surgery, Basic and VSP- CAD/CAM Craniomaxillofacial Reconstruction, Basic and Advanced Rhinoplasty, Advanced Laser Applications and Basics of Craniofacial Surgery.

To conclude, I thank my mother Zakie— my ardent supporter and my father Mohammad Reza, MD, FACS— my mentor. I also thank my wife Maryam— my companion who patiently put-up with me during the lengthy hours while I sat in front of the computer typing-away, sending emails and editing the book chapters 24/7; I would also like to thank my son Mostafa and my daughter Marzieh— both of whom I forgot to thank the last time and Ms. Danijela Duric —Head of Book Publishing at InTech for making all this possible. Again, I hope that the compilation and publication of this text was time well spent; and benefitting all clinicians involved in the practice of Oral and Maxillofacial Surgery.

Mohammad Hosein Kalantar Motamedi, DDS
Professor of Oral and Maxillofacial Surgery
Trauma Research Center, Baqiyatallah University of Medical Sciences,
And Oral and Maxillofacial Surgery Department,
Azad University, Dental Branch,
Tehran, Iran

Section 1

Basic and Advanced Local Anesthesia Techniques and Modifications

Chapter 1

Overview of Local Anesthesia Techniques

Mohammad Ali Ghavimi, Yosef Kananizadeh,
Saied Hajizadeh and Arezoo Ghoreishizadeh

Additional information is available at the end of the chapter

http://dx.doi.org/10.5772/59214

1. Introduction

Down through centuries, efforts have been made to use local anesthesia for treatments. In the ancient times, the Assyrians applied pressure over the carotid artery in order to obtain a certain degree of anesthesia, explaining why this artery is called "the artery of sleep" in the Greek literature. In 1532, the Indians of Peru chewed the leaves of coca shrubs to relieve fatigue and hunger and to produce a feeling of exhilaration. A chemical with some anesthetic property was first introduced in the nineteenth century. A German chemist in 1859, however, reported the anesthetic properties of the coca leaf. In 1859, cocaine was first extracted in its pure form by Albert Neimann, a German chemist. In the mid-1860s, Sir Benjamin Ward Richardson introduced the effect of ether spray for skin anesthesia. Around the same time the adverse effects of cocaine on the mood and psyche were demonstrated. As known today, side effects of cocaine include cardiac stimulation, peripheral vasoconstriction, excitation of the central nervous system (CNS) and addiction. In 1943, lidocaine-the first amide local anesthetic was introduced with greater potency, more rapid onset and less allergenicity as compared to the previously introduced esters.

Pain control in dentistry presents one of the greatest challenges. Pain leads to increased stress, release of endogenous catecholamines and unexpected cardiovascular responses. Before anesthetization, dentists should evaluate the medical history of each patient and document data on the systemic and psychological status of the patients in order to determine whether the patient is able to tolerate the treatment with no risk from the systemic and psychological points of views. Before the injection of the local anesthetic, the dentist should recognize the potential risks. However, most adverse reactions to local anesthetics are not related to the drug itself, but to the injection of the drug. The injection of the local anesthesia is the most reported cause for fear and discomfort of dental patients. Vasodepressor syncope and hyperventilation syndrome are the most common reactions. Others include tonic-clonic spasm, bronchospasm and angina pectoris. Continual research in the field of pain control is still being done in the quest for novel techniques and safer drugs. [1-4].

2. Anatomy

Management of pain in dentistry requires knowledge about the fifth cranial nerve anatomy- the trigeminal nerve. It is the largest of the cranial nerves and has three major divisions: ophthalmic, maxillary and mandibular.

The trigeminal nerve is the major sensory nerve of the face containing both motor fibers for masticatory muscles and sensory fibers. This nerve exits the brain through the area between the pons and the middle cerebellar peduncles.

The ophthalmic branch runs through the lateral wall of the cavernous sinus and, through the superior orbital fissure, enters the orbit, branching again to provide sensation of the lacrimal apparatus, cornea, iris, forehead, ethmoid and frontal sinuses and the nose. The ophthalmic nerve –V1- is the smallest of the three divisions, dividing in to three main branches: the nasociliary, frontal and lacrimal nerves (Figure 1).

The maxillary branch is **the** second branch of the trigeminal nerve – V2 – passes horizontally forward, through the lateral wall of the cavernous sinus, exiting the cranium through the rotundum foramen which is located in the greater wing of the sphenoid bone. Once outside the cranium, this nerve crosses between the pterygoid plates of the sphenoid bone and the palatine bone. As the maxillary nerve crosses the pterygopalatine fossa, it gives off branches to the posterior–superior alveolar nerve, the sphenopalatine ganglion and the zygomatic region. Branches of this nerve continue through the inferior orbital fissure and infraorbital foramen, providing sensation of the maxillary sinuses, upper jaw, sides of the nose and the cheek (Figure 2). [5, 6]

The branches of the maxillary nerve are given off in four regions:

1. **Cranium**
2. **Pterygopalatine fossa**
3. **Infraorbital canal**
4. **Face**

The branch entering the cranium –the middle meningeal nerve– travels with the middle meningeal artery to provide sensory innervation of the dura mater.

Several branches are given off in the pterygopalatine fossa namely the zygomatic nerve, the pterygopalatine nerve and the posterior superior alveolar nerve.

The greater palatine nerve descends through the pterygopalatine canal and through the greater palatine canal emerges on the hard palate, coursing anteriorly between the osseous hard palate and the mucoperiosteum supplying sensory innervation to the bone and palatal soft tissues as far anterior as the first premolar.

The lesser palatine nerve travels along with the posterior palatine nerve emerging from the lesser palatine foramen.

The posterior superior alveolar nerve (PSA) branches from the main trunk of the maxillary division into the pterygopalatine fossa just before the maxillary division enters the infraorbital canal.

The maxillary division (V2) gives off two significant branches namely the anterior superior (ASA) and middle superior (MSA) alveolar nerves.

The ASA nerve – given off from the infraorbital nerve – descends within the anterior wall of the maxillary sinus, providing pulpal innervation of the central and lateral incisors, canine and the sensory innervation of periodontal tissues, buccal bone and the mucous membrane of the gums.

The MSA nerve provides sensory innervation of maxillary premolars and, perhaps, the mesiobuccal root of the first molar, periodontal tissues, buccal soft tissues and the bone and gums in the premolar region.

Branches of the face: through the infraorbital foramen, the infraorbital nerve emerges into the face dividing into its terminal branches: the inferior palpebral, external nasal and superior labial.

The mandibular branch (V3) is considered a motor-sensory nerve innervating masticatory muscles, lower jaw and teeth, parotid and sublingual gland, two third of the tongue and the ear canal and exits the skull through the ovale foramen. The mandibular division: The mandibular division – the largest branch of the trigeminal nerve – descends between the medial ramus and the medial pterygoid muscle, entering the mandible through the mandibular foramen (Figure 2.).

The inferior alveolar nerve has the largest diameter of 2.4±0.4 mm at the lingula.

The anterior division of the V3 branch provides sensory innervation of the cheek, mucous membrane in the buccal of the mandibular molars and motor innervation of the masticatory muscles.

The buccal nerve, passing through the two heads of the lateral pterygoid, reaches the external surface of the lateral pterygoid muscle, continuing in an anterolateral direction.

The auriculotemporal nerve passes through the upper part of the parotid gland crossing the posterior portion of the zygomatic arch.

The lingual nerve travels downward and medial to the lateral pterygoid muscle, lying between the ramus and the medial pterygoid muscle in the pterygomandibular space as it descends. The sensory tract of the anterior two-third of the tongue, the mucous membrane of the mouth floor and mandibular lingual gingiva is provided by the lingual nerve.

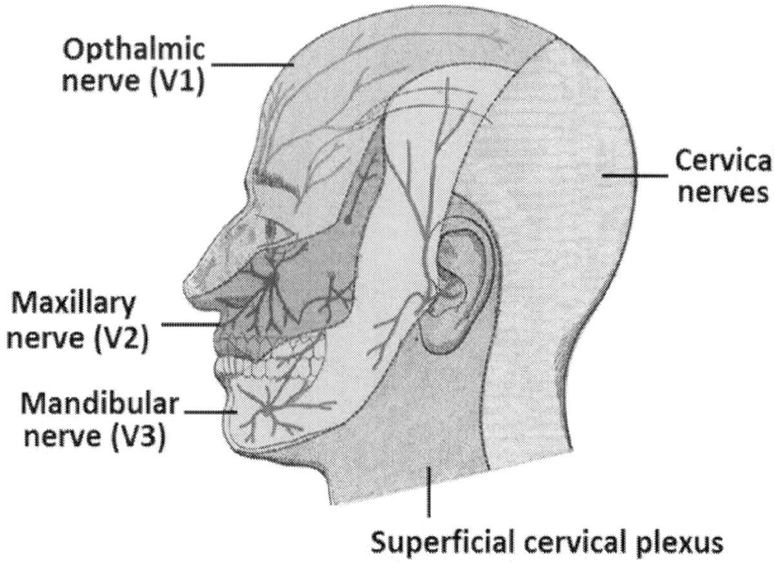

Figure 1. The superficial branches of the trigeminal nerve

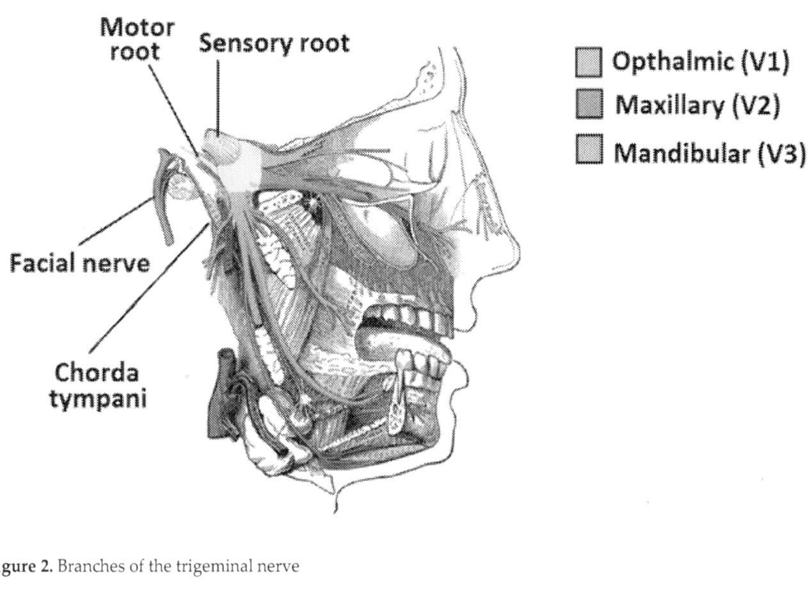

Figure 2. Branches of the trigeminal nerve

The mylohyoid nerve branches off the inferior alveolar nerve just before the entrance of the inferior alveolar nerve into the mandibular canal. This is a mixed nerve providing sensory innervation of the mandibular incisors, and portions of mandibular molars in some. It also provides the motor innervation of the anterior belly of the digastrics and the mylohyoid muscle.

At the mental foramen, the inferior alveolar nerve branches into its terminal branches-- the incisive and the mental nerves:

The incisive nerve, remaining within the mandibular canal, forms a nerve plexus innervating the pulpal tissues of the mandibular first premolar, canine and incisors via the dental branches.

The mental nerve innervates the skin of the chin and the mucous membrane of the lower lip. [1-6]

3. Mandibular anesthesia

There is a great variety of techniques for anesthetizing different regions of the mandible, the most common and useful ones are described in this section.

3.1. Inferior alveolar nerve block

The inferior alveolar nerve block (IANB) is one of the most important and commonly used techniques in dentistry. Unfortunately it is also the most frustrating with the highest percentage of failure even when properly administrated [1].The IANB anesthetizes the IAN (a branch of mandibular division of the trigeminal), incisive nerve, mental nerve and commonly (but not always) the lingual nerve of the injected side. This block effects the sensation of all the teeth on one side of mandible, the bone from the inferior portion of ramus to the midline, the lingual soft tissue and periosteum of the mandible, buccal soft tissues anterior to the mental foramen and anterior two thirds of the tongue and floor of the oral cavity [2].

In one technique, the patient is positioned supine (recommended) or semi-supine. The thumb of the free hand is placed on the coronoid notch retracting the soft tissues. The insertion point of the needle is about 6 to 10 mm above the occlusal plane and at the 3/4 of the anterior posterior distance from the coronoid notch to the pterygomandibular raphe (visual in the oral cavity). The syringe is advanced from across the lower premolar teeth of the opposite side. A long dental needle is used; the bone must be touched while advancing about 25mm of the 35 mm needle into the tissue. After contacting bone the needle is withdrawn slightly, aspiration performed and if negative in two directions 1.5 to 1.8 ml of solution is deposited over a minimum of 60 seconds (Figure 3).. [1]

Two problems occur very commonly with this technique [7]:

1. Contacting the bone too soon: to solve this problem the needle is withdrawn halfway, still remaining in the soft tissue, then the barrel of the syringe is swung over the mandibular

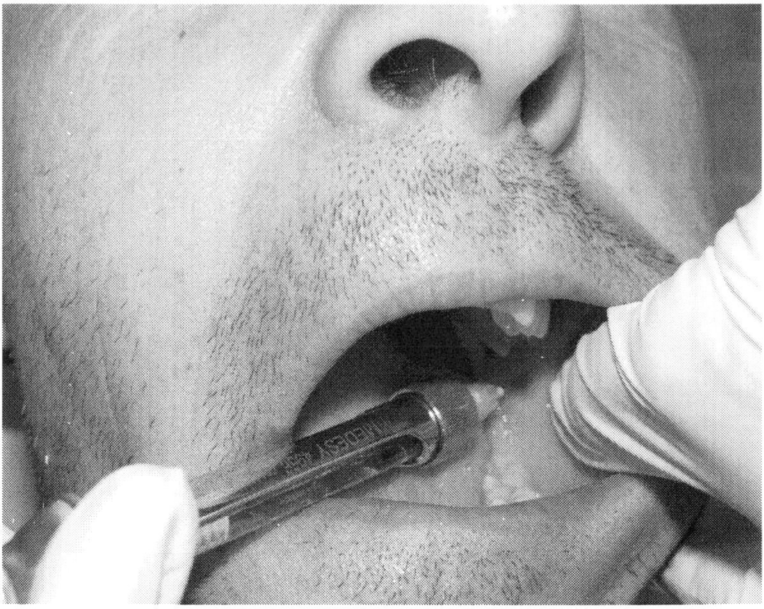

Figure 3. The Inferior Alveolar Nerve Block

teeth of the side being anesthetized, then the needle is advanced about 2.5 mm and the solution is deposited. This is a modification of IANB (the indirect technique) [8].

2. The bone is not contacted after 30 mm of needle insertion: the needle should be withdrawn halfway back then the barrel of the syringe is swung over the molar teeth of the opposite side being anesthetized, and then advanced to touch the bone and then continued as described. When the bone is not touched the solution should not be deposited because the needle could be in the parotid gland near the facial nerve and an injection there could lead to transient paralysis of the facial nerve [1].

One of the most common causes of failure of IANB is depositing the solution too low (below the mandibular foramen) in this case it can be corrected by re-injecting at a higher site, approximately 5 to 10 mm above the previous site.

Mylohyoid nerve is the most common nerve which provides mandible teeth with accessory sensory innervation (most commonly the mesial portion of mandibular first molar). A supplemental injection at the apical region of the tooth in question on the lingual side will solve the problem [9].

Incomplete anesthesia of the central and lateral incisors is due to overlapping fibers of the contralateral inferior alveolar nerve. In this case a supplemental injection with infiltration technique or PDL injection should be done [1].

Olsen reported that in children the mandibular foramen is situated at a level lower than the occlusal plane [10]. Therefore in pediatric patients the injection must be made slightly lower and more posteriorly than for an adult patient.

3.2. Vazirani-Akinosi (closed mouth) mandibular block

Dr. Joseph Akinosi described a close-mouth approach in 1977 [11]. This technique became a successful alternative for inferior alveolar and Gow-Gates mandibular nerve blocks. In 1960 a very similar technique was described by Vazirani, there for the term "Vazirani-Akinosi" is used for the approach. It is also known as "Close-mouth mandibular nerve block" and "Tuberosity approach". Although this technique can be used whenever mandibular anesthesia is desired, its primary indication is in situations where the patient has a limited mouth opening range such as patients with trismus or when spasm of the masticatory muscles on one side of the mandible occur due to several unsuccessful attempt to anesthetize it with IANB, the Vazirani-Akinosi anesthesia approach provides successful anesthesia and a motor blockade (of V3 division of trigeminal nerve) to relieve trismus if it is produced secondary to muscle spasm.

In 1992, Wolfe described a modification of the Vazirani-Akinosi technique, in which the needle is bent at a 45 degree angle to adapt better with the lingual aspect of the ramus. But due to the increase risk of needle breakage this technique cannot be recommended [12]. If the Vazirani-Akinosi technique administered successfully anesthesia of inferior alveolar, incisive, mental, buccal, lingual and mylohyoid nerves is obtained.

For administration of this technique a 25 or 27 gage needle is used. The patient should be positioned supine or semisupine. The index finger or thumb is placed on the coronoid notch reflecting the tissue on the medial side of the ramus laterally. The patient is asked to occlude gently with cheeks and muscles of masticatory relaxed. The syringe is held parallel to the maxillary occlusal plane, with the needle at the mucogingival junction of maxillary third molar (or second molar). The bevel of the needle should be held toward the bone. The needle is inserted to the soft tissue overlying the medial border of the mandible ramus at the point described, and is advanced 25mm (for an average-sized adult) posteriorly and slightly laterally. After negative aspiration in two planes the anesthesia solution can be deposited. Motor nerve paralysis is the first sign to occur so a patient with trismus will notice increased ability to open the jaw. After 1 to 1.5 minute anesthesia of the lip and tongue is noted, and the dental procedure usually can start within 5 minutes.

It is shown in studies that the Vazirani-Akinosi technique has the same success rate of conventional IANB. But with fewer complications and a lower aspiration rate (<10%) [1].

3.3. Gow-Gates mandibular nerve block

In 1973, George Albert Edwards Gow-Gates described a new approach to mandibular anesthesia which he had experience with and reported a success rate of 99% [13]. In this technique the anesthesia solution is deposited on the medial side of the condylar neck just below the insertion of the lateral pterygoid muscles and truly anesthetizes the entire distribution of V3, including the inferior alveolar, lingual, mylohyoid, mental, incisive, auriculotemporal and buccal nerves (in 75% of patients). The Gow-gates technique has a higher success rate and a lower incidence of positive aspiration in comparison to IANB.

In this technique the patient is positioned supine or semisupine and is asked to open his mouth widely, then the syringe, fitted with a long needle, is introduced into the mouth through the corner of the mouth on the opposite side. Insertion point is distal to the second molar and in a height of the mesiopalatal cusp of the second molar. The needle is inserted into the tissue and aligned with the plane extending from the corner of the mouth on the opposite side to the intertragus notch on the side of injection, then advanced about 25mm (two third of the needle) until the bone is touched. Then it is withdrawn about 1mm and after negative aspiration in two directions about 1.8 ml of the solution is deposited. If the bone is not contacted, either the patient has partially closed his mouth or the needle is deflected medially (most common cause). In this situation ask the patient to hold his mouth completely open and after withdrawing the needle half way realign the needle anteriorly by swinging the barrel of the syringe somewhat more distally and then advance the needle to contact the bone and continue the process of anesthesia [1, 9](Figure 4).

Due to greater diameter of the mandibular nerve it may require a larger volume of the anesthesia solution, so if the depth of the anesthesia is inadequate after the first injection deposit up to 1.8 ml in the second injection [9].

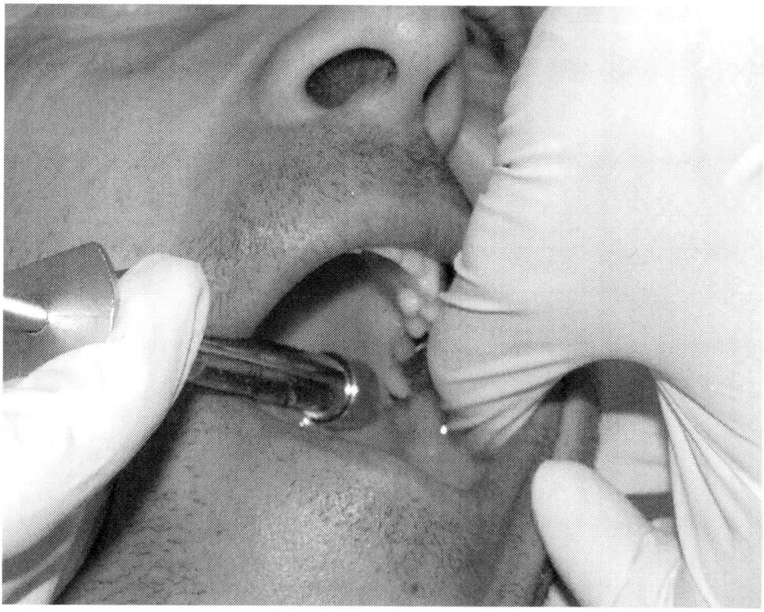

Figure 4. The Gow-Gates technique

3.4. Buccal nerve block

The buccal nerve provides sensory innervation to the buccal gingiva, mucosa and part of the cheek in mandibular molar region. This nerve is consequently not anesthetized during IANB, so if required this nerve most be separately anesthetized. Because the buccal nerve lies immediately beneath the mucous membrane it can be anesthetized easily by depositing about 0.5ml of solution at the coronoid notch (the area distal and buccal to the last molar in the arch). And this nerve block has a success rate of approximately 100% [9].

3.5. Mental and incisive nerve block

The mental nerve and incisive nerve are the terminal branches of the inferior alveolar nerve and provide sensory innervation to the buccal soft tissues lying anterior to the foramen and the soft tissues of the lower lip and chin and those teeth located anterior to the foramen (premolar, canine and incisors) on the injection side. To administer this technique the mental foramen should be located with finger palpation near the apex of the second premolar. The bone immediately around the foramen is rougher to the touch and the patient might feel some soreness when you press your finger against the mental nerve. The needle bevel should be directed toward the bone and the mucosa is penetrated near the mucobuccal fold and the needle is advanced until it reaches the mental foramen, then about 0.6 ml of solution (one third of a cartridge) is deposited. After injection the tissue should be massaged to facilitate entry of the solution into the mental foramen. In the early literature it was emphasized to enter the foramen for a successful nerve block but now it has been shown that this action is completely unnecessary and only increases the risk of damaging the nerve or vessels of the area. Bilateral mental block is very useful when procedures are to be done on anterior or premolar teeth on both sides. [1]

4. Maxillary anesthesia techniques

Different regional blocks and infiltration injections can be used for anesthetizing the maxilla. Some are described herein.

4.1. Supraperiosteal injection (infiltration)

This is the most common technique used for obtaining pulpal anesthesia and is more commonly known as local infiltration. In this technique the patient is asked to partially open his mouth and the syringe is held parallel to the long axis of the tooth. The needle is inserted in the mucobuccal fold above the apex of the tooth and advanced until it touches the bone then withdrawn a little and the solution is deposited at a rate of 30 s/ml (Figure 5). If the solution is deposited while the needle touches the bone the solution is injected below the periosteum which is more painful and may cause post injection discomfort.

This is a very easy technique and has a high success rate but when several teeth require anesthesia or there is an infection or acute inflammation in the area of the injection regional

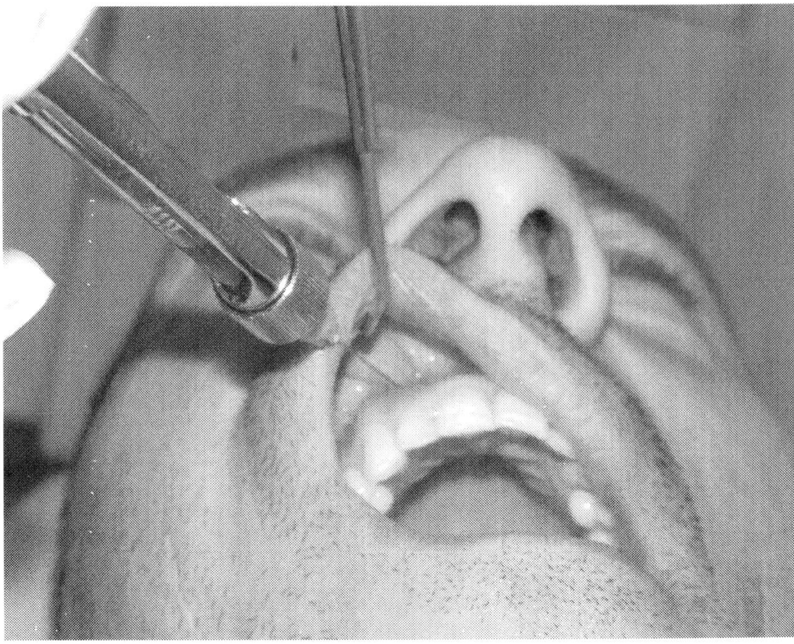

Figure 5. The infiltration technique

nerve blocks are preferred. In pediatric patients infiltration technique can also be used for anesthetizing mandibular primary teeth and in several studies it has been shown that in these patients infiltration technique has a comparable effectiveness to mandibular nerve block for dental procedures [14].

4.2. Maxillary nerve block

The Maxillary (v2) nerve block is an effective method for achieving anesthesia of the hemi-maxilla. With a single injection you can anesthetize all maxillary teeth of one side, buccal periodontium and bone overlying these teeth, soft tissue and bone of hard palate and part of the soft palate, skin of the lower eyelid, side of nose, cheek and upper lip. This nerve can be blocked through several approaches:

4.3. High-Tuberosity approach

The patient is positioned supine or semisupine and the patient's mouth partially open, the mandible is pulled toward the side of the injection and the soft tissues are retracted with the index finger. Then injection is done into the mucobuccal fold distal to the second molar at an angle of 45 degrees; next the needle is advanced posteriorly, superiorly and medially about 30mm and the solution is deposited [9].

4.4. Greater foramen approach

In this approach we attend to insert the needle to the pterygopalatine fissure through the greater palatine foramen and affect the maxillary nerve as it passes through the fossa. We ask the patient to hold his mouth wide open. Palpate the greater palatine foramen medial to the distal aspect of the second molar. Insert the needle at an angle of 45 degree superiorly and distally to the foramen. After advancement about 30mm we deposit the anesthesia solution. This technique is painful and may be dangerous is rarely needed if ever and thus, is not recommended.

4.5. Posterior superior alveolar nerve block

By blocking the posterior superior alveolar (PSA) nerve the molar teeth of maxilla, the associated bone and buccal gingiva will be anesthetized. It is shown that only in 28% of patients the middle superior alveolar nerve provides the mesiobuccal root of the first molar with sensory innervation, in this situation an extra injection (usually infiltration) is necessary to anesthetize the accessory innervations.

To block the PSA, we partially open the patient's mouth and pull the mandible to the side of injection. A short needle is used to prevent distal insertion of the needle which can produce a temporary (10 to 14 days) hematoma. The needle is inserted into the mucobuccal fold over the second molar and advanced about 16mm upwards, inwards and backwards. Then, the anesthesia solution is slowly deposited (Figure 6). [1]

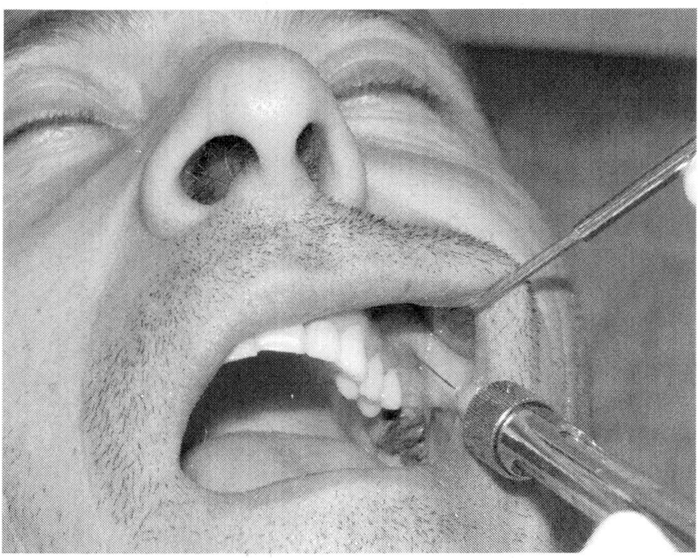

Figure 6. The PSA nerve block

In pediatric patients with primary or early mixed dentition, the thick bone of zygomatic process lies over the buccal roots of the second primary and first permanent molars, attenuating the effectiveness of infiltration injection in this region. So in this situations a PSA nerve block may be used instead [15].

4.6. Middle superior alveolar nerve block

As mentioned before the MSA exist only in 28% of people and provides sensory innervation to maxillary premolars and mesiobuccal root of the first molar. The MSA block is performed by delivering a buccal infiltration at the apex of the second premolar tooth.

4.7. Anterior superior alveolar nerve block

The Anterior Superior Alveolar nerve (ASA) supplies the maxillary incisors and canine teeth on one side and the soft and hard tissue adjacent to it. On the other hand the infraorbital nerve provides sensory innervation to the mucosa and skin surface of one half of the upper lip and part of the skin on lateral aspect of the nose; but because these two nerves can be anesthetized with one approach, the technique is either known as "ASA block" or "Infraorbital nerve block".

To perform this technique we locate the infraorbital foramen; to do so the infraorbital notch is palpated with the index finger then moved downward from the notch, the bone immediately inferior to the notch is convex, which is the roof of the infraorbital foramen, as we continue inferiorly a concavity is felt, this is the infraorbital foramen. When we press against it the patient senses a mild soreness. After the foramen is located we retract the lip and cheek of the patient, a syringe with a long needle is inserted into the mucobuccal fold at the apex of the first premolar. The syringe is held parallel to the long axis of the tooth and is advanced till it reaches near the foramen. The average depth of insertion into the tissue is 16mm (half of the length of a long needle) for an adult of average height. When the needle is in the target area, slowly deposit 0.9 to 1.2ml of the solution. You would be able to "feel" the anesthesia solution as it is deposited beneath the finger on the foramen. Maintain firm pressure with your finger over the injection site for 1 or 2 more minutes to increase the diffusion of the solution into the infraorbital foramen. For decreasing the pain on insertion of the needle and tearing of the periosteum insert the needle with an angled position (away from the bone) and solution is deposit while the needle is advanced through soft tissue [1].It is in no way necessary to enter the foramen.

4.8. Greater palatine nerve block

It is possible to anesthetize palatine tissue by palatal infiltration technique at any place needed but by performing a greater palatine nerve block the posterior portion of the hard palate and the overlying soft tissue anteriorly as far as the first premolar on one side will be anesthetized. The foramen creates a depression in the palate usually distal to the maxillary second molar, which can be located by palpating the area. Deposition of 0.5ml of anesthesia solution in the region of the greater palatine foramen will block the nerve [9].

A very rare complication is ischemia and necrosis of soft tissue of the injection region and it only happens when highly concentrated vasoconstrictor solution is used for hemostasis over a prolonged period [1]. It is in no way necessary to enter the foramen.

4.9. Nasopalatine nerve block

This block anesthetizes the anterior portion of the hard palate (soft and hard tissue) bilaterally mesial to the first premolars. The technique can be performed by depositing 0.2 to 0.5 ml of anesthetic solution adjacent to the incisive papilla. Because the soft tissue in this area is dense, firmly adherent to underlying bone, and quite sensitive the injection in this area is very painful, so several methods are suggested to decrease the pain. One is anesthetizing the dental papilla between centrals labially and inserting the needle through it to the palatal side near the foramen and depositing a little solution to partially anesthetize the soft tissue overlying the nasopalatine nerve before the main injection [1].

4.10. Anterior middle superior alveolar nerve block

This is a relatively new technique, first demonstrated by Friedman and Hochman during development of a computer-controlled local anesthetic delivery (C-CLAD) system [16, 17]. This technique relies on the slow delivery and penetration of anesthetic solution through the porous cortical bone and the nutrient canals.

About 1.4 to 1.8ml of solution (one cartridge) should be deposited very slowly (0.5ml per minute) into the tissue halfway between the palatal midline and the premolar palatal gingival margin. This method is best performed with a C-CLAD. This method blocks the ASA and MSA so it anesthetizes the palate and the teeth anterior to the first molar and adjacent buccal attached gingiva. In studies the AMSA block is shown as effective as multiple maxillary infiltrations [18].

4.11. Palatal anterior superior alveolar nerve block

This method like the AMSA block relies on slow delivery of anesthetic solution via a C-CLAD system and was defined by Friedman and Hochman in the mid1990s [8, 17, 19]. In this approach 1.4 to 1.8ml of solution is deposited in the incisive canal at a rate of 0.5 ml per minute. This block anesthetize the pulp of the incisors and canine bilaterally, facial periodontal tissue associated with these same teeth and anterior hard palate. You should keep in mind that also the injection with a C-CLAD system is not painful but it will take about 3 or 4 minutes which some patients may be reluctant to tolerate.

5. Supplemental anesthesia techniques

These techniques include intraosseous, intrapulpal, intraseptal and intraligamentary methods.

1. **Intraosseous technique:** This is done through a special tool such as X-TIP. The advantages of this method are rapid onset (less than 30 seconds), mild side effects, without the

numbness of the lips and tongue and an atraumatic technique. Contraindications for this method are infection and severe inflammation at the injection area. In this technique, first, a point is recorded distal to the teeth in 2 mm apical to confluence of two lines consisting of a horizontal line from the gingival margin and a vertical line from the interdental papillae. The perforation of the soft tissue and bone is done at this point and the anesthetic drug is injected into the cancellous bone. In this method, depending on the number of teeth ¼ to 1 cartridge is used for the anesthesia. Vasoconstrictors should not be used except where required. The duration of pulpal anesthesia in this technique will be from 15 to 30 minutes [1].Sixon's study in 2008 revealed the effectiveness of this technique as a primary technique. For a total of 181 children and adults, 225 intraosseous injections were done with 4% articaine. The success of this technique was reported to be 95% for primary teeth and 87.9% for permanent teeth and it was shown that the use of this technique could be an appropriate alternative method to classic infiltration anesthetic techniques in children and adults [20]. Wood compared intraosseous and infiltration anesthetic techniques for changes in heart rate and serum concentrations of the drug in 2005. For both techniques lidocaine 2% with epinephrine 1/100000 was used. Pulse oximetery was used to assess heart rate and blood samples were taken to check the amount of lidocaine in the serum. Results showed significant changes in HR for intraosseous compared to the infiltration technique but in the evaluation of lidocaine in serum, no significant difference was found between the two methods [21].

2. **Intraligamentary technique:** Advantages include minimal anesthetic drug requirements, rapid onset and the lack of tongue and lip numbness. This technique can be used as an adjunct method after a nerve block. Contraindications include infection and primary teeth (due to possible damage to permanent teeth). In this technique, a 27 gauge short needle with its long axis parallel to the tooth is inserted at the mesial or distal of the dental root. If the injection is not possible in the mesial or distal surfaces because of tight proximal contacts, it should be applied into the buccal and lingual surfaces parallel with the long axis of the tooth. The infusion rate must be 0.2 ml over 20 seconds. The duration of anesthesia produced by this method is between 5 to 55 minutes [1]. In a 2005 study on 54 patients in whom IAN block did not provided appropriate anesthesia for treatment, it was found that PDL injection provided successful anesthesia in 56% of patients (30 patients) showed this to be a reliable method [22]. A modified technique is recommended for PDL injection with a needle angle of 30 degrees relative to the longitudinal axis of the tooth and the entrance point in the mesiobuccal and distobuccal area; which is a time-tested method (Figure 7) [23].

3. **Intraseptal technique:** This method is indicated when there is a need for pain control and hemostasis of soft and hard tissue simultaneously. Infection in the injection area is a contraindication for this technique. The benefits are similar to the previous techniques. The short duration of pulpal anesthesia and the requirement of the numerous tissue punctures are in the context of its disadvantages. In this technique, a short 27-gauge needle is inserted into the center of the interdental papilla. The entrance point is 2 mm below the tip of the papilla and the direction of the needle will be towards the apex of the tooth. The

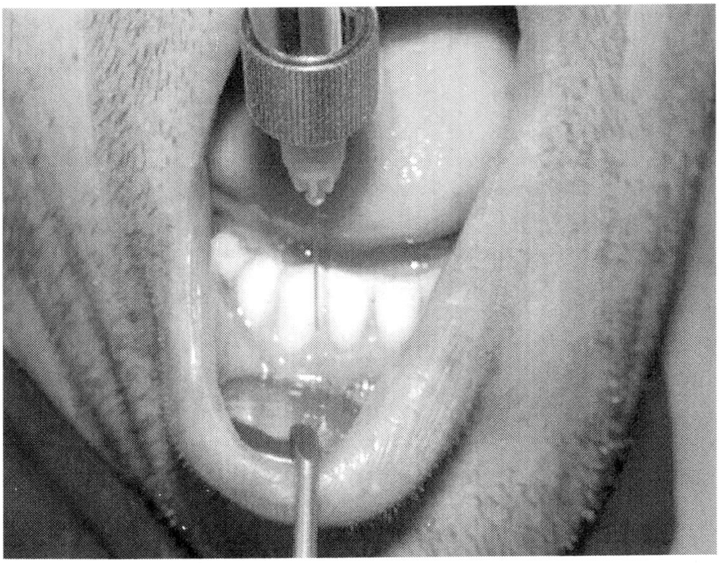

Figure 7. Intraligamentary (PDL) technique

angle of the needle in the frontal plane must be 45 degrees relative to the long axis of the tooth. Then 0.2 to 0.4 ml is injected [1] (Figure 8). This technique can be used for anesthesia in the posterior mandible with dense bone and is comparable to the inferior alveolar nerve block injection [24].

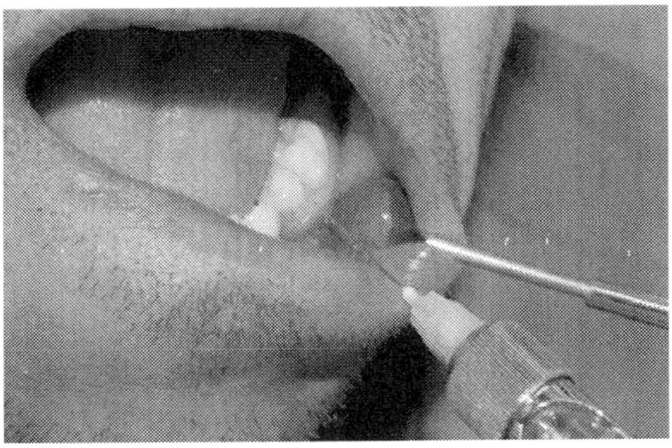

Figure 8. Intraseptal technique

4. **Intrapulpal technique:** In the absence of adequate anesthesia methods, this method can be used for the endodontic treatment of teeth. The benefits consist of fast onset, mild side effects and the lack of lip and tongue numbness. A major disadvantage is that it requires

exposure of the pulp which limits the ability to use this method only in endodontic therapy [1] or in the course of removal of impacted teeth.

5. **Mandibular infiltration technique:** This has a high success rate in children with primary teeth but its success is reduced when children grow and the teeth change from primary to mixed dentition and mandibular cortical thickness increases. Studies have shown that this technique is more successfully with articaine 4% rather than lidocaine 2% but the mechanism is yet unknown. One theory suggests that there is a thiophene loop in articaine that provides greater penetration compared to lidocaine, which has a benzene loop [25].

6. **Topical anesthesia:** The use of topical anesthesia in dentistry or the treatment of laceration is very useful especially in children. The skin needs a larger amount of drugs for topical anesthesia because of less blood supply than mucosa. Due to the poor solubility in water and thus reducing the systemic absorption, benzocaine is the drug of choice for use on mucosal surfaces. Benzocaine Ointment (20%) is used for this purpose. The onset time is 2 to 3 minutes and the duration of anesthesia is 15 minutes. Lidocaine 5% is another common drug in this category with a similar onset and duration of anesthesia to benzocaine. Tetracaine is the strongest surface anesthetic drug that has be presented in a cold spray type in combination with 14% Benzocaine. Tetracaine is also used for endoscopic procedures and gag control [1, 2]. Topical anesthesia will not cause a completely painless injection and that depends more on the needle gauge and duration of the injection. Topical anesthesia will be helpful for periodontal examinations and very conservative treatments [27].

6. New local anesthetics

1. **LMX:** This consists of liposomal capsules containing lidocaine. Liposomes increase lidocaine absorption in a controlled pattern and prevent its systemic toxicity. This drug should be given 30 minutes before surgical intervention on the area in the amount of 1 to 2 mg, sufficient for an area of skin measuring 10 square centimeters [2]. In a study in 2002, liposomal capsules of ropivacaine were compared to EMLA for topical anesthesia of the palatal mucosa during needle entrance into the tissues in which EMLA was significantly more successful than encapsulated ropivacaine [28].Studies have shown that other anesthetic drugs such as bupivacaine provide a greater duration of anesthesia into the liposomal formulation as compared to the normal [29].

2. **EMLA:** This cream is used widely for topical anesthesia to treat laceration and lumbar punctures (Figure 9). This medication contains lidocaine 2.5% and prilocaine 2.5% that penetrate well into tissues due to its micron-sized droplets. Its onset time of action depends on blood supply for the area. On the face it starts to work within 15 minutes. Its maximum depth of anesthesia is 5 mm and can be achieved within 120 minutes. So if more depth is needed we should use the usual anesthetic injection techniques. The amount of 1 to 2 mg of this drug is sufficient for an area of 10 square centimeters of skin and should be placed on the area. At least 1 hour before starting the treatment process. Use of this

http://dx.doi.org/10.5772/59214

medication on the mucosa due to its systemic absorption has not yet been approved [2]. Studies have reported that the analgesic effect of EMLA for periodontal probing and scaling is more than 5% prilocaine ointment. The use of 4 g of EMLA for the creation of analgesia is recommended for the removal of arch bars [30]. The study of Hassio in 1990 showed no difference between 10% lidocaine spray and EMLA for topical anesthesia of the gums. The level of anesthesia at 13-14 minutes measured by EMLA-apparatus was equal in both. The sensitivity of the gums returns to normal within 30 minutes. No toxic reactions were observed but it is said that the absorption of EMLA is faster than lidocaine spray [31].

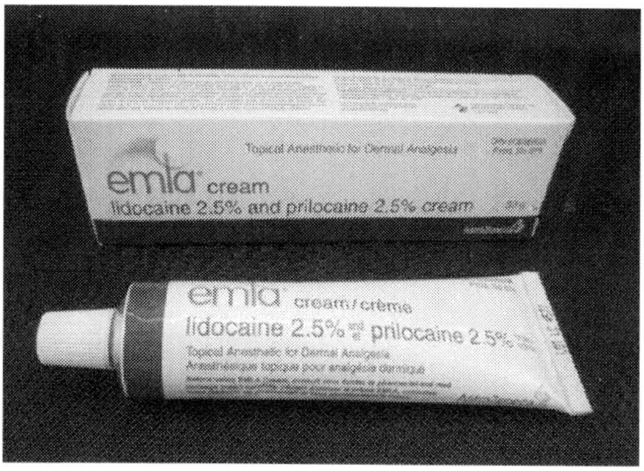

Figure 9. EMLA

3. **LET:** This drug is a combination of lidocaine 4%, epinephrine 0.1% and tetracaine 5% which is available in two types including methylcellulose gel or an aqueous solution. Often used to repair lacerations in children and because of the presence of epinephrine; this drug should not be used in extremities such as fingers, ears or the nose. LET should be given on the area 20 minutes before the start of the treatment and its duration is 40 minutes [2].

4. **Microparticulate formulations:** In this formulation, to increase the duration of anesthesia and reduce the side effects, various drugs and combinations are added to the local anesthetic drugs. For example, the addition of dexamethasone to lipid - protein - sugar particles containing bupivacaine caused the doubling of the nerve block time. These techniques can be used for chronic facial pain or to facilitate physiotherapy in muscle dysfunction [2].

5. **TAC:** TAC is the combination of cocaine 4-11 %, epinephrine 0.025-0.05 % and tetracaine 0.25-0.5 % which begins to work in 10 to 15 minutes and has a duration of 15 to 25 minutes. It can be used to treat children lacerations but has complications such as hypertension, seizures and systemic toxicity [32].

6. **Drug Combination:** The combination of local anesthetic drugs with systemic analgesic drugs such as morphine can reduce the amount of pain during and after the surgery [33]. In general, the combination of opioid with anesthetic drugs reduces the need for analgesics after surgery and increases the duration of anesthesia but has side effects such as nausea and vomiting. The combination of alpha-2 adrenergic agonists such as clonidine, especially with medium-acting anesthetic medications, increases the potential of these drugs. The drug side effects include bradycardia, hypotension and dryness of the mouth, which of course are caused by doses greater than 2 micrograms per kilogram. Ketamine, midazolam and magnesium can increase the power of anesthetic drugs but they must also be considered for their neurotoxic properties. Symptoms such as hallucination and sedation occur following the use of these drugs [34].

7. New techniques

1. **Electronic dental anesthesia (EDA):** This technique is based on the TENS (transcutaneous electronic nerve stimulation) and the electronic waves are used to disrupt neural pain transmission to the brain. Research on this technique continues for use in the dental field [1].
2. **Needle-free injection:** The injection system is based on a piston-pressure system and several systems are introduced such as PED-O-JET, SYRIJET and MED-E-JET. These techniques are widely used for daily injections of insulin in diabetics. In studies, these systems showed less pain compared to conventional injections with a needle gauge of 25 (Figure 10).[1]

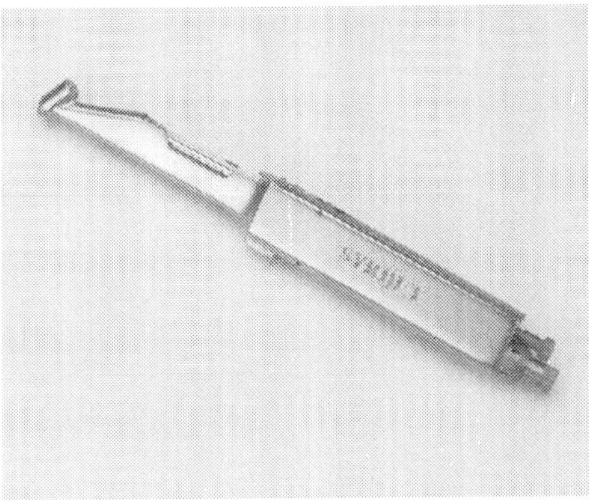

Figure 10. SYRIJET needle-free injection.

1. **Computer controlled injection:** In this technique, computer controls the speed and injection pressure. C-CLADS (computer controlled local anesthetic delivery system) has

less pain and discomfort for patients than conventional syringe injections, but requires greater facilities, more space and higher costs [1].

2. **Ionthophoresis:** This is a new technique for the transdermal administration of lidocaine. In this way, the two external electrodes on the skin are used to make the transition of ionized lidocaine from the stratum corneum layer to the dermis layer to block the nerve ends. Drug penetration rate in this technique is higher than the passive diffusion. The 0.6 to 1 mL of lidocaine 2% with 0 to 4 mA electrical current is used during 10 minutes which causes 5 to 7 mm of drug penetration to the tissue and provides anesthesia [2].

3. **Thermal:** Ice can be used to create a temporary anesthesia for injection or treat small lacerations. For this purpose, the ice should remain on the skin for more than 10 seconds. Ethyl chloride spray as an alternative method can be used for 1-2 seconds, but the duration of anesthesia will be less than caused by ice. These techniques with the saline containing benzyl alcohol are used in hair transplantation [1].

4. **STA system device:** This is an auxiliary system for injection especially made for PDL injections where the dynamic pressure sensory system improves the quality and reduces the side effects of injections. Low-pressure dynamic injection in this technique prevents tissue damage and pain during the injection. In addition, the injected anesthetic drug leakage is detected and prevents creation of an unpleasant taste in the patient's mouth. However, this technique requires the computer system tools [1].

5. **Intranasal local anesthesia:** In the past, the use of nasal mucosa was conventional due to the high blood supply and ability to achieve the systemic effects of drugs. Nowadays for the nasal mucosa and even upper teeth numbness, anesthetic drugs (especially tetracaine) are used on the nasal mucosa. Studies have shown that the use of intranasal tetracaine with a vasoconstrictor such as oxymetazoline can provide tooth anesthesia for the first molar on one side to the first molar on the other side and dental procedures can be performed for the teeth, without need to inject anesthetic drugs [1].

6. **Phentolamine mesylate (Oraverse):** The injectable form of phentolamine (alpha adrenergic receptor antagonist) can be used to terminate drug-induced local anesthesia when it is not required. Especially in high risk populations, where children and the elderly can inadvertently damage the tissues inside the mouth. Soft tissue numbness causes problems with normal functions such as talking, laughing, eating and drinking and can sometimes cause tissue damage. To prevent this situation, a 1.7 mL dental cartridge containing 0.4 mg phentolamine mesylate is used. In this way, the approximate time for the return of normal sensation will be about half. For example, the normal sensation of the tongue will return within 60 minutes with phentolamine mesylate and 125 minutes without it [1].

7. **Electrospun drug-eluting suture:** Contains absorbable sutures with PLGA chemical structures that are combined with bupivacaine. The sutures can slowly release the drug to the surgical site within 12 days and provide appropriate analgesia. Higher concentrations of the anesthetic drug cause a decrease in the suture tensile strength. The suture tissue reaction is comparable to regular PLGA sutures without the combination of anesthetic drugs [35].

8. **Intraoral lidocaine patch (dentipatch):** This patch contains 10-20% lidocaine which is placed on dry mucosa for 15 minutes and provides suitable anesthesia for the mandible and maxilla [36].

9. **Jet–injection:** In this technique, a small amount of anesthetic drug driven into the submucosa without a needle. The air pressure is used for the infiltration of the drug into the mucosa through tiny pores. This method is particularly useful for topical anesthesia for palatal injection [36].

10. **Vibrajet:** It is a device that provides high frequency vibrations in the dental injection syringe which causes a relative decrease in pain during the injection [37].

11. **Accupal:** This is a tool to create pressure and vibration at the injection site. These mentioned irritate the larger nerve fibers and cause the lack of sensitivity during the penetration of the needle [37].

12. **TENS (transcutaneous electronic nerve stimulation):** The result of this method in patient comfort and it provides less pain during the injection. This has been demonstrated especially for IAN nerve block techniques, while topical anesthesia does not cause significant changes to reduce pain during the injection. This technique stimulates the nervous system and it starts before injecting and the pulse rate increases to make a good shake to the patient. The needle is inserted at an area between the electrodes of TENS while generated impulses are continuing at the same level. After withdrawing the injection and removing the needle, pulses are slowly reduced and stopped (Figure 11). [38]

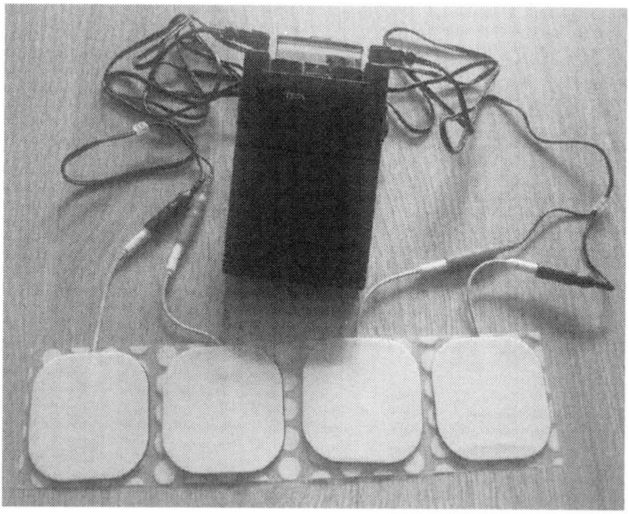

Figure 11. Transcutaneous electronic nerve stimulation

http://dx.doi.org/10.5772/59214

8. Complications

The complications of the injection of local anesthetic drugs can be divided into two parts namely systemic and local complications, explained below.

8.1. Local complications

1. **Pain during injection:** The main reason for this is high-speed injection which can be avoided by injecting each cartridge slowly within a minute. The temperature of the drug also causes pain. The ideal temperature for injection is room temperature. The use of sharp needles, topical anesthesia before injecting and regulating the pH of the drug at 7.4 can help to reduce pain during injection [1].

2. **Trismus:** Its causes include damage to muscles and blood vessels at the infratemporal fossa, damage of the pterygoid muscle, hemorrhage caused by injection and massive volumes of anesthetic drugs. The use of sterile needles, refraining from repeated injections in one area and the use of the minimum effective dose can prevent it. In the case of trismus, it's recommended to use a warm wet towel and physiotherapy for opening the mouth, with the use of anti-inflammatory drugs, analgesics and muscle relaxant drugs such as diazepam. It is important that the patients with continued trismus be referred to a maxillofacial surgeon [1, 2].

3. **Hematoma:** This occurs mostly due to the damage of mental vessels or pterygoid venous plexus. Injections for blocking the inferior alveolar nerve and PSA can cause a large hematoma. The knowledge of the area's anatomy, changes in injection techniques based on patient-specific anatomy and the reduction of frequent needle penetration into the tissues can be helpful in preventing hematoma. Injection for the PSA block is the most common type of anesthetic technique leading to a hematoma. If the hematoma occurs, it is recommended to apply direct pressure on the area, analgesic, anti-inflammatory drugs and placement of ice on the swelling [1]. A study by Bajkin conducted in 2010 showed that there is little risk of hemorrhage and hematoma even in patients taking oral anticoagulant if the correct injection technique is used. Undoubtedly PDL and intraseptal techniques reduce the risk of hematoma more than routine IAN block techniques. Vasoconstrictors and thin needles may help the clinician prevent it [39].

4. **Infection:** This is a very rare complication with contaminated injection needles as the most common cause. The use of sterile needles, disposable cartridges and application of topical antiseptics can be effective in preventing it. Infections have symptoms such as pain and dysfunction. When it occurs, the prescription of antibiotics (penicillin V 500 mg every 6 h for 7-10 days), analgesics, heat, drainage and physiotherapy are recommended for treatment [1, 2].

5. **Breakage of injection needles:** Excessive force during injection, bent needles and unfamiliarity with anatomy are the causes of this rare event. The thin needles (30 gauge) break more often than thicker needles. In case of an accident the patient should be referred immediately to a maxillofacial surgeon. The routes of preventing this in-

clude not using a 30 gauge needle for IAN block injection, not bending the needles, preventing full penetration of the needle into the tissues and precision during injection for young patients or children that can make sudden moves resulting in needle breakage [1].When the needle breakage occurs during the inferior alveolar nerve block injection, it can often be found in the pterygomandibular space, but can migrate to adjacent vital structures and cause damage to them (Figure 12). An unusual case of broken needle displacement during the IAN block injection into the external auditory canal is reported for a 25-year-old woman [40].

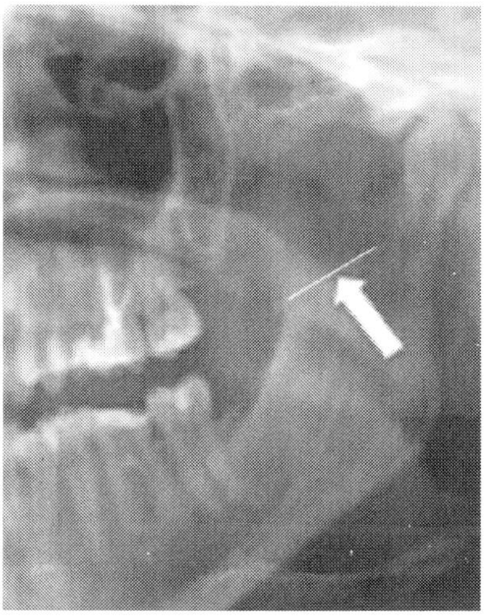

Figure 12. Broken needle shown in the panoramic radiograph

6. **Long-term sensory changes:** This can be due to direct damage to nerves and the contamination of local anesthetic drugs with alcohol that has a neurolytic effect. The most common sensory change is paresthesia. Direct damage is the most common cause of long-term sensory changes, which happens through three mechanisms. Firstly, injury to the nerve fibers. Secondly, the destruction of small vessels in epineurium and the creation of interneural hemorrhage. Finally, the destruction of connective tissue and creation of edema sets in. The dose and concentration of the local anesthetic drugs are contributing factors in this process. According to studies, high concentration drugs such as 4% articaine and prilocaine can cause long-term sensory changes more than other drugs. During injection, the lingual nerve is affected more than other nerves by direct damage. Sensory changes usually resolve within 8 weeks during which the patient should be informed and re-injection of the drug in the affected area should be avoided [2].

7. **Facial nerve paralysis:** Temporary damage to the facial nerve can occur as a result of the spread of local anesthetic drugs to the parotid capsule. Great penetration of the needle in the Akinosi-Vazirani technique or the inappropriate posterior direction of the needle in

the IAN block injection can cause this complication. Prevention is the best cure. When it occurs, inform the patient of the incident, removal of eye lenses and eye protection should be carried out. It must be explained that nerve function will return to normal within a few hours [2].

8. **Soft tissue damage:** After injection, children often bite their lips and cheeks, followed by numbness in these areas (Figure 13). Avoidance of anesthetics with long-term effects, placement of cotton rolls between the teeth and lips, informing the patient to not use warm materials and not bite the oral tissues are effective ways of preventing soft tissue damage. If this happens we need to check for the appropriate use of antibiotics, analgesics and overlying creams on the injury site [1]. In cases of soft tissue injury following numbness, correct diagnosis is very important. Sometimes misdiagnosis causes incorrect treatment such as hospitalization, unnecessary surgical interventions and administration of systemic antibiotics due to improperly suspected bacterial infections. Effective communication between dentists and other medical staffs can help prevent these events [41].

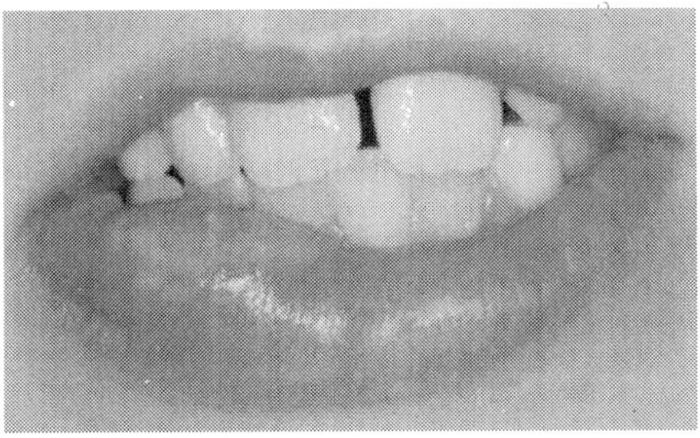

Figure 13. After injection, children often bite their lips and cheeks, because of numbness in these areas.

9. **Burning during the injection:** Burning during injection is a relatively common condition due to low pH and acidity of the local anesthetic with vasoconstrictors, rapid drug injection and contamination of anesthetic drugs with alcohol or sterilizing solutions. To prevent it, the pH of anesthetic drugs should reach 7.4 by buffering the solution before injection. The reduction of injection speed and the maintenance of drugs at room temperature, away from alcohol or sterilizing solution are the other preventing factors. Burning during the injection is transient and does not require specific care [1].

10. **Tissue sloughing:** This occurs due to prolonged use of topical anesthesia drugs or ischemia caused by prolonged use of vasoconstrictor drugs on palatal tissue, of which sterile abscess and epithelial desquamation are symptoms. For prevention, topical anesthetic drugs should only be used for one to two minutes and the use of high concentration vasoconstrictor solutions should be limited. If it occurs, it is not necessary to do anything specific except for pain relief. This condition will resolve spontaneously within 7 to 10 days [1, 2].

11. **Intraoral lesion occurrences after injection:** Recurrent aphthous stomatitis and herpetic lesions originate from this type of lesion that can occur two days after the injection due to the trauma of the needle at the injection site. Treatment will be palliative and the lesions will resolve spontaneously within 7 to 10 days [1].

12. **Eye complications:** Eye complications can occur following the injection of anesthetic drugs in the maxilla and mandible. A permanent loss of vision is reported following a prilocaine injection for tooth extraction in a 73-year-old man prior to surgery for the mitral valve. Visual injury following the injection of anesthetic in dentistry is extremely rare and its mechanism is unknown. A possible etiology is retinal and choroid artery occlusion following the intra-arterial injection which strongly emphasizes the need for aspiration prior to the injection [42]. The next case is a report of paralysis of the right lateral rectus muscle and blurred vision after IAN block and infiltration injections were done in the right maxilla to extract the number 8 tooth in the right mandible and maxilla in a 22-year-old woman who had been normal in terms of systemic health. In this patient, blurred vision and diplopia resolved 6 hours after the injection. The mechanism of this condition is deep anesthetic injections in the retromaxilla, drug diffusion through the greater palatine channel and the lack of the bony barrier between the orbit and this area [43]. In general, the most common ocular complications due to anesthetic injection include: diplopia, mydriasis, eyelids ptosis and abduction disorder and damaged eye. These complications can occur several minutes after the injection and can resolve spontaneously without causing permanent injury and a known mechanism for them is anesthetic drug diffusion to the orbital area [44].

13. **Rare complications:** There are reports of osteonecrosis following the intraosseous injection probably due to the heat of bone drilling done to make a perforation hole for the injection (Figure 14). In addition, systemic disease, such as diabetes and HIV can also have an effect in creating this phenomenon [45].

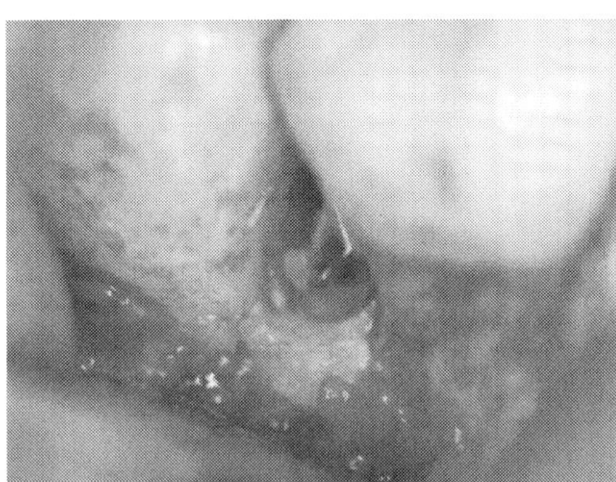

Figure 14. Osteonecrosis following the intraosseous injection

8.2. Systemic complications

1. **Overdose:** Due to a low dose of local anesthetic drugs in dentistry, its prevalence is low. Early symptoms include muscle twitching, shivering, tremor and tonic-clonic seizures. The next symptom that occurs with increased blood toxicity doses is sedation. Respiratory depression and lethargy and ultimately cardiovascular dysfunction will lead to arrhythmias and bradycardia. Some prognostic factors such as very high and very low ages (because of a lower metabolic rate and increase in the half-life of the drug), patient weight, medications (antidepressant, H2 blocker, anti-dysrhythmia drugs), gender (due to the impairment of renal function the risk of overdose increases during pregnancy) and, genetics (genetic deficiency in serum cholinesterase enzyme) should warn us about the risk of overdose. High drug concentration (> 2%), the absence of vasoconstrictors, high-speed injection and the vascularity of the injection area can increase the risk of overdose. Aspiration in at least two planes before the injection, slow injection, dosage adjustment and review of the patient's age, sex, weight, diseases and medications can prevent or reduce the risk of overdose. If the symptoms of overdose occur, the necessary measures are taken including PABCD protocol (position – airway – breathing – circulation – definitive cure). Definitive cures include oxygen prescription, vital signs monitoring, application of anti-seizure medications such as midazolam and stopping the dental procedure. The overdose of vasoconstrictors (such as epinephrine) can result in a rapid increase in blood pressure (primarily in systolic pressure). Tachycardia and cardiac dysrhythmia which will have symptoms such as tremor, anxiety, dizziness, weakness, fatigue and difficulty in breathing may be seen. Treatment will include PABCD protocol, prescription of oxygen (except in hyperventilation) and monitoring of vital signs [2].Unfortunately, a large percentage of dentists do not have enough information about how to determine and calculate the dose of anesthetic drugs (87%) and about 53% of them do not aspirate when injecting [46].

2. **Allergy:** Because of the presence of Para Amino Benzoic Acid (PABA), this occurs more for ester anesthetic drugs. Allergy to an amide local anesthetic drug does not prevent the use of other types of amid anesthetic drugs because the cross-sensitivity to these drugs is not seen. If there is a sensitive reaction to both types of local anesthetic drugs, diphenhydramine solution (0.5 – 1 %) should be used for anesthesia. Allergic reactions include dermatitis, respiratory symptoms (respiratory distress, dyspnea, cyanosis, tachypnea) and generalized anaphylaxis that is a life-threatening condition. Symptoms of anaphylaxis include skin reactions, gastrointestinal smooth muscle spasm (muscle cramps), respiratory distress and cardiovascular collapse. In case of allergies, the PABCD protocol should be implemented. Definitive cure includes prescription of oxygen (5-6 liters per minute), intramuscularly epinephrine in the vastus lateralis with a dose of 0.3 mg for patients weighing more than 30 kg and 0.15 mg for patients weighing less than 30 kg, histamine blocker drugs (50 mg Diphenhydramine or 10 mg Chlorpheniramine), Corticosteroids (100 mg Hydrocortisone) and the cricothyrotomy if needed [2].

3. **Methemoglobinemia:** It occurs due to the oxidation of the iron atoms in hemoglobin by local anesthetic drugs such as prilocaine that causes a defect in the transportation of

oxygen and leads to cyanotic conditions in patients 1 to 3 hours after the injection of anesthesia. The symptoms of cyanosis are created when levels of methemoglobin reach 10 to 20 percent. Increase of methemoglobin levels causes various symptoms such as dyspnea and tachycardia. Children, with methemoglobin reductase and G6PD enzyme deficiency are at a higher risk than other people to methemoglobinemia. The treatment of methemoglobinemia is the intravenous injection of 1-2 mg/kg methylene blue [1].

4. **Malignant Hyperthermia:** MH is determined by the increase in body temperature, muscle stiffness and increased oxygen consumption. The role of anesthetic drugs in the creation of MH is still controversial. This condition is more common in children than adults [2].

5. **Drug interactions:** There are no absolute contraindications to the use of medicinal drugs together with local anesthesia and vasoconstrictors but sometimes there is a need to reduce or adjust the dose of drugs. The chieftains of these drugs are the blood pressure lowering medications. For example, epinephrine in combination with beta-blocker drugs can greatly increase the systolic blood pressure and calcium channel blockers can cause hyperkalemia related to epinephrine. Also beta-blockers reduce hepatic blood flow and decrease the metabolism of anesthetic drugs leading to their increased toxicity [1, 2].

6. **Hemodynamic alterations:** Following the injection of anesthetic drugs in the presence or absence of vasoconstrictors, diastolic blood pressure increases slightly. In the presence of vasoconstrictors, systolic blood pressure increases more than anesthetic drugs without them. Blood glucose increases by administering anesthetic drugs containing vasoconstrictors [47]. However, changes in blood pressure in the presence of an anesthetic were not significant and do not jeopardize the patient's hemodynamics but studies have shown that if you do not inject anesthetic drugs hypertension will be noticeable during dental treatment [48].

Author details

Mohammad Ali Ghavimi*, Yosef Kananizadeh, Saied Hajizadeh and Arezoo Ghoreishizadeh

*Address all correspondence to: m_ghavimi@yahoo.com

Faculty of Dentistry, Tabriz University of Medical Sciences, Tabriz, Iran

References

[1] Malamed SF. Handbook of local anesthesia: Elsevier Health Sciences; 2013.

[2] Fonseca RJ, Frost DE, Hersh EV, Levin LM. Oral and maxillofacial surgery: Saunders Philadelphia, PA; 2009.

spray. The British journal of oral & maxillofacial surgery. 1990;28(2):99-101. Epub 1990/04/01.

[32] Ramamurthi R, Krane EJ. Local anesthetic pharmacology in pediatric anesthesia. Techniques in Regional Anesthesia and Pain Management. 2007;11(4):229-34.

[33] Kaczmarzyk T, Stypulkowska J. Assessment of the effectiveness of peripheral administration of morphine with local articaine anaesthesia for surgery in inflamed oral and maxillofacial tissues. Pain. 2005;115(3):348-54. Epub 2005/05/07.

[34] Biyani G, Chhabra A, Baidya DK. Adjuvants to local anaesthetics in regional anaesthesia e Should they be used? Part II: Cons. Trends in Anaesthesia and Critical Care. 2014:1-6. Epub 2014/05/03.

[35] Weldon CB, Tsui JH, Shankarappa SA, Nguyen VT, Ma M, Anderson DG, et al. Electrospun drug-eluting sutures for local anesthesia. Journal of controlled release : official journal of the Controlled Release Society. 2012;161(3):903-9. Epub 2012/05/23.

[36] Sharma SS, Sharma SA, Saravanan C, Sathyabama. Newer Local Anaesthetic Drugs and Delivery Systems in Dentistry – An Update. Journal of Dental and Medical Sciences. 2012;1(4):10-6.

[37] Saxena P, Gupta SK, Newaskar V, Chandra A. Advances in dental local anesthesia techniques and devices: An update. National journal of maxillofacial surgery. 2013;4(1):19-24. Epub 2013/10/29.

[38] Meechan JG, Gowans AJ, Welbury RR. The use of patient-controlled transcutaneous electronic nerve stimulation (TENS) to decrease the discomfort of regional anaesthesia in dentistry: a randomised controlled clinical trial. Journal of dentistry. 1998;26(5-6):417-20. Epub 1998/08/12.

[39] Bajkin BV, Todorovic LM. Safety of local anaesthesia in dental patients taking oral anticoagulants: is it still controversial? The British journal of oral & maxillofacial surgery. 2012;50(1):65-8. Epub 2010/12/07.

[40] Ribeiro L, Ramalho S, Geros S, Ferreira EC, Faria e Almeida A, Conde A. Needle in the external auditory canal: an unusual complication of inferior alveolar nerve block. Oral surgery, oral medicine, oral pathology and oral radiology. 2014;117(6):e436-7. Epub 2013/10/31.

[41] Chi D, Kanellis M, Himadi E, Asselin ME. Lip biting in a pediatric dental patient after dental local anesthesia: a case report. Journal of pediatric nursing. 2008;23(6): 490-3. Epub 2008/11/26.

[42] Rishiraj B, Epstein JB, Fine D, Nabi S, Wade NK. Permanent vision loss in one eye following administration of local anesthesia for a dental extraction. International journal of oral and maxillofacial surgery. 2005;34(2):220-3. Epub 2005/02/08.

[43] Steenen SA, Dubois L, Saeed P, de Lange J. Ophthalmologic complications after intraoral local anesthesia: case report and review of literature. Oral surgery, oral medicine, oral pathology and oral radiology. 2012;113(6):e1-5. Epub 2012/06/09.

[44] Penarrocha-Diago M, Sanchis-Bielsa JM. Ophthalmologic complications after intraoral local anesthesia with articaine. Oral surgery, oral medicine, oral pathology, oral radiology, and endodontics. 2000;90(1):21-4. Epub 2000/07/08.

[45] Woodmansey KF, White RK, He J. Osteonecrosis related to intraosseous anesthesia: report of a case. Journal of endodontics. 2009;35(2):288-91. Epub 2009/01/27.

[46] Khalil H. Local anesthetics dosage still a problem for most dentists: A survey of current knowledge and awareness. The Saudi Journal for Dental Research. 2014;5(1): 49-53.

[47] Akinmoladun VI, Okoje VN, Akinosun OM, Adisa AO, Uchendu OC. Evaluation of the haemodynamic and metabolic effects of local anaesthetic agent in routine dental extractions. Journal of maxillofacial and oral surgery. 2013;12(4):424-8. Epub 2014/01/17.

[48] Gortzak RA, Oosting J, Abraham-Inpijn L. Blood pressure response to routine restorative dental treatment with and without local anesthesia. Continuous noninvasive blood pressure registration with a finger manometer. Oral surgery, oral medicine, and oral pathology. 1992;73(6):677-81. Epub 1992/06/01.

Chapter 2

Crestal Anesthesia for Dentoalveolar Surgery

Koroush Taheri Talesh, Shiva Solahaye Kahnamouii,
Mohammad Hosein Kalantar, Motamedi,
Shahram Mehrzad and Javad Yazdani

Additional information is available at the end of the chapter

http://dx.doi.org/10.5772/59162

1. Introduction

Predictable anesthesia is an essential requirement for both the patient and the dentist. The patient's opinion about the dental treatment is closely related to the local anesthesia (LA) experience and the proper use of LA techniques and pain management which are indispensable for successful dental treatment. In modern dentistry, creating favorable local anesthesia is an important factor in patient satisfaction and relaxation, the general view of the most successful dentist is one who can do without pain and anxiety for patients. Local anesthesia is a technique that is indispensable for dental professionals. Preventing pain during dental treatment is the ultimate goal of all dentists who are working in their profession. Sometimes problems can prevent them from achieving this goal. These problems include: lack of anesthesia in patients with possible aberrations, inner fears, infections etc. There are many causes for the occurrence of these problems, including: biological diversity in response to medications, anatomical differences between patients and considerable fear and anxiety associated with the injection of local anesthesia. Although this problem may arise in any part of the oral cavity, it most often occurs in the mandibular second molars. In the absence of complete anesthesia, performing dental treatment cannot be done and a significant number of cases of medical emergencies have arisen during dental treatment without LA. Although pain control is accomplished successfully in most cases, some anesthesia techniques like mandibular block are accompanied by drawbacks including difficulty in achieving anesthesia because of anatomic variations, deep and invasive needle penetration, paresthesia, trismus, paralysis, transportation of oral microbial flora to anatomic spaces, delayed onset of anesthesia, hematoma formation, high incidence of positive aspiration, undesired soft and/or hard tissue anesthesia with possible patient-induced injury, and difficulty in hemostasis in those with bleeding disorders. [1]

The inferior alveolar nerve block (IANB) is the most commonly used injection technique for achieving local anesthesia for mandibular restorative and surgical procedures. However, the IANB does not always result in successful pulpal anesthesia. Failure rates of 7 to 75% have been reported in experimental studies.

Supplementary anesthetic injection methods have evolved to circumvent the above disadvantages. These include intrapulpal, intraosseous, intraseptal and intraligamentary injections. Giffin introduced crestal anesthesia (CA) as a new variation of intraosseous anesthesia, which he claimed was tested for different dental procedures ranging from simple restorations to extractions. The technique relies on alveolar crestal perforations formed by canals of Zuckerkandl and Hirschfeld, which provide gingiva with innervation and circulation. Since then some have commented on the technique and approved it. However, to the best of our knowledge, no systematically designed case-controlled study has been done to evaluate its benefits and disadvantages. This chapter assesses our experience with this technique in the mandible.

Mandible anatomy the mandible, the largest and strongest bone of the face, encases the lower teeth. It consists of a curved, horizontal portion, the body, and two perpendicular portions, the rami, which unite with the ends of the body nearly at right angles.

2. Mandibular canal

In human anatomy, the mandibular canal is a canal within the mandible that contains the inferior alveolar nerve, inferior alveolar artery, and inferior alveolar vein. It runs obliquely downwards and forwards in the ramus, and then horizontally forward in the body, under the alveoli and communicates with them by small openings. On arriving at the premolar teeth, it exits via the mental foramen; a small branch known as the mandibular incisive nerve continues to the incisor teeth (Figure 1).

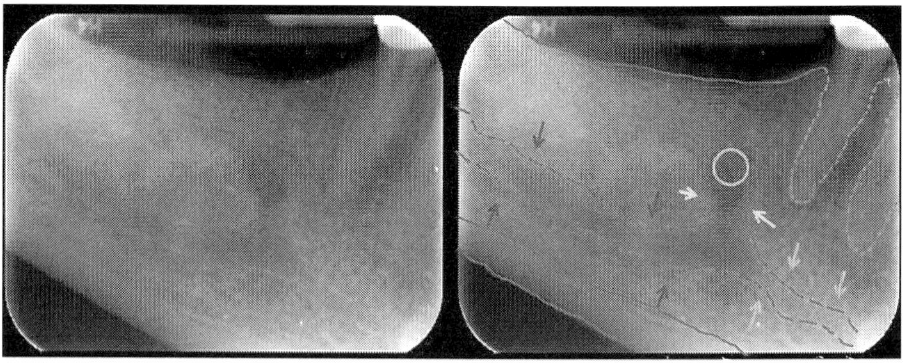

Figure 1. On arriving at the premolar teeth, the IAN exits via the mental foramen; a small branch known as the incisive nerve continues to the incisor teeth through the bone.

The lamina dura is the part of the alveolar bone that lines the socket; it is a thin layer of dense cortical bone called the lamina dura made of immature bone that lies adjacent to the periodontal ligament; lamina dura surrounds the tooth socket and provides the attachment surface which Sharpey's fibers of the periodontal ligament perforate. On an x-ray the lamina dura appears as a radiopaque line surrounding the tooth root. An intact lamina dura is seen as a sign of healthy periodontium. The lamina dura, along with the periodontal ligament, plays an important role in bone remodeling and thus in orthodontic tooth movement. The bone that underlies the lamina dura is cancellous bone. Under the lamina dura is the less dense cancellous bone. Trabeculii are tiny spicules of bone crisscrossing the cancellous bone that make it look spongy. These trabeculii separate the cancellous bone into tiny compartments which contain the blood producing marrow.

The alveolar process is the thickened ridge of bone that contains the tooth sockets in the maxilla and the mandible. It is also referred to as the alveolar bone. The mineral content of the alveolar bone is mostly hydroxyapatite, which is also found in enamel as the main inorganic substance. The buccinator muscle attaches to the alveolar processes of both the maxilla and mandible.

The periodontal ligament (PDL) is a group of specialized connective tissue fibers that essentially attach a tooth to the alveolar bone within which it sits.[1] These fibers help the tooth withstand the substantial natural compressive forces which occur during chewing. It consists of cells, and extracellular compartments of fibers. The cells are fibroblast, epithelial, undifferentiated mesenchymal, bone and cementum cells. The extracellular compartment consists of collagen fiber bundles embedded in ground substance. The PDL substance has been estimated to be 70% water and is thought to have a significant effect on the tooth's ability to withstand stress loads. The PDL is a part of the periodontium that provides for the attachment of teeth to the surrounding alveolar bone by way of the cementum. The PDL appears as the dark space (0.4 to 1.5 mm on radiographs), or radiolucent area between the radiopaque lamina dura of the alveolar bone proper and the radiopaque cementum.

In modern dentistry, providing an efficient and localized anesthesia is a must. The reality is that without anesthesia, one cannot perform safe treatment. In some occasions the anesthetizing techniques are accompanied by some drawbacks especially in mandibular block anesthesia such as: difficulty in achieving anesthesia (due to anatomic variations); deep and invasive needle penetration, paresthesia, trismus, paralysis, transportation of oral microbial flora to anatomic spaces, delayed onset of anesthesia, hematoma formation, high incidence of positive aspiration, undesired soft and/or hard tissue anesthesia with possible patient induced injury and difficulty in hemostasis in patients with bleeding disorders.(3-20)

Supplementary anesthetic injection methods have evolved to circumvent the abovementioned disadvantages. These include intrapulpal, intraosseous, intraseptal and intraligamentary injections. Giffin introduced a new variation of intraosseous anesthesia -Crestal Anesthesia (CA) - which he claimed was tested on more than 6000 teeth for different dental procedures ranging from simple restorations to extractions. The technique relies on alveolar crestal perforations formed by foramina of Zuckerkandl and Hirschfield (17), which provide gingiva with innervation and circulation (Figure 2).

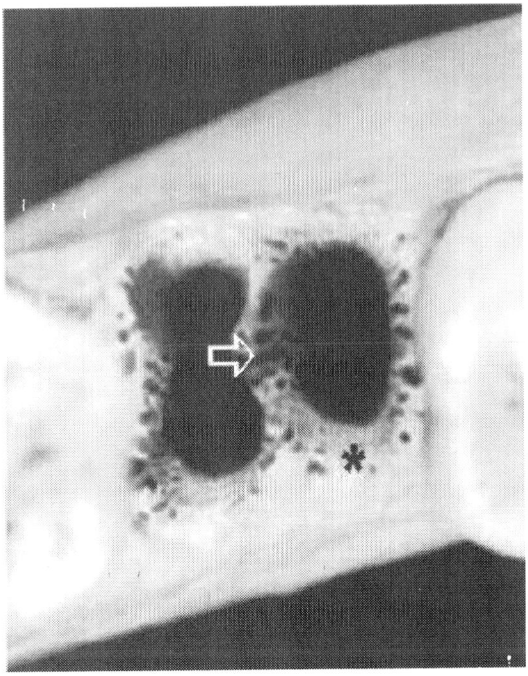

Figure 2. Alveoli of mandibular teeth. Note that the foramina of the nutrient canals are greater both in number and size in the interdental bone (arrow) comparing to marginal bone (*)

Since, then some have commented on the technique and approved it. (9) We also assessed this technique on 69 systemically and mentally healthy individuals between 18 and 47 years randomly selected from patients referring to the department of oral and maxillofacial surgery in Tabriz during 2003-2005. We did a split-mouth case-control clinical trial.

Crestal anesthesia technique: A regular dental anesthetic syringe and a standard short 27 gauge needle are used. Then an interdental gingival papilla is selected adjacent to the tooth or area to be anesthetized. A topical anesthetic agent (in this study benzocaine) is applied with a cotton-tipped applicator and the syringe is positioned so that as the papilla is penetrated, needle bevel and orifice are positioned subperiosteally adjacent to bone and crestal nutrient canals (Figure 3).

Then, using significant pressure the anesthetic agent is injected. This procedure should last at least 20 sec. usually 1/8 of a standard anesthetic cartridge suffices per papilla. One or both of the papilla (in case of inadequate numbness) can be used for the procedure. In this study, we used both papillae to get adequate anesthesia required for extraction. A classic direct Inferior Alveolar Nerve Block (IANB) plus long buccal nerve block was performed on the contralateral side for purpose of comparison. All of the extractions were completed in less than 10 minutes.

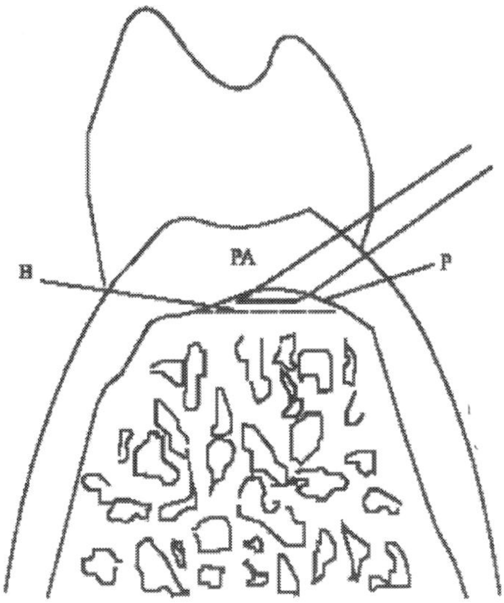

Figure 3. CA technique. Note the pooling of the injectate in subperiosteal area (P). B = alveolar bone, PA =interdental papilla

All had 2 bilateral posterior teeth (premolars, first and second molars) to be extracted. All patients were asked to rate the injection pain based on a scale of 0-5, where 0 represented no pain, 1 mild pain, 2 moderate pain, 3 moderate to severe pain, 4 severe and 5 intolerable pain. The contralateral canine was used as the unanesthetized control to ensure that the pulp tester was operating properly and that the subject was responding appropriately during the experiment. At the beginning of each appointment and before any anesthetic, the experimental tooth and the control canine were tested 3 times using a pulp tester (Gentle-Pulse, Parkell, Farmingdale, NY, USA) to record baseline vitality. The criterion for pulpal anesthesia was an absence of response by the patient to the maximum output (10). To record the changes (increase) of blood pressure an automatic digital blood pressure monitor (Omron HEM-711AC, Omron Healthcare Inc, Bonnockbum, Il, USA) was used. The blood pressure was recorded 5 sec prior to the penetration of syringe's needle to record the baseline blood pressure. Then we recorded the pressure immediately after the injection was initiated terminated and immediately before its termination. Again an average of 2 recordings was used to compare the difference of blood pressure in the 2 techniques. In order to compare, the administered volume of the anesthetic solution, anesthetic cartridges were stamped with milliliter marks and the used volume was recorded. CT scan of the lower jaw after the CA injection (using the mentioned combination of anesthetic solution and radiopaque agent previously tested on rabbits) to show the solution's penetration; the diffusion of the anesthetic solution can be seen in Figure 4 a-e; note the opaque area in the injection site that is a result of the instant diffusion of the injected contrast medium (anesthetic agent + opaque media).

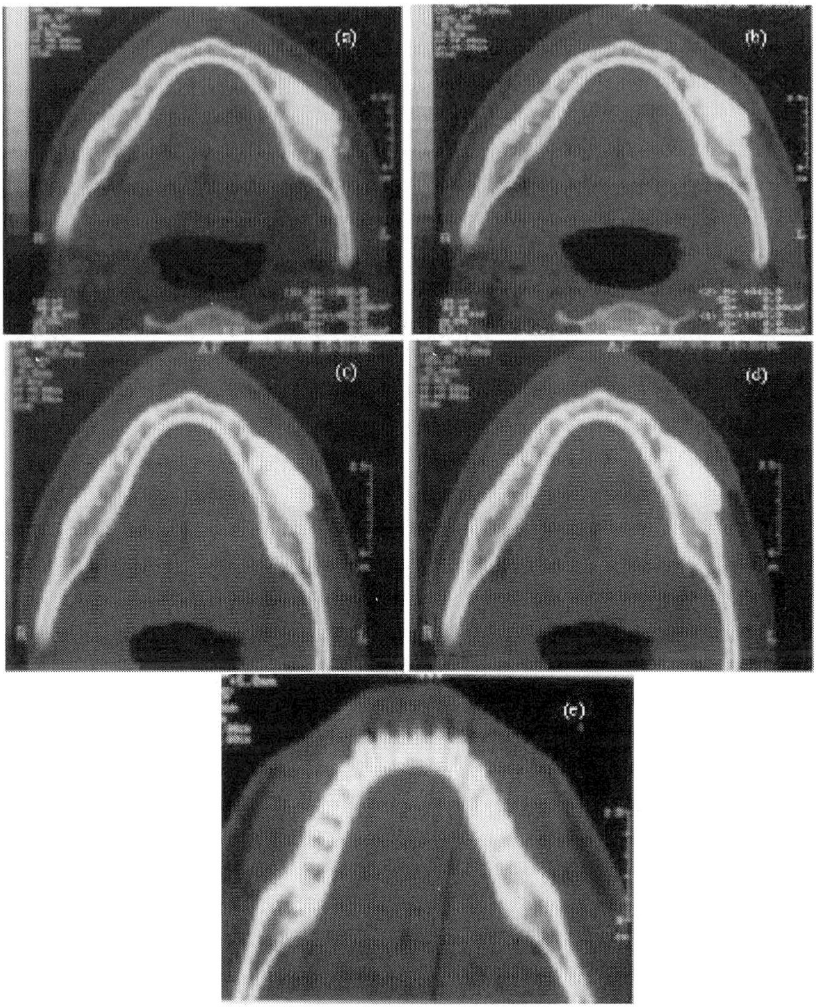

Figure 4. a-e: Penetration of radiopaque contrast media in cancellous bone shows penetration after crestal injection on axial CT scan.

Our study showed there was a statistically significant difference ($p<0.001$) in the onset of anesthesia between CA (7.00+0.71 sec) and IANB (3.30+0.67 min). A statistically significant difference was also present ($p<0.05$) between the duration of anesthesia in CA and IANB which lasted 23.10+2.13 min and 32.10+2.02 min respectively. Thus, the anesthesia was virtually instantaneous for CA and more lasting in IANB. The anesthetic success rates are presented in Table 1.

Tooth	CA	IANB
1st premolar	94 (15)	81 (13)
2nd premolar	95 (21)	81 (18)
1st molar	100 (12)	83 (10)
2nd molar	100 (8)	87 (7)
3rd molar	100 (11)	91 (10)

Table 1. Percentage (No.) of successful anesthesia gained by Crestal Anesthesia (CA) and Inferior Alveolar Nerve Block (IANB) techniques

There were no significant differences in heart rate increase between CA (0.58+0.32 beat min') and IANB (0.97+0.00 beat min') (p> 0.05). Blood pressure increased 0.00+0.07 mmHg in CA and 0.97+0.00 mmHg in IANB. There was no statistically no difference between them (p>0.05). Only about a 5th of an anesthetic cartridge (0.40+0.07 mL) was used in CA. On the other hand, IANB needed about five times more anesthetic solution (1.99±0.06 mL) for initiating the anesthesia. Most of the pain ratings were in the moderate to severe and severe categories for IANB (3.44+0.22) and only in the moderate to severe category for CA (1.45+0.18) and there was a statistically significant difference between them (p<0.001).

The majority of patients receiving CA appreciated not having discomfort and incapacitation often experienced with IANB anesthesia.

One patient with IANB anesthesia developed dry socket she was not a smoker and no other reasonable rationale was found for this occurrence. By the end of three month follow up we found no problems that could be attributed to CA.

3. Conclusion

Although, the CA method or other similar methods of injection such as the intraseptal method (utilizing the alveolar bone nutritional canals) are traditionally considered as supplementary injections, they are successfully used by numerous clinicians as a primary route of anesthetic administration and high success rates of anesthesia and satisfaction both by patients and dentists have been obtained.

The benefits of conventional Intraosseous Injections (I0I) are clearly known. With the advances in this area and introduction of new instruments and techniques patients and dentists benefit from profound anesthesia without unnecessary lip and tongue anesthesia. Unfortunately above facts have not made IOI as popular as the infiltration and block techniques.

Unsuccessful injections in the premolar region may be due to dense cortical bone of mental foramen that acts like a dam and reduces the diffusion rate of anesthetic solution. Also reduced diameter and fewer nutrient canals compared to posterior region may play a role. Reported primary intraligamentary anesthesia success rates of 74-92% were <99% observed in CA. (10)

It seems that the high success rate of CA is due to fast (or even immediate) diffusion of anesthetic agent through the very porous region of the tooth socket.

Longer duration of anesthesia in IANB compared to CA was an expected finding. CA produced duration of anesthesia similar to those of reported intraligamentary injection (2).

Another advantage of CA is its 0% of positive aspiration. The above facts might explain the reason for the statistically lesser readings of blood pressure and the heart (pulse) rate. As with intraosseous types of injections, the CA allows bilateral treatment of mandibular areas without complete mandibular numbness or lack of tongue control.

CA injections penetrate the uncomplicated tissue structures aseptically that probably account for mild post injection discomfort (gingival soreness). The presence of anatomical anomalies such as tori at the proposed site of injection would preclude the dentist from using the CA effectively.

Crestal anesthesia is an efficient, fast, and reliable technique in posterior mandibular dental restorative procedures and may be considered as a reliable and safe primary injection method in posterior mandibular teeth for exodontias or restorative dental procedures.

Author details

Koroush Taheri Talesh[1], Shiva Solahaye Kahnamouii[1*], Mohammad Hosein Kalantar, Motamedi[2], Shahram Mehrzad[3] and Javad Yazdani[1]

*Address all correspondence to: shiva.kahnamouii@gmail.com

1 Tabriz University of Medical Sciences, Tabriz, Iran

2 Trauma Research Center, Baqiyatallah University of Medical Sciences and Azad University of Medical Sciences, Tehran, Iran

3 Private Practice, Country

References

[1] Certosimo, A.J. and R.D. Archer, 1 996. A clinical evaluation of electrical pulp tester as an indicator of local anesthesia. Oper. Dent, 21 (1): 25-30.

[2] Dower, J.S. Jr. and Z.M. Barniv, 2004. Periodontal ligament injection: Review and recommended technique. Gen. Dent, 52 (6): 537-542.

[3] J. Weaver, 1987. An evaluation of electric pulp tester as a measure of analgesia in human vital teeth. J. Endod., 13: 233-238.

[4] Fish, L., D. McIntire and L. Johnson, 1 989. Temporary paralysis of cranial nerves III, IV and VI after a Gow-Gates injection. JADA., 119: 127-30.

[5] Giffin, K.M., 1 994. Providing intraosseous anesthesia with minimal invasion. JADA, 125: 1119-11121.

[6] Goebel, W., 1 983. Multiple techniques of mandibular analgesia. Gen. Dent, 31: 216-220.

[7] Gow-Gates, G., 1973. Mandibular conduction anesthesia: A new technique using extraoral landmarks. Oral. Surg. Oral. Med. Oral. Pathol., 36: 321-328.

[8] Kafalias, M., G. Gow-Gates and G. Saliba, 1 987. The Gow-Gates technique for mandibular block anesthesia: A discussion and a mathematical analysis. Anesth. Prog., 34: 1 42-1 49.

[9] Kama, J.C., 1994. Intraosseous pressure anesthesia. JADA, 125 (11): 1420-1421.

[10] Kaufman, E., L. LeResche, E. Sommers, S. Dworkin and E. Truelove, 1 984. Intraligamentary anesthesia: A double-blind comparative study. JADA, 108: 175-178.

[11] Khedari, A., 1982. Alternative to mandibular block injections through intraligamental anesthesia. Quintessence Int., 2: 231-237.

[12] Kleber, C.H., 2003. Intraosseous anesthesia: Implications, instrumentation and techniques. JADA,134 (4): 487-491.

[13] Malamed, S., 1981. The Gow-Gates mandibular block. Oral. Surg. Oral. Med. Oral. Pathol., 51: 463-467.

[14] Malamed, S., 1982. The Periodontal Ligament (PDL) injection: An 0alternative to inferior alveolar nerve block. Oral. Surg. Oral. Med. Oral. Pathol., 53: 117-1721.

[15] Malamed, S., 2005. Hand Book of Local Anesthesia.5th Edn. Mosby, St. Louis.

[16] Reams, G. and J. Tinkle, 1989. Supplemental anesthetic techniques. J. Ore. Dent. Assoc., 58: 34-39.

[17] Schroeder, H. and R. Page, 1990. The normal periodontium. In: Shluger, S., R. Youdelis, R. Page, R. Johnson (Eds.). Periodontal diseases. Philadelphia: Lea and Febiger, pp: 31-77.

[18] Walton, R., B. Abbott, 1 981. Periodontal ligament injection: A Clinical Evaluation. JADA, 103: 571-575.

[19] Watson, J. and G. Gow-Gates, 1992. Incidence of positive aspiration in Gow-Gates mandibular block. Anesth. Pain Control Dent, 1: 73-76.

[20] Watson, J., 1973. Some anatomic aspects of Gow-Gates technique for mandibular anesthesia. Oral. Surg. Oral Med. Oral. Pathol, 36: 328-330.

Chapter 3

Modified Jorgensen and Hayden Approach to Intraoral Mandibular Anesthesia

Flaviana Soares Rocha, Rodrigo Paschoal Carneiro,
Aparecido Eurípedes Honório Magalhães,
Darceny Zanetta-Barbosa,
Lair Mambrini Furtado and
Marcelo Caetano Parreira da Silva

Additional information is available at the end of the chapter

http://dx.doi.org/10.5772/59163

1. Introduction

There is a wide gap between the success rates of maxillary nerve block anesthesia and inferior alveolar nerve (IAN) block. Clinically acceptable anesthesia in the maxilla rarely represents a problem, except in cases of anatomical abnormality or pathological conditions. [1] For maxillary surgical procedures, in the vast majority of cases infiltration anesthesia is all that is required because the cortical plate of the alveolus of the upper jaw is almost always thin and porous enough to make infiltration anesthesia effective.

Procedures on the lower jaw will most often require nerve block anesthesia of the inferior alveolar, lingual, and buccal nerves. The IAN block is the most commonly used block in dentistry, having widespread applications in all fields of dentistry. Unfortunately, anesthetic block of the IAN has high failure rates, varying between 15% and 35%. [1,2] The high failure rate is frequently attributed to differences in the morphology of the mandibular ramus and also the position of the mandibular foramen, however inadequate technique is the most common cause for failure. [3,4] Specifically, improper mouth opening allows the IAN to stay relaxed preventing the close approximation of the nerve with the medial wall of the ramus. Incorrect anterior, posterior or inferior placement of the needle also leads to failure. Because the target for the conventional IAN block is very near the neurovascular bundle, this technique also has a high frequency of positive aspiration, and intravascular injection is possible. [5]

Achieving excellence in pain control is an intrinsic, yet challenging, goal of dentistry. Traditionally, the inferior alveolar nerve block (IANB), also known as the "standard mandibular nerve block" or the "Halsted block," has been used to provide anesthesia in mandibular teeth. This technique, however, has a success rate of only 80 to 85 percent, with reports of even lower rates. Investigators have described other techniques as alternatives to the traditional approach, of which the Gow-Gates mandibular nerve block and Akinosi-Vazirani closed-mouth mandibular nerve block techniques have proven to be reliable but each of which have merits and draw backs [5].

2. Standard Inferior Alveolar Nerve Block (SIANB)

There are many reasons why the success rate of SIANB is low. One is that the dentist can make mistakes during the technique. These problems are easily resolved by reviewing the anatomical landmarks and the steps to perform the technique involved. Another important reason is the presence of inflamed or infected tissue. Infection areas are acidic, which can influence the beginning of anesthesia. When infection occurs, it is necessary to administer an injection into a deeper location away from infection to avoid this problem. A third reason is that a patient's anxiety often can cause local anesthetic failure. [6] This problem can be solved by the discussion with his fear of injections patient and, if necessary, considering the use of minimal sedation such as that provided by nitrous oxide. Intravascular injection may be another reason for failure because the local anesthetic can be taken away from the site of action. This problem can be avoided by careful aspiration before any injection [7].

Anatomical variability and accessory innervation can also be a problem in providing successful mandibular anesthesia. Once the needle has penetrated the oral mucosa, the dentist is essentially proceeding in a blind mode and assuming that the patient has the same anatomy learned in the dental school. All patients anatomy, however, are not the same and this anatomic variability can lead to failure of SIANB. [8]

Accessory innervation occurs when the main inferior alveolar nerve trunk is not the only source of innervation to the pulp. This accessory innervation may arise from various sources such as a distinct branch from alveolar nerve [8], mylohyoid nerve, as well as the buccal, lingual or auriculotemporal nerves. This situation can be diagnosed when the patient has signs of a successful mandibular nerve block such as a dormant lip, but the tooth is still sensitive when stimulated with a drill [8,9].

Although some researchers report that the success rates for alternative blocks are higher than those reported for SIANB [8,10]' others reported comparable rates [11,12]. However, researchers of the latest study reported that the best rate for SIANB was probably due to the experience of dentists who administer the anesthetic blocks. [12]

The main objective of each block of the mandibular nerve is the inferior alveolar nerve anesthesia, which innervates the pulps of the lower teeth, as well as the buccal periodontium anterior to the mental foramen. This is achieved by depositing the anesthetic within pterygomandibular space. This anatomic space encloses the inferior alveolar nerve and the lingual nerve. The pterygomandibular space also contains the inferior alveolar artery and vein and sphenomandibular ligament. This space is limited laterally by the mandibular ramus, medially and inferiorly by the medial pterygoid muscle, superiorly by the lateral pterygoid muscle,posteriorly by the parotid gland and anteriorly by the buccinator muscle [10,11].

The Gow-Gates and Akinosi-Vazirani methods are indicated when there is anatomical variation or accessory innervation. The Akinosi-Vazirani method is also indicated when the patient has limited mouth opening or whose tongue persistently obstructs the view of the soft-tissue landmarks used in the IANB. These three techniques have similarities, and each has advantages and disadvantages [11].

3. Gow-Gates mandibular nerve block

Gow-Gates initially described what became known as the "Gow-Gates mandibular nerve block" in 1973. The aim of the technique is to place the needle tip and administer the local anesthetic at the neck of the condyle. This is in proximity to the mandibular branch of the trigeminal nerve after it exits the ovale foramen. Before looking inside the patient's mouth it is necessary to establish the extra-oral reference points. An imaginary line is drawn from the intertragus notch (the point immediately inferior to the tragus of the ear) to the corner of the mouth. Then we align the syringe parallel to this plane during insertion.. Inside the mouth, we have to find the bony landmark by palpating the external oblique ridge of the anterior surface of the ramus in the coronoid notch. The temporal muscle attaches onto the coronoid process, and it is important to feel this muscle when inserting the needle. After palpating the landmarks, we must keep the syringe at the correct angle, as determined previously, with the needle tip aiming for the neck of the condyle. The barrel of the syringe usually is over the contralateral mandibular canine or premolars [12,13].

The intraoral insertion point is lateral and superior when compared with that of the SIANB. This point is on the lateral margin of the pterygotemporal depression and just medial to the attachment of the temporal muscle. The upper boundary of the insertion point is the maxillary occlusal plane. Usually, the needle lies just below the mesiopalatal cusp of the maxillary second molar, which can be a reliable landmark [13].

Just before the needle insertion, we ask the patient to open his mouth as widely as possible. The wide opening is critical to the success of this technique. Once the needle is inserted, is moved forward slowly until it contacts bone (the condyle neck). This contact should occur at a depth of 25 millimeters. If bone is not contacted, we should not apply the injection, but instead redirect the needle until we feel the neck of the condyle. Once contact is made, we remove the needle 1mm and administer a full cartridge of local anesthetic after a negative aspiration. We should not administer less than a full cartridge [12,13].

The final position of the needle tip is just anterior to the neck of the condyle, inferior to the lateral pterygoid muscle, lateral to the medial pterygoid muscle and medial to the ramus. The nerves anesthetized by Gow-Gates technique include the inferior alveolar and its branches (incisors and mental), lingual, mylohyoid, auriculotemporal and buccal (about 75 percent of the time). Anesthesia of the mylohyoid and auriculotemporal nerves resolve the concern with accessory innervation, as would be the uppermost position of the anesthetic administration. The gow-gates technique resulted in a rate of about 2% positive suction compared with 10 to 15% SIANB. [1] This rate may be lower because the inferior alveolar vein and artery are further away than the target site are to SIANB [9, 10,12,13].

After the injection is administered, we should ask patients to keep their mouths open for at least 20 seconds, if possible, to keep the inferior alveolar nerve closer to the site of injection and improve onset of anesthesia. The onset of anesthesia is usually five to 10 minutes, which is longer than that for the SIANB (usually three to five minutes) [13].

4. Akinosi-Vazirani closed-mouth mandibular nerve block

Two dentists independently described the closed mouth mandibular nerve block as an alternative to the IANB. In 1977, Akinosi [14] brought this method to the attention of educators, but they soon realized that this technique had been published by Vazirani in 1960. [15] This is indicated particularly if the patient has trismus or the dentist has difficulty seeing the intraoral landmarks used for the SIANB.

What makes this technique unique is that the patient's mouth is closed. The aim is to place the needle tip between the ramus and the medial pterygoid muscle. Since the mouth is closed, seeing the intraoral landmarks can be difficult. A curve at approximately 15° to 30° angle toward the ramus can help minimize the chance of the needle being inserted into the medial pterygoid muscle [15].

Inside the mouth, the bone reference is essentially the same as it is for the SIANB and Gow-Gates methods. We palpate the external oblique ridge of the anterior surface of the ramus and then move the thumb superiorly to palpate the coronoid. The temporal muscle attaches here, and the needle should not enter this sensitive structure. Thus, in a lateral plane, the insertion point is medial to the coronoid process and lateral to the maxillary tuberosity. In superoinferior plane, this insertion point is at the height of the mucogingival junction of the upper teeth, with the tissue retracted laterally, the dentist should insert the needle in a posterior direction [14, 15].

The syringe should be at the level of the mucogingival junction of the upper molars, parallel to maxillary occlusal plane and as close to the maxillary mucosa as possible without touching it. We move the syringe such that the needle moves laterally and posteriorly. Once the needle is inserted 25 mm (for an average adult patient) to stop the advancement of the syringe and administer one full cartridge after a negative aspiration [10,15].

The purpose of using the Akinosi-Vazirani technique is to fill the pterygomandibular space with local anesthetic, bathing the inferior alveolar, lingual and mylohyoid nerves with anesthetic solution. Using Akinosi-Vazirani technique should result in no bony references being hit. The nerves anesthetized by the Akinosi- Vazirani technique include the inferior alveolar and its branches (incisive and mental), lingual, mylohyoid and buccal (approximately 75 percent of the time). A separate buccal nerve block is not needed because successful anesthesia of the buccal nerve is common when this technique is used. The begining of anesthesia is intermediate (five to seven minutes) compared with that of the SIANB and the Gow-Gates technique [10,14,15].

5. Modified Jorgensen & Hayden technique

To achieve mandibular anesthesia, many dentists use an injection technique targeting the mandibular sulcus, similarly described by Jorgensen and Hayden in 1967. [16] This injection remains a proven method for the delivery of local anesthetic safely with minimal discomfort to the patient. However, there are disadvantages associated with standard inferior alveolar nerve block, usually associated with the identification of anatomical landmarks [14,16]. Therefore, we propose a modified Jorgensen - Hayden technique to achieve mandibular anesthesia.

6. Anatomical aspects for modified Jorgensen - Hayden technique

A thorough knowledge of the anatomy of the pterygomandibular space is essential for the successful administration of the inferior alveolar nerve block. Anesthetic solutions deposited low in the pterygomandibular space will not diffuse up to where the inferior mandibular nerve enters the mandibular canal. In addition to the neural aspects of the pterygomandibular space, there are vascular pathways, fibrous tissue elements, muscular structures, and glandular tissue that need to be considered to improve the predictability, effectiveness, and safety of block anesthesia. Greater understanding of the nature and extent of variation in intraoral landmarks and underlying structures should lead to improved success rates, and provide safer and more effective IAN anesthesia.

Pterygomandibular space: The pterygomandibular space is a small fascial-lined cleft containing mostly loose connective tissue. [17] It is bounded medially and inferiorly by the medial pterygoid muscle and laterally by the medial surface of the mandibular ramus. Posteriorly, the parotid gland curves medially around the posterior border of the mandibular ramus to form a posterior boundary of the space, whereas anteriorly, the buccinator and superior constrictor muscles come together to form a fibrous junction, the pterygomandibular raphe. Important structures are positioned in this space: the inferior alveolar nerve (IAN), the inferior alveolar artery (IAA), inferior alveolar vein (IAV), lingual nerve (LN), mylohyoid nerve and the sphenomandibular ligament.

Pterygomandibular raphe: The pterygomandibular raphe (pterygomandibular ligament) is a ligamentous band of the buccopharyngeal fascia, attached superiorly to medial pterygoid plate, and inferiorly to the posterior end of the mylohyoid line of the mandible (Figure 1). It is formed by the junction of the buccinators muscle and pharynx superior constrictor muscle. [16]

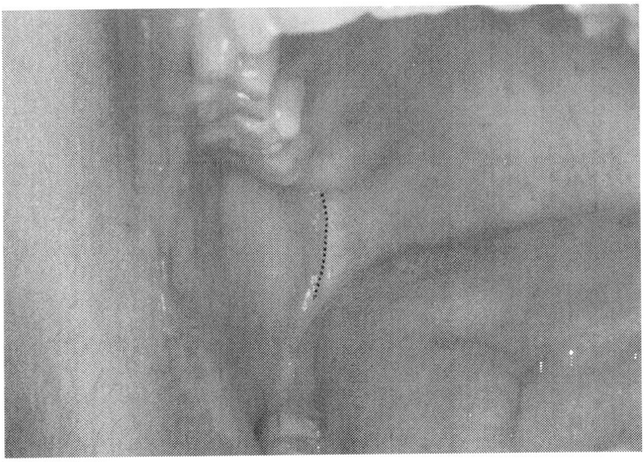

Figure 1. Pterygomandibular raphe location.

Coronoid fossa/notch: The coronoid fossa/notch is the region of greatest concavity of the anterior border of the ramus of the mandible (Figure 2). [1]

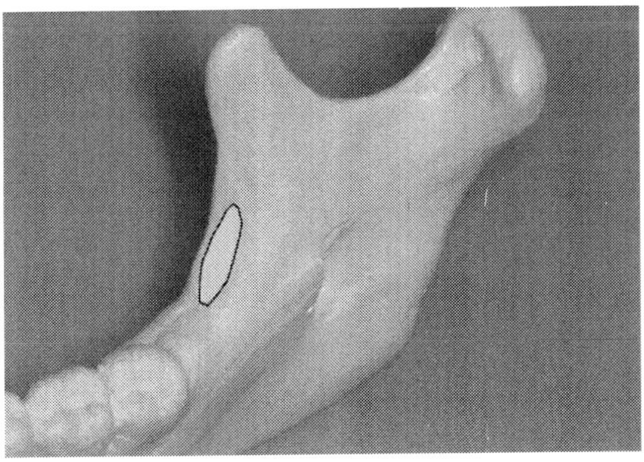

Figure 2. Coronoid fossa location.

Temporal crest: The temporal crest is an extension of the coronoid process, which ends in the retromolar area. [18] An extremely important technical aspect is that on the temporal crest the deep temporal muscle tendon is inserted (Figure 3).

Sphenomandibular ligament: The sphenomandibular ligament is a flat, thin band which is attached superiorly to the spine of the sphenoid bone, and, becoming broader as it descends, is fixed to the lingula of the mandibular foramen. [19] The sphenomandibular ligament has a very important influence on the diffusion of anesthetic solution injected into the area.

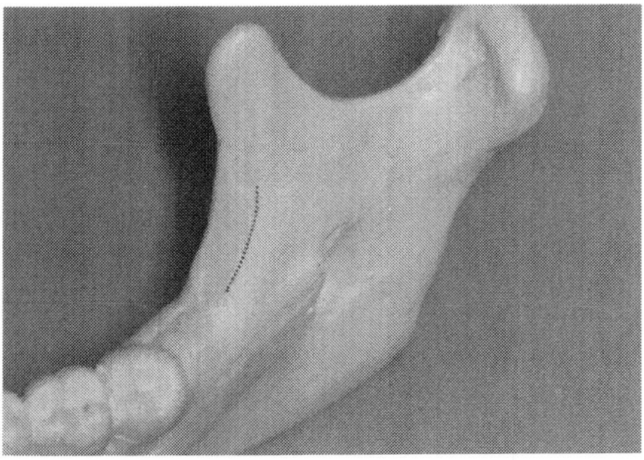

Figure 3. Temporal crest location.

Mandibular foramen: In the center of the medial ramus of the jaw there is a large hole, the foramen of the mandible, which continues inside with the mandibular canal. Serve as a passage way to IAN, IAA and IAV (Figure 4). [18]

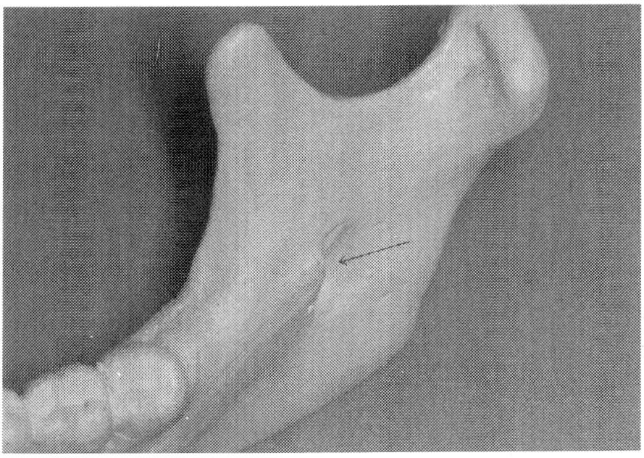

Figure 4. Mandibular foramen location.

Mandibular lingula and mandibular groove: The margin of the mandibular foramen is irregular; presented in front of a prominent ridge, topped by a sharp spine, the mandibular lingula, which gives attachment to sphenomandibular ligament; at its lower and back part there is a notch from which the mylohyoid groove runs obliquely downward and forward, and allocates the vessels and mylohyoid nerve (Figure 5). [19]

Occlusal plane: In 1972 Jorgensen and Hayden [16] reported that if we could trace a line parallel to the occlusal plane, passing through the center of the coronoid fossa, we could reach

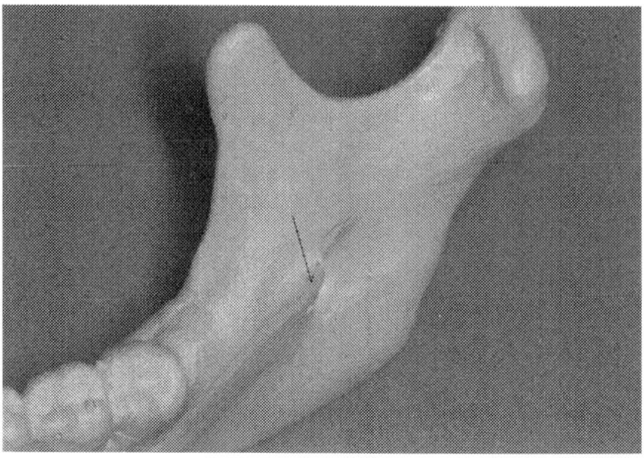

Figure 5. Mandibular lingula position.

a point immediately above the mandibular foramen. According to the literature, a needle inserted 5 mm above the occlusal plane and parallel to it would lie above the lingula in 64% of mandibles and below it in 36%. A needle placed 11 mm above the occlusal plane would be above the lingula in 96% of mandibles. [20]

Contralateral premolars: The premolars on the opposite side of injection are used to help direct the syringe (Figure 6).

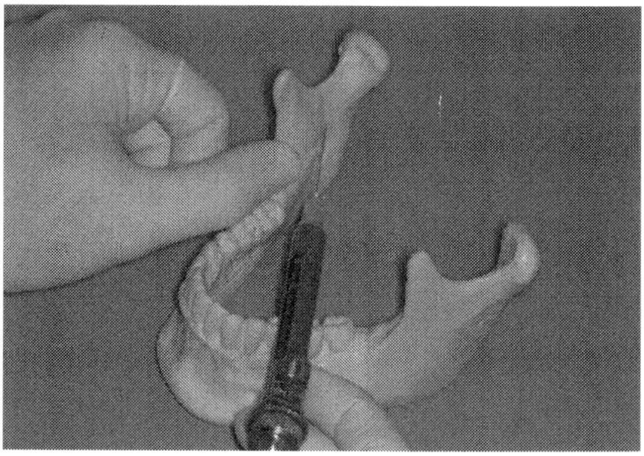

Figure 6. Position of the syringe in relation to the opposite premolar teeth.

7. Modified Jorgensen & Hayden technique

Patient positioning and maintenance of aseptic conditions are prerequisites to avoid complications with local anesthesia. The technique is performed with a long needle gauge (25 mm).

http://dx.doi.org/10.5772/59163

We use the index finger to palpate the point of greatest depression of the Coronoid fossa/notch. This will give us a notion of the height of the puncture. We then move the index finger posteriorly, maintaining the cheek and the deep temporal muscle tendon retraction while feeling the temporal crest (Figure 7).

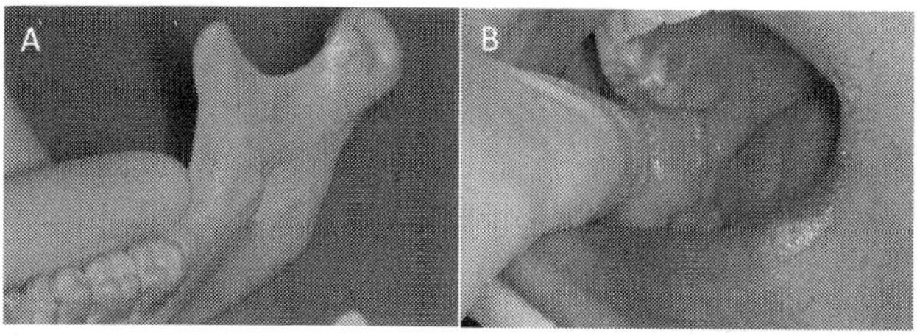

Figure 7. Palpation on the coronoid fossa, delimitating the area of puncture.

This modification is proposed to ensure better delimitation and also narrow the area of puncture, facilitating IAN block. We maintain this position during the technique. The needle is inserted medially to the temporal crest, and laterally to the pterygomandibular raphe. The height of the puncture is center of the fingernail, which corresponds to the center of the Coronoid fossa/notch (Figure 8).

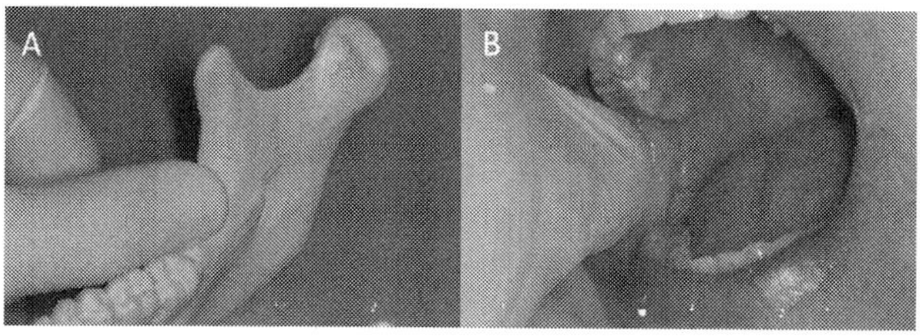

Figure 8. Palpation on the temporal crest.

The syringe is positioned parallel to the occlusal plane and directed between the premolars of the opposite side. The needle is inserted until hitting the bone (Figure 9).

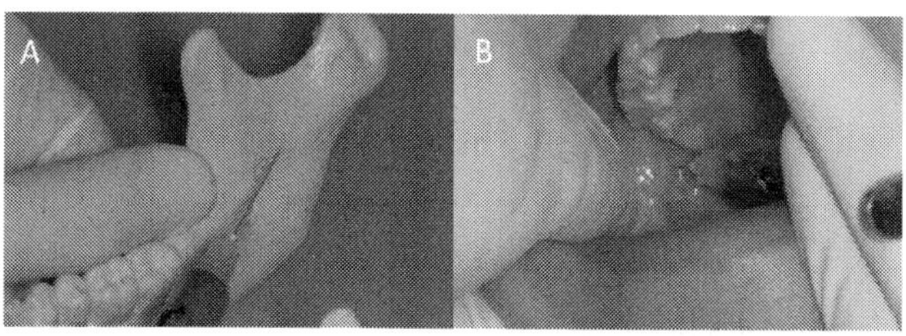

Figure 9. Needle insertion until hitting the bone.

This area is immediately over the mandibular lingula and near the mandibular foramen. The next step is to pull back 1mm to avoid intravascular injection. Then we aspirate and slowly inject almost all of the anesthetic solution. We then withdraw the needle halfway and inject the remainder of the anesthetic solution to block the lingual nerve. The buccal nerve must be anesthetized separately.

8. Discussion

Anatomical knowledge of pterygomandibular region is very important when we want to perform a successfully IAN block. The correct palpation of the coronoid fossa gives us the appropriate height of the puncture and along with other anatomical references, permits the delimitation of a compartment located between the mandible and sphenomandibular ligament. If we respect the anatomic points, the anesthetic solution will be deposited at a point immediately above the mandibular lingula. The proposed modification of Jorgensen - Hayden Technique facilitates the correct puncture. Also, the restriction in the horizontal plane avoids both excessive and insufficient introduction of the needle - a common cause of failures. Another important aspect of this modified technique is the anesthetic block of the inferior alveolar nerve and also the lingual nerve in a single injection.

9. Summary

The anesthesia of the inferior alveolar nerve is a basic procedure in clinical practice and Dentistry. In order to enhance their practice, every contribution is welcome, allowing achieving a higher success rate in implementation. This chapter draws attention to anatomical guidelines that are easily found in all patients, making it a safer and successful procedure.

Author details

Flaviana Soares Rocha*, Rodrigo Paschoal Carneiro, Aparecido Eurípedes Honório Magalhães, Darceny Zanetta-Barbosa, Lair Mambrini Furtado and Marcelo Caetano Parreira da Silva

*Address all correspondence to: flavianasoares.rocha@gmail.com

Department of Oral and Maxillofacial Surgery and Implantology – School of Dentistry - Federal University of Uberlândia, Brazil

References

[1] Malamed SF. Handbook of local anesthesia.Elsevier Editora Ltda. Rio de Janeiro, 2013; 428p.

[2] Gautam A, Madan GA, Sonal G, Sonal G. Failure of inferior alveolar nerve block: exploring the alternatives. J. Am. Dent. Assoc. 2002; 843-846.

[3] Madan GA, Madan SG, Madan AD. Failure of inferior alveolar nerve block: exploring the alternatives. J Am Dent Assoc. 2002 Jul;133(7):843-6.

[4] Perin CP, Suzuki AMM, Fernandes A, Westphalen FH, Schussel JL. Importância das variações anatômicas dos canais mandibulares e suas implicações clínicas. J Bras Clin Odont Int. 2004; 8 (44): 144-6.

[5] Johnson TM1, Badovinac R, Shaefer J. Teaching alternatives to the standard inferior alveolar nerve block in dental education: outcomes in clinical practice. J Dent Educ. 2007 Sep;71(9):1145-52.

[6] Kaufman E, Weinstein P, Milgrom P. Difficulties in achieving local anesthesia. JADA 1984;108(2):205-208.

[7] Palti DG, Almeida CM, Rodrigues Ade C, Andreo JC, Lima JE. Anesthetic technique for inferior alveolar nerve block: a new approach. J Appl Oral Sci. 2011 Jan-Feb;19(1): 11-5

[8] Afsar A, Haas DA, Rossouw PE, Wood RE. Radiographic localization of mandibular anesthesia landmarks. Oral Surg Oral Med Oral Pathol Oral Radiol Endod 1998;86(2): 234-241.

[9] Blanton PL, Jeske AH; ADA Council on Scientific Affairs; ADA Division of Science. The key to profound local anesthesia: neuroanatomy. JADA 2003;134(6):753-760.

[10] Malamed SF. The Gow-Gates mandibular block: evaluation after 4,275 cases. Oral Surg Oral Med Oral Pathol 1981;51(5):463-467.

[11] Aggarwal V, Singla M, Kabi D. Comparative evaluation of anesthetic efficacy of Gow-Gates mandibular conduction anesthesia, Vazirani-Akinosi technique, buccal-plus-lingual infiltrations, and conventional inferior alveolar nerve anesthesia in patients with irreversible pulpitis. Oral Surg Oral Med Oral Pathol Oral Radiol Endod 2010;109(2):303-308.

[12] Robertson WD. Clinical evaluation of mandibular conduction anesthesia. Gen Dent 1979;27(5):49-51.

[13] Montagnese TA, Reader A, Melfi R. A comparative study of the Gow-Gates technique and a standard technique for mandibular anesthesia. J Endod 1984;10(4):158-163.

[14] Gow-Gates GA. Mandibular conduction anesthesia: a new technique using extraoral landmarks. Oral Surg Oral Med Oral Pathol 1973;36(3):321-328.

[15] Akinosi JO. A new approach to the mandibular nerve block. Br J Oral Surg 1977;15(1):83-87.

[16] Vazirani SJ. Closed mouth mandibular nerve block: a new technique. Dent Dig 1960;66:10-13.

[17] Jorgensen NB, Hayden JJr. Local and Sedation Anesthesia in dentistry. 2 Ed. Lea & Febierg Ed. Philadelphia. 1972: 163p.

[18] Berns JN, Sadove NS. Mandibular block injection: a method of study using an injected radiopaque material. J Am Dent Assoc, 1962 Dec; 65: 735-745.

[19] Madeira MC. Anatomia da Face, 7a ed., São Paulo: Sarvier, 2010.

[20] Sicher H, ed. Sicher and DuBrul`s oral amatomy. 5th ed. St. Louis; Ishyaku Euro America; 1998; 273-280.

[21] Ogle OE, Mahjoubi G. Local anesthesia: agents, techniques, and complications. Dent Clin North Am. 2012 Jan;56(1):133-48.

Chapter 4

Novel Modifications in Administration of Local Anesthetics for Dentoalveolar Surgery

Esshagh Lassemi, Fina Navi,
Mohammad Hosein Kalantar Motamedi,
Seyed Mehdi Jafari, Kourosh Taheri Talesh,
Kamal Qaranizade and Reza Lasemi

Additional information is available at the end of the chapter

http://dx.doi.org/10.5772/59235

1. Introduction

The importance of pain management during dental procedures cannot be over-emphasized, but without proper anesthesia, the treatment plan may not be feasible or may result in potential harm to some of the patients. Anesthetic injections should be as painless as possible, especially in the palate which is the most sensitive area of the oral cavity for injection [1].

The conventional nasopalatine nerve block is commonly used to obtain anesthesia in the anterior portion of the palate. The painful nature of this approach, however, has led investigators to seek alternative methods to obtain an anesthesia. Labial infiltration of the maxillary central incisors can be considered an effective anesthetic substitute for procedures of the anterior palate. This chapter presents the anesthetic effect of a modified labial infiltration method for anesthetizing the nasopalatine nerve. The authors have reported this method of labial infiltration to be an effective alternative to the painful conventional nasopalatine nerve block to obtain efficient anesthesia of the anterior palate ($p < 0.001$).

1.1. Modified labial infiltration method to obviate nasopalatine nerve block or lessen pain of injection

1.1.1. Clinical anatomy

Anesthesia of the nasopalatine nerve is a mandatory prerequisite to perform surgical procedures on the soft and hard tissues of the anterior palate and for extraction of upper anterior teeth [1].The nasopalatine nerve passes through the Incisive fossa which is posteroinferior to anterior nasal spine and finally enters the oral cavity via the incisive foramen and innervates the anterior palate, maxillary central incisors and nasal floor (Figure 1). [1-3]

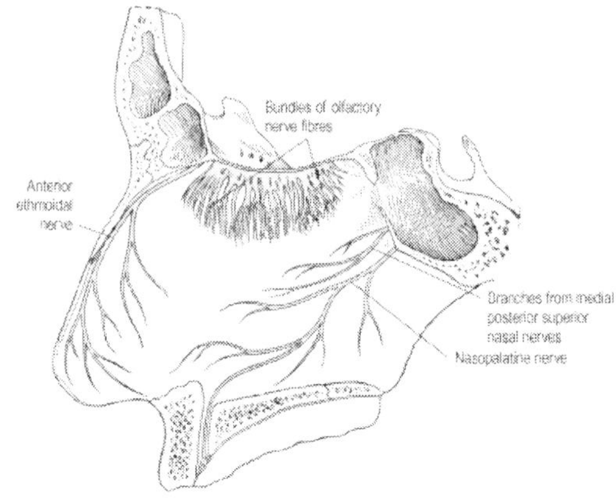

Figure 1. Diagram of the nasopalatine and surrounding nerves

Labial tissues are anaesthetized by labial infiltration. Obtaining anesthesia for the relevant palatal soft tissue is however, not possible this way and necessitates direct injection of an anesthetic agent in the palatal area (incisive papilla). Palatal soft tissues, especially in the vicinity of the hard palate, are tightly attached to the underlying bone. Injection in this area is thus, painful when the conventional method for injecting the anesthetic agent directly into or aside the incisive papilla is used [4].Therefore removal of maxillary teeth without a palatal injection is desirable.

1.2. Technique

In this technique two injections at two sites should be done.

1. Anesthesia of the maxillary hard and soft tissue of the labial area is obtained by injection of 1 cc of local anesthetic agent in the labial vestibule, with the syringe parallel to the long axis of the lateral incisor tooth and the needle bevel toward the bone. This is a nerve block because local anesthetic is deposited close to the main nerve trunk [2] (Figures 2, 3 and 4).With this injection the canine, lateral incisor, central incisors, hard and soft tissue of the alveolar area to the midline are anesthetized.

2. After 2-3 minutes and relative anesthesia of the labial area, infiltration of about 0.6 ml of the remaining solution is administered via a needle inserted superior to the apices of central incisors in the vicinity of the superior border of the base of the anterior nasal spine near the nasal floor at a 45 degree angle to the long axis of the central incisor, to obtain anesthesia in the anterior palate (Figure 5).

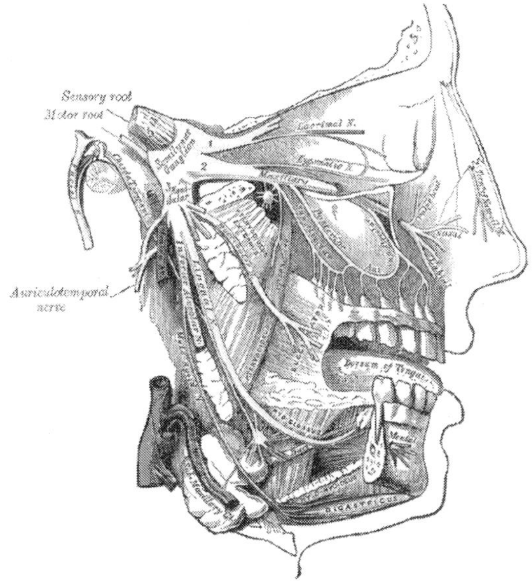

Figure 2. Diagram of the nasopalatine and surrounding nerves (from Gray's Anatomy, 37th Ed.).

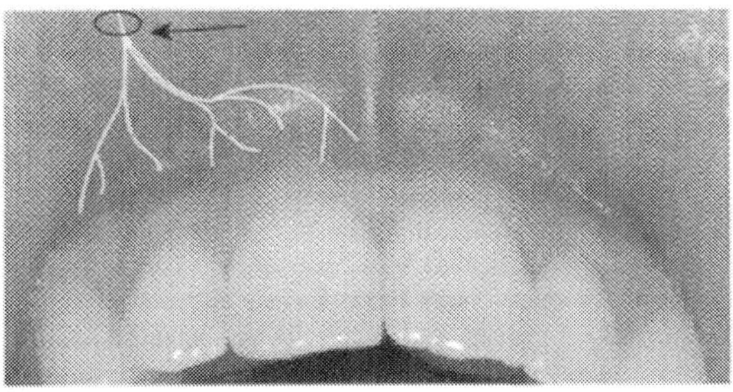

Figure 3. Nerve block (from Malamed 2013, 5th ed.)

Five to six minutes following the second injection, the extension and efficiency of anesthesia in the anterior palate is assessed by an explorer or periosteal elevator and if pain-free the nasopalatine nerve need not be injected from the palate and there is no need for another injection for extraction or dentoalveolar surgery. In the case of mild pain, severe pain, moderate pain or no anesthesia, a complementary injection in the palate is needed. The authors assessed this via a clinical trial that included 60 patients referring for the extraction of maxillary incisors and canine. They showed complete anesthesia of the anterior area of the palate in 76.7% of patients using this method; 23.3% needed a conventional nasopalatine nerve block to complement the effect of anesthesia prior to treatment. In controls we used the conventional technique.

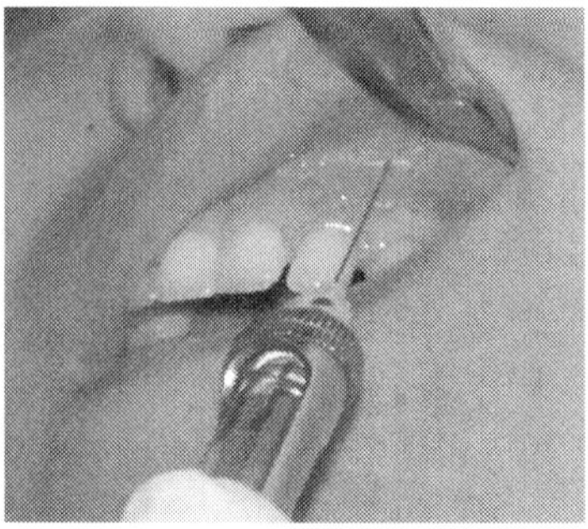

Figure 4. The anesthesia of the maxillary hard and soft tissue of the labial area is obtained by injection of 1 cc of local anesthetic agent, with the syringe parallel to the long axis of the tooth. Orient the needle bevel toward the bone.

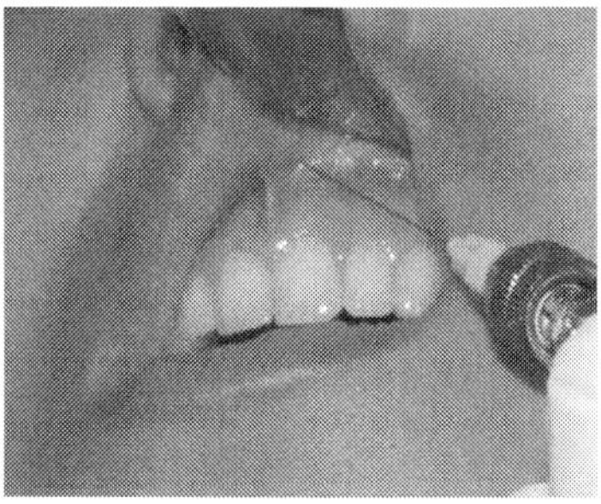

Figure 5. Needle inserted superior to the apices of central incisors in the vicinity of the superior border of the base of the anterior nasal spine near the nasal floor at a 45 degree angle to the long axis of the central incisor, to obtain anesthesia in the anterior palate.

The level of anesthesia obtained by our method in the anterior palate is satisfactory. The labial infiltration method resulted in total anesthesia in the majority of the cases. Failures may be the result of anatomic and physiologic variations. An eight minute wait or longer may be more effective than five minutes following the second injection. The amount of pain experienced by the patients during the injection in the labial infiltration approach is less than the conventional approach in most cases. [5]

2. Modified mental incisive nerve block technique

2.1. Overview

- The mental-incisive nerve block can be used where lower premolars and anterior teeth require treatment. In this chapter we present our method of mental-incisive nerve block for extraction of the lower premolars and anterior teeth or dentoalveolar surgery.

- The authors reported a 95% success rate with the modified injection distal to the second lower premolar, while the success rate was 72.5% when the injection was done traditionally between lower premolars.
- This modified mental-incisive nerve block with injection done distal to the second premolar is more successful than between premolars

2.2. Background

The Inferior Alveolar Nerve Block (IANB) is the most important injection technique in dentistry. Unfortunately it also proves to be the most frustrating; with the highest percentage of clinical failure [6]. Potocnik and Bajrovic reported that even when a proper technique is employed, clinical studies show that IANB fails in approximately 30% to 45% of cases [7]. When dental treatment involved procedures on mandibular premolars and anterior teeth the incisive nerve block can be administered with greater success [6]. However, the injection technique for mental-incisive nerve block (MINB) may also influence the success rate.

2.3. Clinical anatomy

The target is the mental foramen located on external surface of the body of the mandible below the first and second premolars where the IAN divides into terminal (incisive and mental) branches. The incisive branch continues forward in a bony canal or in a plexiform arrangement, giving off branches to the first premolar, canine and incisor teeth, and the associated labial gingiva. The lower central incisor teeth receive a bilateral innervation, fibers probably cross the midline within the periosteum to re-enter the bone via numerous canals in the labial cortical plate. The mental nerve passes upward, backward and outward to emerge from the mandible via the mental foramen between and just below the apices of the premolar teeth [8].

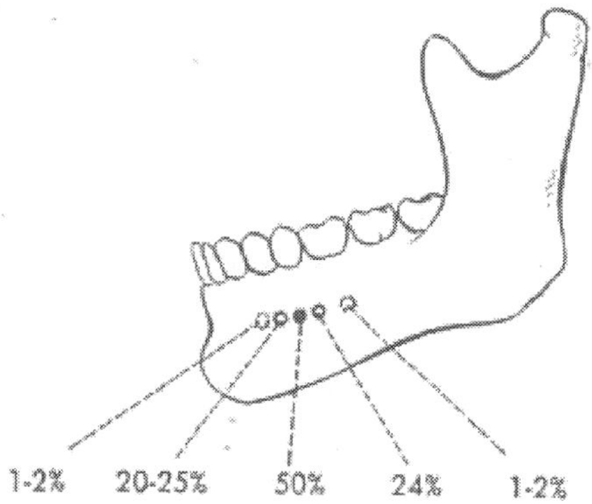

Figure 6. In 24% of individuals the mental foramen is located distal to the root of the second premolar; in 20 to 25%, between the premolars roots, in 50% at the site of the second premolar root and in 1% to 2% anterior to the first premolar or mesial to the first molar.

However, the location of mental foramen varies in different people [8-13]; in 24% of individuals the mental foramen is located distal to the root of the second premolar; in 20 to 25%, between the premolars roots, in 50% at the area of the second premolar root and in 1% to 2% anterior to the first premolar or mesial to the first molar (Figure 6). [13] This variability in location may cause problems in obtaining anesthesia [8, 10, 13-15].

2.4. Technique

There are different methods for MINB; the authors compared 2 mental–incisive nerve block techniques for the extraction of lower premolars and anterior teeth bilaterally. One method was to inject between the first and second premolar so that the needle passed between the two premolars vertically. In the other method, the injection was performed distal to the second premolar.

This randomized double blind, split-mouth clinical study was done; in the case group, the needle penetrated the depth of the vestibule distal to the second premolar using a 27 gauge needle. Entry was from behind the patient at the ten O′ clock and the opposite side at the 2 O′ clock position. The needle entered the soft tissue about 5-8 mm supraperiosteal, with mouth half-open and lip and buccal tissues retracted. When standing behind the patient, the anatomical landmarks were the second premolar and buccal vestibule (Figure 7).

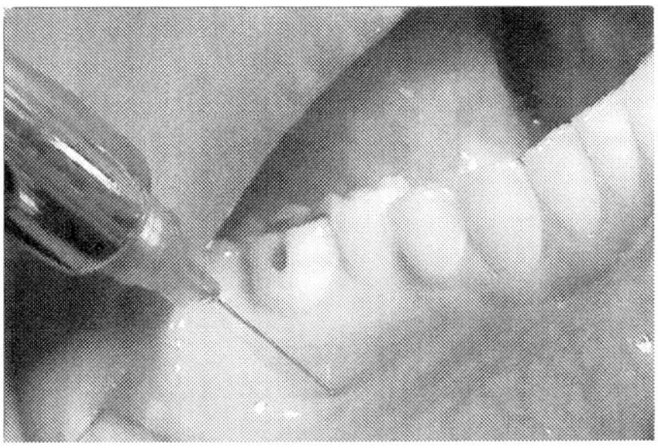

Figure 7. The injection administered distal to the second premolar. The syringe should be from posterior to anterior, from above to below and from lateral to medial while standing behind the patient.

In the control group an injection was done in the depth of buccal mucosa between two premolars at a depth of 5-6 mm using a 27 gauge needle with the mouth half open standing behind the patient (Figure 8). [16]

In both groups the local anesthetic solution was lidocaine 2% (1 cc) with epinephrine (1/80000). It is not necessary for the needle to enter the mental foramen. Data was statistically analyzed using the chi-square test. All patients had a lingual injection (0.5 cc) which was administered 5 mm distal to the tooth in the floor of the mouth.

The MINB with needle entrance distal to the second premolar from behind had a 95% success rate and MINB with needle entrance between premolars had a 72.5% success rate respectively

http://dx.doi.org/10.5772/59235

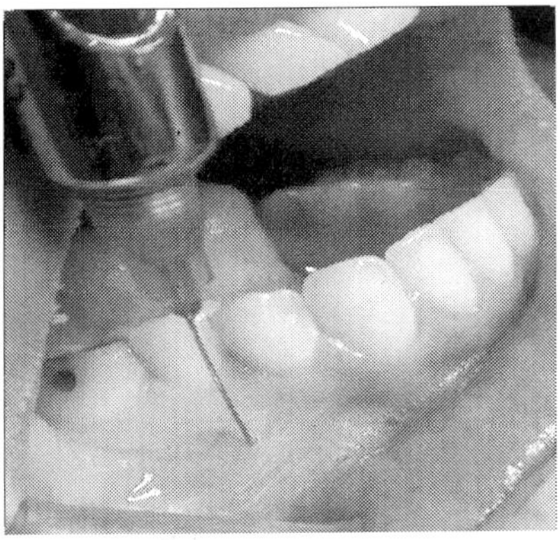

Figure 8. The injection administered in the depth of buccal mucosa between two premolars at a depth of 5-6 mm using a 27 gauge short needle with the mouth half open while standing behind the patient.

($p<0.01$). Thus, if the mental nerve block injection is administered with the needle entrance between premolars, the chance of failure is greater (R.R=5.5).

2.5. Discussion

The MINB can be an alternative to the IANB when dental procedures requiring pulpal anesthesia on mandibular teeth anterior to the mental foramen (e.g. canine to canine or premolar to premolar) are treated. According to the result, we found that MINB with needle penetration distal to second premolar was more effective (95%) than injection between two premolars (72.5%). Al Yasser and Al Nwoku [15] showed that the mental foramen location on both sides of the mandible in 80% of cases is symmetrical and in 46.2% of cases the mental foramen is located between the longitudinal axes of the two premolars. Moiseiwitch [10] reported that anterior-posterior positions of mental foramens in most cases are symmetrical. In most studies on mental foramens in different cases, researchers reported that most mental foramens are in line with second premolars [11, 14]. What most scientists agree with is the presence of mental foramen in range of the long axis of the second premolar [10-12] with about 50% of cases at the level of the root of second premolar, between the two premolars in about 20% to 25% and posterior to the second premolar in about 24%, and in approximately 1% to 2% it lies as forward as the first premolar or as far back as the first molar [13]. This may be why the technique in which the needle penetrates mucosa distal to second premolar may yield the success rate of MINB higher. According to the results, the success rate of anesthesia administered distal to second premolar was 95% and with needle penetration between premolar was 72.5% [6, 9]. According to Malamed the correct position of the dentist is in front of the patient so that the syringe may be placed into the mouth below the patients line of sight and the thumb or index finger in the mucobuccal fold against the body of the mandible in the first molar area and moved slowly anteriorly until feeling the bone become irregular and somewhat concave [6] while in our technique there is no need to palpate the area and produce discomfort for patients. Mucosal penetration done from the distal of the second premolar hides the needle from the line of sight of the patient. When standing in front of the patient it is easier for the patient to see the needle whereas when standing behind the patient it is unlikely for him or her to visualize the needle. [17]

2.6. Conclusion

Mental-incisive nerve block injection distal to the second premolar from behind the patient was more successful than between premolars from the front.

3. Modified direct inferior alveolar nerve block technique

3.1. Overview

This modified direct technique is easier and more practical than the conventional technique described by Malamed in the handbook of local anesthesia [18]; also it is easier to learn and teach dental students. We have used this technique in practice for many years with a high success rate (up to 98%).

3.2. Technique

a. A 27 gauge short or long needle is recommended.

b. The mouth should be open wide.

c. Placement of the syringe barrel at the first molar of the opposite side.

d. Needle penetration occurs at the point one centimeter above the occlusal plane of the mandibular molar and parallel to it just at the lateral border of pterygomandibular raphe. In this situation, the needle touches the medial aspect of the ramus at about a 90 angle. When entering the pterygomandibular space injury to the medial pterygoid muscle should be avoided. The pterygomandibular fold may serve as a landmark for the anterior border of the muscle. The needle pierces the mucous membrane lateral to the pterygomandibular fold and injury to the medial pterygoid muscle is avoided easily [18-21]

e. While slowly advancing, the needle contacts bone; then we withdraw the needle about 1 mm to prevent subperiosteal injection. If aspiration is negative, we slowly deposit 1.5 ml of anesthetic within 60 seconds; the remaining solution is deposited for lingual nerve anesthesia while withdrawing the needle. The average depth of needle penetration to bony contact depends on soft tissue thickness of the area on the medial aspect of the ramus. This will be approximately 8-10 mm or less, it is not necessary to advance the needle in the posterior direction at all or you will be far from the exact injection site. In this technique using the thumb or finger is not necessary, a dental mirror or Minnesota retractor can be used; however there is really no need to use these instruments. With this technique the inferior alveolar and lingual nerves are anesthetized. The long buccal nerve should be anesthetized separately for molar extraction (Figure 9).

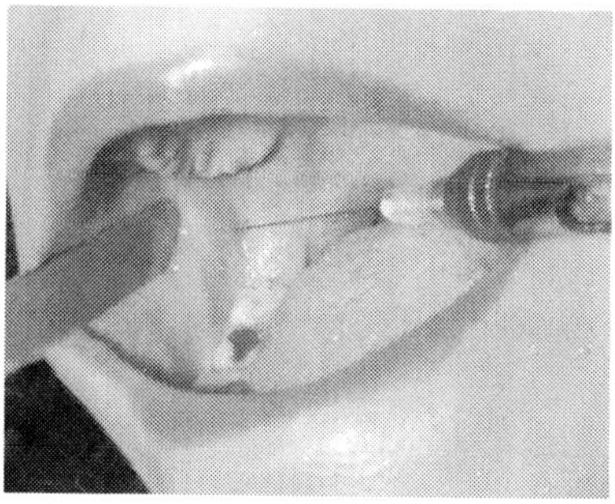

Figure 9. The modified direct technique.

4. Conclusion

With regard to the high success rate of the technique and because of simplicity and easy learning curve by dental students it can be placed into the academic curriculum.

Author details

Esshagh Lassemi[1], Fina Navi[1*], Mohammad Hosein Kalantar Motamedi[1,2], Seyed Mehdi Jafari[1], Kourosh Taheri Talesh[1,3], Kamal Qaranizade[1] and Reza Lasemi[4]

*Address all correspondence to: fina_navi@yahoo.com

1 Department of Oral and Maxillofacial Surgery, Dental School, Azad Islamic University of Medical Sciences, Tehran, Iran

2 Trauma Research Center, Baqiyatallah University of Medical Sciences, Tehran, Iran

3 Department of Oral and Maxillofacial Surgery,Dental School, Tabriz University of Medical Sciences, Tabriz, Iran

4 Medical University of Vienna, Austria

References

[1] Uckan S, Dayangac E, Araz K. Is permanent maxillary tooth removal without palatal injection possible? *Oral Surg Oral Med Oral Pathol Oral RadiolEndod*2006; 102: 733-735.

[2] Malamed (2013) Local Anesthesia. (5thed), Elsevier Mosby Publications, USA, and Chap13:190-191

[3] Meechan J G, Day P F, McMillan A S. Local anesthesia in the palate: a comparison of techniques and solutions. *AnesthProg*2000; 47: 139-142.

[4] Meechan J G, Howlett P C, Smith B D. Factors influencing the discomfort of intraoral needle penetration. *AnesthProg*2005; 52: 91-94.

[5] Lassemi E, Motamedi M. H. K., Jafari S. M, TaleshK. T., Navi F. Anesthetic efficacy of alabial infiltration method on the nasopalatine nerve.Br Dent J. 2008 Nov 22; 205(10):E21. doi: 10.1038/sj.bdj.2008.872.

[6] Malamed S (2004) Hand book of local anesthesia (5thedn), Mosby Publications, Missouri, USA 14: 228-252.

[7] Potocnik I, Bajrovic F (1999) Failure of inferior alveolar nerve block. Endod Dent Traumatol 15: 247-251.

[8] Williams D, Bannister L, Berry M (2008) Gray's Anatomy(39thedn) Churchill Livingstone Publications 33: 601.

[9] Joyce A, Donnely J (1992) Evaluation of effectiveness and comfort of incisive nerve anesthesia inside or outside the mental foramen. J Endod 18: 409-411.

[10] Moiseiwitsch JR (1998) Position of the mental foramen in North American white population. Oral Surg Oral Med Oral Pathol Oral Radiol Endod 85: 457-460.

[11] Green R (1987) The Position of the mental foramen: A comparison between the southern Chinese and other ethnic and racial groups. Oral Surg Oral Med Oral Pathol 63: 287-290.

[12] Phillips JL, Weller RN, Kulid JC (1992) The mental foramen: Part 3, size and position on panoramic Radiographs, J Endod 18: 383-386.

[13] Henry Hollinshead. Anatomy For Surgeons: The Head and Neck. (3rd ed) Harper & Row, Publishers Philadelphia 1: 358.

[14] Wesley E Shankland (1994) The position of the Mental Foramen in Asian Indians. J Oral Implantology 20: 118-122.

[15] Al Jasser NM, Al Nwoku (1998) Radiographic study of the mental foramen in a selected Saudi population. Dento maxillofacial Radiology 27: 341-343.

[16] Sicher H (1970) Oral Anatomy. (5thedn), Mosby Publications, USA, chap 1: 44-48.

[17] Lassemi E, Kalantar Motamedi MH, Alemi Z (2013) Anesthetic Efficacy Assessment of Two Mental Nerve Block Techniques for Tooth Extraction. Anaplastology S6: 003. doi: 10.4172/2161-1173.S6-003

[18] Malamed (2013) Local Anesthesia. (5thedn), Elsevier Mosby Publications, Chap14: 228

[19] Gray`s Anatomy (2008).(39thed), Elsevier Ltd,USA,Chap 32:574

[20] Gray `s Anatomy (1989). (37thedn), Churchill Livingstone Publications, UK, Chap 7:1101

[21] DuBrul and Sicher, Oral anatomy (1970). (5thedn), Mosby company, USA, Chap 10:416-417

Section 2

Basic and Advanced Surgical Orthodontics

Chapter 5

Orthodontic Considerations in Surgical Interventions for Impacted Teeth

Massoud Seifi and
Mohammad Hosein Kalantar Motamedi

Additional information is available at the end of the chapter

http://dx.doi.org/10.5772/59143

1. Introduction

Parallax is the effect whereby the position of a tooth or similar structure appears to differ when viewed from different positions of the X-ray tube.[1] This method (Image/Tube Shift Method, Buccal Object Rule or Clark's Rule) has been the technique of choice to localize impacted teeth anterior to the molars in both jaws using Vertical or Horizontal Tube Shift (VTS /HTS).[2] With the continued technologic advances, the role of Cone Beam Computed Tomography (CBCT) is changing in orthodontic workup and should be viewed as complementary to plain X-rays or 2D X-rays in effective diagnosis, especially in impaction cases as a 3D evaluation. Effective dose of radiation measured in micro-Sievert (μSv)) is decreased from full field of view (FOV) to both jaws (13 cm) and single jaws (6 cm), from large-volume to small-volume and from high resolution (HR) to conventional.[3] Therefore, as the effective dose is of foremost concern, it can be decreased by appropriate selection of exposure parameters, FOV and resolution (only for impacted tooth/teeth) to be comparable from a "dose" perspective with several periapical and occlusal radiographs (parallax). However, the results of dosimetry on a specific CBCT scanner may not be transferable to another CBCT scanner and every image involving ionizing radiation, including CBCT, must be justified and optimized.

The treatment (including decision makings) of impacted teeth can be categorized into five steps:

1. Cost-Benefit Analysis/ Cost-Effectiveness Analysis
2. Space preparation/Barrier removal
3. Selection of the method for eruption (Closed vs. Open)

4. Selection of the appropriate (effective) biomechanical approach
   a. Anchorage preparation (Direct vs. Indirect)
   b. Force application
5. Alignment/ Leveling Torque/Angulation (ALTA) corrections

2. Cost-Benefit Analysis (CBA)/ Cost-Effectiveness Analysis (CEA)

Cost-benefit analysis (CBA) or Cost-effectiveness analysis (CEA) requires quantifiable input data; both methods are accounting techniques that have been applied to medical decision-making. Using Standard CEA, benefits are expressed either directly or indirectly in terms of "quality of life" improvement, and costs are expressed in monetary values and in morbidity and mortality. Using CBA, benefits and costs are all converted into monetary equivalents.[4] The CBA is also defined as a systematic process for calculating and comparing benefits and costs of a project or decision i.e. exposure of impacted tooth and ALTA correction versus alternative treatment modalities. Results must be treated with caution, making it difficult to make robust claims about the comparative cost-effectiveness of either treatment plan.

Systemic conditions or metabolic disturbances may be related to multiple impacted teeth. To achieve optimum results, an interdisciplinary teamwork is needed between the orthodontist, oral surgeon, prosthodontist and possibly some other specialties. The patient shown in Figure 1 an active social person, had several impactions in both jaws but was seeking a swift procedure to get his anterior teeth. The facial profile, esthetic smile, and time spent for each appointment in a nonprofit dental center were also among his concerns. It seems that the selected option for the patient had more benefit gain in comparison to cost (time, pain, inconveniences, and risks and...etc.).

In the first step clinicians should make a decision from the CBA/CEA perspective to select the best option appropriate for the individual looking for treatment of the impacted tooth/teeth.

2.1. Early intervention for impaction prevention

Space deficiency has been mentioned as the first etiologic factor for a palatal impaction. Many other contributing factors are associated with a palatal impaction such as over-retention of the primary canines, abnormal position of the tooth bud, disturbances in tooth eruption, localized pathologic lesions, abnormal sequence of eruption, missing lateral incisors or abnormal form of the lateral incisor roots (e.g. dilacerations), presence of an alveolar cleft, supernumerary tooth, and idiopathic factors.[5]

Crowding, thick soft tissue, supernumerary tooth/teeth, and tipped tooth/teeth situations are considered as barriers to eruption. During the regular orthodontic examination of a patient (Figure 2) an impaction was discovered on panoramic radiography suspected to be an abnormal position of the tooth bud but proximity of developing root of tooth 14 and crown of #13 (FDI Two-Digit Notation- ISO 3950) in addition to their abnormal route are the major

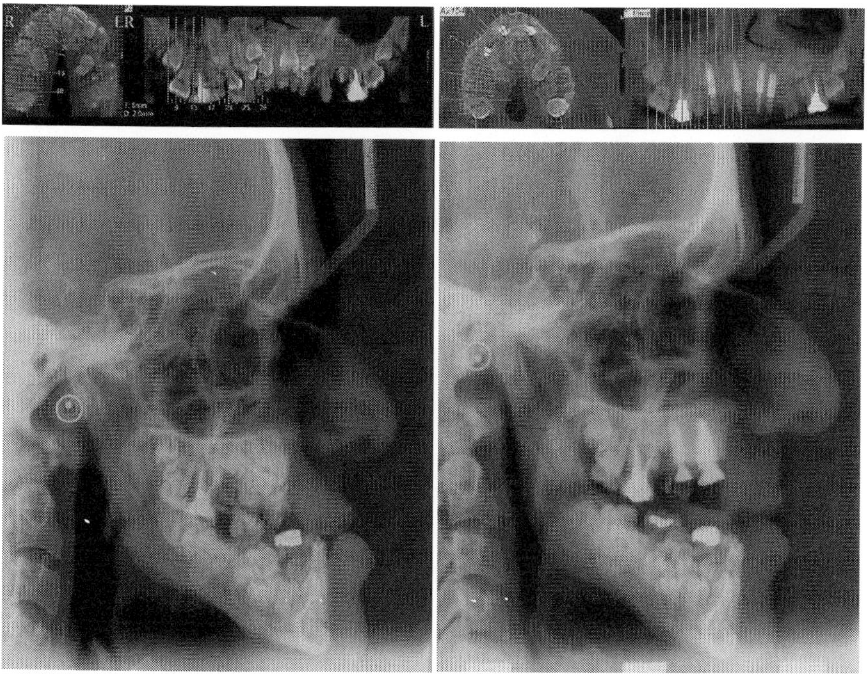

Figure 1. Cost versus benefit appraisal for the above patient was considered according to the duration of the treatment versus time needed to receive anterior implants and reliability of this option. Multiple impacted teeth were extracted and after placement of allograft-based bone graft substitute, four dental implants were inserted. The patient continued his treatment and the implants were used as anchorage for extruding mandibular impacted teeth.

concerns. It was postulated that rapid developing root with differentiating cells of the dental papilla plus vascular pressure toward malposed erupting crown of tooth 13 had caused both teeth to deviate from their normal route. After extraction of the upper right first primary molar, the pressure was relieved. By using a banded expander and extraction it seems that more space was provided for erupting teeth and the impacted canine is getting more vertical relative to the initial radiograph.

2.2. Difficulty index as a tool for expression of the "Cost"

The canine is the second most commonly impacted tooth (after the third molar), with the rate of maxillary canine impaction ranging from approximately 1% to 3% [6] and incidence of approximately 20% in orthodontic clinics. Should you ALTA correction of tooth at the expense of extra time and money or extract the impacted tooth, saving time and orthodontic payments for the patient but perhaps at the expense of esthetics and long-term function.

When treating impacted teeth, duration of treatment or chairtime, success rate or risks, and complcations (root resorption of impacted or adjacent teeth, ankylosis,..) can be converted to

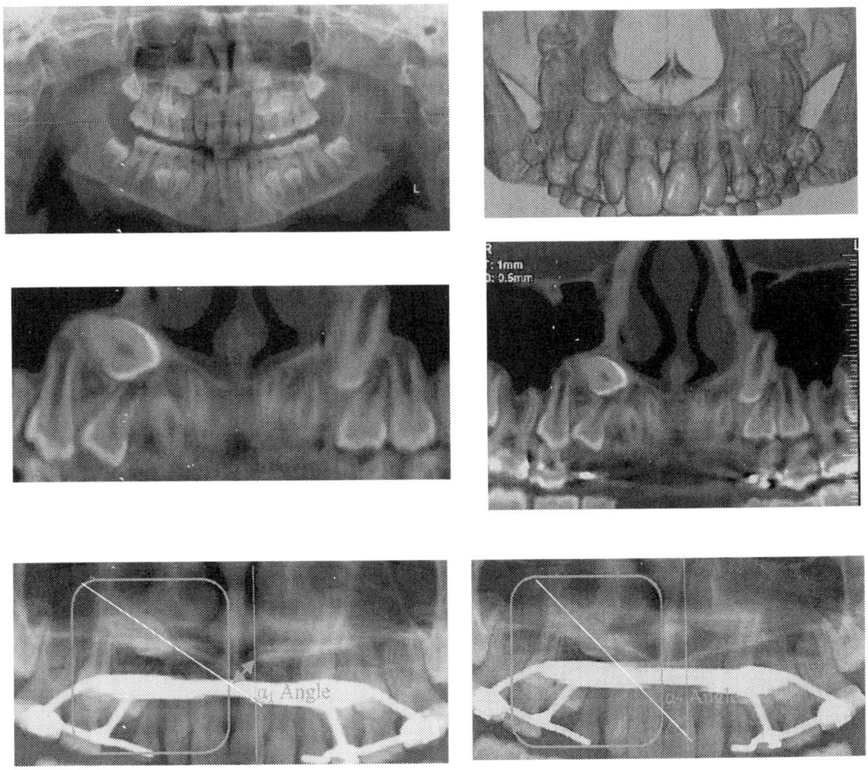

Figure 2. Impacted canine has angulated towards the horizontal (Top-right) and made the management more challenging and difficult. Impacted tooth 13 has tipped toward a better vertical position (bottom left to bottom right) in other words Alpha (α) angle is decreased after banded expander installed and tooth 54 (D) was extracted ($\alpha_1 > \alpha_2$).

a single score that would be compared to the benefits. However, sensitivity and specificity of these scores or methods are uncertain and questionable. Many variables have role in determination of difficulty for impaction cases including age (over 25 requires longer time), distance of impacted tooth from occlusal plane, mesiodistal location of the crown, angulation of the tooth, transverse relationship of the crown to the midline, location of the impacted tooth cusp/incisal tip and its relationship to the adjacent teeth (lateral incisor in canine impaction cases), apex position, and transposition with adjacent teeth (lateral incisor and first premolar in canine impaction cases).[7] Angular measurements on lateral cephalometry are Omega (ω) angle and Delta (δ) angle and linear measurement is d2 (Distance to Occlusal Plane) (Figure 3). Angular measurements in panoramic views are the canine inclination (C.I.) to midline or Alpha (α) angle and its inclination to the lateral incisor (or first premolar) or Beta (β) angle (Figure 4-second row). Mesiodistal position of the canine cusp tip in relation to adjacent lateral and central incisors on panoramic radiographs is called "Zone" and numbers 1 to 5 are assigned to its position as it gets closer to the midline (Figure 4-third row).[6] Inclination of the canine in the horizontal plane or the degree of mesial orientation of the canine is analyzed by measuring the Gamma (γ) angle between projection of long axis of the canine and the midline of the maxilla in axial CBCT slice of maxilla (Figure 4-bottom left)

In quantitative terms, the larger the relative risk, the more likely the association is causal. When studying causative factors, it is very important to analyze the strength of the association in addition to the significance. More advanvce canine development, a more medial position of the canice cusp, considering the zones [1-5], and mesial inclination of the canine to midline exceeding 25° (α angle) are powerful factors.[8]

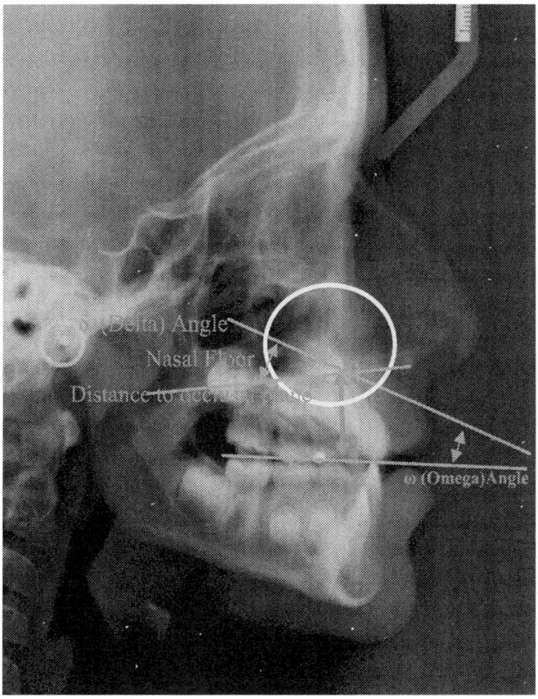

Figure 3. Angular measurements or inclinations of the canine in the sagittal plane are Omega (ω) angle and Delta (δ) angle (path of eruption) and linear measurement is d2 (Distance to Occlisal Plane).

Regression analysis indicated that horizontal position, age of patient, vertical height and bucco-palatal position, in descending order of importance, are the factors which determine the difficulty of canine alignment.[9]

Sector location and angulation of the unerupted tooth have been analyzed previously as predictors of canine eruption after deciduous extraction. Additionally, sector location has been studied as an indicator of eventual impaction, resulting in good predictive success (Figure 5).[10] Different indices provide useful treatment planning aid for the management of impacted maxillary canines like treatment difficulty index (TDI) [9] and 3D cone beam CT based classification system for canine impactions (the KPG index).[11]

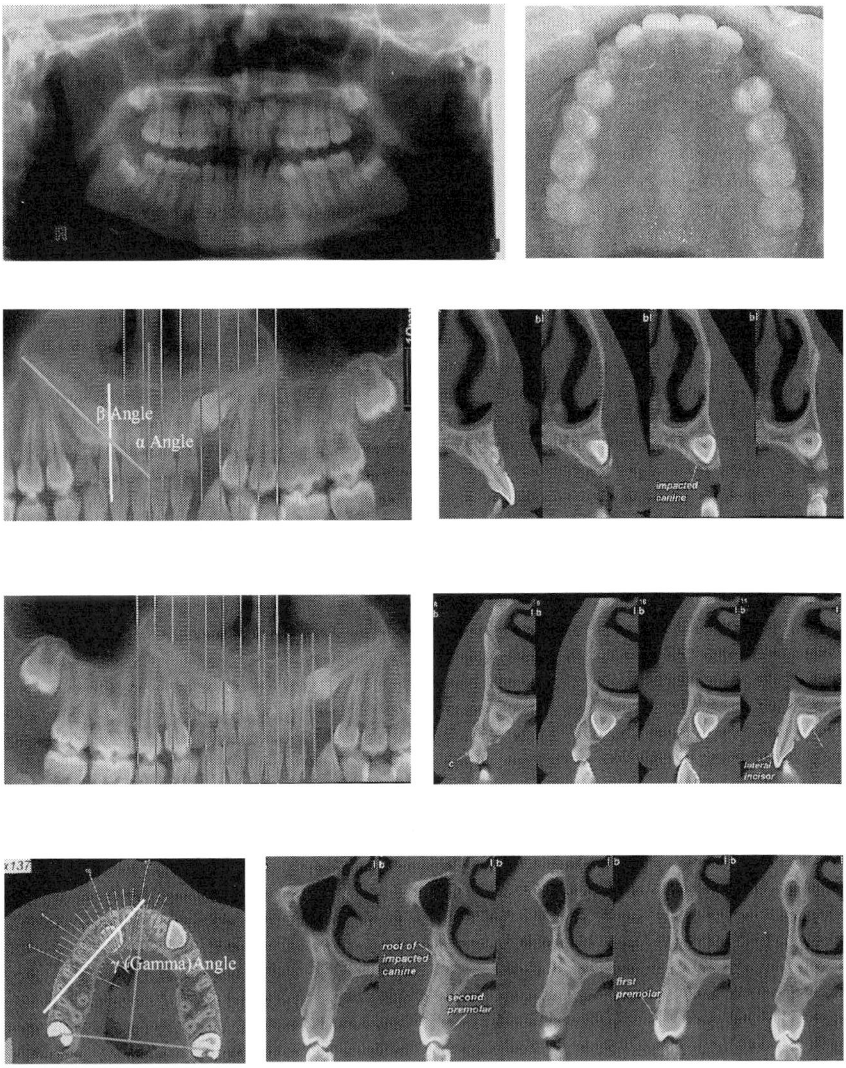

Figure 4. Angular measurements in panoramic views are the canine inclination to midline or Alpha (α) angle and its inclination to the lateral incisor or Beta (β) angle (second row). Mesiodistal position of the canine cusp tip in relation to adjacent lateral and central incisors on panoramic radiographs is called "Zone" (third row). Inclination of the canine in the horizontal plane or the degree of mesial orientation of the canine is analyzed by measuring the Gamma (γ) angle between projection of long axis of the canine and the midline of the maxilla (bottom left).

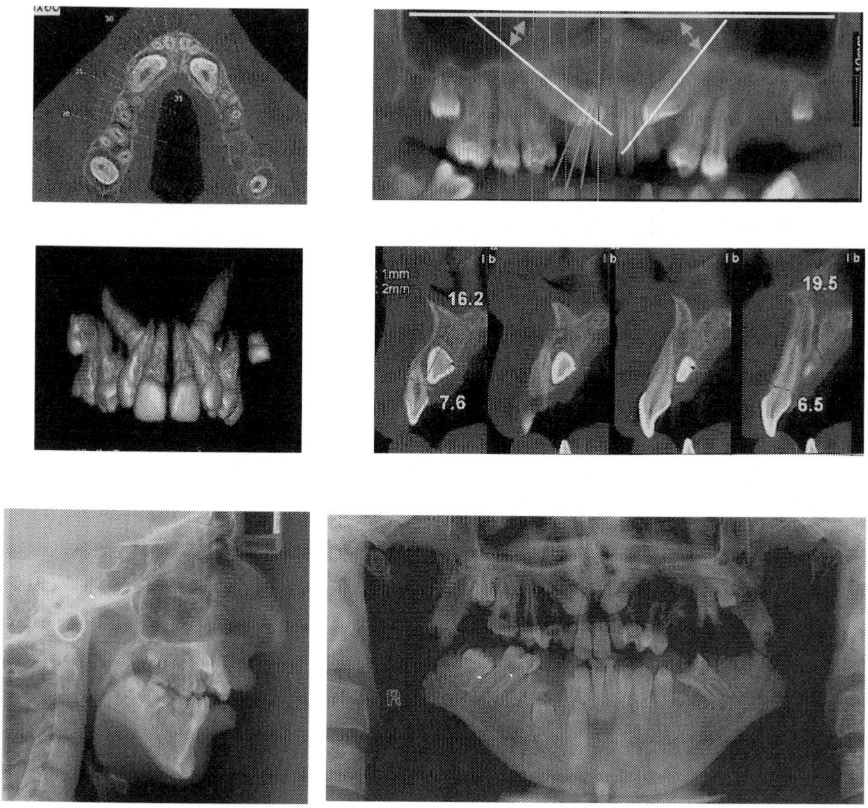

Figure 5. Sector I represents area distal to line tangent to distal heights of contour of lateral incisor crown and root. Sector II is mesial to sector I, but distal to bisector of lateral incisor's long axis. Sector III is mesial to sector II, but distal to mesial heights of contour of lateral incisor crown and root. Sector IV includes all areas mesial to sector III (3 red line-Top right). The most superior point of the condyle was selected as a landmark; a bicondylar line was then drawn and used as a constructed horizontal reference line. The measurement was taken of the mesial angle formed by using the constructed horizontal and the long axis of the unerupted tooth (Top right).

3. Space preparation/Barrier removal

Space is needed (space available) for bringing teeth (teeth materials) into the dental arch. Many mechanisms exist for creating the adequate space including Stripping mesial or distal enamel of the teeth (proximal) with condition of existing Bolton discrepancies between upper and lower dentition, Extraction of premolars, incisors with condition of Bolton ratio considerations, or decayed teeth, Derotation or Uprighting of the posterior teeth after extractions or in the missing teeth conditions, proclination of anterior teeth, distalization of the posterior teeth, Orthopedic (Maxilla) or Orthodontic Expansion of dental arches.

Constricted arches, dental irregularities, proclinations of teeth relative to jaw bases or patient profile, deep bites and open bites with tight contacts between the teeth should be considered as space deficiency or crowding. Reproximation or proximal stripping produces up to 3.5 mm of space and 1 mm of expansion in the posterior part of maxilla is capable to produce 0.7 mm increase in arch perimeter that can be used for crowding resolution.

Upper dental arch expansion and lower dental arch uprighting (from lingual side to buccal side) produce space for bringing the impacted teeth to the dental arch. After full bonding of the arches, by incremental increase in wire diameter plus changes in cross sections (from round to rectangular) and material (from NiTi to Stainless Steel); dental arches begin to get adapted to final wire shape and size from its lingually collapsed cases to the consequent expanded arch.

Maxillary expansion can be skeletal or orthopedic if it is conducted in appropriate time i.e. before fusion of palatal suture. For maxillary expansion, banded expander (with Hyrax screw and acrylic free palate), banded+bonded (occlusal acrylic coverage) expander, and banded +palatal acrylic (Haas type) expander can be used for both dental and skeletal expansions.

In addition to space regaining in dental arches, physical barriers as supernumerary teeth, odontomas, or other pathologic lesions that inhibits tooth eruption; should be removed. Apart from hard tissue lesions, soft tissue fibrotic hyperplasia or thick fibrotic gingiva can prevent regular tooth eruption and they can be treated surgically or by laser beam.

4. Selection of the method for eruption of impacted tooth (Closed versus Open)

Method of exposure is very important to be practical for the surgeon, to be useful for application of biomechanical forces for the orthodontist, and to be beneficial for the patient. Benefits for the patient consist of several immediate and future outcomes; including periodontal health, esthetics, and stability of treatment. Facio-lingual and vertical position of the impacted teeth are very important in determining an appropriate approach for exposure. Buccally/Labially impacted teeth can be accessed after apically positioned flap or closed eruption technique. Excisional uncovering or gingivectomy necessitates special conditions including superficial position of tooth (vertically and facio-lingually), and adequate width of keratinized gingiva. An example of inappropriate surgical approach for uncovering the impacted central is conducting the procedure apical to the mucogingival junction and removing the keratinized gingiva (Figure 6).

Apically positioned flap (Open) or closed eruption technique is an aid for maintenance of the biologic width. The biological width is comprised of epithelial attachment and connective tissue attachment (both dimensions added) coronal to the crest of the alveolar bone. It should be planned to preserve an adequate apico-coronal height of keratinized gingiva (2-3 mm), especially in the presence of thin gingival biotype (transparency of the periodontal probe through gingival margin). In some cases impacted teeth are superficial and coronal or near mucogingival junction, in these circumstances, an apically positioned flap or open approach

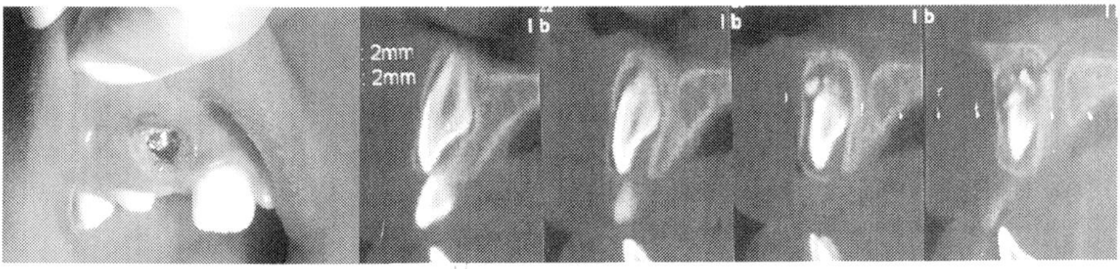

Figure 6. An inappropriate way to expose the impacted left central incisor. Incorrect technique is independent of tools i.e. laser beam or scalpel; a required width of attached gingiva (necessary for periodontal health) has been removed to create a buttonhole window (Left) as an unaccepted procedure with a bonded attachment. On the first right slice of CBCT, an odontoma-like malformation is obvious but has been neglected during the surgical intervention (red arrow).

is indicated but the author suggests minimum apical repositioning of the flap equal to the amount needed for bonding of an orthodontic bracket in proper position for avoiding future apical migration of the gingival margin. Uneven gingival contours can be corrected by cosmetic periodontal plastic surgery (laser, scalpel, or radiosurgery) if adequate soft tissue exist. Uncontrolled tipping toward labial/buccal can produce gingival/bone recession plus a long clinical crown that should be avoided.

When impacted teeth need a facial (labial or buccal) approach, and the position of tooth is deep, closed eruption is an option. In the aforementioned situation, an apically positioned flap will not be stable and rebound of soft tissue may occur in addition to unwanted exposed parts of the bone that should be covered by a flap (Figure 7).

During tooth exposure, care should be given to protect root surface, for example; by avoiding the usage of sharp or rotary instrument if possible because bone and the unerupted tooth are color matched and any damage to the root leads to periodontal ligament breakdown, increased risk of ankylosis, and increased risk for future bone and gingival recession (deleterious effects to periodontal health and esthetics). Thin layers of bone can be removed by periosteal elevator or similar instruments e.g. curette to reach the coronal part of the tooth (Figure 7).

Soft tissue covering the hard palate is called masticatory mucosa and it consists of keratinized stratified squamous epithelium. Since the palate is covered with keratinized mucosa or attached gingiva, problems with alveolar mucosa are not part of this operational area. If the bulge of an impacted canine is obvious from the palatal aspect, the cuspid tooth should be located superficially and accessible after soft tissue removal plus removal of covering bone. The patient shown in Figure 8, had no canine bulge on the left side on facial aspect (top row-left and center slides) but it was seen on the palatal aspect clinically (top row-right slide) and also in CBCT (bottom- left and center). Uncovering the tooth and bonding through a small window can be hectic using a scalpel a palatal flap may help in achievement an isolated and dry environment for the bonding and open or close eruption technique. Again sufficient bone removal is recommended without damage to the tooth root because PDL is the interface for tooth movement and the enamel of the crown has no potential for participating in bone remodeling and consequent tooth movement. Absolute anchorage was used for eruption of

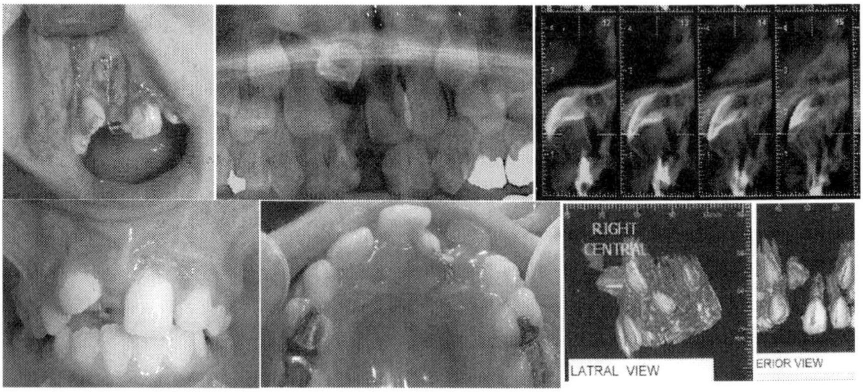

Figure 7. Upper right central incisor is positioned horizontally. An apically positioned flap is not indicated in the present situation and a closed eruption surgical approach may be used. Thin overlying bone can be removed with a periosteal elevator instead of rotary instrument (burs) and bonding performed in an isolated dry environment (top row). After wound healing, tooth 11 can be pulled towards the dental arch by means of absolute anchorage (mini-screws) or after bonding upper dental arch (continuous wire). In this case, an orthodontic attachment was bonded in the lingual fossa of tooth 11 and ligature wire was placed out of the flap for biomechanical extrusive forces (bottom row).

tooth #23 by means of Seifi Twin Screws (STS) for protecting other teeth from early unwanted orthodontic forces (Figure 8).

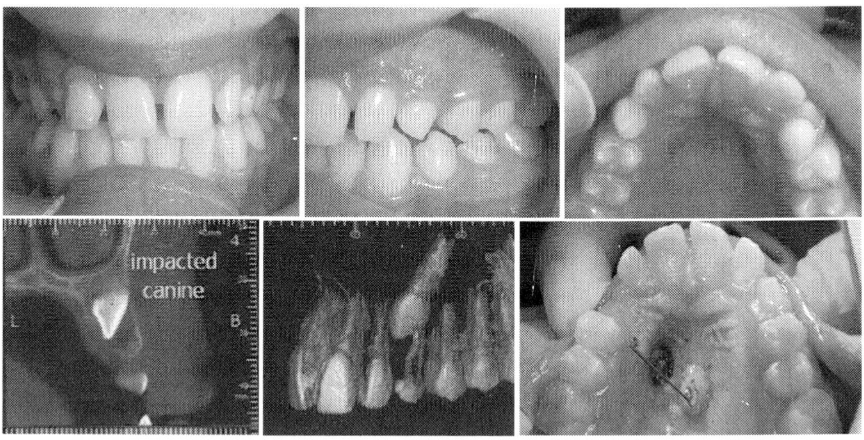

Figure 8. Patient with an impacted tooth #23 underwent a surgical uncovering of a palatal left canine (mirror image after surgery-bottom right). An absolute anchorage by combination of two miniscrews and a cantilever helical loop (Seifi Twin Screws/STS) was used for forced eruption or extrusion of impacted canine without exerting unwanted orthodontic force to the adjacent teeth. Miniscrews were covered by composites for better performance of springs and sustained stability.

http://dx.doi.org/10.5772/59143

5. Selection of the appropriate (effective) biomechanical approach

After selection of the proper approach to reach the impacted tooth, an appropriate biomechanical approach should be selected. A proper biomechanical system is capable of protecting periodontium and avoiding any unwanted tooth movement or root damage of the adjacent teeth.

a. Anchorage preparation (Direct vs. Indirect)

In contrast to dental implants, orthodontic miniscrews are loaded immediately, and most authors suggest the use of light forces early on.[12] Only a few studies, mostly on animals, have dealt with the investigation of tissue reaction to immediate loading of miniscrew implants. Miniscrew implants can be immediate loaded (there is no need for a waiting period for osseointegration, in contrast to orthodontic implants), reducing the total treatment time. There is no need for complicated clinical and laboratory procedures (i.e., fabrication of acrylic splints by taking imprints with additional implant copying systems to accurately transfer the implant position to cast models) to facilitate safe and precise implant insertion.[13]

Direct anchorage screws are useful when prognosis of the eruption (impacted tooth) is questionable. If the impacted tooth is ankylosed, by applying force from a continuous arch, the dental arch could be deflected towards the ankylosed tooth (sometimes creating open bites); but, an absolute anchorage could be a valuable tool to determine the sensitive stage of tooth eruption without endangering the adjacent anchored teeth (Figure 8). Direct anchorage can be used for anterior retraction in protrusion cases or non-extraction treatment of the Class III malocclusions (retraction of lower anterior sextant) and cases who have midline shift toward previous extraction sites (Figure 9).

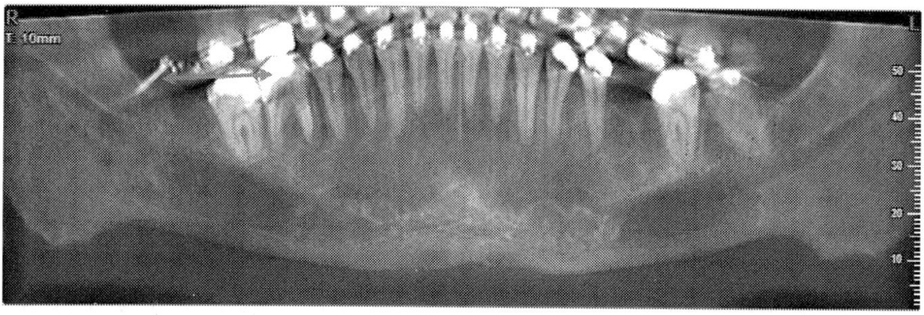

Figure 9. Patient with Class III open bite with midline deviation towards the left side, a prvious extraction site. A miniscrew was inserted in the right retromolar area for midline correction ; meanwhile retraction of anterior teeth to correct class III relationship and establishment of proper overjet and overbite was done.

Protraction of the upper dentition is possible by using miniscrews in anterior or palatal parts. Better results in protraction of the upper dentition can be expected by using miniscrews in combination with miniplates. In some situations transpalatal arch (TPA) is used for eruption of impacted teeth as a direct anchorage unit; resistance to displacement depends on the number of teeth and the root surface area (Figure 10).

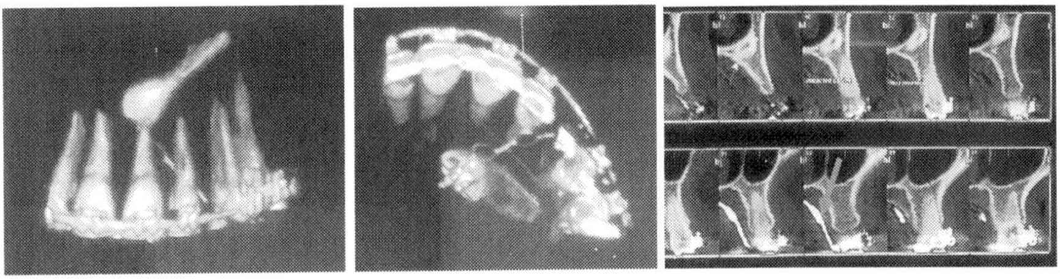

Figure 10. Transpalatal arch (TPA) has served as indirect anchorage (contributing role of root surface area of upper first molars) in addition to a full size rectangulet wire that resists reactive forces produced by traction force on the impacted upper right canine.

Following force application, some mobility or movement of teeth will be noticeable and on X-ray examination, disappearance of the lamina dura plus widening of PDL will be evident; these are sequel of force dispersion in the dental anchorage units. In maximum anchorage cases (Group A), mesial movement of posterior teeth (protraction) should be less than 25% of the extraction site, in moderate anchorage cases (Group B), posterior protraction is almost equal to anterior retraction, and in minimum anchorage cases (Group C), posterior protraction is more than 75% of the extraction site.

Indirect anchorage miniscrew stabilizes dental units, which in turn serve as the anchor units, and opens absolute anchor possibilities that can be even more flexible than direct-anchor setups. Indirect-anchor setups will entail an implant, or TAD, placed in a non-dental location, which is then used to stabilize teeth, rendering them as indirect absolute anchors, on which orthodontic force is placed. Locations for indirect anchors include retromolar, buccal vestibule, and midpalatal areas (Figure 11). As they are not destined for restoration or any functional use after serving as anchor units, all indirect-anchor devices are explanted at some time after the completion of orthodontics. Consequently, all indirect-anchor devices, be they endosseous implants or mini-screws, must be considered TADs.[14]

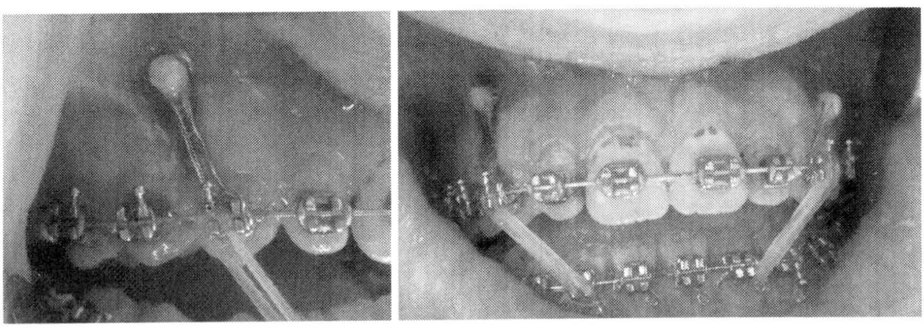

Figure 11. Miniscrews as an indirect anchorage resist against vertical pull of elastics for open bite closure. In the present condition eruption of lower anterior teeth has a major role for establishment of proper overbite. Vertical movement of the maxillary dentition is controlled by ligating both upper canines to miniscrews as indirect anchorage.

http://dx.doi.org/10.5772/59143

b. Force application

After anchorage preparation, a pivotal phase of treatment begins i.e. force application for eruption of the impacted tooth into the dental arch. Any root damage to the impacted tooth is not acceptable e.g. ligating ligature wire around the cervical part of the tooth may destroy PDL and have a deleterious effect on periodontal health of the future leveled/aligned tooth. In addition, the author does not prefer enamel drilling for canine traction (EDCT) over accessory bonding for canine traction (ABCT) i.e. bonding orthodontic attachment for loading because of its inherent characteristics in enamel destruction. A clean, etched surface of enamel is a prerequisite for successful bonding but before force application, a recheck of bonded attachment by manual traction is a prerequisite for wound closure.

Description of tooth movement for an impacted tooth is intricate and difficult. Only 3-dimensional analysis that contains information on both rotation and translation of the tooth movement has potential to evaluate and explain the nature of the exact movement. However, coordinate systems are used in orthodontics for better understanding of clinicians. Application of force to the center of resistance of a rigid body can produce translation without rotation. If the vector of the force is out of the center of resistance (C_{Res}), according to its distance to the C_{Res} it can produce a moment of the force (M_F) with an expression of rotation for free-bodies or rotation tendency for teeth. In Figure 12, a 100 gram force plus 1000 g mm of moment equals the 100 gram force applied to the bracket with 10 mm distance. By addition of counterbalancing moment (M_C) i.e. insertion of rectangular archwire in the bracket slot and its engagement to the walls, the bracket system will act like the system in the green box of Figure 12 (the green box is hypothetical) and depending on the proportion of M_C/M_F, a controlled tipping ($0<M_C/M_F<1$), translation or bodily movement ($M_C/M_F=1$), and torque ($M_C/M_F>1$) can be produced. The relationship between the orthodontic force and counterbalancing moment is also expressed in the "moment to force ratio" or M/F ratio. M/F ratio 1 to 7 produce controlled tipping; ratios of 8 to 10 (according to root length) produce bodily movement, and ratios greater than root length produce root torque movement.

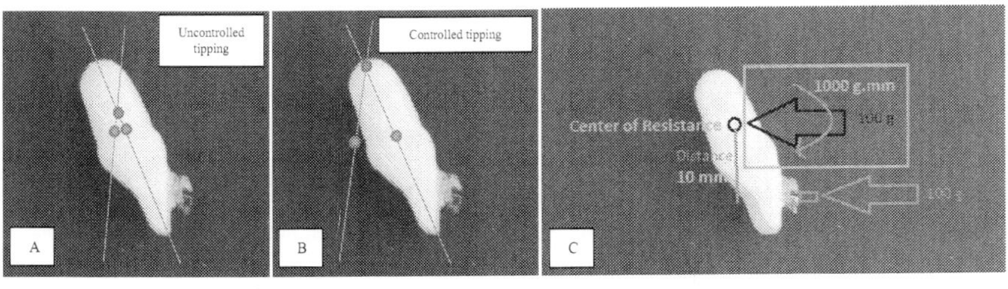

Figure 12. Application of force to the bracket without any tools to exert moment (like round wire in bracket or labial bow in removable appliances) produce a type of "uncontrolled tipping" movement (slide A). In this type of movement, the center of rotation (red circle) is near the center of resistance (blue circle). The similar or equivalent force system can be produced by exerting force (100 g) plus moment (100x10=1000 g mm) to the center of resistance (green box-slide C). If 100 g force is applied to the bracket (slide A) and a counterbalancing moment (M_C) is produced by rectangular wire (slide C) but less than 1000 g mm, it can move the center of rotation near to the apical area and create a type of "controlled tipping" (slide B) type of movement.

The correct M/F ratio should be obtained for bringing the impacted tooth into the dental arch but it is important to maintain the ratio for a constant center of rotation. By using rectangular loop (R-loop) in a cantilever spring, load-deflection rate will be decreased i.e. make the spring more flexible (relative to straight wire), and the configuration of the spring leads to a better maintenance of M/F ratio for a constant center of rotation. Segmented R-loop has long range action with minimal force decrease during tooth movement and acceptable control of force magnitude. If the spring is distorted by the patient, it can significantly move the tooth in an unwanted direction (Figure 13).

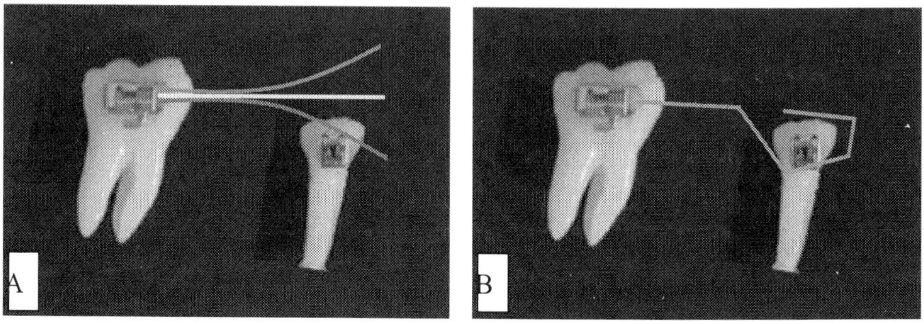

Figure 13. A straight wire is used in (A) to erupt the bicuspid. When the wire is bent (blue line) and engaged in the bracket, the root apex tends to go to distal, in the next yellow line position, the root is upright and moment drops off, and in red line position; roots tends to go to the mesial while the crown is depressed. With this configuration, several centers of rotation exist and constancy of the moment to force ratio is affected (inconsistent force system). Slide B demonstrates preactivated rectangular loop (R-loop) which provides constant control of M/F ratio. The R-loop is made from 0.018x0.025 inch Stainless Steel or 0.017x0.025 inch Titanium Molybdenum Alloy (TMA).

Treating a clinical case of a maxillary canine in infralabioversion by means of the straight archwire technique used to level the tooth is a harmful procedure for adjacent teeth. Canine extrusion would occur regardless of the type of bracket, whether conventional or self-ligating; however, it would be followed by undesired intrusion and moment on the lateral incisor and first premolar (Figure 14). Many authors believe that these side effects can be solved with intermaxillary rubber bands, arch bends or wire progression. Conversely, with the aid of the segmented arch technique (SAT) and after preparation of the anchorage unit, only the canine is extracted by a cantilever or a rectangular loop (Figure 14).

Differently from the conventional techniques, which normally use an archwire made of one single alloy, connecting all brackets and adjacent tubes, the SAT uses arch segments connected to each other, but not necessarily connected to brackets and adjacent tubes. This allows a combination of wires made of different alloys, dimensions and hardness to be used. Rigid and thick archwires can connect groups of teeth to anchorage units, whereas flexible archwires are used to exert forces between these units. [15]

http://dx.doi.org/10.5772/59143

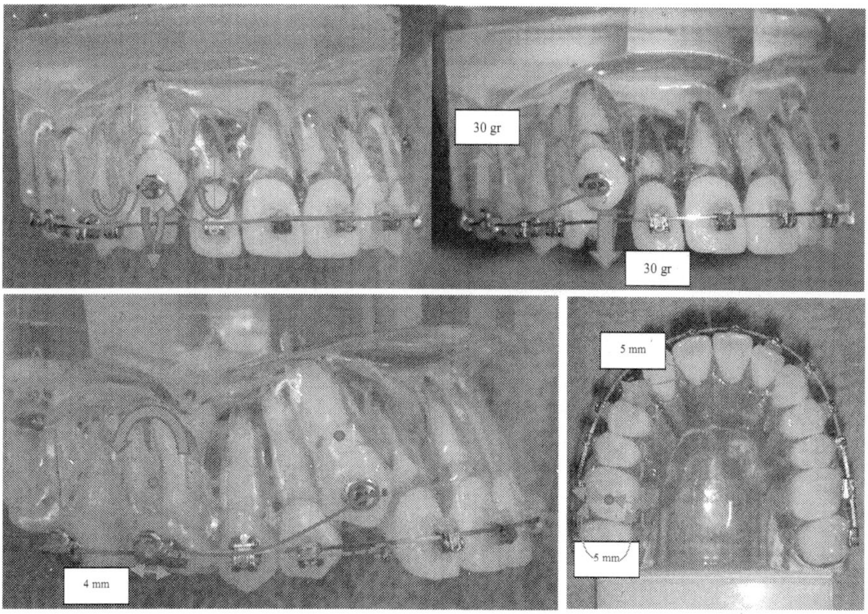

Figure 14. Top-left) Continuous arch wire (NiTi or CuNiTi) or straight archwire technique can be used to level the impacted canine/high buccal canine (infralabioversion canine); but canine extrusion would be followed by intrusive force and positive and negative moment on the first premolar and lateral incisor. A lingual moment is created for the upper canine that will lead it to the dental arch. Top-right) with the cantilever mechanics or segmented arch technique (SAT), a cantilever rectangular spring is inserted into a rectangular tube and tied to one point on the other side to produce "determinate one-couple system". Bottom-left) Sectional cantilever spring is used to extrude the impacted canine (force 30 grams, and distance between canine and first molar, presumably, about 20 mm). Extrusive force on canine (30 grams) will produce 30 gram intrusive force on upper first molar plus 600 g mm moment (M=Fxd=30x20=600) to create distal root movement (blue arrow). The moment may be created by a couple (molar tube, presumably, 4 mm in length) with 150 grams force (600/4=150g) upward on the mesial end of the tube and 150 grams downwards on the distal end. Bottom-right) the abovementioned force system from the occlusal view. Consider the moment created by the rectangular archwire in molar tube (torque) and moment on the canine. If center of resistance of the canine tooth is, presumably, about 5 mm lingual to the bonded button on the crown, a 150 g mm (30x5=150g.mm) moment rotates the tooth lingually. At the first molar, if the center of resistance is 5 mm lingual to the tube, a 30 g intrusive force can create 150 g mm moment to rotate it buccally. If the center of resistance of the impacted canine is, presumably, 10 mm palatal to the buccal surface of the first molar, activation of spring to tie to the canine, can twist it and create 300 g mm (30x10=300g mm) moment to rotate the molar crown palatally. The result at the molar is a net 150 g mm (300 g mm palatal – 150 g mm buccal =150 g mm palatal) palatal crown torque. (Bracket type and existence of continuous archwire of the model are not related to the biomechanical explanations.)

5.1. Biomechanical alternatives for forced tooth eruption

The orthodontist should avoid mechanics that draw the tooth labially, which could produce a bony dehiscence and accelerated migration of the labial gingival margin, resulting in labial recession. A "Ballista" loop is a simple, convenient, unobtrusive method of applying a vertical vector of force to a labially impacted tooth to erupt the crown into the center of the alveolus. When the canine crown is displaced mesially and lies over the root of the permanent lateral incisor, an apically positioned flap is the appropriate surgical uncovering technique. Exposure of the crown facilitates attachment of an elastomeric chain directed toward the center of the edentulous alveolar ridge to gradually guide the canine crown into the dental arch. [16] A "Vertical spring" bent into 0.14 inch stainless steel wire that faces downward before activation is another alternative. It can be activated by pushing the vertical legs toward the impacted canine. This kind of round wire has the benefit of increased length and springiness but needs some kind of anti-rotation bent for avoiding rotation of round wire inside bracket slot that neutralizes the activity of the spring. Another alternative is an "Overlaid Auxiliary NiTi wire" on the rectangular stabilizing arch. These auxiliary arch wires are very efficient to bring an impacted tooth into dental arch. "Cantilever springs" can be used, either soldered to a heavy base arch or from auxiliary tube on the first molar. Some have used headgear tube plus an anti-rotation bend on wire and a helix around main arch wire for forced eruption of impacted teeth.

5.2. Molar uprighting in impacted cases

A dental arch with aligned teeth and heavy main archwire can serve as an anchorage unit to be used for uprighting posterior second or third molar teeth by a NiTi or sectional Stainless Steel wire incorporating loops e.g. T-loop. Absolute anchorages i.e. miniscrews or titanium miniplates are other alternatives for distalizing or uprighting impacted molar teeth (Figure 15).

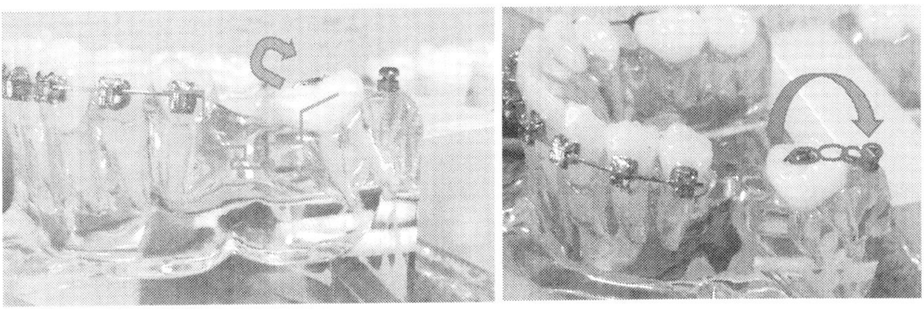

Figure 15. T-loops have efficient control on angulation and torque of an inclined tooth (left). An alternative to absolute anchorage can help in uprighting the tilted impacted second or third molars without endangering other teeth as anchorage units that may be affected with orthodontic force and tooth movement or root resorption.

Molar uprighting is generally associated with extrusion of antagonist teeth, reduction in edentulous space, bone dehiscence in the mesial surface of tipped molars, gingival recession of tipped molars, early contact in centric relation and occlusal interference on excursion of the mandible. With regard to integrated planning, clinicians must decide whether the tooth subject to uprighting will undergo movement for space closure, opening of space for prosthetic rehabilitation or implant placement. Mesial movement of molars may be rendered difficult due to the following: alveolar bone resorption resulting from tooth loss, which causes the molar mesial bone to become too thin; unfavorable root morphology for movement of lower molars; greater mandibular bone density in relation to the maxilla; and thin buccolingual bone thickness from distal to mesial in the mandibular arch. Using straight wires to upright tipped molars is considered unfeasible, given that, in these cases, there is a strong tendency towards extrusion of molars, especially due to the short distance between brackets. Additionally, incorporating a T-loop spring into the arch will lead to extrusion of premolars. A cantilever, extended up to the anterior region, may be used to reduce the effects of extrusion on molars. Researchers have proved a moment of 1200 gf.mm to be appropriate for molar uprighting. Should a 30-mm cantilever be used, an activation of 40 gf is enough for molar uprighting, in which case 40 gf corresponds to intrusive forces in the anterior region and extrusive forces in the region of molar teeth. Mesocephalic or brachycephalic patients are able to eliminate or reduce this effect of extrusion by their own muscular pattern. [15, 17]

6. Alignment/ Leveling/Torque/Angulation (ALTA) corrections

The root apices are located in the apical portion of the jaws and malposition almost always develops as the eruption paths of teeth are deflected; for impacted teeth the problem is more complicated and both apex and crown are usually misplaced. ALTA corrections have been considered for the time that impacted tooth has been brought near to the dental arch. Light and continuous force is recommended for the beginning of the treatment i.e. "Alignment", through tipping movement for impacted teeth in facio-lingual direction. As a general rule, heavy wires should be avoided at this stage. A minimum of 0.004 inch clearance is needed for sliding mechanics, in other words, in 0.018 slot an archwire with 0.014 inch stainless steel can be accepted for sliding but for severe crowding or malposition situation, more length of wire in the form of loop or helices should be incorporated. Although resilient wire with rectangular shape like A-NiTi or CuNiTi (Damon system) could be used, but because they produce unwanted root movement, possible root resorption, and possible delay in alignment progression, rectangular resilient wires are not advisable. Wires should have excellent strength and springiness, long range of action and low load deflection rate. NiTi wires are springier and stronger (in small section) than beta-titanium (TMA), for these reasons, A-NiTi and CuNiTi wires are recommended for initial stages of aligning.

In addition to alignment, impacted teeth should be "Leveled" in occluso-gingival direction. Leveling can be obtained by absolute intrusion or by relative intrusion and sometimes by differential elongation or extrusion of teeth. Utility arches e.g. 2x4 appliance, reverse curve for lower arch, intrusion arch and combination of sectional wires, segmented arches and titanium miniscrews are used for leveling the dental arch.

After establishment of proper alignment and leveling, two other crown position characteristics should be achieved i.e. "Torque" and "Angulation". Torque is in facio-lingual direction and usually involves root movement and moment (increased M/F ratio) is needed for its correction. Angulation is related to mesio-distal characteristics of crown positioning and like the amount of torque degree, is considered in bracket prescription in straight wire appliances (SWA). Wire bending like what is performed in "Standard Edgewise" for finishing and establishment of correct torque and angulation, is needed for severe impacted cases for obtaining the proper ALTA correction and accepted occlusion (according to ABO scores).

7. Conclusion

Bone-impacted canines of the hard palatal are more likely to respond to surgical exposure and orthodontic management if angulation to midline is less than 45 degrees on the OPG; there is no root anomaly found on OPG, periapical (PA), and maxillary occlusal (MO) radiographs; and overlap of the adjacent lateral incisor root (OALIR) by the canine crown is nonexistent or less than grade 2 (half the root) on the OPG.[18] Researchers have tried to predict impaction of a maxillary canine using geometric measurements made on panoramic radiographs. Diagnosis of an outcome can be performed cross-sectionally, however; for prediction, two separate prospective data sets should be used. [19]

Deimpaction of the impacted teeth can be accelerated by means of thick soft tissue removal with laser application. Laser-assisted surgical removal of the fibrous tissue over erupting premolars (DTE) with appropriate irradiation parameters appears to be a promising adjunct to orthodontic treatment for bringing them to the aligned and leveled dental arch.[20] Orthodontic tooth movement and root resorption of impacted teeth can be influenced by laser [21] and administration of different drugs.[22,23]

Author details

Massoud Seifi[1*] and Mohammad Hosein Kalantar Motamedi[2]

*Address all correspondence to: seifimassoud@gmail.com

1 Dentofacial Deformities Research Center, Department of Orthodontics, Shahid Beheshti University of Medical Sciences, Tehran, Iran

2 Trauma Research Center, Baqiyatallah Medical Sciences University, Tehran, Iran

References

[1] CA C. A Method of ascertaining, the Relative Position of Unerupted Proc R Soc Med 1910;3((Odontol Sect)):87-90.

[2] Jacobs SG. Radiographic localization of unerupted teeth: further findings about the vertical tube shift method and other localization techniques. American journal of orthodontics and dentofacial orthopedics : official publication of the American Association of Orthodontists, its constituent societies, and the American Board of Orthodontics. 2000;118(4):439-47.

[3] Roberts JA, Drage NA, Davies J, Thomas DW. Effective dose from cone beam CT examinations in dentistry. The British journal of radiology. 2009;82(973):35-40.

[4] Trobe JD KJ. Cost-benefit analysis in screening. Unexplained visual loss.. Surv Ophthalmol 28(3):189-93.

[5] Bahreman A. Early-age orthodontic Treatment: Quintessence Publishing Co, Inc; 2013.

[6] Stewart JA, Heo G, Glover KE, Williamson PC, Lam EW, Major PW. Factors that relate to treatment duration for patients with palatally impacted maxillary canines. American journal of orthodontics and dentofacial orthopedics : official publication of the American Association of Orthodontists, its constituent societies, and the American Board of Orthodontics. 2001;119(3):216-25.

[7] Zuccati G, Ghobadlu J, Nieri M, Clauser C. Factors associated with the duration of forced eruption of impacted maxillary canines: a retrospective study. American journal of orthodontics and dentofacial orthopedics : official publication of the American Association of Orthodontists, its constituent societies, and the American Board of Orthodontics. 2006;130(3):349-56.

[8] Ericson S KJ. Resorption of maxillary lateral incisors caused by ectopic eruption of the canines. A clinical and radiographic analysis of predisposing factors. American journal of orthodontics and dentofacial orthopedics : official publication of the American Association of Orthodontists, its constituent societies, and the American Board of Orthodontics.94(6):503-13.

[9] Pitt S, Hamdan A, Rock P. A treatment difficulty index for unerupted maxillary canines. European journal of orthodontics. 2006;28(2):141-4.

[10] Warford JH, Grandhi RK, Tira DE. Prediction of maxillary canine impaction using sectors and angular measurement. American Journal of Orthodontics and Dentofacial Orthopedics. 2003;124(6):651-5.

[11] Kau CH, Pan P, Gallerano RL, English JD. A novel 3D classification system for canine impactions--the KPG index. The international journal of medical robotics + computer assisted surgery : MRCAS. 2009;5(3):291-6.

[12] Melsen B, Verna C. Miniscrew implants: The Aarhus anchorage system. Seminars in Orthodontics. 2005;11(1):24-31.

[13] Papadopoulos MA, Tarawneh F. The use of miniscrew implants for temporary skeletal anchorage in orthodontics: a comprehensive review. Oral surgery, oral medicine, oral pathology, oral radiology, and endodontics. 2007;103(5):e6-15.

[14] Celenza F. Implant Interactions with Orthodontics. Journal of Evidence Based Dental Practice. 2012;12(3):192-201.

[15] Caldas SG, Ribeiro AA, Simplício H, Machado AW. Segmented arch or continuous arch technique? A rational approach. Dental Press J Orthod. 2014 Mar-Apr;19(2): 126-41.

[16] Kokich VG. Surgical and orthodontic management of impacted maxillary canines. Am J Orthod Dentofacial Orthop. 2004 Sep;126(3):278-83.

[17] Romeo DA, Burstone CJ. Tip-back mechanics. Am J Orthod. 1977 Oct;72(4):414-21.

[18] Motamedi MH, Tabatabaie FA, Navi F, Shafeie HA, Fard BK, Hayati Z. Assessment of radiographic factors affecting surgical exposure and orthodontic alignment of impacted canines of the palate: a 15-year retrospective study. Oral Surg Oral Med Oral Pathol Oral Radiol Endod. 2009 Jun;107(6):772-5. doi:10.1016/j.tripleo.2008.12.022.

[19] Sabour S, Vahid Dastjerdi E. Early prediction of maxillary canine impaction from panoramic radiographs. Am J Orthod Dentofacial Orthop. 2012 Oct;142(4):428; author reply 428-9. doi: 10.1016/j.ajodo.2012.08.010.

[20] Seifi M, Vahid-Dastjerdi E, Ameli N, Badiee MR, Younessian F., Amdjadi P. The 808 nm Laser-Assisted Surgery as an Adjunct to Orthodontic Treatment of Delayed Tooth Eruption: J Lasers Med Sci 2013; 4(2):70-4

[21] Seifi M, Atri F, Yazdani MM. Effects of low-level laser therapy on orthodontic tooth movement and root resorption after artificial socket preservation. Dent Res J (Isfahan). 2014 Jan;11(1):61-6.

[22] Seifi M, Eslami B, Saffar AS. The effect of prostaglandin E2 and calcium gluconate on orthodontic tooth movement and root resorption in rats. Eur J Orthod. 2003 Apr; 25(2):199-204.

[23] Seifi M, Badiee MR, Abdolazimi Z, Amdjadi P. Effect of basic fibroblast growth factor on orthodontic tooth movement in rats. Cell J. 2013 Fall;15(3):230-7. Epub 2013 Aug 24.

Chapter 6

Surgical Exposure and Orthodontic Alignment of Impacted Teeth

Mohammad Hosein Kalantar Motamedi

Additional information is available at the end of the chapter

http://dx.doi.org/10.5772/58956

1. Introduction

Tooth impaction is a condition in which the tooth is embedded in the tissues such that its eruption is prevented.[1, 2] Management of impactions is usually either by surgical exposure and forced eruption or surgical extraction; the decision depends upon a multitude of factors that need to be assessed via clinical and radiographic evaluations of the patient before formulating the overall treatment plan. The clinical evaluation includes assessment of:

- Patient age
- Oral hygiene and dental caries
- Depth of the impaction
- Displacement of the impaction and associated pathologies
- Esthetics and morphological suitability of the impaction
- Functionality of the impacted tooth
- Length of orthodontic and surgical treatment and costs
- Worthiness of salvaging the impacted tooth
- Treatment options for the impaction
- Feasibility of surgical exposure and orthodontic alignment

These factors are among the issues that are influential in deciding whether to expose or to extract the impacted tooth. Patient cooperation and compliance are additional determinants which should be considered before commencing treatment. [3, 4]

2. Clinical evaluation

2.1. Patient age

The best age for tooth exposure and forced eruption or surgical extraction is in childhood and adolescence; because as age increases, the impacted tooth often develops ankylosis (fusion to bone) precluding the possibility to move it into the dental arch orthodontically. The inability to move the impaction may not be readily diagnosed preoperatively; and may become evident only when the tooth fails to move after it has been exposed and orthodontic traction has been applied for several weeks or more. Aside from age, ankylosis may occur following dentoalveolar trauma in childhood or adolescence. Trauma to the primary dentition in childhood can lead to damage to the dental germ resulting in deformation or displacement. Premature loss of a primary tooth may also result in delayed or barred eruption of the permanent tooth due to bone or dense fibrous tissue formation in the normal path of eruption.

2.2. Oral hygiene and dental caries

Tooth exposure, forced eruption and orthodontic therapy of an impaction may not be indicated if the patient has rampant caries, poor oral hygiene, lacks motivation or is uncooperative. If the impacted tooth is decayed, it may be an indication for removal of the impaction.

2.3. Depth of the impaction

Impactions that are very deep may not be amenable to exposure and orthodontic therapy. Sometimes even surgical removal of such teeth is not indicated especially when harm may be inflicted upon vital structures or teeth in the course of the procedure. Such cases may be left alone and followed periodically with radiographs every 6-12 months for changes in the follicle of the impaction. Removal of the crown only (coronectomy) is another option.

2.4. Displacement of the impaction and associated pathologies

Displacement of adjacent teeth and pathological lesions associated with an impacted tooth may mandate removal of the impaction. However, eruption cysts, dentigerous cysts and benign lesions (i.e. adenomatoid odontogenic tumor, giant cell lesions, aneurysmal bone cysts etc.) may be exceptions. In these cases it may be possible to just remove the pathology and salvage the impacted tooth (discussed later in this chapter). [5-13]

2.5. Esthetics and morphological suitability of the impaction

Esthetics and morphological suitability of the impaction are among the issues that may influence the decision to expose or to extract the impacted tooth. The canine tooth for example is very strategic because it is usually visible when the patient smiles; therefore, it merits salvage; whereas, a deformed, unsightly or nonfunctional canine may not be worth saving unless it can be restored.

2.6. Functionality of the impacted tooth

A severely deformed or short-rooted impacted tooth deemed unlikely to be functional is more likely to require removal rather than surgical exposure and orthodontic alignment.

2.7. Length and costs of orthodontic and surgical treatment

The length of orthodontic and surgical treatment and expenses are additional sideline issues to be considered and discussed with the patient, parents or guardians before formulating a treatment plan. The length of orthodontic treatment to guide the impaction into the dental arch and into occlusion, usually takes 1-3 years (depending on patient age, bone density, the amount of root formation and dilaceration, depth and angulation of the impaction, available arch space etc.). Expenses are directly correlated to the aforementioned parameters (the longer it takes to bring the impaction into position the more it will cost). An estimate should be made prior to commencing treatment.

2.8. Worthiness of salvaging the impacted tooth

The third molar is commonly impacted because of arch-length tooth-size discrepancy. Wisdom teeth often require extraction due to of lack of arch space, periodontal pockets, a blocked path of eruption, malocclusion, caries or pericorontitis. Thus, third molars are rarely surgically exposed or uprighted; however, up-righting the mandibular third molar may be indicated when a distal abutment is needed for anchorage of a prosthesis.

Second molars and premolars are less commonly impacted and treatment is dictated by factors such as occlusion, arch space, caries, strategic value of the tooth and costs. The decision to salvage or extract is case-specific. Decisions are made after clinical assessment, consultation and collaboration with the orthodontist.

The permanent incisors are rarely impacted; however, when they are, they often merit salvaging in both jaws because they are esthetically important and readily seen when the patient smiles. They also play a major role in the dental midline which is very important esthetically; because deviation of the dental midline is conspicuous and readily noticed by others.

The permanent canine of the maxilla is the second most commonly impacted tooth. It is the tooth with the longest root and is important in cuspid-rise type occlusions. The canine is usually seen when the person smiles. It is thus, esthetically important and merits salvaging whenever possible.

2.9. Treatment options for the impaction

The treatment options open to a patient with a permanent impacted canine include:

1. *Interceptive removal:* Interceptive removal of the deciduous canine to enhance eruption of the permanent canine is done when the root has not formed completely and space is available for eruption.

2. *No treatment:* No treatment, except periodic radiographical evaluation for pathological changes, is done when there are limitations to surgically expose or extract.

3. *Surgical removal:* Surgical removal of the impacted canine and prosthetic replacement is done when there are limitations for salvaging the tooth.

4. *Surgical exposure:* Surgical exposure of the impacted canine and orthodontic alignment is done when indicated and deemed feasible. [3, 4]

Data such as age and sex, space for alignment, presence of the primary canine, migration of the first premolar in the site of the canine, and other aforementioned issues must be assessed and documented. If the tooth is strategic and should it be desired to save it, then a feasibility study must also be done to see whether the impacted canine can respond to surgical exposure and forced eruption or if it has to be surgically removed.

2.10. Feasibility of surgical exposure and orthodontic alignment

Salvaging the bone-impacted canine of the palate usually requires a combination of both surgical and orthodontic management. To ascertain if exposure and orthodontic treatment is feasible, first arch space assessment followed by the radiographic evaluation is necessary.

2.11. Arch space assessment

A comprehensive evaluation must be done In order to assess whether or not space is available in the arch or has to be made available for eruption and alignment of the impacted tooth, or if the impaction must be removed. Sometimes the primary tooth has not exfoliated and should be extracted. Arch space and tooth size measurements have to be done. More often than not, space has to be made orthodontically to accommodate the canine in the dental arch.

2.12. Radiographic evaluation

In addition to clinical assessments, predicting the feasibility to expose and move an impacted permanent canine from the hard palate into the alveolar arch can be done radiographically. Radiographic records are used to assess depth of the impaction, root morphology and the degree of difficulty.

2.13. Radiographic records

Radiographic records (orthopantomogram [OPG], periapical [PA], and maxillary occlusal [MO]) must be taken, assessed and documented. Preoperative radiographs of each patient have to be viewed and examined using a light box. Digital images can be viewed on an LCD monitor. Root anomalies and radiographic measurements are sought prior to treatment.

2.14. Root anomaly

The presence or absence of root anomaly must be recorded when apparent on the OPG, PA, and MO radiographs. Root angulation or dilaceration must also be assessed from the radiographs. Severe dilaceration or bulky roots may render forced eruption and alignment unfeasible.

2.14.1. *Radiographic measurements*

Several angles and measurements of impacted canine position can be made from the OPG radiograph namely:

- canine angulation to the midline (CAM),
- ratio of root formation (RRF),
- lateral incisor root overlap (LIRO) and
- degree of vertical impaction (DVI)

The aforementioned measurements may aid in the decision making process.

2.14.2. *Canine angulation to the midline (CAM)*

A midline is constructed as shown in Fig. 1 and a second line is drawn through the canine root apex and canine tip to the midline. The angle formed between the 2 lines is the impacted canine angulation to the midline, and is graded as follows:

- **Grade1** (0-15°), Easy
- **Grade2** (16-30°), Moderate
- **Grade3** (31°+), Difficult

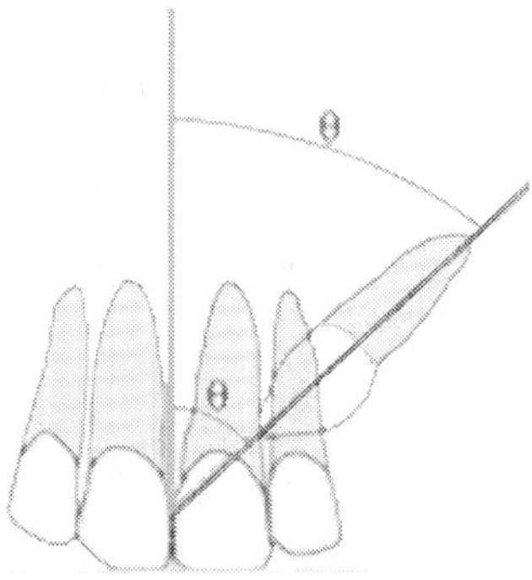

Figure 1. The angulation of the palatally-impacted canine to the midline. The more obtuse the angle the more difficult it will be to expose and align and the poorer the prognosis.

The more obtuse the angle the more difficult it will be to expose and align the impacted canine and the poorer the prognosis.

2.14.3. Ratio of Root formation (RRF)

The canine root formation ratio is graded from 1 to 3 depending upon the amount of root formed:

- **Grade 1** (1/3 formed), Easy
- **Grade 2** (2/3formed), Moderate
- **Grade 3** (completely formed) Difficult

The more the root has formed the more difficult it will be to expose and align the impacted canine and the poorer the prognosis.

2.14.4. Lateral incisor root overlap (LIRO)

The position of the canine(s) on the OPG helps predict the feasibility and prognosis for alignment of the canine by reference to the amount by which its crown overlaps the incisor roots in both the horizontal and vertical planes. The degree of overlap of the adjacent lateral incisor root via the crown of the palatally-impacted canine is assessed and graded as follows:

- **Grade 1**: No horizontal overlap; Easy
- **Grade 2**: Overlap less than half the root width; Moderate
- **Grade 3**: Overlap more than half, but less than the whole root width; Difficult
- **Grade 4**: Complete overlap of root width or more; Very difficult.

The closer the canine is to the midline in the horizontal plane the greater the difficulty and the poorer the prognosis (Fig. 2).

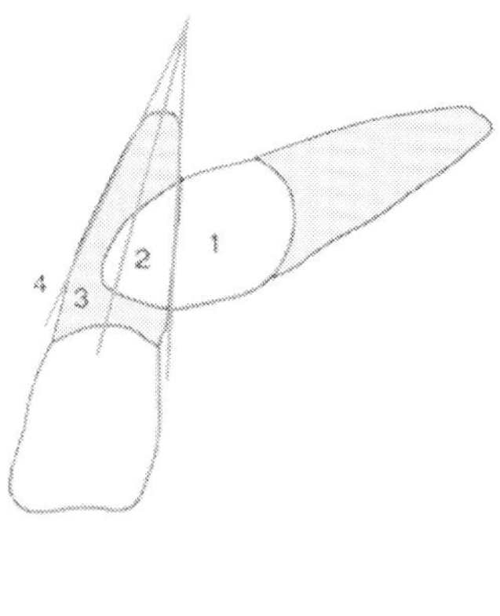

Figure 2. Grades of overlap of the adjacent lateral incisor root via the crown of the impacted canine in the palate. The greater the overlap the more difficult the procedure will be.

http://dx.doi.org/10.5772/58956

2.14.5. Degree of vertical impaction (DVI)

The vertical depth of the canine(s) on the OPG also helps predict the feasibility and prognosis for alignment of the canine by reference to the amount by which it lies in respect to the apical third of the lateral incisor root in the vertical plane:

- **Grade 1** Easy (canine crown at the coronal segment of the lateral incisor root).
- **Grade 2** Moderate (canine crown below the coronal segment of the lateral incisor root but above half the root).
- **Grade 3** Difficult (canine crown below half the root of the lateral incisor root but above the apex).
- **Grade 4** Very difficult (canine crown at the apical segment of the lateral incisor root).

The higher the impaction lies the greater the difficulty and the poorer the prognosis for surgical and orthodontic treatment (Fig. 3). [5, 6]

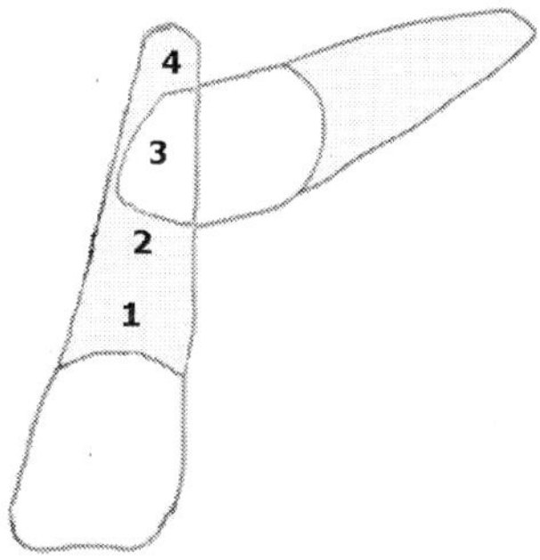

Figure 3. Besides the amount of overlap of the adjacent lateral incisor root via the crown of the impacted canine in the palate, the higher the impaction lies vertically the more difficult the surgical and orthodontic procedure will be.

The influence of increased canine angulation to the midline, the greater lateral tooth overlap and the deeper the vertical depth means a deep horizontally positioned impaction and thus, a more difficult canine to expose and align orthodontically. There is an increased probability that such canines will require removal instead of exposure.14-17 However, although a large amount of information may be obtained regarding impacted canine position from radiographs, this was not a major influence on our decision to surgically expose or remove impacted canines. Our study showed impacted canine angulation and depth correlated with difficulty in alignment and eruption. Age may be an influencing factor; however, all our cases were adolescents.

When there is a primary canine remaining in place of the permanent canine impacted in the palate, the patient does not have much to lose if the impaction is exposed surgically and orthodontic alignment is attempted. However, if the space is occupied by the permanent first premolar then extracting the premolar to make space for the palatally bone-impacted permanent canine is risky because the canine may be fused and defy forced eruption. Thus, in such cases it should be attempted to expose and move the impaction before the premolar is extracted. If the impacted tooth responds favorably to forced eruption then the premolar is extracted.

3. Surgical exposure techniques

3.1. Exposure technique for a palatally-impacted canine

The surgical technique used to expose a palatally-impacted canine is relatively uncomplicated. After local anesthesia, a window is made in the palate at the site where the crown of the impaction is anticipated to be using an electrosurgery knife; the electrosurgery knife is used to remove the tissue overlying the tooth. Then, the palatal mucoperiosteum is dissected off the bone and discarded. The bony covering of the tooth is removed with a rose bur and handpiece under copious saline irrigation. The follicular tissue is scraped off the palatal surface of the crown and removed. The cavity is enlarged if necessary by further soft tissue and/or bone removal as required to expose the entire palatal or buccal surface of the impaction (depending on the orientation of the impaction). The cementoenamel junction is left undisturbed. After hemostasis, the tooth is dried and after acid etching and resin bonding a bracket is fixed to the labial or palatal surface of the crown; then the wound is packed using periodontal dressing.

Alternatively, orthodontic brackets may be bonded 3 to 7 days postoperatively by the orthodontist (instead of intraoperatively). Seven to 10 days postoperatively 50 to 60 g elastic traction is applied (Fig.4).

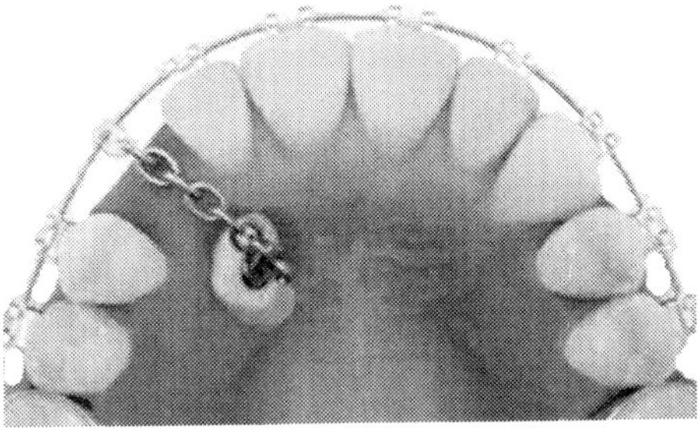

Figure 4. A palatally-impacted canine is exposed through a round window and a bracket is attached to the palatal surface of the crown.

3.2. Exposure technique for a buccally-impacted canine

Buccally-oriented impacted canines are generally easier to treat. The surgical technique used to expose a buccally-oriented impacted canine after local anesthesia, includes reflection of a small trapezoid flap at the site where the crown of the impaction is anticipated using a scalpel

http://dx.doi.org/10.5772/58956

and no.15 blade. The underlying bone is removed using a round bur and handpiece. Then, the follicle is removed exposing the crown. The flap is then repositioned apically at the CEJ of the impaction and sutured in the vestibule leaving the crown exposed for bracket bonding. In due time the tooth erupts (or is forced to erupt) bringing attached gingiva along with it (Fig. 5).

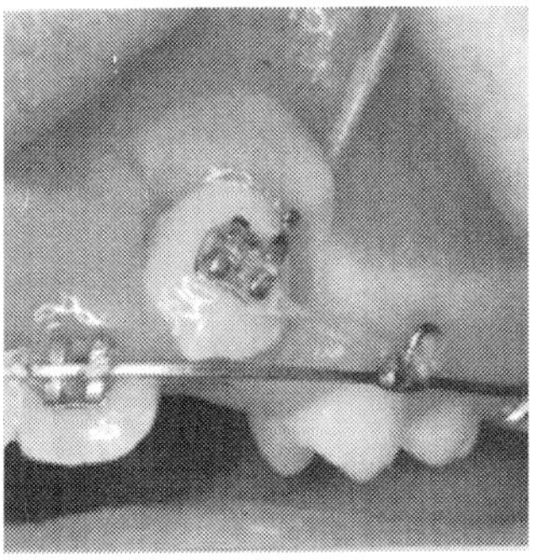

Figure 5. A buccally-impacted canine is exposed through a trapezoid flap sutured apically so that it erupts along with the attached gingiva; a bracket has been attached and elastic traction has been applied.

Follicular enlargement or cystic change around an impacted canine should be sought and this factor is taken into consideration when planning treatment for impacted canines. However, this per se does not mean that the impacted canine must be extracted (discussed later in this chapter).5,6

3.3. Severely-displaced impacted maxillary canine

Sometimes the impacted canine is displaced in the jaws; this is often due to a pathologic lesion most commonly a dentigerous cyst (Fig. 6).

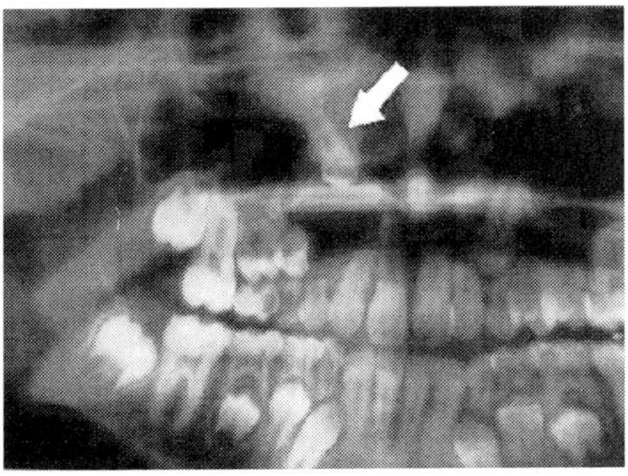

Figure 6. Impacted canine displaced high up in the maxilla adjacent to the orbital floor due to a dentigerous cyst.

In such cases the exposure has to be made through the mucosa. Impediments (cyst, tumor, teeth, fibrosis etc.) must be removed, sent to the pathologist and the tooth be given time to descend (Fig.7).

When the tooth is accessible in the vestibule it is then exposed and bonded (Fig. 8). [18]

After 2 years the tooth was finally in the dental arch (Fig. 9).

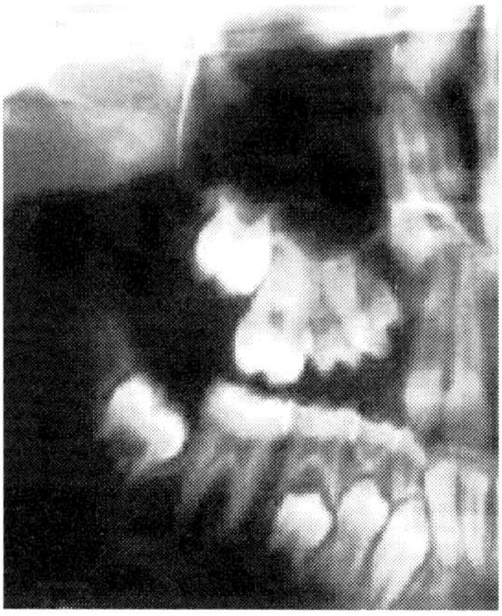

Figure 7. The tooth has descended after cyst removal.

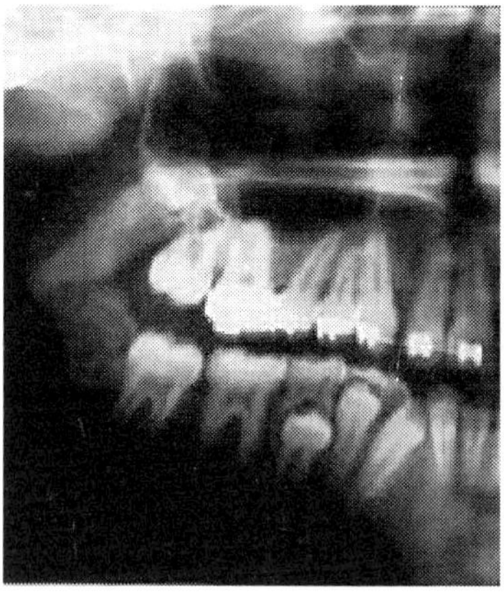

Figure 8. The tooth has descended 3-4 cm and brought into occlusion.

http://dx.doi.org/10.5772/58956

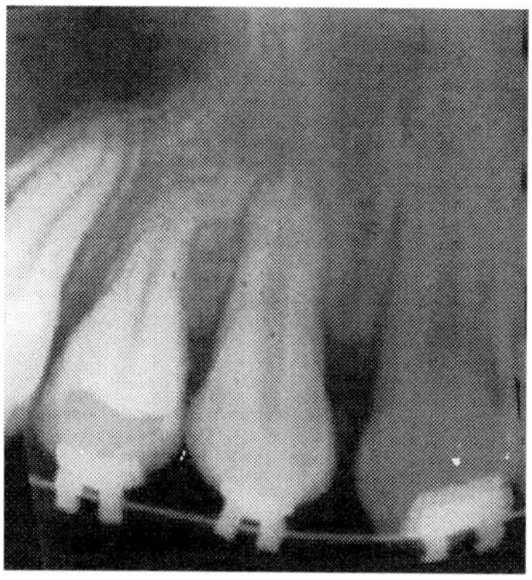

Figure 9. The canine tooth has been brought into the dental arch. (Orthodontist: Dr. Jabari)

3.4. Severely-displaced impacted mandibular canine

A cyst may also displace an impaction in the mandible to a great extent. Enucleation of the cyst without extraction of the impacted tooth may be indicated for children and adolescents if the involved tooth is strategic. There may be swelling in the vestibular area of the mandibular canine region. A common cause is a dentigerous cyst. Aspiration of the lesion must be performed first; in many cases, aspiration reveals a clear yellow fluid in dentigerous cysts. Next, the entity must be confirmed by a pathologist. In our case, excisional biopsy was performed under local anesthesia via a submarginal mucoperiosteal trapezoid flap reflected from the right canine tooth to the left premolar from below the attached gingiva; the cystic lesion was removed after it was separated from the bone and incised off the tooth surface using a #15 scalpel. The flap was sewn in the vestibule, which left the crown exposed for bracket bonding. Orthodontic treatment was started 2 weeks postoperatively. (Figs. 10 and 11).

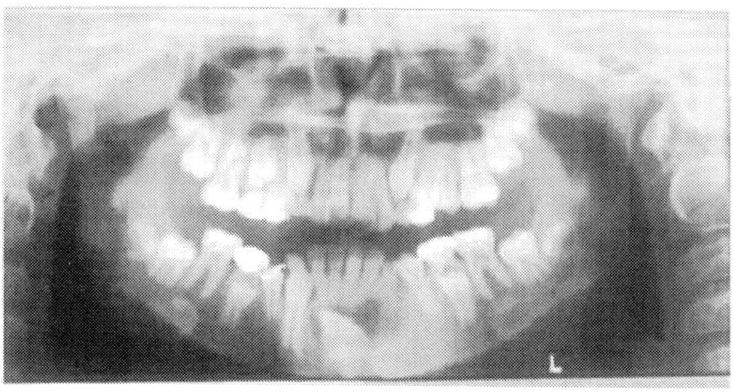

Figure 10. Orthopantomogram of an impacted canine displaced to the inferior border of the chin by a large dentigerous cyst of the mandible extending from the right canine to the left first premolar tooth

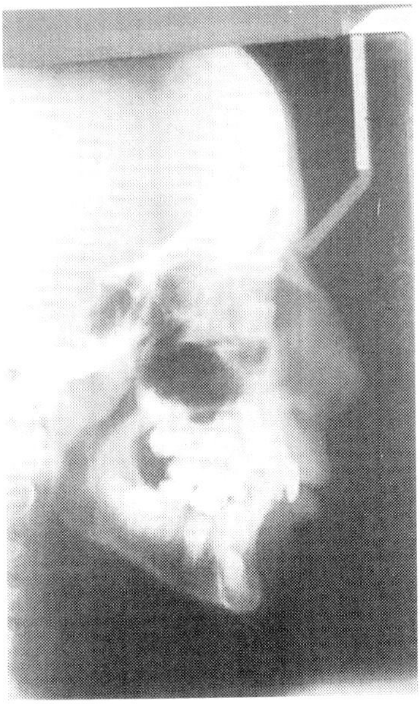

Figure 11. Lateral cephalogram obtained at the same time.

The canine was brought into occlusion orthodontically within 4 years (Figs. 12 and 13). [19]

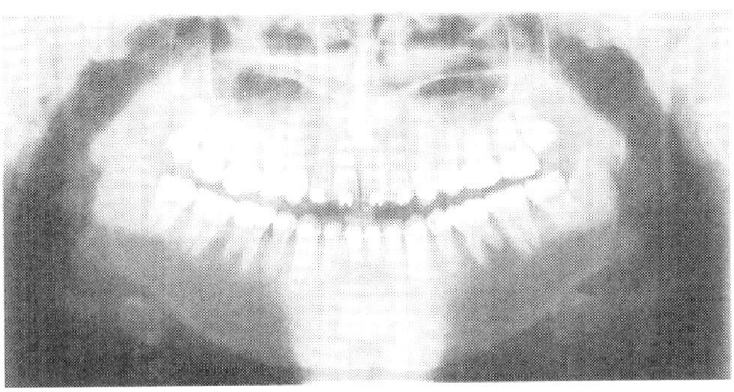

Figure 12. Orthopantomogram 4 years after surgery. The tooth has been brought into occlusion after surgical exposure and orthodontic guidance; the vitality of all of the teeth has been preserved.

http://dx.doi.org/10.5772/58956

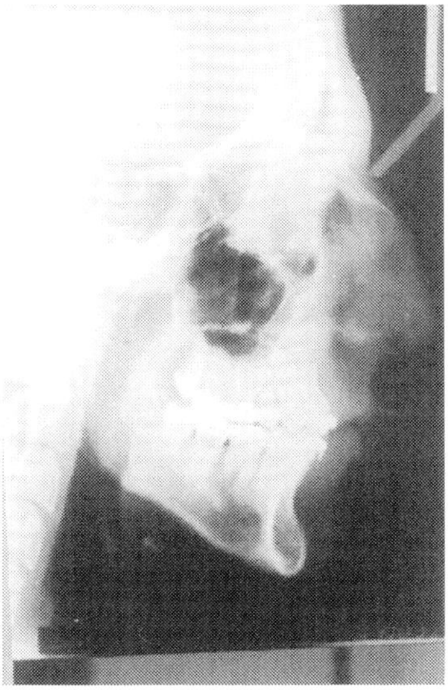

Figure 13. Lateral cephalogram obtained at the same time. This bone has healed in the chin.

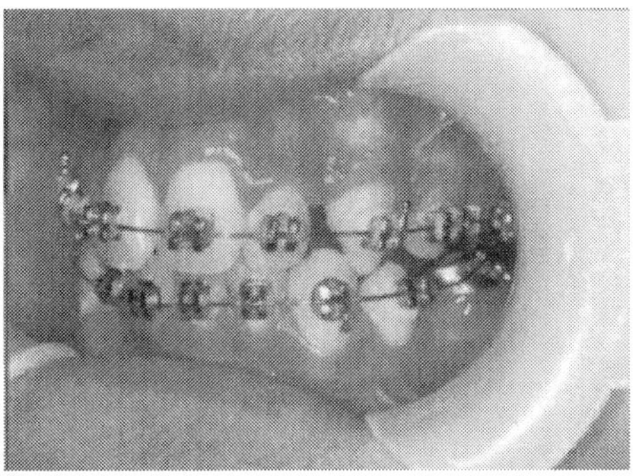

Figure 14. Oral view (Orthodontist Dr. Masoud Seifi).

3.5. Impacted teeth associated with benign tumors

The surgical technique used to expose an impacted tooth associated with a benign tumor is similar. Aspiration of the lesion is negative for fluid. An excisional biopsy under local anesthesia is done. A trapezoid flap is reflected from the mesial and distal aspects of the involved tooth. The lesion is completely removed after separating the capsule from the bone and excising it off the canine tooth surface. Minimal bone removal in the bed of the lesion is done with a rose bur. Clinically, nothing is left attached to the tooth surface. The wound is irrigated and the flap is sutured apically leaving the crown exposed for bracket bonding. Orthodontic treatment is started 1-2 weeks postoperatively depending on the case (Figs. 15 and 16). [6]

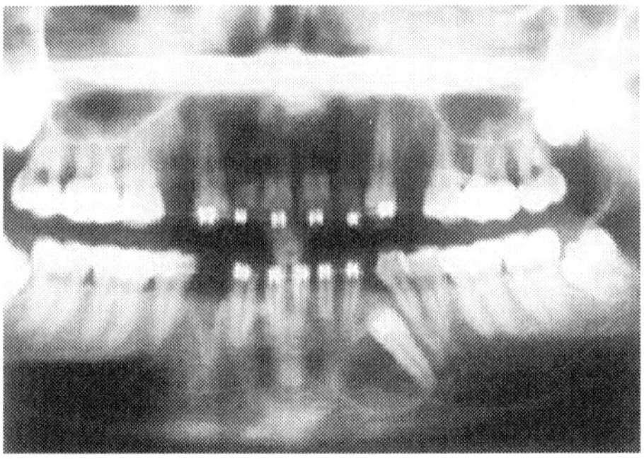

Figure 15. A 13-year-old female with an impacted left mandibular canine tooth and a relatively well-defined radiolucent lesion (AOT) on the mesial aspect spanning the length of the crown and root. Care was taken not to devitalize the tooth.

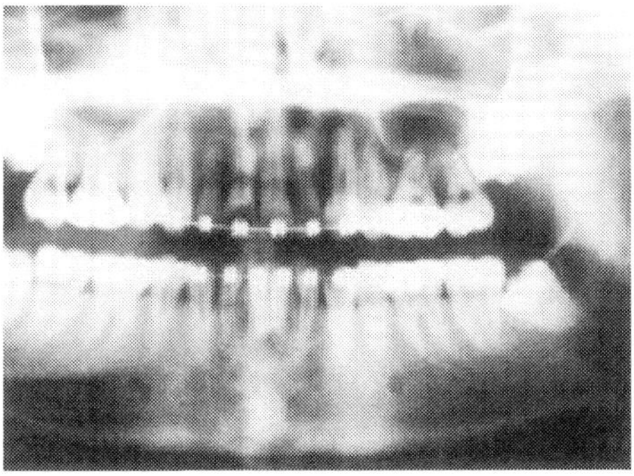

Figure 16. The 3-year postoperative radiograph showing complete bone formation and canine alignment (Orthodontist: Dr. H.A. Shafeie).

Such cases require periodic follow-up after completion of treatment. Our cases had no recurrences to date.

4. Conclusion

The decision to expose or remove a bone-impacted permanent tooth is based on clinical and radiographic information as well as surgical and orthodontic judgment.

Author details

Mohammad Hosein Kalantar Motamedi

Trauma Research Center, Baqiyatallah Medical Sciences University and Azad University of Medical Sciences, Dental College, OMFS department, Tehran, Iran

References

[1] Kasander T. The impacted canine: diagnosis and treatment. J Clin Orthod 1994;5:13-21.

[2] Ericson S, Kurol J. Radiographic assessment of maxillary canine eruption in children with clinical signs of eruption disturbances. Eur J Orthod 1986;8:133-40.

[3] Ericson S, Kurol J. Early treatment of palatally erupting maxillary canines by extraction of primary canines. Eur J Orthod 1988;10:283-95.

[4] Bishara SE. Impacted maxillary canines: a review. Am J Orthod Dentofacial Orthop 1992;101:159-71.

[5] Motamedi MH, Talesh KT. Management of extensive dentigerous cysts. Br Dent J 2005;198:203-6.

[6] Motamedi MH, Shafeie HA, Azizi T. Salvage of an impacted canine associated with an adenomatoid odontogenic tumor: a case report. Br Dent J 2005;199:89-90.

[7] Motamedi MH, Behroozian A, Azizi T, Nazhvani AD, Motahary P, Lotfi A. Assessment of 120 Maxillofacial Aneurysmal Bone Cysts: A Nationwide Quest to Understand This Enigma. J Oral Maxillofac Surg. 2014, joms.2013.12.032. [Epub ahead of print]

[8] Motamedi MH, Navi F, Eshkevari PS, Jafari SM, Shams MG, Taheri M, Abbas FM, Motahhari P. Variable presentations of aneurysmal bone cysts of the jaws: 51 cases treated during a 30-year period. J Oral Maxillofac Surg. 2008 Oct;66(10):2098-103.

[9] Motamedi MH. Destructive aneurysmal bone cyst of the mandibular condyle: report of a case and review of the literature. J Oral Maxillofac Surg. 2002 Nov;60(11): 1357-61. Review.

[10] Kalantar Motamedi MH. Aneurysmal bone cysts of the jaws: clinicopathological features, radiographic evaluation and treatment analysis of 17 cases. J Craniomaxillofac Surg. 1998 Feb;26(1):56-62.

[11] Motamedi MH, Stavropoulos MF. Large radiolucent lesion of the mandibular condyle. J Oral Maxillofac Surg. 1997 Nov;55(11):1300-4.

[12] Motamedi MH, Yazdi E. Aneurysmal bone cyst of the jaws: analysis of 11 cases. J Oral Maxillofac Surg. 1994 May;52(5):471-5.

[13] Motamedi MH, Khodayari A. Aneurysmal bone cyst mimicking a malignancy. J Oral Maxillofac Surg. 1993 Jun;51(6):691-5.

[14] Zuccati G, Ghobadlu J, Nieri M, Clauser C. Factors associated with the duration of forced eruption of impacted maxillary canines: a retrospective study. Am J Orthod Dentofacial Orthop 2006;130:349-56.

[15] Baccetti T, Crescini A, Nieri M, Rotundo R, Pini Prato GP. Orthodontic treatment of impacted maxillary canines: an appraisal of prognostic factors. Prog Orthod 2007;8:6-15.

[16] Ferguson JW, Parvizi F. Eruption of palatal canines following surgical exposure: a review of outcomes in a series of consecutively treated cases. Br J Orthod 1997;24:203-7.

[17] Stivaros N, Mandall NA. Radiographic factors affecting the management of impacted upper permanent canines. J Orthod 2000;27:169-73.

[18] Motamedi MH, Tabatabaie FA, Navi F, Shafeie HA, Fard BK, Hayati Z. Assessment of radiographic factors affecting surgical exposure and orthodontic alignment of impacted canines of the palate: a 15-year retrospective study.Oral Surg Oral Med Oral Pathol Oral Radiol Endod. 2009;107:772-5.

[19] Motamedi MH, Seifi M: Is it possible to salvage impacted strategic teeth associated with extensive dentigerous cysts? JCDA 2005, 71:633-635.

Chapter 7

Orthodontic Preparation for Orthognathic Surgery

Abdolreza Jamilian, Alireza Darnahal and
Letizia Perillo

Additional information is available at the end of the chapter

http://dx.doi.org/10.5772/58957

1. Introduction

Orthodontic treatment goals can be divided into five categories: facial esthetics, dental esthetics, functional occlusion, periodontal health, and stability.[1] Nevertheless, when a severe skeletal deformity exists in non-growing teen and adult patients with significant skeletal jaw discrepancy, the goals of treatment are often impossible to achieve by orthodontics alone. In these circumstances, both orthodontics and surgery are required to correct the dental malposition and the skeletal disharmony. This corrective jaw surgery, also called orthognathic surgery, is performed by oral and maxillofacial surgeons to correct a wide range of minor and major skeletal and dental irregularities, including the misalignment of jaws and teeth, which, in turn, can improve chewing, speaking and breathing. Orthodontics in conjunction with orthognathic surgery can do wonders in improving the appearance of the face. Combined orthodontic and surgical treatment usually requires about 18-24 months to complete. The treatment may be divided into four stages:

a. Treatment Planning

b. Presurgical Orthodontics

c. Surgical Treatment

d. Post-Surgical Orthodontics

2. Treatment planning

Proffit and Ackerman [2] introduced the concept of envelope of discrepancy to graphically illustrate four ranges of correction for any characteristics of malocclusion: (A) an amount that can be accomplished by orthodontic tooth movement alone; (B) a larger amount that can be accomplished by orthodontic tooth movement aided by absolute anchorage; (C) an additional amount that can be achieved by functional or orthopedic treatment to modify growth;[3-5] and (D) a still larger amount that requires surgery as part of the treatment plan.

People who can potentially benefit from orthognathic surgery include those with jaws that are positioned incorrectly. Orthognathic surgery is also the treatment of choice in patients who have not had the benefit of dentofacial orthopedics for growth guidance, or in cases where the deformity is so severe that orthodontics alone is not enough to correct it. Achieving successful treatment outcomes in these patients requires implementing an effective treatment plan. It should be considered that treatment planning is one of the most important stages because once the treatment is started it is hardly possible to reverse or suspend it. At this stage, the patient should be verified to have no potential of growth. If the patient is still growing he or she should be examined annually until growth is complete. Once facial growth cessation is verified the patient should be referred to a multidisciplinary clinic for joint treatment planning with the maxillofacial surgeon and orthodontist. In the beginning information about patient's general health state and previous diseases is evaluated and if there are no contraindications for surgery and general anesthesia a thorough examination of the face including evaluation of facial and dental photographs, cephalometric radiographs, and dental casts should be done. Subsequently, the orthodontist and maxillofacial surgeon should make a joint decision concerning the treatment approach. One of the aspects for consideration is whether the surgery is required in the mandible, maxilla or both and whether the jaw is to remain in one piece or to be segmented.

3. Presurgical orthodontics

Orthodontic preparation for surgery is different from orthodontic correction alone. Achievement of optimal facial esthetics requires integrated cooperation of orthodontists and maxillofacial surgeons. Routine preoperative orthodontics involve dental alignment, incisor decompensation, and arch coordination for the purpose of obtaining maximum intercuspal interdigitation when the jaws are surgically aligned. In short the aims of presurgical treatment are to decompensate lower and upper incisors, level and align both arches and relieve the crowding. In general these corrections will make the malocclusion look worse presurgically, but it will show the true magnitude of the skeletal problem thus allowing an optimal correction at surgery.[6] To sum up, the essential steps in orthodontic preparation for orthognathic surgery are to align the arches individually, achieve compatibility of the arches or arch segments, and establish the proper anteroposterior and vertical position of the incisors.

3.1. Dental alignment

Dental crowding, spacing, misalignment and rotations of the teeth should be corrected before orthognathic surgery. The key is to get the teeth in proper position and angulation. In this phase of the treatment, extractions might be needed to relieve moderate to severe crowding and make needed space for teeth alignment. Extraction can also help remove dental compensations. It should be taken into consideration that extraction should be avoided if the space of the jaw permits favorable dental alignment. Incisor inclination, crowding, type of malocclusion and surgical procedure are among the determining factors in deciding which teeth should be extracted.

3.2. Decompensation

Most severe skeletal jaw discrepancies are partly compensated. This natural phenomena called"dentoalveolar compensation" is a system which attempts to maintain normal interarch relationship.[7]

Compensations can be dental or skeletal in nature. Dental compensations can be vertical, transverse and/or sagittal. The factors responsible for dentoalveolar adaptation include: a normal eruptive system, surrounding soft tissue pressures and the influence neighboring and opposing teeth during occlusion. For example in class II skeletal malocclusions the upper anteriors retrocline to compensate for maxillary prognathism and lower incisors procline to compensate for mandibular retrognathism. While in class II skeletal malocclusion the upper anteriors procline to compensate for maxillary retrognathism and lower incisors retrocline to compensate for mandibular prognathism.

In contrast to dental camouflage, in preparation for orthognathic surgery, it is necessary to remove any dental compensations present and to place the teeth in a favorable position with their supporting bone. This is called presurgical decompensation. Presurgical orthodontic decompensation is essential to enable the surgeon to make a considerable amount of surgical correction. Failure to fully remove anterior incisor compensations presurgically will limit the surgical correction, leading to compromised facial esthetics and occlusion. Such anteroposterior dental decompensation may involve specific extractions, anchorage needs, or use of class II/class III elastics. For example, decompensation of skeletal class II malocclusion will often require the use of class III elastics to upright lower incisors and decompensation of skeletal class III malocclusion necessitates the use of class II elastics to procline lower incisors and establish adequate reverse overjet.

Decompensation accentuates the patient's deformity but is necessary for achievement of normal occlusal relationships when skeletal bones are properly positioned at surgery.

3.3. Arch coordination

Arch coordination refers to coordinating the widths of the dental arches so that there is a normal transvers relationship following sagittal jaw movements. Coordination often involves arch expansion, arch contraction, and occlusal plane leveling and alignment. Orthodontic expansion or contraction to coordinate the upper and the lower arches should be carried out prior to the surgical procedure in order to provide correct post-operative occlusal interdigitation. Poor arch coordination, particularly in the transverse or vertical plane, will restrict or destabilize jaw movements at the time of surgery and compromise postsurgical stability.

3.4. Presurgical orthodontics objectives in the transverse plane

Ideally, the width of maxilla should be slightly more than the mandible in order to produce normal buccal overjet. Transverse discrepancy happens when there is a defect in the widths of the arches. The maxilla is more commonly affected in this discrepancy which can be either unilateral or bilateral. This discrepancy is often combined with sagittal or vertical problems.

Pre-surgical orthodontic treatment consideration of transverse discrepancy:

i. The problem is the skeletal or dental

Dental discrepancies are usually treated by means of buccal tipping of the posterior teeth while skeletal discrepancies are corrected by bodily movement of the posterior teeth. If the posterior teeth are tipped lingually, presurgical orthodontic expansion (buccal tipping) should be used; however, the tipping should not exceed 4 to 6 mm total. Bodily movement of the posterior teeth should be done by means of segmental osteotomy, without the need for orthodontic expansion.

ii. Is the problem relative or absolute

Articulation of the casts into a class I occlusion allows the clinician to easily distinguish between relative and absolute maxillary constriction. If the occlusion is proper when the casts are brought into class I canine relationship the discrepancy is relative; otherwise, if a crossbite still exists, then the discrepancy is absolute. Absolute skeletal transverse discrepancy requires planning for segmental osteotomies or surgically assisted rapid palatal expansion (SARPE).[5]

SARPE technique is used in cases with a severe discrepancy or when the transverse defect of the maxillary bone is an isolated skeletal anomaly. While, segmental maxillary osteotomy is used for more modest defects (up to 7 mm) or when the transverse deficit is one of a number of maxillary skeletal deficits, including sagittal and vertical defects that would require surgical attention.[8]

3.5. Presurgical orthodontics objectives in the vertical plane

3.5.1. Open bite cases

Treatment of anterior open bite has always been a great challenge in orthodontics. Extrusion of anterior teeth and orthognathic surgery are among the possible options for treatment of open bite in non-growing patients. However, dental extrusion of skeletal open bite will be unstable in the long run. Furthermore, it may also create an excessive display of gingiva. Unaesthetic results and lack of stability of dental correction make surgery the treatment of choice for skeletal open bite cases. One of the chief considerations for treatment of these patients is the choice between one piece or segmented maxillary osteotomy. The decision for or against segmentation is made based on the patient's baseline skeletal deformity. These patients generally have an excessive curve of Spee in the upper jaw which is an indication of skeletal problem rather than a dental one. The severity of the curve of Spee indicates the need for segmental osteotomy. In other words, the more severe the curve of Spee, the more obvious the need for segmental osteotomy. When surgical segments are planned, the orthodontist's role is to level presurgically within the segments but not across the osteotomy sites and to make sure that there is enough space between the roots of the involved teeth to allow interdental osteotomies.

Pre-surgical orthodontic treatment considerations in open bite cases:

i. Avoid closing the anterior open bite presurgically by extruding the anterior teeth

ii. Avoid closing the anterior open bite presurgically by intruding the posterior teeth

iii. Accentuated or reversed curve of Spee should be levelled

a. Leveling the maxillary arch:

In the presence of a flat curve of Spee with no vertical discrepancies within the arch, leveling is done with a continuous arch wire and the open bite can be corrected by a 1-piece Lefort I osteotomy. However, if a segmental Le Fort I osteotomy is planned for open bite correction, presurgical dental leveling and alignment should be carried out separately in each segment.

b. Leveling the mandibular arch:

Since patients with open bite generally do not have severe reverse curve of Spee in the lower arch, continuous arch wire is used for complete leveling.

3.5.2. Deep bite cases

In patients with deep bite, there is nearly always an excessive curve of Spee in the lower arch and occasionally a reverse curve in the upper arch. In these cases, the curve of Spee is leveled intruding the incisors or extruding the posterior teeth. The decision to level by intrusion of the incisors or extrusion of the posterior segment depends on the initial facial height of the patients. As a general rule, the shorter the face height, the greater the need for extrusion.

3.6. Presurgical orthodontics objectives in the sagittal plane

3.6.1. Class II malocclusion

Skeletal class II malocclusion is naturally compensated to mask the skeletal discrepancy. This natural dental compensation involves retroclination of the upper incisors and proclination of lower incisors. The goals of presurgical orthodontics for these cases involve decompensation of these natural compensations along with alignment of teeth and establishing compatible arch forms.

Orthodontic decompensation of skeletal class II malocclusion cases involve proclining of retroclined upper incisors and uprighting the proclined lower incisors. This decompensation will increase the amount of overjet, which allows the maxillofacial surgeon to carry out maximum mandibular advancement and subsequently establish class I canine relationship after the surgery. (Figure 1)

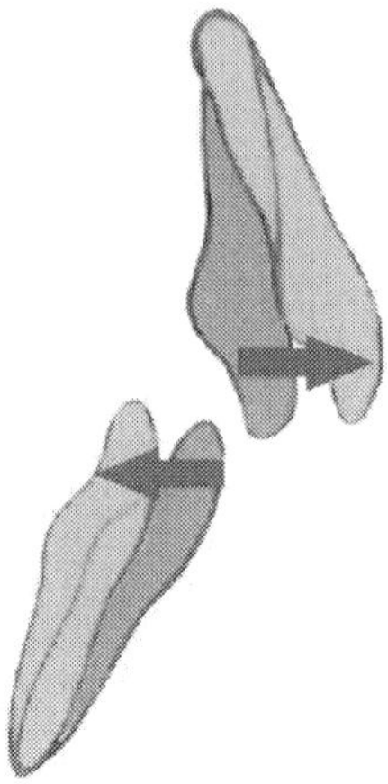

Figure 1. Orthodontic presurgical decompensation of class II malocclusion.

Alignment and leveling and the need for extraction in skeletal class II malocclusion cases depends on the degree of crowding. In crowded cases, extraction of upper second premolars and lower first premolars is a common orthodontic plan in preparation for surgical correction. The extraction of upper second premolars prevent further retroclination of upper incisors and the extraction of lower first premolars facilitate uprighting of lower incisors and subsequently establish enough overjet for surgery. We should bear in mind that extraction space should be closed before surgery

3.6.2. Class III malocclusion

In skeletal class III malocclusion cases the natural dental compensation involves proclination of the upper incisors and retroclination of lower incisors. Therefore, in these cases, orthodontic decompensation is achieved by uprighting the upper incisors and proclining the lower incisors and thereby increasing the reverse overjet to the maximum which would allow the surgeon to carry out maximum mandibular setback.

Similar to skeletal class II patients, in these cases also the alignment and levelling and the need for extraction depends on the degree of crowding. The usual pattern of extraction in these cases involves the extraction of upper first premolars in order to facilitate the uprighting of upper incisors and extraction of lower second premolars in order to prevent further retroclination of the lower incisors. These extractions also help to establish enough reverse overjet for the surgical procedure. Extraction space should also be closed before surgery. (Figure 2)

http://dx.doi.org/10.5772/58957

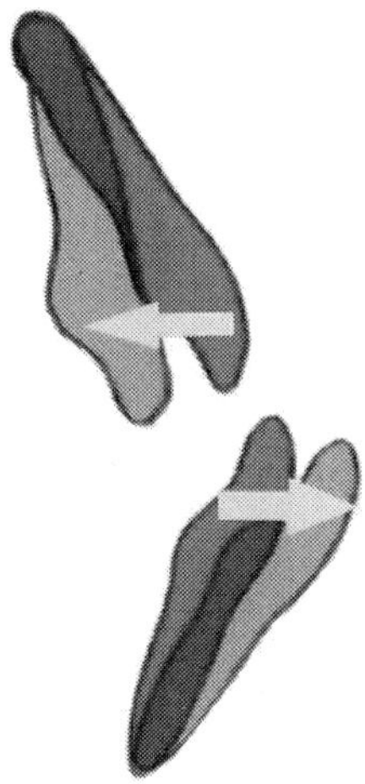

Figure 2. Orthodontic presurgical decompensation of class III.

4. Orthognathic surgery

Skeletal dentofacial deformities are associated with numerous problems including: esthetic, functional, psychological, speech, mastication, digestion, and possible temporomandibular joint dysfunctions.

Orthognathic surgery is a hospital based operation in which the elements of the facial skeleton are manipulated to restore the proper anatomic and functional relationship in patients with skeletal dentofacial deformities and overcome the above mentioned problems. The results of orthognathic surgery can have dramatic and positive effects on many aspects of the patient's life.

Orthognathic surgery is done through a variety of osteotomies including maxillary segmental osteotomies, Le Fort I maxillary osteotomy, Le Fort II osteotomy, Lefort III osteotomy, sagittal split osteotomy of the mandibular ramus, vertical ramal osteotomy, inverted L and C osteotomies, mandibular body segmental osteotomies, and mandibular symphysis osteotomies.

After the surgery, patients should expect the following:

- Swelling
- Nasal and sinus congestion
- Difficulty eating and chewing food for several weeks following surgery.

5. Post-surgical orthodontics

Approximately four to six weeks after surgery the patient should return to the orthodontist to begin post-surgical treatment. This short phase of orthodontic treatment postoperatively is necessary to detail the final occlusion and improve the stability of surgery. The goal is to settle the teeth in good occlusion and alignment and correct any possible skeletal relapse following surgery. Post-surgical orthodontics usually takes about six months and may involve use of intermaxillary elastics.

It is noteworthy to mention that precise and proper presurgical orthodontics minimalize post-surgical orthodontics. After debanding and debonding the patients should be provided with upper and lower retainers.

5.1. Common mistakes in presurgical orthodontics

The orthodontist should avoid:

- Masking skeletal discrepancies by dental camouflage
- Closing the anterior open bite presurgically by extruding the anterior teeth in open bite cases
- Closing the anterior open bite presurgically by intruding the posterior teeth in open bite cases
- Aligning dental midlines in transverse plane discrepancy cases
- Correction of overjet in class II malocclusion cases
- Correction of reverse overjet in class III malocclusion cases

6. Summary

Successful treatment of patients who are candidates for orthognathic surgery requires close cooperation between the orthodontist and surgeon. Prior to surgery, the patients undergo orthodontic treatment in order to be prepared for corrective jaw surgery. Presurgical orthodontics involves dental decompensation, alignment of the dentition within the arches, leveling of the curve of Spee, and coordination of the maxillary and mandibular dentition. These steps vary from case to case based on the type of malocclusion and its severity.

7. Case report

7.1. Case summary

A 17 year-old boy with marked high angle skeletal class III malocclusion with severe maxillary retrognathia and mandibular prognathism. The patient had crowding in the upper jaw and the lower incisors were tipped lingually due to Class III malocclusion compensation. Class III molar and canine relationship with posterior cross bite with high maxillary-mandibular plane angle and incompetent lips were noticeable. The patient did not complain from any TMJ signs or symptoms.

Examination of head and face

In the frontal plane the face of the patient had an elongated shape. Skeletal Class III pattern with severe maxillary retrusion, mandibular prognathism and concave profile.

Functional examination

The patient's path of closure showed no deviation. Maximum jaw opening was normal at 49 mm.

Intraoral examination

Severe Class III molar and canine relationship with 9 mm of reverse overjet. Anterior and posterior cross bite could be detected. Crowding was also seen in the upper jaw. The lower incisors were retroclined.

Mandibular arch: Good arch form; Lingual displacement of lower incisors.

Maxillary arch: Good arch form; crowding in the upper anterior segment

Occlusion (Sagittal): Severe Class III with reverse overjet of 9 mm; Very severe Class III molar and canine relationship on both sides

Occlusion (Vertical): Anterior open bite of 2 mm

Occlusion (Transversal): Upper midline coincided with facial midline; lower midline deviated 1 mm to the left

Cephalometric assessment

Cephalometric assessment shows skeletal Class III malocclusion with excessive growth of the mandible and reduced growth of the maxilla. The mandible was elongated. It also shows a degree of dento-alveolar compensation present in the lower anterior region. Upper incisors are positioned labially (Figure 3).

The patient's chief complaints:

- Severe maxillary deficiency
- Severe mandibular prognathism
- Crowding of upper arch

Treatment Plan:

Considering the severity of the malocclusion, the underlying skeletal discrepancy, age of the patient, a surgical-orthodontic approach was chosen.

The treatment plan was as follows:

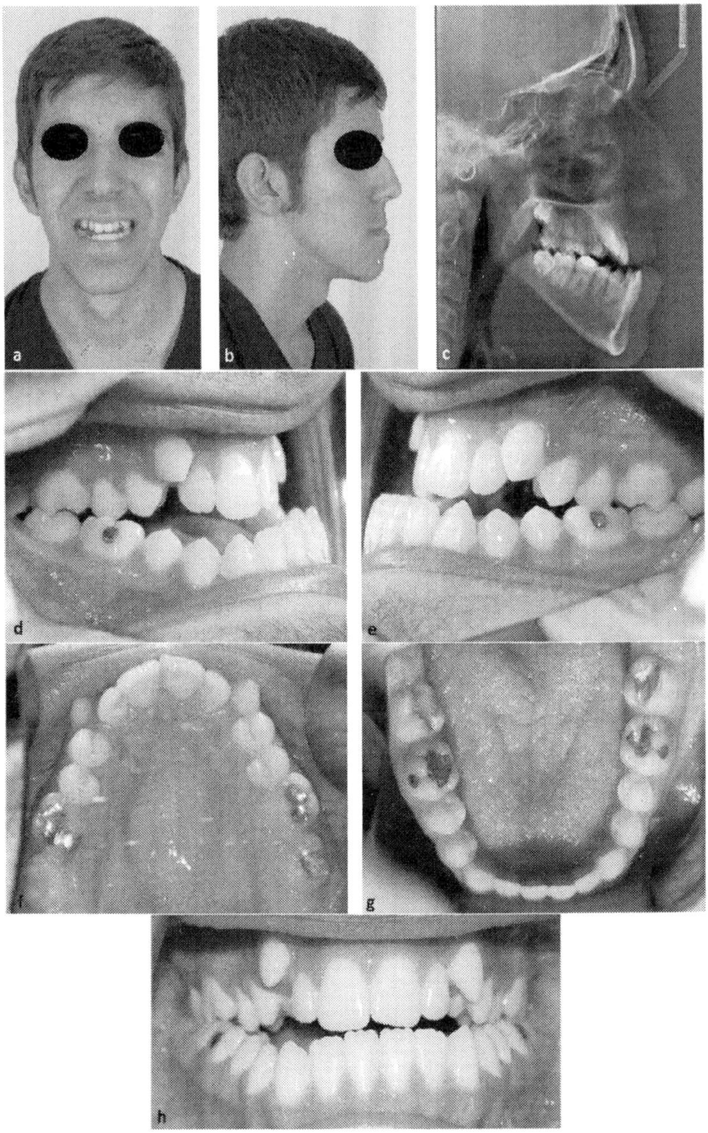

Figure 3. Before treatment records of an orthognathic surgery case with high angle skeletal class III malocclusion, severe maxillary retrognathia, lingually tipped lower incisors, upper crowding and mandibular prognathism.

- Levelling and aligning
- Decrowding

- Incisor decompensation by means of fixed appliance
- Bimaxillary surgery involving a maxillary advancement and impaction (Lefort 1), and a mandibular setback (bilateral sagittal split ramus osteotomy). Chin Augmentation.
- Post-surgical orthodontics: Arch coordination, detailing, suitable interdigitation
- Debonding
- Retention

8. Presurgical orthodontics

Upper removable appliance with a screw was fitted in the midline to expand the maxillary dentition and create space to relieve upper crowding. Upper and lower 0.018 standard edgewise fixed appliances were placed and the teeth were levelled and aligned. Class II elastics were used for decompensation of upper and lower incisors. At this stage the reverse overjet of the patient increased from 9 mm to 11 mm. Surgical wires were placed in the upper and lower jaws. After levelling, alignment, decrowding, decompensation and achieving increased reverse overjet, the patient was referred to the maxillofacial surgeon. (Figure 4)

9. Orthognathic surgery

- Maxillary advancement (6 mm)
- Maxillary impaction (4 mm)
- Mandibular setback (6 mm)
- Chin augmentation with Medpor ®

10. Post-surgical orthodontics

After the surgery the patient had very mild paraesthesia in the lower lip. One month after the surgery postsurgical orthodontics was started by replacing surgical wires with 0.016 stainless steel wires. Class III elastics were placed and Torque adjustment was done in the upper and lower jaws. After debanding and debonding upper and lower Hawley appliances were placed.

The post-surgical cephalogram of the patient showed significant improvement of the upper and lower jaws. Facial profile was more balanced and had improved significantly. Advancement of the Maxilla and setback of the mandible were obvious in the cephalogram. Chin augmentation with Medpor® could also be seen in the cephalometric image. The patient had satisfactory positive overjet and overbite. Overall, a pleasing Class 1 occlusion had been achieved in the patient. (Figure 5)

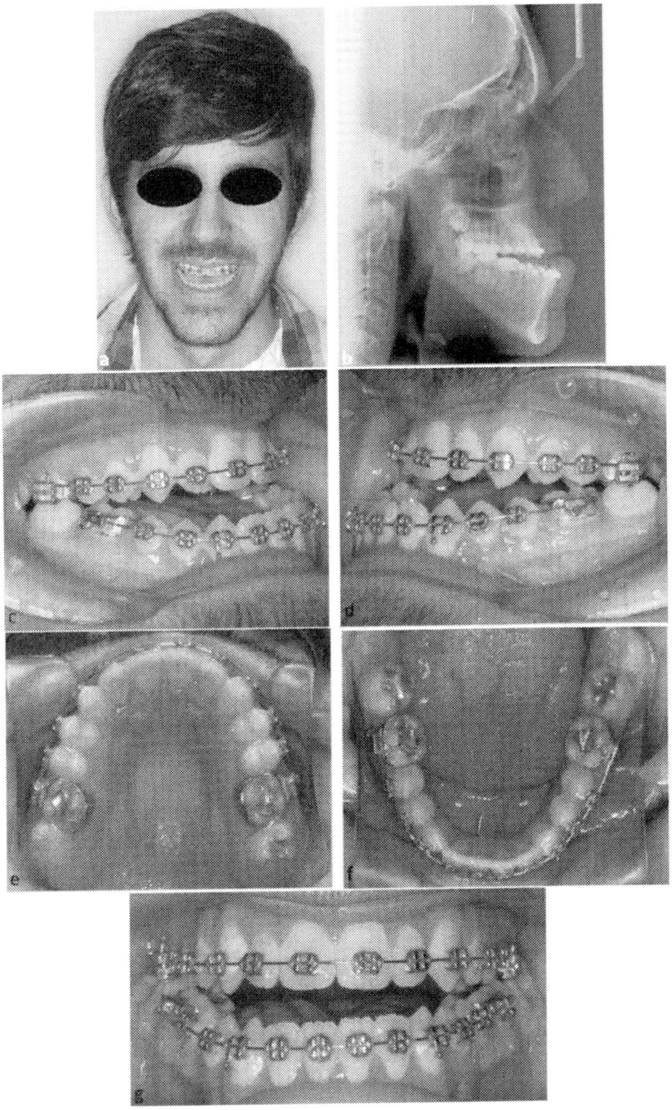

Figure 4. Presurgical orthodontics of the same patient. Upper and lower 0.018 standard edgewise fixed appliances

Intraoral examination showed that the patient had molar and canine class I relationship with no discrepancy between the jaws.

The intercuspation was satisfactory and no signs of bruxism or other dysfunction was detected. The lips were competent and the patient was very satisfied with his appearance. No clicking or no signs and symptoms of temporomandibular dysfunction were noted.

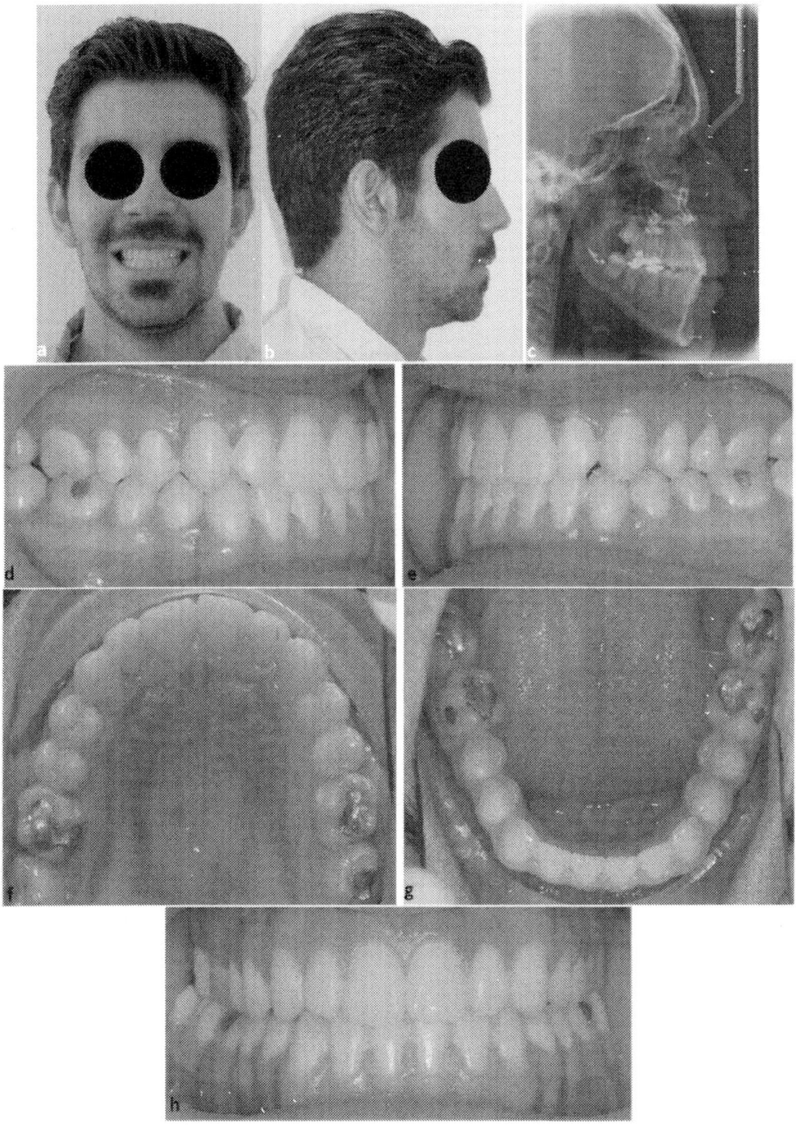

Figure 5. Same patient after surgery and retention

Author details

Abdolreza Jamilian[1*], Alireza Darnahal[1] and Letizia Perillo[2]

*Address all correspondence to: info@jamilian.net

1 Tehran Dental Branch, Department of Orthodontics, Islamic Azad University, Tehran, Iran

2 Departments of Orthodontics, Second University of Naples, Naples, Italy

References

[1] Roth R. Roundtable: Diagnosis and treatment planning. J Clin Orthod 1992;26:585.

[2] Ackerman JI, Nguyen T, Proffit WR. The Decision-Making Process in Orthodontics. In: Graber TM, Vanarsdall Jr. RL, editors. Orthodontics : current principles and techniques. St. Louis, [Mo.]: Mosby; 2012.

[3] Jamilian A, Haraji A, Showkatbakhsh R, Valaee N. The effects of miniscrew with Class III traction in growing patients with maxillary deficiency. International journal of orthodontics. 2011;22(2):25-30.

[4] Showkatbakhsh R, Jamilian A, Ghassemi M, Ghassemi A, Taban T, Imani Z. The effects of facemask and reverse chin cup on maxillary deficient patients. Journal of orthodontics. 2012;39(2):95-101.

[5] Suri L, Taneja P. Surgically assisted rapid palatal expansion: a literature review. American journal of orthodontics and dentofacial orthopedics : official publication of the American Association of Orthodontists, its constituent societies, and the American Board of Orthodontics. 2008;133(2):290-302.

[6] Sabri R. Orthodontic objectives in orthognathic surgery: state of the art today. World journal of orthodontics. 2006;7(2):177-91.

[7] Solow B. The dentoalveolar compensatory mechanism: background and clinical implications. British journal of orthodontics. 1980;7(3):145-61.

[8] Marchetti C, Pironi M, Bianchi A, Musci A. Surgically assisted rapid palatal expansion vs. segmental Le Fort I osteotomy: transverse stability over a 2-year period. Journal of cranio-maxillo-facial surgery : official publication of the European Association for Cranio-Maxillo-Facial Surgery. 2009;37(2):74-8.

Chapter 8

Surgically Assisted Maxillary Expansion

Sertaç Aktop, Onur Gönül, Hasan Garip and
Kamil Göker

Additional information is available at the end of the chapter

http://dx.doi.org/10.5772/59285

1. Introduction

An adequate transverse maxillary dimension is a critical component of a stable and functional occlusion. [1] Orthopedic rapid maxillary expansion in skeletally immature patients is the procedure of choice to correct this condition in that age group. However, as skeletal maturity approaches, bony interdigitation increases as the sutures fuse. [2,3] After suture closure or completion of transverse growth, orthopedic transverse maxillary expansion is largely unsuccessful because the expansion is primarily composed of no basal skeletal movement. [4] This phenomenon leads to difficulty separating the maxilla with orthopedic forces alone and bending of the alveolus, dental tipping and minimal maxillary expansion. The result is relapse despite overcorrection, periodontal defects, and malocclusion. [5]

Rapid maxillary expansion can produce unwanted effects when used in a skeletally mature patient, including lateral tipping of posterior teeth [6,7], extrusion [8-10], periodontal membrane compression, buccal root resorption [11-13], alveolar bone bending [7], fenestration of the buccal cortex [13-16], palatal tissue necrosis [17], inability to open the midpalatal suture, pain, and instability of the expansion [7,10,18-20]. Several reasons have been speculated regarding factors that limit orthopedically induced maxillary expansion in skeletally mature patients.

However, a few reports in the literature contradict these findings and state that nonsurgical maxillary expansion is as successful in adults as it is in children [21, 22]. Experiencing more complications, after attempts to orthopedically alter the transverse dimension of the maxilla with advancing age, surgical procedures have been recommended to facilitate correction of transverse discrepancies by Perrson [23], who found evidence of bony union at 17 years in the midpalatal suture. Burston [24], however, found no evidence of synostosis in the same suture by the age of 18 years.

2. Correction of transverse discrepancy via orthodontics

This is successful until the age of approximately 14–15 years depending on the gender of the patient. After this age, orthodontic widening becomes virtually impossible and very painful. In general, it is assumed that closure of the midpalatal suture prevents this type of expansion [25-27].

On the other hand, Mommerts outlined a basic treatment strategy for patients with maxillary constriction, based on age that rapid maxillary expansion should be completed to treat maxillary constriction in patients under the age of 12. From age 14 on, surgically assisted palatal expansion is indicated to release areas of bony resistance in the midface [28].

3. Surgically Assisted Rapid Maxillary Expansion (SARME)

The areas of resistance to lateral forces in the midface are the pyriform aperture (anterior), the zygomatic buttress (lateral), the pterygoid junction (posterior) and the midpalatal synostosis suture (median). Many surgical interventions and techniques have been developed by the identification of these areas of resistance. Surgery assisted maxillary expansion procedures have conventionally been grouped into 2 categories:

1. Segmenting the maxilla during a LeFort osteotomy to reposition the individual segments in a widened transverse dimension, and
2. Surgically assisted rapid maxillary expansion (SARME).

Advantages of SARME over orthodontic therapy and segmental Le Fort procedures include decreased risk of periodontal damage, improved esthetics when smiling, improved nasal air flow, and decreased risk of avascularity. SARME is also a relatively simple procedure and is associated with minimal morbidity. Intraoperative complications are uncommon and there is also less chance of avascularity leading to aseptic necrosis than with segmental Le Fort I procedures. [29, 30] Brown [12] was probably the first who described a technique of SARME with midpalatal splitting. [31] In 1961, Haas described the downward and forward movement of the maxilla that occurs during rapid maxillary expansion because of the location of the craniomaxillofacial sutures. He believed that the hemimaxillas separated from each other develop tipping rather than separating in a parallel fashion due to the strength of the zygomatic buttresses. [32]

Most methods consider the zygomaticomaxillary junction the major site of resistance and perform a corticotomy through the zygomatic-maxillary buttress from the pyriform rim to the maxillopterygoid junction. The midpalatal suture is historically considered the major place of resistance. The pterygoid plates are also a considerable site of resistance but because of the increased risk of injuring the pterygoid plexus by the osteotomy, some chose not to, without losing much mobility. By not releasing the pterygoid junction, the pattern of opening of the maxillary halves is more V-shaped with the point of the V located dorsally [33-37].

Isaacson and Ingram [38] and Isaacson et al. [39] mention that historically, the midpalatal suture was thought to be the area of resistance to expansion, but the facial skeleton increases its resistance to expansion as it ages and matures, and that the major site of resistance is not the midpalatal suture but the remaining maxillary articulations. Wertz stated that resistance of the zygomatic arch prevents parallel opening of the midpalatal suture [40]. Many surgeons release the midpalatal suture to improve mobility and to prevent deviation of the nasal septum. Several authors describe two paramedian palatal osteotomies from the posterior nasal spine to a point just posterior to the incisive canal [41-43].

In 1975 and 1976 Bell and Epker demonstrated that the area of increased facial skeletal resistance to expansion was indeed not the midpalatal suture, but the zygomaticotemporal, zygomaticofrontal and zygomaticomaxillary sutures. [44, 45] On the other hand, Shetty concluded that exclusive use of bilateral zygomaticomaxillary buttress osteotomies to facilitate SARME was inadequate. They therefore concluded that complete midpalatal and pterygo-maxillary osteotomies were essential for predictable maxillary expansion in adults. [46]

There is a lack of consensus among orthodontists and surgeons about the indications for SARME. Although maxillary expansion may be required for many patients, an accurate diagnosis of maxillary transverse distraction is somewhat ambiguous. This is further complicated by case reports in the literature about orthodontic maxillary expansion or other forms of expansion in adults. The following have been reported in the literature as indications for SARME, all applying to a skeletally mature patient with a constricted maxillary arch.

4. Indications for SARME

1. To increase maxillary arch perimeter, to correct posterior crossbite, and when no additional surgical jaw movements are planned.
2. To widen the maxillary arch as a preliminary procedure, even if further orthognathic surgery is planned. This is to avoid increased risks, inaccuracy, and instability associated with segmental maxillary osteotomy.
3. To provide space for a crowded maxillary dentition when extractions are not indicated.
4. To widen maxillary hypoplasia associated with clefts of the palate.
5. To reduce wide black buccal corridors when smiling.
6. To overcome the resistance of the sutures when OME has failed. [47]

Several authors have shown that surgically assisted maxillary expansion can be carried out using only sedation and local anesthesia when a more conservative surgical technique is chosen. General anesthesia is preferred for invasive techniques. [48-50] Considering all these surgical techniques and discussions of advantages of one technique to another, most surgeons prefer to perform osteotomies on all four areas of resistance.

5. SARME technique

In our clinic, we perform the following protocol routinely. A horizontal incision is made through the mucoperiosteum above the mucogingival junction in the depth of the buccal vestibule, extending from the canine region to the mesial of the first molar. Keeping the incision more distally than the first molar region may cause damage to the pterygoid plexus or Bichat fat sometimes due to abnormal anatomic variations. Damage to pterygoid plexus may not be noticed intraoperatively. The vasoconstrictor effect of local anesthetics could curtail the bleeding during the operation and a postoperative bleeding may occur.

This incision is made in two layers as a safety precaution to any leak after suturing. Any gap or rupture of suture may cause exposure of the surgical bony area. The first layer incision is made on the epithelium and the periosteum is reached with dissection of connective tissue inferiorly, creating a pocket like formation of tissue. The second layer of the incision is then made on the periosteum 6-8 mm below the first layer. This technique forms a two level wound. Suturing this incisions layer by layer creates a more secure postoperative wound (Figure 1).

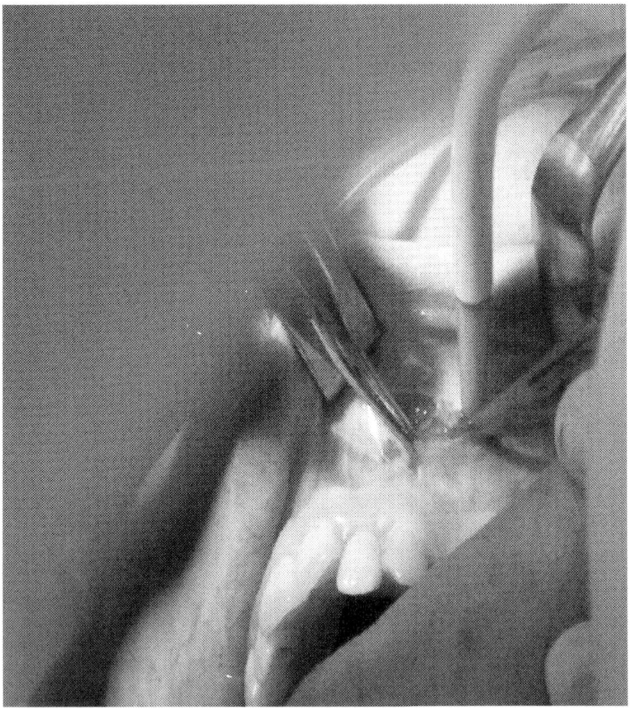

Figure 1. Dissection through the connective tissue from epithelial incision to periosteal incision beveled in order to create a pocket-like tissue wound.

Nasal mucosa should be elevated gently from the lateral nasal wall. Because the SARME is not a down fracture procedure, nasal bleeding can be easily controlled with nasal tampons which should be considered as a minor complication if patient has no coagulopathy. The maintenance of the blood supply requires an appropriate surgical procedure, with careful manipulation of soft tissues and ensuring the periosteum remains intact. [51]

A horizontal low-level osteotomy is made through the lateral wall of the maxilla 5-6 mm superior to the apices of the anterior and posterior teeth with tiny round burs (Figure 2) and then an osteotome, microsaw or piezo-surgery device, on the same level is used to make the bone cuts; the osteotomy extends from the inferolateral aspect of the pyriform rim posteriorly to the inferior aspect of the junction of the maxillary tuberosity and pterygoid plate (Figure 2). Working with piezo-surgery devices would clearly be more secure but take more operative time. At this point, retractors should be used gently to prevent infraorbital nerve damage.

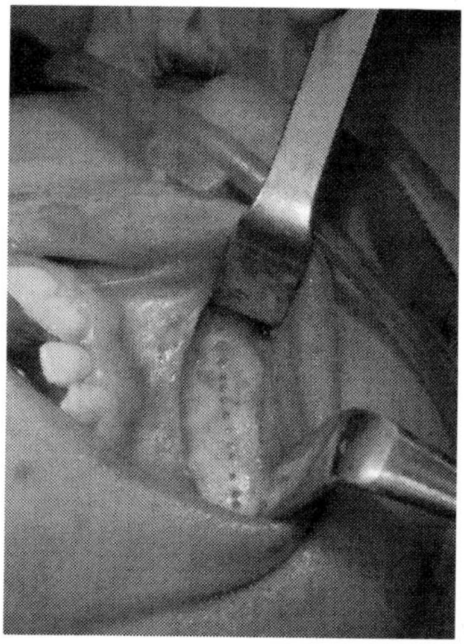

Figure 2. After marking the osteotomy route with a tiny round bur

The maxilla is separated from the pterygoid plate with a curved osteotome (Figure 4).

The risk of bleeding increases if the pterygoid plates are separated from the maxilla. If the pterygoid plates are separated from the maxilla, the most common sources of hemorrhage after SARME are the terminal branches of the maxillary artery, especially the posterior superior alveolar artery, and the pterygoid venous plexus. Turvey and Fonseca showed that the mean distance from the most inferior part of the pterygomaxillary junction to the most inferior part of the internal maxillary artery is 25 mm. During pterygomaxillary separation, pterygoid osteotomes should be correctly positioned and variations of this anatomy should be taken into account. [52] The pterygoid region should always be packed with moistened gauzes until suturing to avoid excessive blood loss and less postoperative swelling or hematoma.

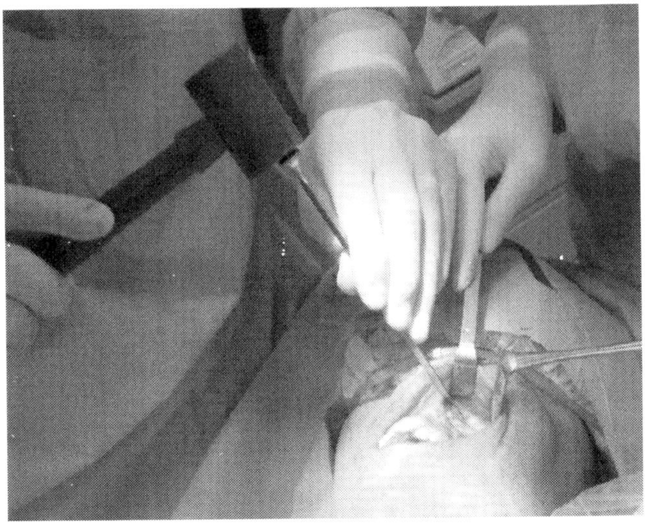

Figure 3. Osteotomy with an osteotome through the marked osteotomy line

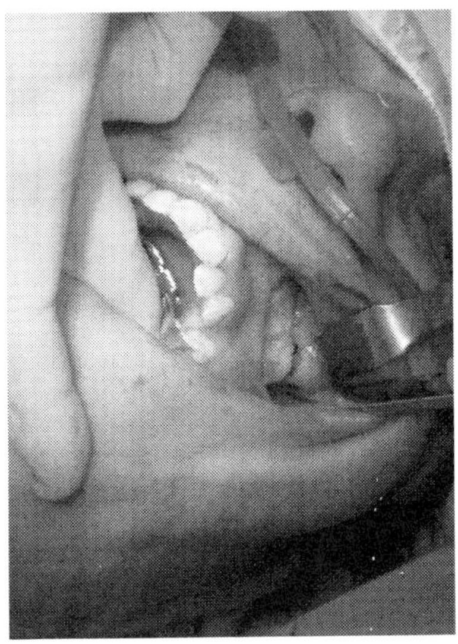

Figure 4. Separation of the pterygoid plate with a curved osteotome. Note the position of the finger to feel the osteotome intraorally

In conjunction, a sagittal palatal osteotomy is carried out, running from the midline of the alveolar bone, between the central incisors, to the posterior nasal spine. First a vertical incision is made along the labial frenulum between the central incisors. Then an osteotome is positioned in the central incisor interradicular space and manipulated to achieve equal and symmetric mobilization of the anterior maxilla. The forefinger is positioned on the incisive papilla to feel the redirected osteotome as it transects the deeper portion of the midpalatal suture (Figure 5).

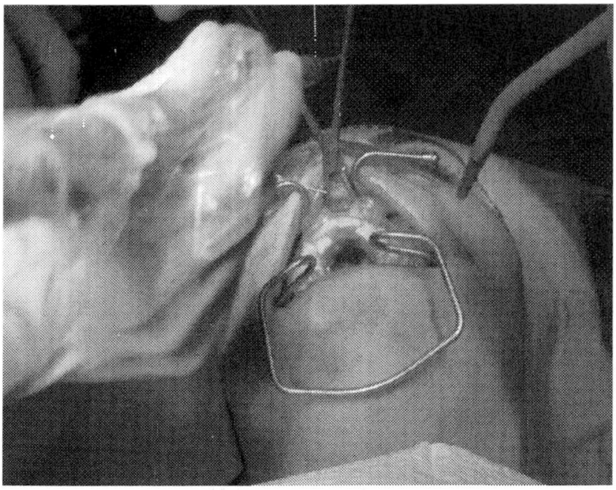

Figure 5. An easy way of traction of midline incision to reach and perform midpalatal osteotomy

Releasing the anterior nasal spine to improve mobility and to prevent deviation of the nasal septum is useful. Lateral nasal walls on both sides should be checked and released with osteotomes. A lateral nasal wall osteotomy might cause damage to the descending palatine artery and this could be minimized by limiting the extent of the osteotomy posterior to the pyriform rim to 35 mm in men and 30 mm in women [52].

Before the osteotomies the Hyrax appliance is activated to obtain easy palatal separation for about 8-10 turns, for maximum aperture and diastema formation. An immediate gap between central incisors should be observed intraoperatively after the osteotomies are performed. This is followed by immediate regression, leaving a 1 mm gap. Patients should receive postoperative prophylactic antibiotics and analgesics for 7 days postoperatively (Figure 6).

A surgically assisted maxillary expansion procedure is essentially a combination of osteogenic distraction with controlled expansion of soft tissues. Some principles must be followed to ensure that bone repair occurs in osteogenic distraction namely:

- Preservation of blood supply in the region
- Stability of the distractor and bone fragments
- Adequate latency period
- Adequate rate and frequency of activation and
- Observance of the retention period.

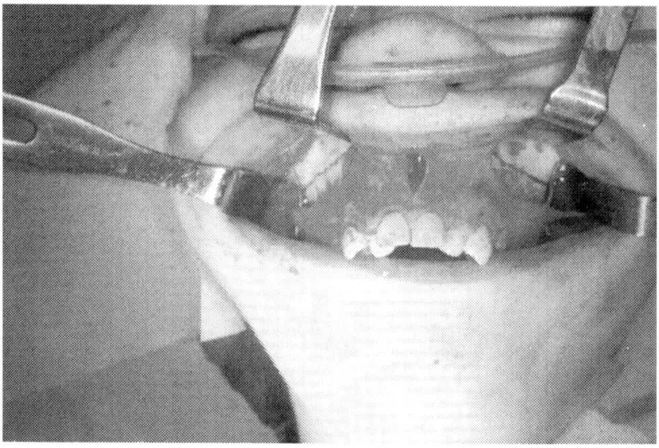

Figure 6. View of a completed osteotomy. Also zygomatic retention plates are implemented for orthodontic purposes.

The technique is based on a 5-day period of rest after corticotomy before the expansion starts. This gives the tissue time to form the first callus but is too short for consolidation.

Four phases of new bone formation can be described.

1. The first is a fibrovascular hematoma; between days 5 and 7 collagen fibers are formed that will arrange parallel to the distraction vector.
2. Second, the bone formation follows the collagen fibers through intramembranous ossification; from the outside to the inside.
3. Third, remodeling phase of the new bone.
4. Fourth, formation of solid compact bone with the same texture as the surrounding (old) bones.

When the distraction is performed too fast, the collagen fibers lose contact and there is no ingrowth of new bone, causing nonunion or malunion. In cases of a too slow distraction premature consolidation can occur and the required elongation cannot be reached [53].

Latency is considered to be the time interval between osteotomy and the appliance start-up and varies from 0 to 14 days in experimental and clinical studies. [54-56]

Activation rate is the amount of daily bone distraction (in millimeters); it varies from 0.25 to 1.0 mm.

Frequency represents the number of times the appliance is activated per day. [57] De Freitas et al recommend the expansion procedure with an overexpansion index of 23% above the desired measurements to compensate for relapse [58].

Retention period at the end of the distraction is necessary for the neoformed bone tissue to acquire the necessary resistance to bear the tipping forces. In experimental and clinical studies this period can vary from one to six months. [54, 59]

SARME procedures have traditionally been reported to have low morbidity especially when compared with other orthognathic surgical procedures. However, many complications have been reported in the literature varying from life-threatening epistaxis to a cerebrovascular accident, skull base fracture with reversible oculomotor nerve paresis and orbital compartment syndrome. [60-64]

Rapid maxillary expansion can produce unwanted effects when used in a skeletally mature patients, including lateral tipping of posterior teeth, extrusion, periodontal membrane compression, buccal root resorption, alveolar bone bending, fenestration of the buccal cortex, palatal tissue necrosis, inability to open the midpalatal suture, pain, and instability of the expansion. [6-8,10-15,17,28,46]

Complications associated with SARME reported in the literature also include significant hemorrhage, gingival recession, injury to the branches of the maxillary nerve, infection, pain, devitalization of teeth and altered pulpal blood flow, periodontal breakdown, sinus infection, alar base flaring, extrusion of teeth attached to the appliance, relapse, and unilateral expansion. [60,61,65-73] Postoperative bleeding starting on the third week due to the rupture of greater palatine artery, rupture of inferior nasal mucosa or any damage of venous plexus during the expansion procedure may even be observed. Segments or sharp prominences of bone in the intrapalatinal region could be considered to abrade or lacerate these tissues while the expansion procedure is processed. Moreover postoperative hemorrhage, pain, sinusitis, palatal tissue irritation/ulceration, asymmetrical expansion, nasal septum deviation, periodontal problems and relapse were reported as minor complications; and although SARME is considered a procedure with little risk of serious complications, several complications were discussed.

Author details

Sertaç Aktop*, Onur Gönül, Hasan Garip and Kamil Göker

*Address all correspondence to: sertacaktop@hotmail.com

Marmara University Dentistry Faculty, Department of Oral and Maxillofacial Surgery, Istanbul, Turkey

References

[1] Vanarsdale R, White R: Three-dimensional analysis for skeletal problems. Int.I Adult Orthod Orthognatb Surg 1994; 9:159,

[2] Melson B: Palatal growth studied on human autopsy material. Am J Orthod 1975; 68:42

[3] Melson B, Melson F: The postnatal development of the palatomaxillary region studied on human autopsy material. Am J Orthod 1982; 82:329

[4] BettsNJ,Vanarsdall RL, BarberHD,Higgins-Barber K, Fonseca RJ. Diagnosis and treatment of transverse maxillary deficiency.Int J Adult Orthod Orthognath Surg 1995; 10:75–96

[5] Haas AJ: Long-term post-treatment evaluation of rapid palatal expansion. Angle Ortho 1980; 50:189

[6] Timms DJ. A study of basal movement with rapid maxillary expansion. Am J Orthod 1980;77:500-7.

[7] Wertz RA. Skeletal and dental changes accompanying rapid midpalatal suture opening. Am J Orthod 1970;58:41-66.

[8] Isaacson RJ, Murphy TD. Some effects of rapid maxillary expansion in cleft lip and palate patients. Angle Orthod 1964;34:143-54.

[9] Mommaerts MY. Transpalatal distraction as a method of maxillary expansion. Br J Oral Maxillofac Surg 1999;37:268-72.

[10] Zimring JF, Isaacson RJ. Forces produced by rapid maxillary expansion. 3. Forces present during retention. Angle Orthod 1965;35:178-86.

[11] Barber AF, Sims MR. Rapid maxillary expansion and external root resorption in man: a scanning electron microscope study. Am J Orthod 1981;79:630-52.

[12] Langford SR, Sims MR. Root surface resorption, repair, and periodontal attachment following rapid maxillary expansion in man. Am J Orthod 1982;81:108-15.

[13] Timms DJ, Moss JP. An histological investigation into the effects of rapid maxillary expansion on the teeth and their supporting tissues. Trans Eur Orthod Soc 1971:263-71.

[14] Moss JP. Rapid expansion of the maxillary arch. II. Indications for rapid expansion. JJPO J Pract Orthod 1968;2:215-23.

[15] Moss JP. Rapid expansion of the maxillary arch. I. Indications for rapid expansion. JPO J Pract Orthod 1968;2:165-71.

[16] Shetty V, Caridad JM, Caputo AA, Chaconas SJ. Biomechanical rationale for surgical-orthodontic expansion of the adult maxilla. J Oral Maxillofac Surg 1994;52:742-9.

[17] Alpern MC, Yurosko JJ. Rapid palatal expansion in adults with and without surgery. Angle Orthod 1987;57:245-63

[18] Greenbaum KR, Zachrisson BU. The effect of palatal expansion therapy on the periodontal supporting tissues. Am J Orthod 1982;81:12-21.

[19] Haas AJ. Long-term posttreatment evaluation of rapid palatal expansion. Angle Orthod 1980;50:189-217.

[20] 18. Moss JP. Rapid expansion. Int J Orthod 1976;14:15-9.

[21] Handelman CS. Nonsurgical rapid maxillary alveolar expansion in adults: a clinical evaluation. Angle Orthod 1997;67:291-305.

[22] Handelman CS, Wang L, BeGole EA, Haas AJ. Nonsurgical rapid maxillary expansion in adults: report on 47 Angle Orthod. 1999;70:129-144.

[23] Persson M. Structure and growth of facial sutures. Odontol Revy 1973: 24(6).

[24] Latham RA, Burston WR. The postnatal pattern of growth at sutures of the human skull. Dent Pract 1966: 17: 61–67.

[25] Melsen B. Palatal growth studied on human autopsy material. Am J Orthod 1975: 68: 42–54.

[26] Ozturk M, Doruk C, Ozec¸ I, Polat S, Babacan H, Bic¸akci A. Pulpal bloodflow: effects of corticotomy and midline osteotomy in surgically assisted rapid palatal expansion. J Cranio Maxillofac Surg 2003: 31: 97–100

[27] Profitt WR. Contemporary Orthodontics. 3rd edn. St. Louis, USA: Penny Rudolph, Mosby Inc. 2000.

[28] Mommaerts MY: Transpalatal distraction as a method of maxillary expansion. Br J Oral Max Surg 1999;37:268-72.

[29] Glassman AS, Nahigan SJ, Medway JM, Aronowitz H. Conservative surgical orthodontic adult rapid maxillary expansion: sixteen cases. Am J Orthod 1984;86:207-13.

[30] Lehman JA, Haas AJ, Haas DG. Surgical orthodontic correction of transverse maxillary deficiency: a simplified approach. Plast Reconstr Surg 1984;73:62-6

[31] Brown GVI. The Surgery of Oral and Facial Diseases and Malformation. 4th edn. London: Kimpton 1938: 507

[32] Haas AJ. Rapid palatal expansion of the maxillary dental arch and nasal cavity by opening the midpalatal suture. Angle Orthod 1961: 31: 73–90

[33] Aziz SR, Tanchyk A. Surgically assisted palatal expansion with a bone-borne self-retaining palatal expander. J Oral Maxillofac Surg. 2008;66(9):1788-93.

[34] Isaacson R, Ingram A: Forces produced by rapid maxillary expansion: Forces present during treatment. Angle Orthod 1964;34:256-60.

[35] Haas AJ: Palatal expansion: Just the beginning of dentofacial expansion. Am J Orthod 1970;57:219-55.

[36] Koudstaal MJ, Poort LJ, van der Wal KGH, Wolvius EB, Prahl-Andersen B, Schulten AJM: Surgically assisted rapid maxillary expansion (SARME): a review of the literature. Int. J. Oral Maxillofac. Surg. 2005; 34: 709–714

[37] Seeberger R, Kater W, Davids R, Thiele OC. Long term effects of surgically assisted rapid maxillary expansion without performing osteotomy of the pterygoid plates. Journal Of Cranio-Maxillo-Facial Surgery (2010) 38, 175-178.

[38] Isaacson RJ, Ingram AH. Forces produced by rapid maxillary expansion I: forces present during treatment. Angle Orthod 1964: 34: 256–260.

[39] Isaacson RJ, Wood JL, Ingram AH. Forces produced by rapid maxillary expansion II. Angle Orthod 1964: 34: 261.

[40] Wertz RA. Skeletal and dental changes accompanying rapid midpalatal suture opening. Am J Orthod 1970: 58: 41–66.

[41] Bierenbroodspot F, Wering PC, Kuijpers- Jagtman AM, Stoelinga PJW. Surgically assisted rapid maxillary expansion: a retrospective study. Ned Tijdschr Tandheelk 2002: 109: 299–302

[42] Booy A, Dorenbos J, Tuinzing DB. Corticotomie een chirurgisch aspect van orthodontie. Ned Tijdschr Tandheelkd 2000: 107: 213–214.

[43] Remmelink HJ. Corticotomie van de bovenkaak: een andere benadering. Ned Tijdschr Tandheelkd 2000: 107: 417 [comment in 418].

[44] Lines PA. Adult rapid maxillary expansion with corticotomy. Am J Orthod 1975: 67: 44–56.

[45] Bell Wh, Epker Bn. Surgical orthodontic expansion of the maxilla. 1976: 70: 517–528.

[46] Shetty V, Caridad JM, Caputo AA, et al: Biomechanical rationale for surgical-orthodontic expansion of the adult maxilla. J Oral Maxillofac Surg 1994; 52:742

[47] Suri L, Taneja P. Surgically assisted rapid palatal expansion: A literature review Am J Orthod Dentofacial Orthop 2008;133:290-302

[48] Berger JL, Pangrazio-Kulbersh V, Borgula T, Kaczynski R. Stability of orthopedic and surgically assisted rapid palatal expansion over time. American Journal of Orthodontics and Dentofacial Orthopedics 1998: 114: 638–645.

[49] Betts NJ, Ziccardi VB. Surgically assisted maxillary expansion. In: Fonseca RJ, ed: Oral and Maxillofacial Surgery Orthognathic Surgery v2. Philadelphia: WB Saunders 2000: 211– 231.

[50] Byloff FK, Mossaz CF. Skeletal and dental changes following surgically assisted rapid palatal expansion. European Journal of Orthodontics 2004: 26: 403–409.

[51] R. R. de Freitas, A. J. Gonc¸alves, N. J. Moniz, F. A. Maciel: Surgically assisted maxillary expansion in adults: prospective study. Int. J. Oral Maxillofac. Surg. 2008; 37: 797–804

[52] Turvey TA, Fonseca RJ. The anatomy of the internal maxillary artery in the pterygopalatine fossa: Its relationship to maxillary surgery. Journal of Oral Surgery 1980; 38(2):92-95.

[53] M. J. Koudstaal, L. J. Poort, K. G. H. van der Wal, E. B. Wolvius, B. Prahl-Andersen, A. J. M. Schulten: Surgically assisted rapid maxillary expansion (SARME): a review of the literature. Int. J. Oral Maxillofac. Surg. 2005; 34: 709–714

[54] do Amaral CMR, Di Domizio G, Tiziani V, Galhardi F, Buzzo CL, Rinco T. Gradual bone distraction in craniosynostosis. Preliminary results in seven cases. Scand J Plast Reconstr Surg Hand Surg 1997: 31: 25-37.

[55] Tavakoli K, Walsh WR, Bonar F, Smart R, Wulf S, Poole MD. The role of latency in mandibular osteodistraction. Journal of Cranio-Maxillofacial Surgery 1998: 26: 209–219

[56] Troulis MJ, Glowacki J, Perrot DH, Kaban LB. Effects of latency and rate on bone formation in a porcine mandibular distraction model. J Oral Maxillofac Surg 2000: 58: 507–513.

[57] Ilizarov GA. The tension-stress effect on the genesis and growth of tissues. Part I. The influence of stability of fixation and soft-tissue preservation. Clinical Orthopaedics and Related Research 1989: 238: 249–281.

[58] R. R. de Freitas, A. J. Gonc¸alves, N. J. Moniz, F. A. Maciel: Surgically assisted maxillary expansion in adults: prospective study. Int. J. Oral Maxillofac. Surg. 2008; 37: 797–804

[59] Cleall JF, Bayne DI, Posen JM, Subtelny JD. Expansion of the midpalatal in the monkey. Angle Orthod 1965: 35: 23– 35.

[60] Mehra P, Cottrell DA, Caiazzo A, Lincoln R. Life-threatening, delayed epistaxis after surgically assisted rapid palatal expansion: a case report. J Oral Maxillofac Surg 1999;57:201-4.

[61] Li KK, Meara JG, Rubin PA. Orbital compartment syndrome following orthognathic surgery. J Oral Maxillofac Surg 1995; 53:964-8.

[62] Kraut RA. Surgically assisted rapid maxillary expansion by opening the midpalatal suture. J Oral Maxillofac Surg 1984: 42: 651–655.

[63] Pogrel MA, Kaban LB, Vargervik K, Baumrind S. Surgically assisted rapid maxillary expansion in adults. Int J Adult OrthodonOrthognath Surg 1992: 7: 37–41.

[64] Messer EJ, Bollinger TE, Keller JJ. Surgical-mechanical maxillary expansion. Quintessence Int 1979: 10: 13–16.

[65] Lanigan DT, Hey JH, West RA: Major complications of orthognathic surgery: Hemorrhage associated with Le Fort 1 osteotomies. J Oral Maxillofac Surg 1990; 48:561

[66] Glassman AS, Nahigan SJ, Medway JM, Aronowitz H. Conservative surgical orthodontic adult rapid maxillary expansion: sixteen cases. Am J Orthod 1984;86:207-13.

[67] Carmen M, Marcella P, Giuseppe C, Roberto A. Periodontal evaluation in patients undergoing maxillary expansion. J Craniofac Surg 2000;11:491-4

[68] Vardimon AD, Graber TM, Pitaru S. Repair process of external root resorption subsequent to palatal expansion treatment. Am J Orthod Dentofacial Orthop 1993;103:120-30.

[69] Ozturk M, Doruk C, Ozec I, Polat S, Babacan H, Bicakci AA. Pulpal blood flow: effects of corticotomy and midline osteotomy in surgically assisted rapid palatal expansion. J Craniomaxillofac Surg 2003;31:97-100.

[70] Harada K, Sato M, Omura K. Blood-flow change and recovery of sensibility in the maxillary dental pulp during and after maxillary distraction: a pilot study. Oral Surg Oral Med Oral Patho Oral Radiol Endod 2004;98:528-32

[71] Cureton SL, Cuenin M. Surgically assisted rapid palatal expansion: orthodontic preparation for clinical success. Am J Orthod Dentofacial Orthop 1999;116:46-59.

[72] Schimming R, Feller KU, Herzmann K, Eckelt U. Surgical and orthodontic rapid palatal expansion in adults using Glassman's technique: retrospective study. Br J Oral Maxillofac Surg 2000;38:66-9.

[73] Woods M, Wiesenfeld D, Probert T. Surgically-assisted maxillary expansion. Aust Dent J 1997;42:38-42.

Chapter 9

Combined Surgical and Orthodontic Management of Maxillofacial Deformities

Sana Alami, Hakima Aghoutan, Samir Diouny,
Farid El Quars and Farid Bourzgui

Additional information is available at the end of the chapter

http://dx.doi.org/10.5772/59164

1. Introduction

The development of orthognathic surgery techniques and materials has allowed surgeons and orthodontists to standardize treatment of maxillomandibular deformities. Multidisciplinary treatment of skeletal deformities by orthognathic surgery in addition to orthodontics has become a routine strategy believed to result in functional and esthetic outcomes in adult patients.

When malocclusion is caused by severe skeletal discrepancies, the orthodontist can propose dentofacial orthopedics in growing children, dental compensation for skeletal deformity or orthognathic surgery combined with orthodontic treatment (when the major growth potential of the patient has been completed). The decision is based on clinical examination and cephalometric analysis, both of which aim to assess the amount of three dimensional discrepancy. Patients with functional and esthetic issues require a multidisciplinary approach involving orthodontic and orthognathic surgery to reposition the maxilla and/or the mandible in three dimensions. Such a therapeutic approach is considered as the best treatment; it corrects dentofacial deformities which cannot be treated by orthodontics alone [1].

The stability of results in addition to the functional well-being and aesthetic appearance approach the level of excellence. The issue of skeletal, dento-alveolar and soft tissue relapse is a matter of discussion, debate and controversy in the orthodontic literature. The aim of this chapter is to define the criteria for stability that must be complied during both preparatory orthodontic and surgery phases in orthognathic surgery, without over-timing the postoperative orthodontic phase.

1.1. Stability criteria of ortho-surgical treatment

The management of dento-skeletal dysmorphosis requires a team of specialists that mainly include orthodontists and maxillofacial surgeons. The ultimate aim of orthodontists is both to meet the patients' expectations, and make effective sustainable interventions. Three treatment objectives, which form the basis in treating patients with dento-facial deformities, are fundamental in orthognathic surgery namely function, esthetics, and stability. Skeletal relapse is the most common complication following orthognathic surgery. Optimal treatment planning for maxillofacial surgery requires an understanding of postoperative skeletal stability, dento-alveolar position and the soft tissue response to skeletal movement. Accurate treatment planning and careful orthodontic and surgical protocols are essential to the achievement of treatment objectives; these have to be planned with collaborating partners upon initial consultation (Figure 1). [1]

Influencing Factors

- Preoperative age
- Soft tissue and muscles
- Presurgical skeletal pattern
- Dental decompensation
- Coordination of dental arcss
- Direction and amount of surgical movement
- Type and material of fixation

Figure 1. Factors influencing stability in orthognthic surgery treatment.[1]

2. Preliminary patient evaluation

A systematic examination is necessary to adequately evaluate and treat patients with dento-facial deformities. Treatment planning should start only when the orthodontist and surgeon have agreed on a final treatment plan. It is mandatory that the patient be well informed about the treatment plan and related possible disadvantages.

Indeed, efficacy is guaranteed when there is clear and effective communication between the orthodontist and the maxillofacial surgeon from the outset.

Routine evaluation includes [1]:

http://dx.doi.org/10.5772/59164

- Evaluation of patient's medical history
- Socio-psychological assessment of the patient's motives and expectations
- Aesthetic facial evaluation involving frontal and profile analysis
- Dental and occlusal oral function evaluation
- Cephalometric radiographic evaluation which forms an important part of the database for orthognathic surgical treatment planning. Soft tissue, skeletal and dental analysis are helpful diagnostic guides.
- Occlusion and study cast evaluation which includes examination for intra and inter- arch relationships.

The initial consultation aims to discuss the possible need for surgical procedure as part of the treatment to achieve optimal results. However, before treatment, it is important to put emphasis on those elements that are directly related to stability; some of these include operative age, the soft tissue and muscles, and mandibular inclination. [2, 3]

2.1. Preoperative age

Growth following surgery may result in relapse; surgical osteotomy and osteosynthesis have little influence on the mandibular jaw growth. The initial growth of the patient's face and continuous remodeling processes may lead to an advantageous or disadvantageous change of position of the mandible after sagittal split osteotomy. [3] The inability to predict the potential growth of the mandible can lead to failure or recurrence when the surgical indication is established before the end of growth. This leads practitioners to adopt a cautious attitude. To minimize the risks of relapse due to continuous growth, surgery should only be recommended to patients when growth is complete.

2.2. Soft tissue and muscles

Although long-term studies of surgical orthodontic stability are sparse, many authors predict the importance of active and /or passive contractions exerted by muscles and/or post surgical skeletal recurrences due to soft tissue. [2] An examination of cervical soft tissues and orofacial muscles (in particular the tongue) at rest and during function requires due attention. This is illustrated in case 1 which was a 19-year-old female admitted for burn injuries following a home accident at the age of 6 yrs. Aesthetic imbalance and significant dento-skeletal deformity is due to post-burn contractures of the neck (Figures 2 and 3). Facial appearance is the patient's main concern. Radiographic evaluation and cephalometric analysis showed the patient presented high values for mandibular length and plane angle (FMA= 38°). The Wits appraisal indicated a large anteroposterior discrepancy between the maxilla and mandible (AO-BO=-6.5mm) (Figure 4). Only surgery can improve the aesthetics. The expected dental and soft tissue changes to be affected by the preoperative orthodontic treatment are illustrates by cephalometric tracing. The surgical plan consisted of two-jaw surgery (Figure 5).

- Lefort I maxillary osteotomy is used to perform advancement and expansion of the maxilla and a slight superiorly repositioning is needed to allow the mandible to auto-rotate and close the openbite.
- Bilateral sagittal split osteotomy for setback of the mandible.

Preoperative orthodontic treatment planning included teeth alignment without extraction and provision of good arch form assisted by maxillary expansion (Figure 6).

But the project initially conceived can only succeed after surgical repair of cervical skin tissue, the only guarantee of stability after orthognathic surgery. Lingual Frenectomy, re-education for tongue position during swallowing are modalities that help stability.

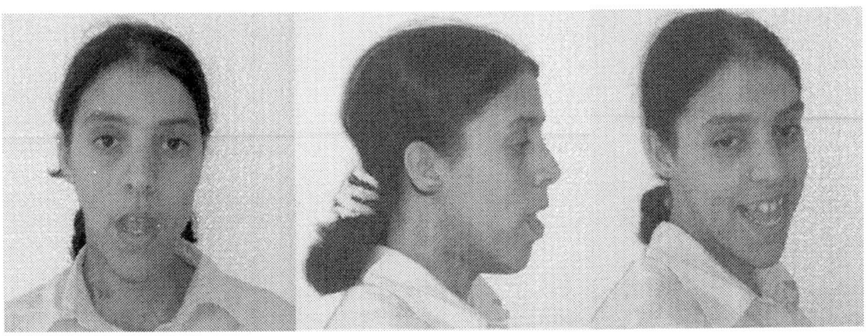

Figure 2. Frontal view, profile and smile of the patient before treatment: Female, 19 years of age, characteristics long face pattern, prognathism and vertical growth pattern, scar contracture due to neck burn and increased interlabial gap.

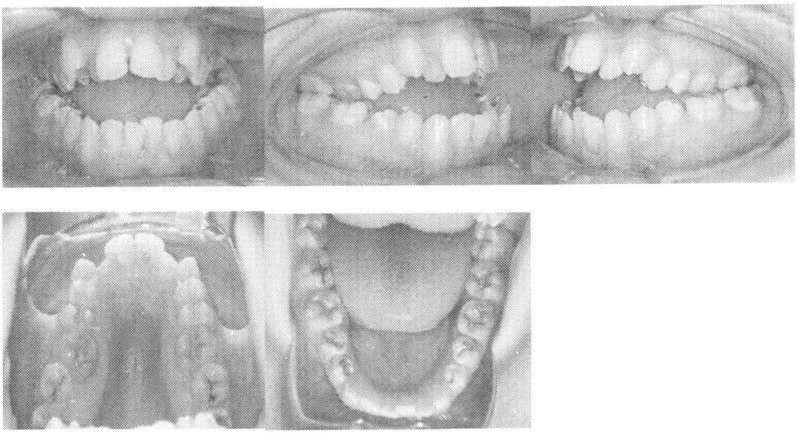

Figure 3. Pre-treatment intra-oral photographs: frontal lateral occlusion shows severe open bite and maxillary antero-posterior and transverse deficiency. Constricted maxillary arch explains the crowding in the anterior maxilla.

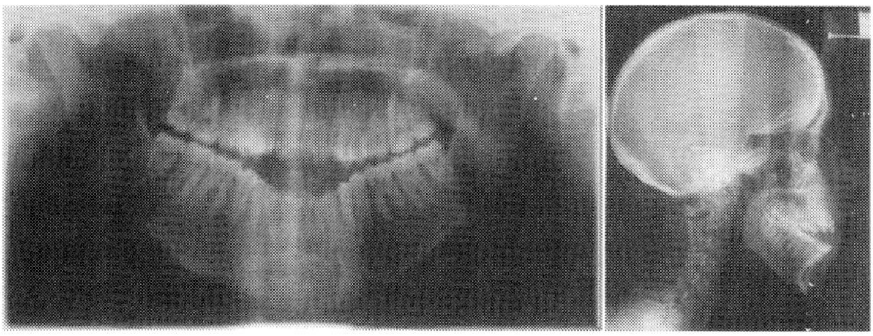

Figure 4. Pre-treatment orthopantomogram and lateral teleradiogram of skull.

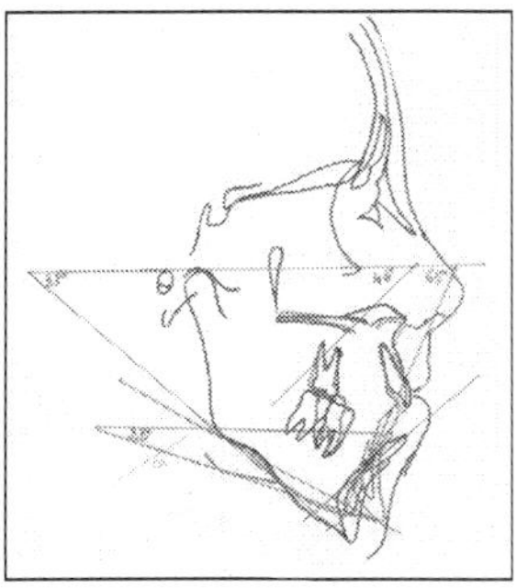

SNA	73°
SNB	78°
ANB	-5°
AO-BO	-6mm
FMA	38°
FMIA	42°
IMPA	100°
Occl. To Fr	15°
I to NA	20°/4mm
I to NB	45°/ 11mm

Figure 5. The orthodontic visual treatment objective illustrates the desired presurgical orthodontic tooth movement and predicts the surgical repositioning of the jaws and subsequent soft tissue changes. It has a key role in choosing dental extractions, if needed.

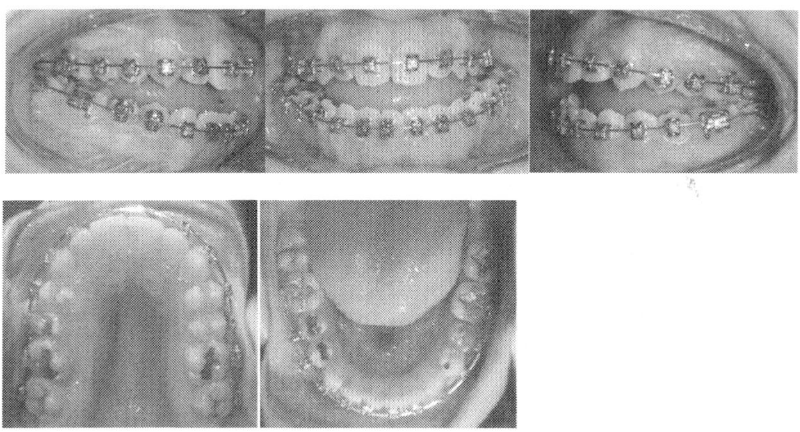

Figure 6. Immediate preoperative intraoral photographs. Treatment did not need dental teeth extraction and the aim of preparatory orthodontic stage was to establish a good arch form in the maxillary and mandibular arches.

2.3. Presurgical skeletal pattern

The influence of the mandibular plane angle on horizontal and vertical skeletal stability has been shown in several studies. [3, 4] High angle patients have a greater risk of relapse after receiving bilateral sagittal split ramus osteotomy than low and normal–angle patients. Patients with a low mandibular plane angle, compared to high and normal angle patients, appear to have a more predictable procedure. Then, patients with a low mandibular plane angle have increased vertical relapse when advancement surgery is indicated; whereas patients with a high mandibular plane angle have more horizontal relapse. [3] Because the muscles of mastication are lengthened in the ramus area, they tend to return to their original positions, rotate the mandible in a clockwise movement, open the bite, and cause relapse. To minimize the risk of relapse, patients should be selected carefully; isolated mandibular advancement or setback should not be performed for patients with high mandibular plane angles. [3]

3. Defining treatment objectives

Therapy planning should be clear and precise and the objectives need to be defined with collaborative partners before a final treatment planning decision:

- Focus of the objective of surgery should center on osteotomy choice and its site;
- Orthodontic objective conditioned by the surgical objective, will consist of determining the necessary strategies to reduce preliminary occlusal obstacles and the rebalancing of the dentoalveolar system.

Starting cases orthodontically and then, if unsuccessful, referring them for surgery often produces compromised results. [5] It is, therefore, important to prioritize problems and think of potential solutions; this way one can define the objectives of each treatment step. The initial treatment plan must be established following a discussion between the different parties responsible for the smooth implementation of the various steps of the treatment plan.In fact, cephalometric and occlusal simulation setup permits the practitioner to project the occlusal dental and facial skeletal result, to ascertain and determine a suitable orthodontic surgical protocol. Those set-up demonstrates the general reharmonization of the teeth, the jaw and the face. It can then be used as a reference instrument in discussions with the surgeon and patient, and can be modified at all times according to the particular needs. The set-up is, and remains, an estimation which supplies simple quantitative proportional and comparative data. We can record all the data in it (Figure 7). [6]

The use of information technology in dental studies and orthodontics in particular, has contributed to the use of set-up scanning. A 3D simulation system has been developed for orthognathic surgery ; it helps integrate the shape data of the teeth, jawbone and face into the same coordinate system on a computer. The movement of bone associated with mandibular osteotomy and the subsequent changes in the facial form can thus be estimated preoperatively. [7]

The three-dimensional setups allow orthognathic surgery simulation through:

- Integration of the dental arch using a three-dimensional digital model and accurate face scan of the patient.
- Simulation of different possible osteotomies (Lefort, Obwegeser genioplasty), and removal of bone fragments.
- Visualization of contact points.
- Realization of a morphing orthognathic surgery

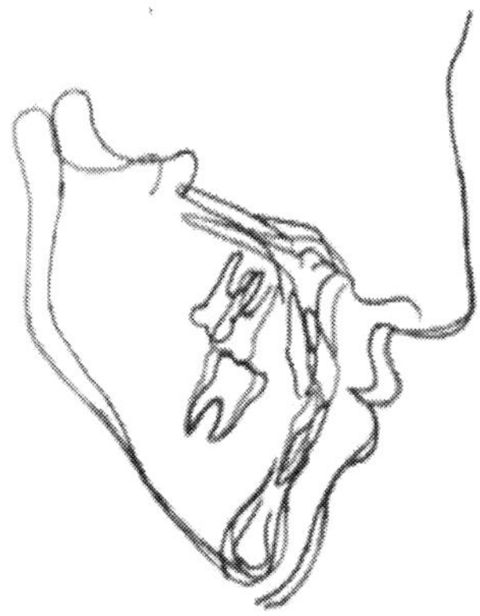

Figure 7. Surgical visual treatment prediction The presurgical setup can assist surgical diagnosis accurate prediction of the postoperative skeletal, dental and facial profile and has become an essential part of the diagnostic and treatment planning procedure of combined surgical-orthodontic therapy.

4. Surgical treatment

The treatment protocol includes three distinct, but successive steps: Orthodontic phases of preparation are enacted prior to surgical treatment. Generally speaking, the stability of expected results depends on both meeting pre-defined objectives for each step as well as on the smooth and proper course of treatment. Otherwise, it could also be compromised by incomplete orthodontic treatment and yield unfavorable outcomes in orthognathic surgery or functional occlusal imbalance following treatment (Figure 8). [8]

Successful surgical correction of dentoskeletal cases is determined by both pre- surgical-orthodontic treatment (which eliminates dental compensation), correct surgical planning, and postoperative orthodontic therapy applied to refine the patient's occlusion. Fixed appliances are normally used in both of these orthodontic stages.

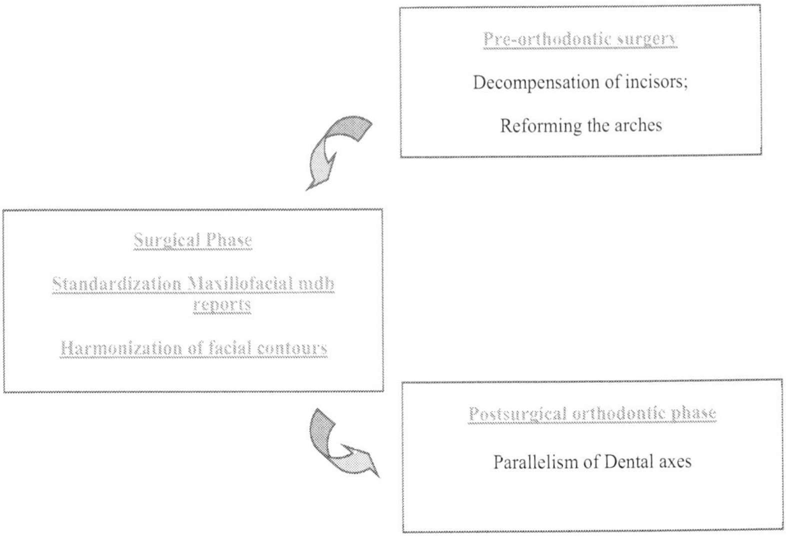

Figure 8. The aim of surgical correction is to achieve the right occlusal and skeletal relationships and correct esthetics simultaneously.

4.1. Preoperative / pre-surgical orthodontic phase

In orthognathic surgery cases, orthodontic treatment objectives are for the most part different from those used in conventional orthodontics. The purpose of pre-surgical orthodontics is to position the teeth to the most desirable position in preparation for surgery, to restore the anteroposterior and vertical positions in addition to coordinating incisors. Two main elements must prevail during this first phase: Incisors decompensation and transverse and dental arch coordination. [1, 9]

4.1.1. Anteroposterior dental decompensation

In the presence of a bone gap, teeth manage to maintain an occlusion with dental compensation in three dimensions.

In the sagittal plane, overjet does not represent magnitudes of bone gap. However, during surgery, bone bases are mobilized to allow dental occlusion [10] in this context, it is clear that the relationship between anterior and posterior bases of incisors determines the magnitude of anterior-posterior relocation of the bone base. [11]

Presurgical orthodontic treatment aims to decompensate incisor inclination toward normal values. It is therefore necessary to define beforehand the objective of the "terminal incisor position". Therefore In the case of skeletal class II, the lower incisors are proclined while the upper incisors are lingual retroclined (Figure 9). In Class III, the reverse pattern is observed; upper incisors are proclined while the lower incisors are retroclined (Figure 13). Bone gap is compensated for by teeth inclination [10] presurgical intra-arch objectives include positioning of the incisors in "ideal" positions, establishment of correct torque, and elimination of tooth-size discrepancies so as to permit the establishment of Class I canine and molar relationships after surgery. In orthognathic surgery cases, extraction patterns, and types of mechanics used are frequently the reverse of those used in conventional orthodontics. [11] Very often in skeletal Class II, the first premolars are extracted in order to cover mandibular incisors and obtain a Class I canine relationship. Extraction of the second premolars allows in recovery of the upper incisors and the mesial movement of upper molars. The ultimate goal is to achieve a Class I molar relationship (Figures 10- 12).

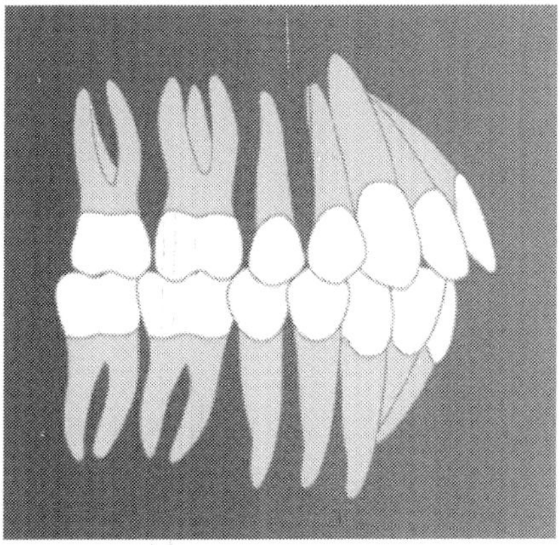

Figure 9. Dental compensation in skeletal Class II malocclusion

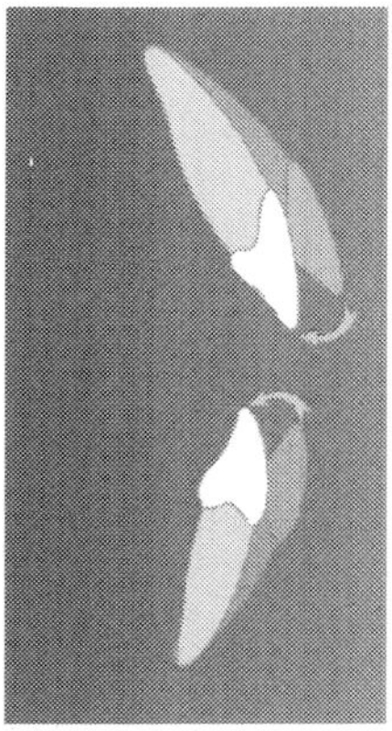

Figure 10. Direction of incisor decompensation in Class II malocclusion: the lingual inclination of the lower incisors is increased and in some cases (Class II.1 malocclusion), the upper incisors retroclined

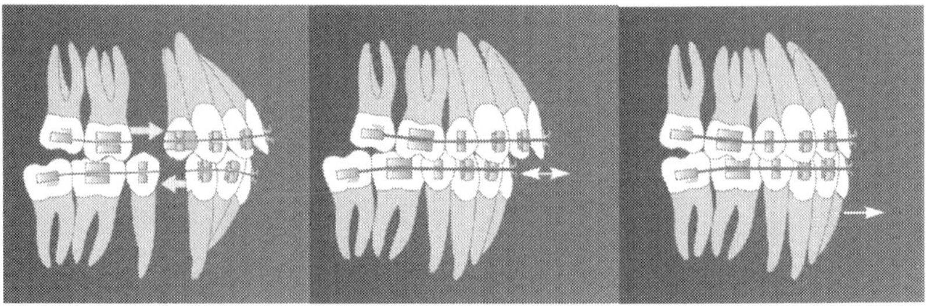

Figure 11. Classic pattern extraction of 15, 25, 34 and 44 in order to increase the overjet and presurgically decompensate for the malocclusion. The presurgical position of the teeth dictates the teeth removal and the surgical movement of the jaws and ultimately the soft tissue facial balance.

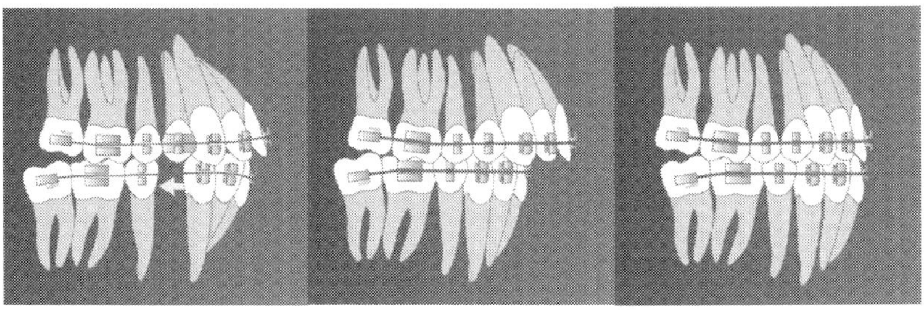

Figure 12. Extraction of 34 and 44 only can be justified

As for skeletal Class III, extraction of upper first premolar is enacted to reposition upper incisors and obtain Class I canine relationship. (Figure 14) Extraction of the 2nd premolars is not systematic given that therapeutic Class II molar is tolerated from an occlusodontic perspective. (Figures 15, 16) In fact, presurgical objectives in the sagittal plane focus on removal of dental compensations. However, decompensation represents security for stable occlusion and improved aesthetics.

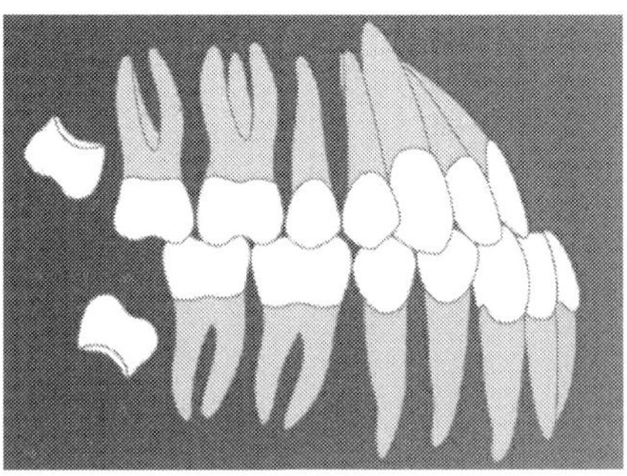

Figure 13. Dental compensation seen in skeletal Class III malocclusion

http://dx.doi.org/10.5772/59164

This may require the use of Class III elastics in Class II cases (and vice versa), thus allowing for maximal surgical correction of the underlying skeletal deformity.

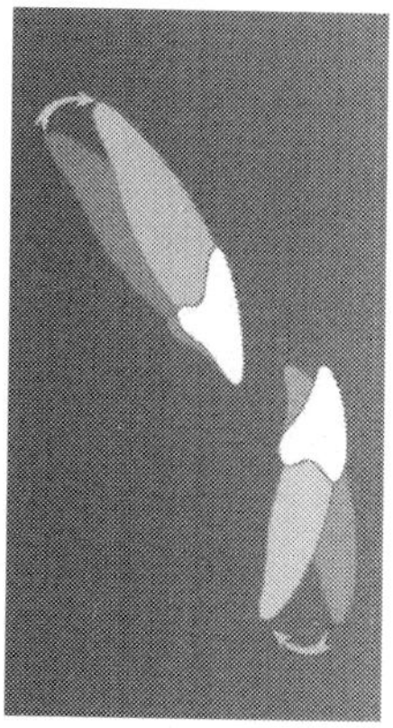

Figure 14. Direction of incisor decompensation in Class III malocclusion: the labial inclination of the lower incisors is increased and the upper incisors reduced

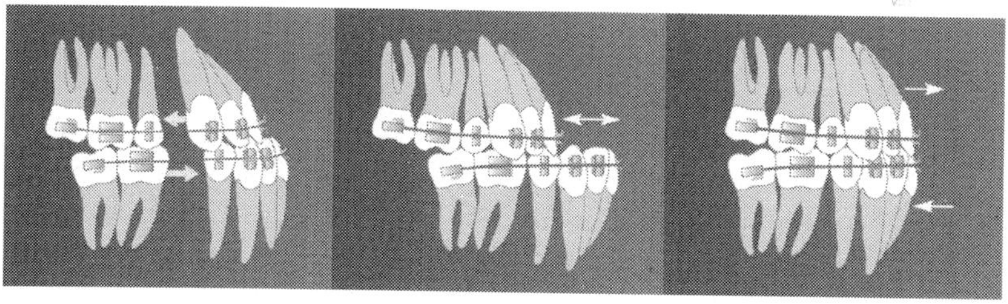

Figure 15. Classic pattern extraction of 14, 24, 35 and 45 in order to increase the negative overjet and presurgically decompensate for the malocclusion. Correct planning of the orthodontic tooth positioning before surgery will enhance the surgical potential and, hence, the esthetic result.

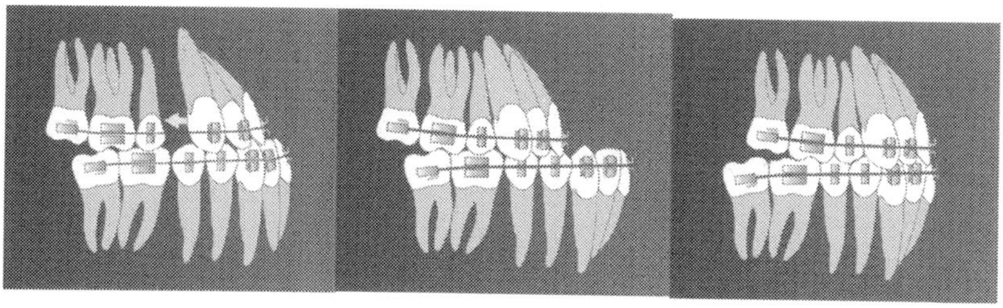

Figure 16. Extraction of 14 and 24 is often sufficient and molar Class II acceptable.

4.1.2. Transverse arch coordination

One goal of presurgical orthodontics is that maxillary and mandibular transverse diameters coincide for a reasonable intercuspation after surgery. [10] It is clearly established that both vertical and horizontal recurrence correlate with dental arches in coordination and the persistence of occlusal interferences. The resulting occlusal imbalance is closely related to orthodontic preparation, sometimes without extraction [12] in the transverse plane; differentiation of skeletal from dental problems as well as identification of relative and absolute discrepancies should be carried out presurgically. Orthodontic or surgical expansion should be used, depending on individual circumstances (Figure 17). [11]

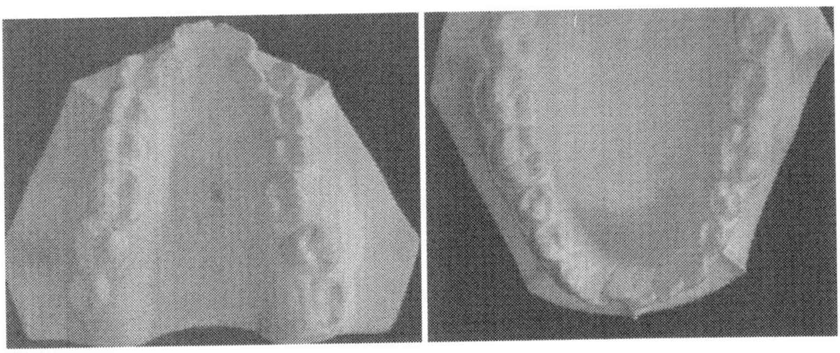

Figure 17. Dental arch width must be assessed preoperatively by measuring and comparing the distance between the mesiolingual cusps of the maxillary first molars versus the central fossae of the mandibular first molars. In this case, there are skeletal transverse deficiencies which must be corrected by surgical maxillary expansion.

In the absence of a major transverse problem, arch compatibility is generally achieved by coordination. [11] This is true for class II cases, where transverse shift goes unnoticed as revealed by the manipulation in the corrected position. This is a favorable orthodontic work so that both arches engage properly when the surgical mandibular advancement is performed.

Surgical disjunction or surgically assisted expansion can help to prevent transverse recurrence related to excessive teeth release. [10] Study casts carried out at the end of orthodontic preparation are essential; they allow rectifying any condition that may potentially lead to complications, and thus affects the success and stability of the surgical procedure. [13]

4.2. Surgical phase

The order of importance begins with the direction and amount of skeletal movement, the type of fixation used, and finally, the surgical technique. [3, 14] Other factors were also stated, namely, the maxillomandibular order or surgery-orthodontics[15- 17]

4.2.1. Direction and amount of surgical movement

In a report on the hierarchy of stability in orthognathic surgery, Proffit ranked isolated maxillary advancement as the second most stable orthognathic surgical procedure after

http://dx.doi.org/10.5772/59164

maxillary upward positioning; the latter was performed more than maxillary advancement with or without mandibular setback. [13, 14]

4.2.1.1. *Maxillary upward*

Maxillary impaction is recommended in the case of patients with dolichofacial condition and vertical maxillary excess. Excellent skeletal stability is achieved in 90% of the cases, irrespective of the type of osteosynthesis used. [14] Such stability is due to the physiological occlusal adaptation related to mandible rotation. Interocclusal space is then maintained. [14, 18]

In asymmetry correction of the maxilla characterized by the inclination of the occlusal plane, surgery combines maxillary impaction and mandibular surgery. The maxillary component of this asymmetry correction is considered stable [19]

4.2.1.2. *Mandibular advancement*

Sagittal split ramus osteotomy (SSRO) is a well-established procedure for correcting mandibular retrognathism. [20] The literature contains a number of studies on postoperative changes after SSRO. At retention phase, relapse occurred due to the increase in mandibular plane and ANB angle, and an increase in overjet. [19, 21] The etiology of relapse is multifactorial, involving the proper seating of the condyles, the amount of advancement, the soft tissue and muscles, the mandibular plane angle, the remaining growth and the skill of the surgeon. [3, 8, 21] It is believed that orthosurgical treatment for the correction of Class II with mandibular advancement could be stable, provided the amount of skeletal movements and the circumjacent soft tissues are respected. Advancements over 10mm lead to horizontal relapse. [14, 21, 22] In systematic review that evaluate horizontal relapse in bilateral sagittal split advancement osteotomy, it was shown that advancements in the range of 6 to 7 mm or more predispose to horizontal relapse. [3]

4.2.1.3. *Maxillary advancement*

Maxillary advancement could be stable, provided that skeletal movements, as recommended by some others, were under 6, 8 or 10mm. In fact, the use of rigid fixation and bone grafting for good stability of maxillary advancement up to 6 mm showed no recurrence. [14, 19, 23-25] For a maxillary advancement of less than 8mm, it was suggested that the maxillary maintain its horizontal postsurgical position (less than 2 mm) in 80% of the cases; a risk of recurrence between from 2 and 4 mm can be seen in 20% of the cases. [25]

4.2.1.4. *Mandibular setback*

The sagittal split ramus osteotomy (SSRO) and the intraoral vertical ramus osteotomy (IVRO) are well-established procedures for correcting mandibular prognathism. Both techniques have advantages and disadvantages; include bony contact between the distal and mesial segments and application for both advancement and retraction and the duration of intermaxillary fixation (IMF). Orthognathic surgeons must weigh up these advantages and disadvantages when deciding which surgical treatment to use in cases of mandibular prognathism. Another important factor for surgeons to consider is postoperative stability. While the literature contains a number of studies on postoperative changes after SSRO, a few reports concern post-operative stability after IVRO.

IVRO is a relatively simple technique, which is applicable for only retraction of the mandible. The postoperative changes and stability tend to be influenced by the surgical techniques employed and the skills of the surgeons. In the short term after IVRO, clockwise rotation was observed due a less bony contact between the proximal and distal segments during surgery. After this period of adaptive rotation, the mandible showed a slight tendency to relapse with forward movement up to 2 years after IVRO. [20] With bilateral sagittal split osteotomy setback (BSSO), the relapse is more frequent than vertical osteotomy. However, it is an effective treatment of skeletal class III and a stable procedure in the short and long term. Analyzing the different relapse rates in systematic review showed that main relapse mostly takes place immediate after surgery and in the short term. [2, 14] From the reviewed literature, it was conclude that skeletal relapse is very frequent and was influenced by the magnitude of surgical correction and the inclination of the ramus after surgery. But, compared with mandibular advancement BSSO, the amount of setback was correlated less frequently with the amount of relapse. Opinions differ and generally speaking, the father the distal segment is set back (more than 10mm), the greater the tendency for the proximal segment to rotate. Furthermore, maintaining the initial inclination of the ramus could therefore reduce the tendency to relapse. [2, 14, 22, 26] Other research suggested that post-operative relapse in mandibular setback surgery may relate to the pre-surgical skeletal pattern of each patient and the perimandibular connective tissue action. Additionally, some vertical mandibular relapse after setback surgery may be affected by the postural changes of the tongue and hyoid bone [26] However, it was reported that the role of suprahyoid muscles is less important after a mandibular setback than after advancement or a closing gap.[26,27] Correcting the open bite by orthognathic surgery directed only at the mandible has a high risk of relapse because of mandibular up-repositioning in a counter-clockwise rotation. A mandibular backward repositioning is equally performed to prevent open bite relapse. [28]

4.2.1.5. Maxillary advancement combined with mandibular setback

The mandibular setback is frequently combined with Le Fort I osteotomy for maxillary advancement when there is a greater discrepancy between the maxilla and mandible and greater labial projection. Surgical correction of Class III malocclusion after combined maxillary and mandibular procedures appears to be a fairly stable procedure for maxillary advance-ments up to 5 mm, independent of the type of fixation used to stabilize the mandible. Likewise, no statistically significant differences have been observed between the procedures conducted on both jaws versus the lower jaw only. [21, 29- 31] Over the past few years, the number of patients with mandibular prognathism as a component of a skeletal Class III problem who were treated with mandibular setback alone decreased remarkably, compared with outcomes in patients with two- jaw surgery. A number of reasons to explain such a tendency are listed below: [32, 33]

- Restricting the amount of mandibular setback by simultaneously advancing the maxilla contributes to stability.

- Facial appearance was better if simultaneous maxillary advancement allowed a smaller mandibular setback;
- Large setbacks lead to airway reduction
- The outcomes of isolated mandibular setback surgery were shown to be less predictable and less stable than desired.
- The better control of the ramus position when 2-jaw surgery is performed

4.2.1.6. Maxillary expansion

Transverse maxillomandibular discrepancies are a major component of several malocclusions. The correction of skeletal transverse deficiency of the maxilla may be achieved surgically. [34]

The segmental maxillary osteotomy (SMO) is recommended when a moderate transverse defect of the maxillary bone in the amount of 5 to 6mm require correction. To increase the transverse diameter of the maxilla, maxillary expansion is simultaneously performed with Lefort I planned to correct all maxilla-mandibular discrepancies (vertical and sagittal repositioning). It consists at least to two osteotomy lines, one on either side of the palatine raphe, performed after orthodontic preparatory stage. [34, 35] Maxillary expansion is relatively simple, but treatment stability remains a common problem. Overcorrection and rigid osteosynthesis are recommended. In addition, the corrected maxilla should be reinforced with intraoral retention provided by a preformed palatal bar or splint. [14, 35]

The Surgically assisted rapid palatal expansion (SARPE) is used in cases of severe deficit estimated at more than 6 to 7mm; surgically-assisted maxillary expansion, which depends on osseous distraction osteogenesis the separating of segments of bone to create new bone and the movement of whole groups of teeth and their periodontium. This technique works by release of the maxilla bone resistances and assures excellent stability.

4.2.1.7. Genioplasty

The chin is subject to morphological anomalies in the sagittal (retrogenia or progenia), vertical (excess or insufficient height), or transversal (laterogenia) axes. Genioplasty, used alone or in conjunction with other maxillomandibular osteotomies, is an important and reliable technique for the esthetic treatment of the lower facial skeleton. It can be a powerful procedure to improve the facial profile by modifying the position of the chin bones in three planes. Genioplasty is a stable surgical procedure when used in conjunction with rigid internal fixation. So there is no significant relapse after genioplasty and bilateral sagittal split osteotomy or genioplasty alone after 12 months. In fact, the changes are minimal and hard to detect clinically. [36]

4.2.2. Osteotomy fixation (type and materials)

Osteotomy fixation technique is one of the factors that determine the horizontal and vertical postsurgical relapse potential. The short- and long-term outcomes of different fixation techniques are a topic of interest in the orthodontic literature. [37] In earlier years, maxillary osteotomies were stabilized using intraosseous wires. In the 1980s, rigid internal fixation of osteotomy segments using miniplates and/or screws were introduced in an attempt to decrease postsurgical relapse and to allow earlier mobilization of the mandible. In fact, miniplates were introduced for fixation in BSSO, and have several advantages compared with bicortical screw osteosynthesis, because of the stretching of the musculature and paramandibular tissues, the bilateral compound joints, the masticatory forces, and occlusion. [27, 37] A number of studies that addressed the value of rigid internal fixation reported that 50% of the total forward relapse of mandible occurred during the 6 weeks after surgery. In contrast, with wire fixation and maxillomandibular fixation, the mandible maintained its position or moved posteriorly during MMF fixation. [33] On the other hand, in study which investigates biomechanical stability of RIF, the relationship between screw placement configurations and stability was demonstrated. It was concluded that bi-cortical screws with a 2.3-mm diameter and triangular configuration were considered as a sufficient fixation tool for BSSO than the linear configuration. [38] However, there is a trend toward increase in relapse from short-term to long-term studies when bicortical screws are used. [3] Bicortical screws of titanium, stainless steel, or bioresorbable material show little difference regarding skeletal stability compared with miniplates in the short term. A greater number of studies with larger skeletal long-term relapse rates were evident in patients treated with bicortical screws instead of miniplates. [3] The use of bicortical screws or monocortical screws, together with plates, is the most demanding fixation procedure of the craniofacial skeleton when used in mandibular advancement patients. [8] It was also shown that the use of BSSO of the mandible with or without counterclockwise rotation of the occlusal plane for anterior open bite correction, increases stability in the vertical direction. [39] Thus, some of the limitations of metal plates and screws used for the fixation of bones have led to the development of plates made from titanium. Such a technique has been in use in orthognathic surgery for about two decades, because of their high biocompatibility and resistance to corrosion. In addition, titanium fixation produces stability for the osteotomy site and allows patients to use their masticatory system functionally immediately after surgery. [40] The development of bioresorbable osteosynthesis devices made it possible to avoid second surgery to remove titanium plates linked sometimes to palpability, infectious complications or allergies; although they are rare. However, concerns remain about the stability which was related to the movements in orthognathic surgery. [26, 40] The systematic reviews of bioresorbable versus titanium fixation for orthognathic surgery, have shown that bioresorbable fixation systems produce reliable skeletal stability. [40] However, it suggested no statistically significant difference for plate and screw fixation using either titanium or resorbable materials. There are a few studies about the stability of biodegradable devices osteosynthesis and it was recommended that these materials should be used with caution for bony movements of greater magnitude until their usefulness is evaluated in studies with large maxillary advancements. [30]

4.3. Postsurgical orthodontics

Postsurgical orthodontic treatment involves finalization of the occlusion and retention. Working wire and light up and down elastics or slightly Class II or Class III elastics ensures the refinement of the occlusion. This final stage is equally important to ensure stable results. It is not enough to place orthodontic retainers at the end of treatment. It is appropriate to finalize and fine-tune the occlusion with a view to achieve stability, function, and facial balance. [1, 41]

4.3.1. Functional balance conditions

Neutralizing the functional matrix at the end of treatment contributes significantly to stability of results. It is important to note that mastery of the neuromuscular environment is an important element of skeletal and dentoalveolar modeling of each patient. The stability of the result after treatment is therefore based on the diagnosis of muscle behavior, and functional rehabilitation.

This final phase of treatment is the best time to prescribe exercises for normalizing orofacial muscles and harmonizing skeletal relationships making rehabilitation more effective.

4.3.2. Occlusion balance conditions

The finishing and detailing phase, the last stage of active orthognathic surgery treatment, makes it possible to improve the occlusion, by adopting a number of criteria as defined by various authors; the ultimate goal is to improve the esthetic result, on the condition that treatment objectives during the pre-planning phase have been met.

Dental balance should be considered both statically and dynamically. Indeed, intra-arch condition inter-arch relationships, and balance provides functional comfort and lasting results.

Treatment stability depends in part on obtaining a "functional occlusion" consistent with the physiology of TMA. The quality of finishing for some researchers (Tweed) is sufficient as a natural retainer tool.

4.3.2.1. The sequence of ortho-surgical treatment

The sequence of steps of ortho-surgical treatment is illustrated through a clinical case: A 16-year-old patient reported aesthetic and psychological discomfort related to severe skeletofacial discrepancy. The patient also complained of functional difficulty during mastication and expressed concern at his inability to bite using the anterior sector of the dentition. In face and profile views, skeletal class III due to underdevelopment of the upper jaw and to mandibular deformity in frontal, vertical and sagittal dimension was noticed (Figure 18).

Intraoral examination showed severe molar and canine Class III, the absence of overbite and the marked negative overjet. The crowding of the superior incisors was confirmed in occlusal view. The position of the incisors had evidently compensated for the skeletal malocclusion (Figure 19).

The lateral teleradiogram and relative cephalometric values confirmed the diagnosis of serious skeletal Class III (Figure 20).

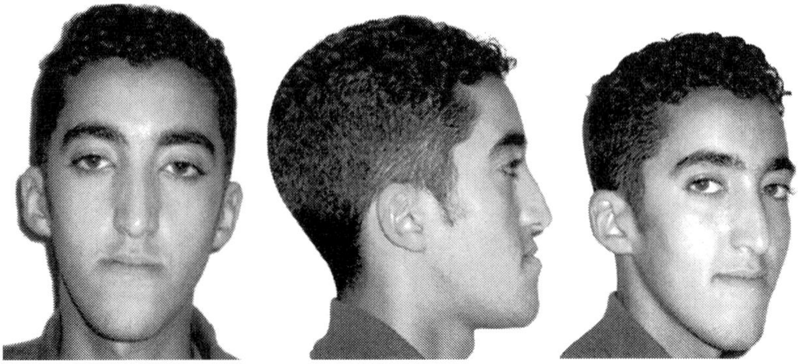

Figure 18. Frontal view, profile and smile of the patient before treatment showing long and narrow face, concave profile, lack of upper lip support, with maxillary anteroposterior deficiency and mandibular anteroposterior excess. Clinically significant deviation of the mandible to the right is present.

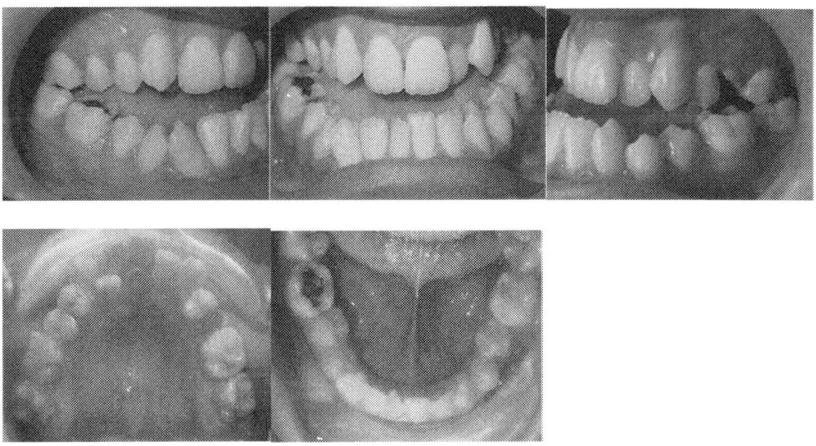

Figure 19. Pretreatment intraoral photographs: frontal, lateral and occlusion The Class III malocclusion is characterized by an anterior and posterior crossbites. Crowding is present in both arches (palate-position of maxillary lateral incisors) due to narrow maxillary dental arch and compensated mandibular incisors

Given the severe skeletal disharmony, the treatment plan suggested was orthognathic surgery to improve both esthetic and functional problems. The surgery was followed by presurgical preparation of dentition. The treatment plan consisted of extraction of the first maxillary premolars to align the anterior arch, eliminate compensations and to establish ideal incisor, and second mandibular premolars position (Figure 21). The outcome of this preparation is evident in the postorthodontic presurgical intraoral and profile photographs and composite cephalometric tracing. The patient felt his profile was getting worse (Figures 22, 23)

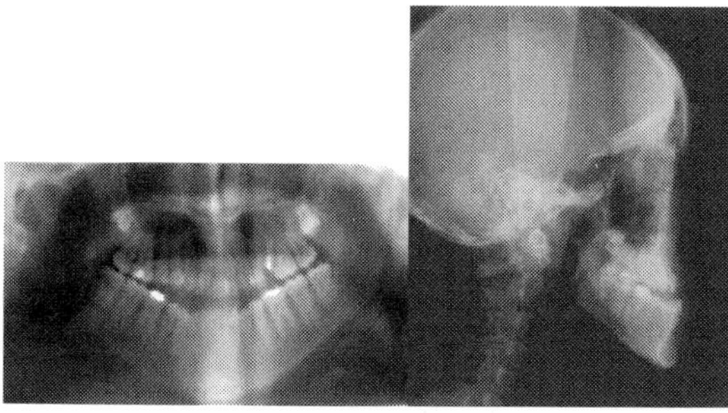

SNA	70°
SNB	77°
ANB	-7°
AO-BO	-18mm
FMA	33°
FMIA	73°
IMPA	74°
Occl. To SN	27°
I to NA	33°/8mm
I to NB	15°/ 2mm

Figure 20. Pretreatment orthopantomogram and lateral teleradiogram of the skull. The orthopantomogram shows and impacted 18 and 28 that must be removed. The maxillomandibular disharmony and incisor compensations were evident. Both teleradiogram and cephalometric values showed lingual inclination of mandibular incisors and protrusion of maxillary incisors.

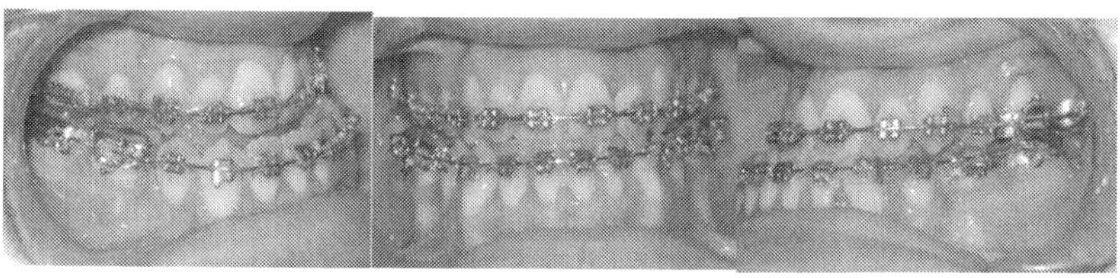

Figure 21. Intraoral views after presurgical orthodontic preparation The objective of presurgical treatment should be to create a harmonious form of the maxillary and mandibular dental arches independently. The use of class III elastics is necessary to increase the labial inclination of the lower incisors and the negative overjet and presurgically decompensate for the malocclusion.

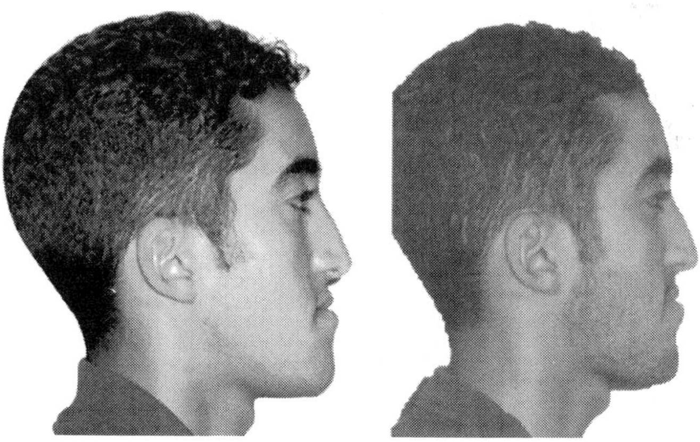

Figure 22. Pretreatment and presurgical profile views: The worsening of the profile was due to dental decompensation, with the incisors positioned on the bony bases as adequately as possible.

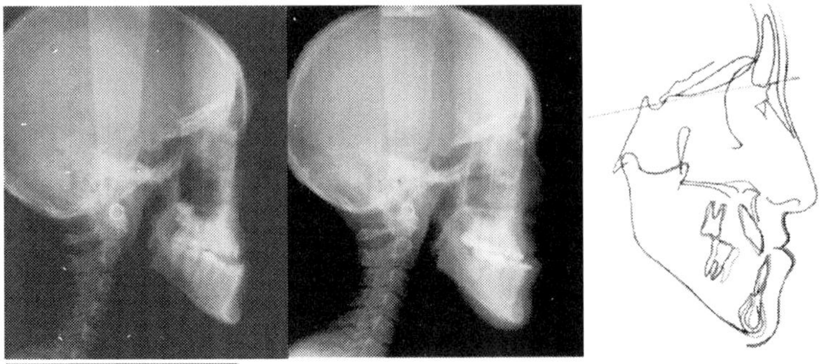

SNA	70°	69°
SNB	77°	78°
ANB	-7°	-9°
AO-BO	-18mm	-20mm
FMA	33°	34°
FMIA	73°	77°
IMPA	74°	69°
Occl. To SN	27°	24°
I to NA	33°/8mm	27°/5mm
I to NB	15°/ 2mm	17°/ 5mm

Figure 23. Pretreatment and presurgical lateral teleradiographies and composite cephalometric tracing of the patient. Note the values illustrating the decompensation of incisors and the increase of Witts.

Surgical visual treatment objectives are shown in Figure 24. Two-jaw surgery was performed in this case. The maxilla was advanced and mandible setback with counterclockwise rotation by means of Lefort I maxillary and sagittal split osteotomies.

The postoperative views show the resolution of the main issues, the establishment of a bilateral molar and canine Class I relationship and correct overjet and overbite. The satisfactory aesthetic result in terms of profile appearance and smile line is evident from the extraoral photographs, which also show correct upper incisor exposure and normalization of the position of the bony bases. The curve in the contour line is more harmonious after surgical advancement of the maxilla and mandibular setback. (Figures 25- 27)

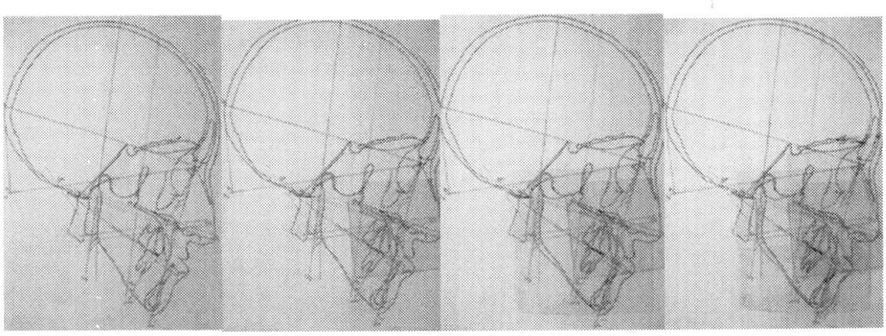

Figure 24. Lefort maxillary osteotomy to superiorly reposition and advance the maxilla to allow the mandible to auto-rotate and close the openbite.

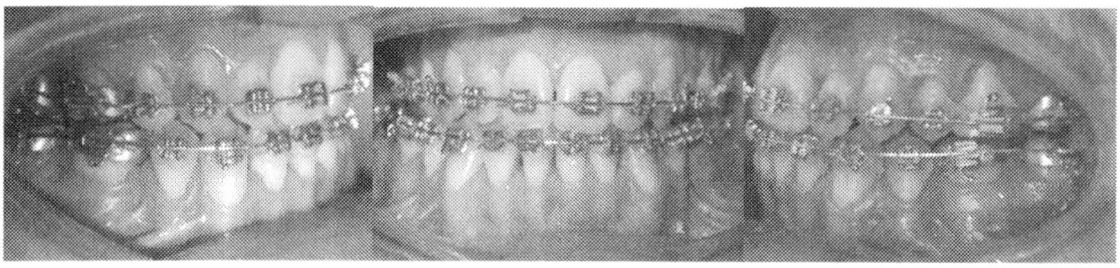

Figure 25. Immediate postoperative intraoral views: the use of surgical arch wires along with controlled elastic therapy and exercise programs after fixation, greatly facilitate treatment.

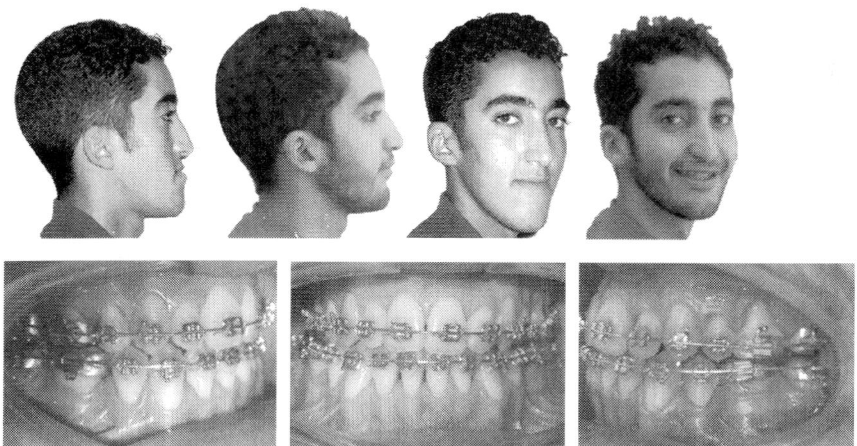

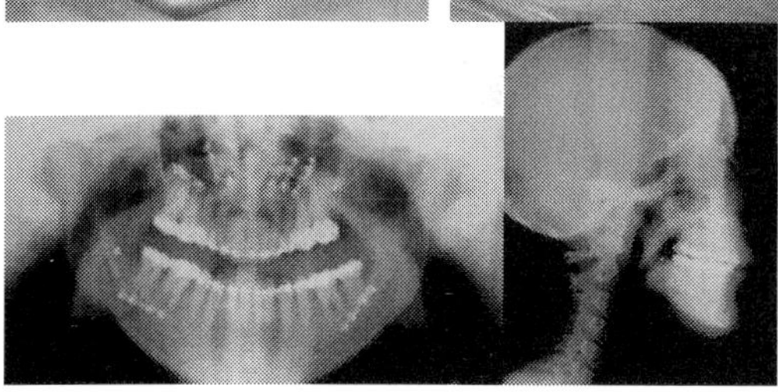

SNA	70°	69°	74°
SNB	77°	78°	73°
ANB	-7°	-9°	1°
AO-BO	-18mm	-20mm	-3mm
FMA	33°	34°	4mm
FMIA	73°	77°	68°
IMPA	74°	69°	80°
Occl. To SN	27°	24°	20°
I to NA	33°/8mm	27°/5mm	23°/4mm
I to NB	15°/ 2mm	17°/ 5mm	20°/ 4mm

Figure 26. Clinical appearance and post surgical orthopantomogram and lateral teleradiogram of skull. Note the immediate postoperative changes and the osteosynthesis of the maxilla and the mandible with titanium miniplates and screws. The Witts and the ANB values illustrate the re-harmonization of the maxillomandibular relationship..

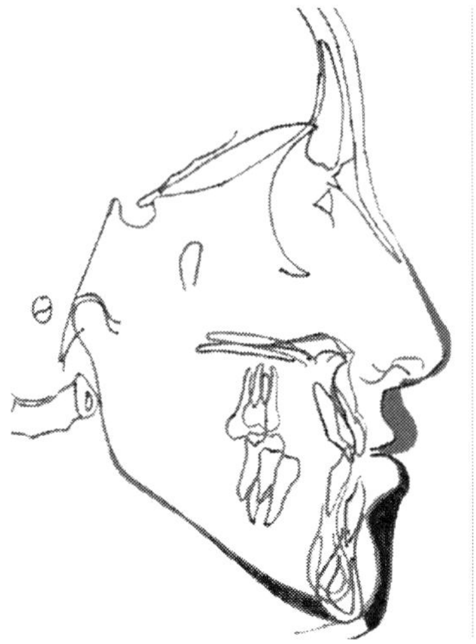

Figure 27. Pretreatment and post-surgery composite cephalometric tracing illustrating the soft tissue, skeletal and dental changes.

The end results of treatment were gratifying (Figure 28).

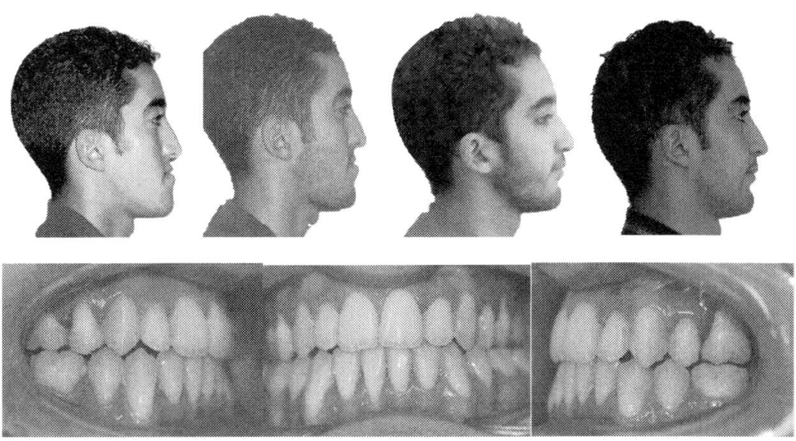

Figure 28. The changing profile during treatment and intraoral views after debonding

5. Conclusion

Stability of results depends on overall treatment plan. Successful treatment depends on a rigorous diagnosis and a treatment, a close collaboration between all the different members involved; all of which deal within predefined objectives using a highly personalized approach. Moderate to severe skeletal deformities often require a combined orthodontic and surgical approach for optimal function and best esthetic results. Indeed, given the development of orthodontic and surgery techniques, this approach becomes a fully-fledged form of treatment which belongs, quite naturally, in the arsenal of treatment we can offer our adult patients. Orthognathic surgery has created new and exciting opportunities in the treatment of patients with dentofacial deformities and has relieved the orthodontist of having only compromised treatment to offer patients with skeletal disharmony.

One needs to be fully convinced that ortho-surgical treatments should be in no way viewed as a game of chance. The main focus of orthodontic treatment should be on obtaining and maintaining long-term clinically satisfactory stability results. Without stability, the achievement of good function and satisfactory aesthetics is obviously not successful.

Author details

Sana Alami[1], Hakima Aghoutan[1], Samir Diouny[2], Farid El Quars[1] and Farid Bourzgui[1*]

*Address all correspondence to: faridbourzgui@gmail.com

1 Department of Dento-facial Orthopedics, Faculty of Dental Medicine, Hassan II Ain Chok University in Casablanca, Morocco

2 Chouaib Doukkali University, Faculty of Letters & Human Sciences, El Jadida, Morocco

References

[1] Reyneke J P. Essentials of orthognathic surgery. China: Quintessence Publishing Co, Inc; 2003

[2] Jos CU, Vassalli IM. Stability after bilateral sagittal split osteotomy setback surgery with rigid internal fixation: a systematic review. J Oral maxillofac Surg. 2008; 66; 1634-43

[3] Jos CU, Vassalli IM, Stability After Bilateral Sagittal Split Osteotomy Advancement Surgery With Rigid Internal Fixation: A Systematic Review. J Oral Maxillofac Surg. 2009; 67; 301-13

[4] Guglielmi M1, Schneider KM, Iannetti G, Feng C, Martinez AY. Orthognathic surgery for correction of patients with mandibular excess: don't forget to assess the gonial angle. J Oral Maxillofac Surg. 2013; 71 (6) 1063-72.

[5] Jacobs JD, Sinclair PM. Principles of orthodontic mechanics in orthognathic surgery cases. American Journal of Orthodontics. 1983, 84 (5) 399-407

[6] Brunel JM, Garcia C. Orthodontic – surgical synergy. International Orthodontics. 2006; 4; 155-97

[7] Noguchi N, Tsuji M, Shigematsu M, Goto V. An orthognathic simulation system integrating teeth, jaw and face data using 3D cephalometry. Int. J. Oral Maxillofac. Surg. 2007; 36: 640–45.

[8] Costa F, Robioni M, Polti M. Stability of sagittal split ramus osteotomy used to correct class III malocclusion : review of literature. Int J Adult Orthod Orthognath Surg 2001;16 (2) 121-29.

[9] Kim CS, Lee SC, Kyung HM, Park HS, Kwon TG. Stability of mandibular setback surgery with and without presurgical orthodontics. J Oral Maxillofac Surg. 2014; 72 (4) 779-87

[10] Sabri R. Objectifs orthodontiques en chirurgie orthognathique. Rev Orthop Dento Faciale 1995;29; 319-35.

[11] Proffit WR, White RP. combined surgical orthodontic treatment: who does, what, when?. Surgical orthodontic treatment: Mosby; 1991.

[12] Nam-Ki Lee, Young-Kyun Kim Jrba. Evaluation of post-surgical relapse after mandibular setback surgery with minimal orthodontic preparation, Journal of Cranio-Maxillo-Facial Surgery. 2013; 41 (1) 47- 51

[13] Ariane Hohoff A, Meier N, Stamm T, Ehmer U, JoosU. Optimizing presurgical orthodontic planning by means of the transverse coordinate simulation system (TCSS). Journal of Cranio-Maxillofacial Surgery. 2002; 30; 75–86.

[14] 56- Proffit WR, Turvey TA, Phillips C. Orthognathic surgery: a hierarchy of stability. International Journal of Adult Orthodontics and Orthognathic Surgery. 1996;11; 191-204.

[15] Béziat JL, Babic B, Ferreira S, Gleizal A. Justification for the mandibular-maxillary order in bimaxillary osteotomy. Rev Stomatol Chir Maxillofac. 2009;110; 323-326.

[16] Kim JY. Postoperative stability for surgery-first approach using intraoral vertical ramus osteotomy: 12 month follow-up. Br J Oral Maxillofac Surg. 2014: 1-6 http://dx.doi.org/10.1016/j.bjoms.2014.03.011

[17] Liou EJW, Wang YC, Huang CS. Surgery-first accelerated orthognathic surgery: postoperative rapid orthodontic tooth movement. J Oral Maxillofac Surg. 2011; 69; 781-85.

[18] Proffit WR, Phillips C, Turvey TA. Stability following superior repositioning of the maxilla by LeFort I osteotomy. American Journal of Orthodontics and Dentofacial Orthopedics. 1987; 92: 151-61.

[19] Bailey LTJ, Cevidanes LHS, Proffit WR: Stability and predictability of orthognathic surgery. Am J Orthod Dentofacial Orthop. 2004; 126: 274-77.

[20] Nihara J, Takeyama M, Takayama Y, Mutoh Y, Saito I. Postoperative changes in mandibular prognathism surgically treated by intraoral vertical ramus osteotomy. Int. J. Oral Maxillofac. Surg. 2013; 42: 62–70.

[21] De Lir ALS, de Moura W L, Ruellas A C O, Souza MMG, Nojima LI. Long-term skeletal and profile stability after surgical-orthodontic treatment of Class II and Class III malocclusion. Journal of Cranio-Maxillo-Facial Surgery. 2013; 41; 296- 302.

[22] Eggensperger N. Skeletal relapse after mandibular advancement and setback in single jaw surgery. J oral maxillofac surg. 2004; 62 pages

[23] Bailey LT, Proffit WR, White RP. Trends in surgical treatment of Class III skeletal rela tionships. International Journal of Adult Orthodontics and Orthognathic Surgery. 1995; 10: 108-18.

[24] Arpornmaeklong P, Heggie AA, Shand JM. A comparison of the stability of single-piece and segmental Le Fort I maxillary advancements. Journal of Craniofacial Surgery. 2003; 14: 3-9.

[25] Proffit WR, Phillips C, Prewitt JW, Turvey TA. Stability after surgical-orthodontic correction of skeletal Class III malocclusion. 2. Maxillary advancement. International Journal of Adult Orthodontics and Orthognathic Surgery. 1991; 6: 71-80

[26] Kim YK, Kim YJ, Yun PY, Kim JW. Evaluation of skeletal and surgical factors related to relapse of mandibular setback surgery using the bioabsorbable plate. Journal of Cranio-Maxillofacial Surgery. 2009; 37: 63-68.

[27] Kraft T, Bouletreau P, Raberin M, Etienne C, Breton P, Freidel M. Severe class III skeletons: long-term stability. Retrospective analysis of 12 cases. Rev Stomatol Chir Maxillofac, 2004 ; 105 (3) 153-59.

[28] Ito G, Koh M, Fujita T, Shirakura M, Ueda H, Tanne K. Factors related to stability following the surgical correction of skeletal open bite. Aust Orthod J. 2014; 30 (1) 61-6.

[29] De Haan IF, Ciesielski R, Nitsche T, Koos B. Evaluation of relapse after orthodontic therapy combined with orthognathic surgery in the treatment of skeletal class III. J Orofac Orthop. 2013; 74: 362-369.

[30] Costa F, Robiony M, Zorzan E, Zerman N, Politi M. Stability of skeletal Class III malocclusion after combined maxillary and mandibular procedures: titanium versus resorbable plates and screws for maxillary fixation. J Oral Maxillofac Surg. 2006; 64 (4) 642-51.

[31] Politi M, Costa F, Cian R, Polini F, Robiony M. Stability of skeletal class III malocclusion after combined maxillary and mandibular procedures: rigid internal fixation

versus wire osteosynthesis of the mandible. J Oral Maxillofac Surg. 2004; 62 (2) 169-81

[32] Proffit WR, Phillips C, Turvey TA. Stability after mandibular setback: mandible-only versus 2-jaw surgery. J Oral Maxillofac Surg. 2012, 70: 408-14.

[33] Proffit WR, Phillips C, Dann Ct, Turvey TA. Stability after surgical-orthodontic correction of skeletal Class III malocclusion. I. Mandibular setback. International Journal of Adult Orthodontics and Orthognathic Surgery. 1991; 6 :7-18.

[34] Suri L, Taneja P. Surgically assisted rapid palatal expansion: A literature review. Am J Orthod Dentofacial Orthop. 2008; 133: 290-302.

[35] Bouletreau P, Paulus C. Surgical correction of transverse skeletal abnormalities in the maxilla and mandible. International Orthodontics. 2012 ; 10 : 261-73.

[36] Talebzadeh N., Pogrel MA. Long-term hard and soft tissue relapse rate after genioplasty. Oral Surg Oral Med Oral Pathol Oral Radiol Endod. 2001; 91(2) 153-6.

[37] Solano-Hernández B, Stylianos Antonarakis G, Scolozzi P, Kiliaridis S. Skeletal Anterior Open-Bite Malocclusion: A Systematic Review on Vertical Stability. J Oral Maxillofac Surg. 2013; 71: 98-109.

[38] Ming-Yih L, Chun-Li L, Wen-Da T, Lun-Jou L. Biomechanical stability analysis of rigid intraoral fixation for bilateral sagittal split osteotomy. Journal of Plastic Reconstructive & Aesthetic Surgery. 2010; 63: 451-55

[39] Nieblerova J, Folta R, Hanzelka T, Pavlìkovà G, Vik M, Klìma K, SamsonyanL. Stability of the miniplate osteosynthesis used for sagittal split osteotomy for closing an anterior open bite: an experimental study in mini-pigs. Int. J. Oral Maxillofac. Surg. 2012; 41; 482–88.

[40] Yang L, Xu M, Jin X, Xu J, Lu J, Zhang C, Li S, Teng L. Skeletal stability of bioresorbable fixation in orthognathic surgery: A systemic review. Journal of Cranio-Maxillo-Facial Surgery. 2013, 1- 6

[41] Fourquet L, Göttle M, Bounoure G. Finishing and detailing, stability and harmony. Orthod Fr. 2014 ; 85 (1) 93-125.

Chapter 10

Advanced Adjunct Orthosurgical Esthetic Prodedures

Seied Omid Keyhan, Seifollah Hemmat,
Peyman Mehriar, Arash Khojasteh and
Mohammad Ali Asayesh

Additional information is available at the end of the chapter

http://dx.doi.org/10.5772/59088

1. Introduction

Changes in the esthetic appearance of the face is highly depended on the bony structures of the facial skeleton, including the malar-midface region, nose, and chin. Alterations of soft tissue and skin alone will not satisfy all of our aesthetic demands. Multiple factors such as skin (texture, color, thickness and...), soft tissue (symmetry, composition, location and...) and facial bony contours (size, shape, location, symmetry and...) contributes to creating esthetically appealing appearance of the face.

Since many years ago numerous surgical and office based techniques have been introduce to augment, reduce or refine the most projected points of the face such as cheek, chin, nose, Para-nasal area, angle of the jaw..According to the literature the techniques can be classified to: 1) Office based or non-invasive techniques; such as fillers injection, facial lipostructure or facial liposuction which modified the soft tissue coverage of the facial skeleton.2) Facial prosthesis. 3) Maxillofacial osteotomies. Based on our knowledge the first and second group have been considered more in the literatures and text book of the Oral and Maxillofacial Surgery (OMFS) or Plastic Surgery, it is perhaps related to the more complications of the osteotomy techniques or easiness of the office –based one. OMFS are familiar with orthognatic surgeries and their skill in this field can help them to plan the third one,especially in cases whom the long term results should be considered. In current chapter we reviewed the esthetic osteotomy techniques of the facial skeleton and introduce a surgical techniques for management of the most projected points of the face namely:

- **Chin modification**

Reduction genioplasty

- **Paranasal modification**

Piriform augmentation osteotomies

- **Mandibular Angle modification**

Angle augmentation osteotomies

Angle reduction oeteotomies

- **Malar modification**

Malar augmentation osteotomies

Malar reduction osteotomies

- **Forehead modification**

Frontal Bossing reduction techniques

2. Chin modification

The creation or restoration of an esthetically pleasing facial contour can encompass many surgical approaches. Several surgical techniques are available for correcting and giving harmony to the lower third of the face.[1] In this respect, some well-known techniques seek to correct the shape and size of the chin using different kinds of chin implants or osteotomies in an effort to move it and change its spatial location, thus determining a new facial contour.

2.1. Augmentation genioplasty

Genioplasty (anterior horizontal mandibular osteotomy) means a plastic procedure on the chin that involves both bony components (ie, anterior portion of the base of the mandible) and the soft tissue component.The procedure can be performed either alone or as an adjunct to other orthognathic and facial plastic surgeries. Either direct osteoplasty and soft tissue correction or implantation of an alloplastic material/cartilage/bone has been recommended for genioplasty. Since 1942, with first sliding advancement genioplasty that was described by Hofer, various genioplasty techniques with various indications, advantages, and disadvantages have been developed for correction of microgenia and macrogenia. In recent chapter we did not focused on augmentation genioplasty techniques.The readers can update their knowledge by reviewing the other chapters or books.

2.2. Reduction genioplasty

In the event of anterior mandibular bony excess different surgical approaches can be used. Each have their own limitations and disadvantages. For instance simple burring down removal of bony excess from anterior mandible through an intraoperative approach will usually result in an abnormal appearance and is not the best choice of treatment.

Reduction genioplasty surgical procedure results in narrowing or shortening of the chin. However, the literature lacks data about the best technique, indications, complications, and long-term results. The soft tissue envelope of the chin area usually follows the genial osseous movement approximately 90% or more, but the predictability ratio of horizontal reduction genioplasty is limited; it follows approximately 50% to 60%.[1]

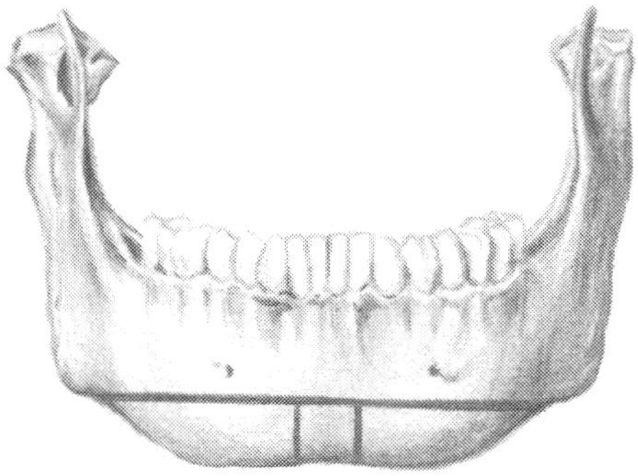

Figure 1. reduction genioplasty technique described by Ukan and park.

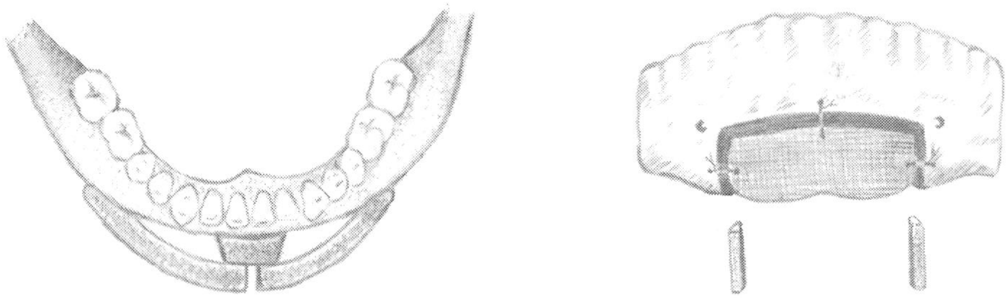

Figure 2. Horizontal T genioplasty and modified reduction genioplasty techniques.

To date, only 2 articles have been published about the narrowing of the chin by use of this technique.Minor step-off at the chin-mandible junction and mild transient numbness of the lower lip, jowls, and bunching of the chin were reported as the most common complications of this technique. Because the lingual muscle is released, there is a risk of avascular necrosis of the distal segments, and the chin prominence should be minimally degloved to prevent this complication. Furthermore, because the mid-symphysis area is removed, the chance of asymmetry or unesthetic results could be increased(fig.1).[1] another techniques such as horizontal T osteotomy were also described but is not used widely(fig.2).[10, 46]In 2013 we described[1, 47] a novel technique to reduce the prominent chin 3-dimentionally(fig.3).This new genioplasty (Zigzag genioplasty) makes it possible to decrease the vertical and transverse dimension of the chin alone or simultaneously, symmetrically or asymmetrically. This genioplasty alsomakesit possible to decrease the mental sagittal projection,if indicated, and simultaneously reduce the mandibular body height. Zigzag genioplasty allows one to properly correct excess of the chin(3-dimensionally), avoiding the need for muscular repositioning (except sometimes in types III and IV)(fig.4).A simple geometric calculation allows one to mobilize the chin in a vertical, horizontal, and sagittal direction,according to the needs of each patient. Furthermore, this design preserves the suprahyoid muscle attachmentsand the most important anatomic portion of symphysis area; narrowing the wide chin by this technique provides an esthetic and natural facial look.[1, 47]

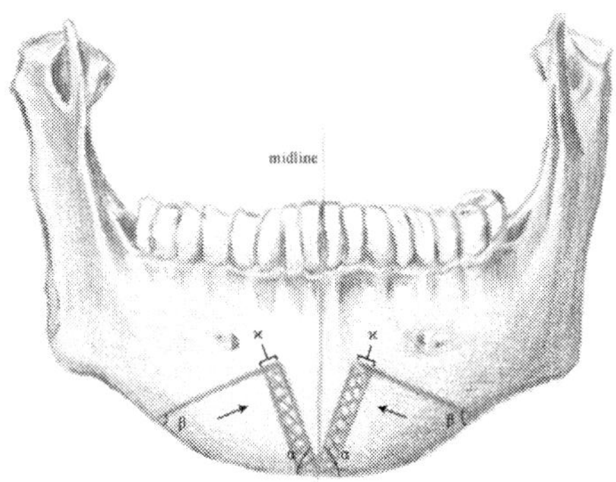

Figure 3. Zigzag osteotomy design is based on the displacement of 2 bone fragments on the slopes of an inclined plane with a superior-medial direction. The degree of inclination for these slopes (the α and β- angles) will be estimated pre-surgically according to ; the extent of the vertical and transverse displacement wanted for a given case, mandibular symphysis height and width, the size of remained bone fragments after ostectomy, the need for conventional or extended (to the mandibular body) reduction, the position of anterior mandibular teeth apices, the position of mental foramina and symmetrical or asymmetrical reduction.The posterior edges of the osteotomy, either could be finished just beneath the mental foramina (obtuse degree of inclination) or extended to the Anti-Gonial notch(acute degree of inclination),especially in such cases that, simultaneous reduction of inferior mandibular body osteotomy must be done, also. The amount of β-angle must be equal bilaterally except in asymmetrical cases.The anterior edge of the osteotomy which is extended medially from canine root apices (with a distance of 5 mm) to the mid-symphysis area, either could be extended above the inferior border(especially; in such cases which simultaneous advancement or set back should be done) or beyond it.As the same manner to posterior edge, the degree of inclination in the anterior part (the α-angle) could be determined pre-surgically,and must be equal in both sides except in asymmetrical cases.[from Keyhan et al. Zigzag genioplasty: a new technique for 3-dimensional reduction genioplasty. *Br J Oral Maxillofac Surg*.2013]

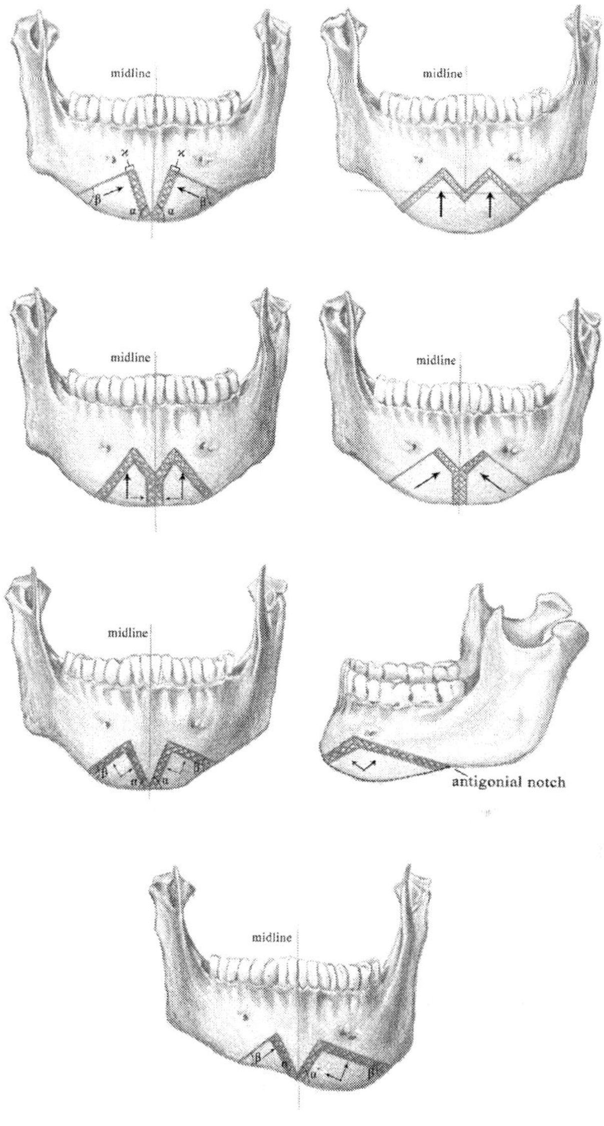

Figure 4. Schematic views of osteotomy design modifications of zigzag genioplasty technique (type I-VII). The anterior edge of the osteotomy could either be extended above the inferior border or beyond it. The posterior edges of the osteotomy, could either be finished just beneath the mental foramina or extended up to the Anti-Gonial notch. For pure chin narrowing with minimal reduction in vertical dimension, bone removal just near the strut of bone in the middle should be done, and if vertical reduction is planned as well, bone strips should be removed above both posterior and anterior slobs. [from keyhan et.al. Zigzag genioplasty; patients evaluation, technique modifications and review of the literature. Br J oral amxillofac surg.2013] Figure reprinted with permission from The Br J oral amxillofac surg.

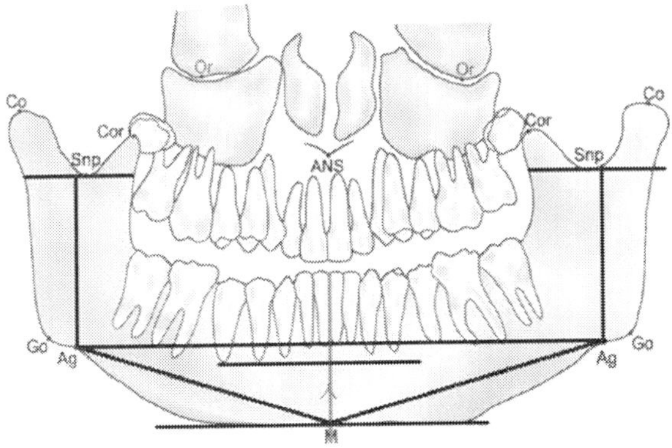

Figure 5. A simple geometric calculation allows one to mobilize the chin in a vertical, horizontal andsagittal direction, according to the needs of each patient the design of the planed osteotomy can be trace on the tracing paper and a surgical guide can be made simply.

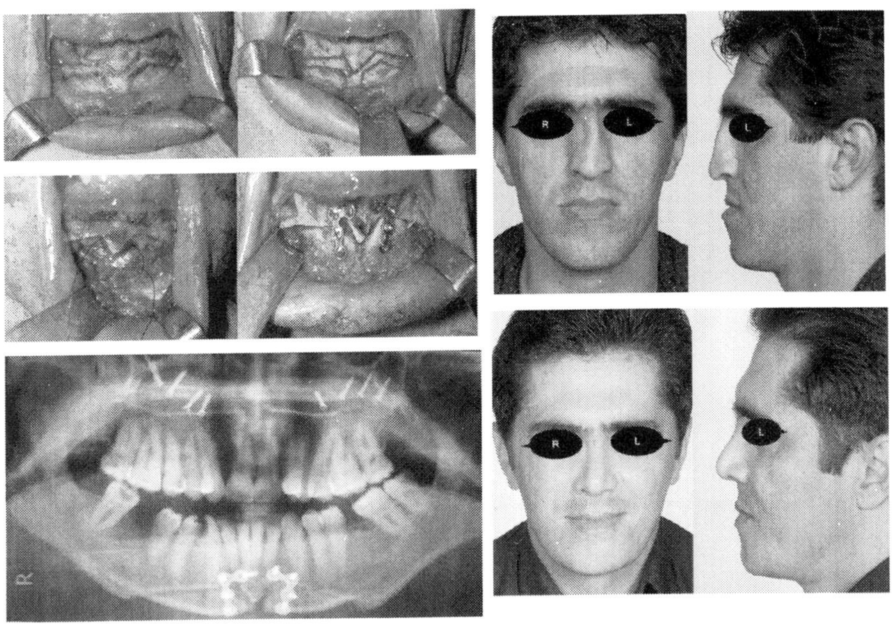

Figure 6. A 29 years old man who underwent zigzag genioplasty(type III) in combination with rhinoplasty,buccal fat pad lifting[48],malar prosthesis and paranasal augmentation.a,b,c,d) Incision of the oral mucosa was performed 5 to 7 mm labial to the depth of the vestibule and directed horizontally. Then, the muco-periosteal flap was released, and the mental nerve was exposed. The chin prominence was degloved, and the lingual muscle attachments were maintained for blood supply. The osteotomy sites (type III) were marked with a surgical marker and the ostectomy was done with reciprocal saw and fissure bur In the next step, bone strips were removed bilaterally and the osteotomy was continued

bilaterally, after down-fracturing, the interferences were removed,with high accuracy in maintain lingual pedicle tissues, detached supra-hyoids muscles was secured to the bone strut and medial and superior displacement was performed with the traction of two 10 centimeter wires.e) 2 L-shape miniplates were used for fixation.Any bone irregularity could be removed with round bur although, most often they could be remodeled post operatively. Vestibular incision was closed with 3-0 vicryl sutures.f,g)pre-operative views.h,i)post-operative views, simultaneous rhinoplasty and malar and para-nasal augmentation were performed also. [from keyhan et.al. Zigzag genioplasty ;patients evaluation,technique modifications and review of the literature. Am J Cosmetic surg,2013].**Figure reprinted with permission from The American Journal of Cosmetic Surgery**.

3. Paranasal modification

Clinical evaluation: There is no specific soft tissue or skeletal cephalometric landmark(s) or values to quantify the "fullness" of this region, so deficiency assessment of para-alar region is mainly based on qualitative profile judgment.[64]

Surgical technique: After general anesthésia and flap incision and elevation the osteotomy is done 2cm above the nasal floor from one side to another side To allow adequate mobilization the junction between septum and bony segment should be cut this can be done by a osteotomy.

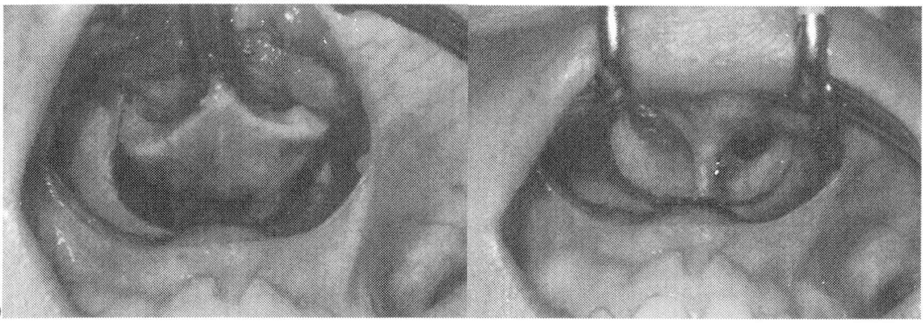

Figure 7. U- shaped osteotomy of piriform aperture. [from Herna´ndez-Alfaro F, Garcıa E, Martı C, Porta A. U-shaped osteotomy in management of paranasal deficiency. Int. J. Oral Maxillofac. Surg. 2006]

4. Angle modification

Caucasians consider a prominent mandibular angle to be unappealing in their populations, and mandibular angle ostectomy has been popular since Baek et al. introduced it in 1989.[66] Standard procedure to correct prominent mandibular angles is mandibular angle ostectomy with anoscillating saw through the intraoral approach, although a number of modifications and improvements in operative techniques have been reported in the last two decades.[68, 69]Kim et al.[70] classified all the patients with prominent mandibular angle according to mandibular angle shape into four classes (I, II, III, and IV).[70]

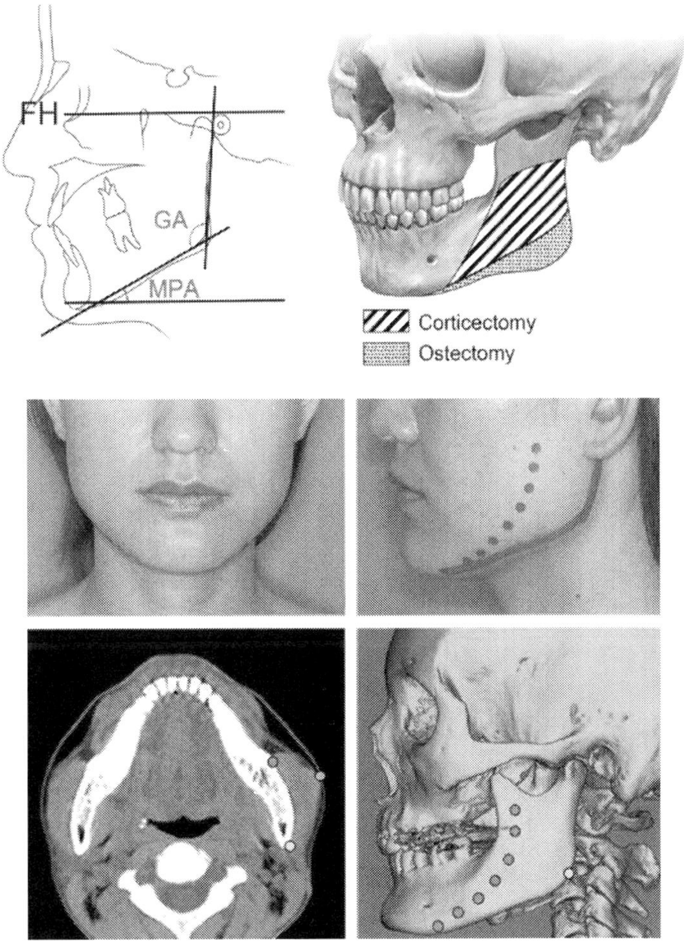

Figure 8. Preoperative evaluation and planning for mandibular angle reshaping. [from Hirohi et al. Lower face reduction with full-thickness marginalostectomy of mandibular corpus-angle followed by corticectomy. J Plast Reconstr Aesth Surg. 2010.]

Clinical evaluation: For patients analysis it is important to consider the plans for correcting the lateral and frontal appearances of the lower face separately, because the ideal correction require two surgical techniques.

Surgical technique: Firstly, the ostectomy of the marginal part of the mandibular corpus-angle was performed, then corticectomy after evaluating the thickness of the resected bone fragment Mandibular corticectomy was performed to improve the frontal appearance.[66] After designing the ostectomy line with a pencil, a groove was hollowed out on the lateral cortex using a round burr. [66]

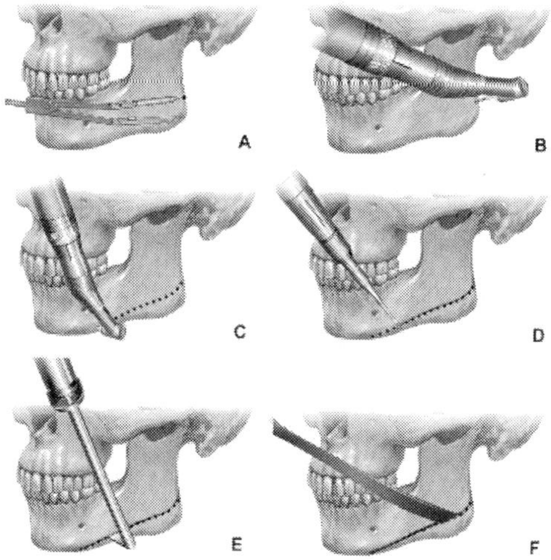

Figure 9. Operative procedures for en-bloc mandibular corpus-angle ostectomy (MCAO) with a contra-angle handpiece. [from Hirohi et al. Lower face reduction with full-thickness marginalostectomy of mandibular corpus-angle followed by corticectomy. J Plast Reconstr Aesth Surg. 2010.]

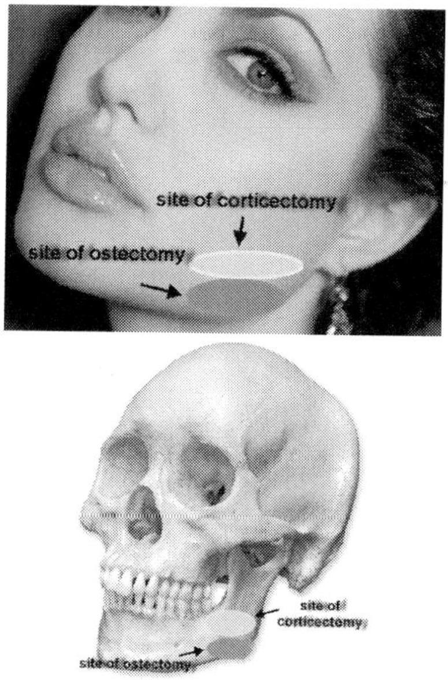

Figure 10. schematic view of sites of corticectomy and ostectomy.

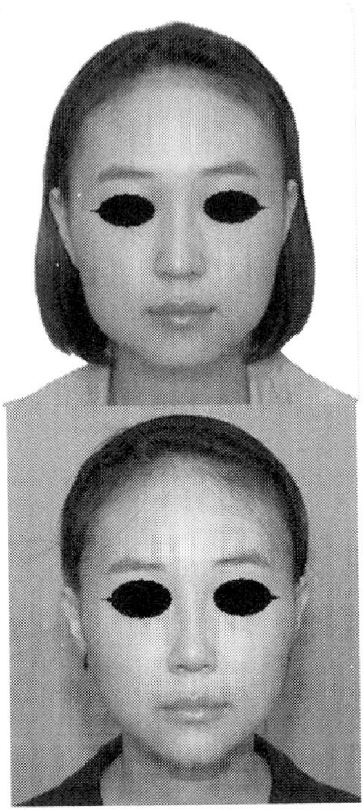

Figure 11. A 28 year-old woman with a muscular and square face desired mandibular reshaping and underwent mandibular corpus-angle ostectomy and corticectomy. The postoperative frontal view shows that the width of his lower face was greatly reduced by ostectomy and corticectomy.

4.1. Reduction malarplasty

Reduction body malarplasty (RBM) can be done for patients with a hyperplastic anterior mid-face. Reduction body and arch malarplasty (RBAM) is suited for patient with a hyperplastic anterior and posterior midface which will soften their square and wide facial appearance.[90, 94, 95]

Surgical techniques: since many years ago numerous surgical technique have been introduce to reduce the prominent malar.which some of these techniques are discussed here.

Zygoma shaving procedure: After intra oral flap elevation the entire zygomatic body and arch is exposed and subperiosteal dissection is carried out. [89] The most prominent portion of the zygoma, including part of the zygomatic arch, is shaved using a broad chisel or a bone bur. [89]

I-shaped osteotomy: Using a reciprocating saw, 2 parallel cuts are made on the zygomatic body from inner cortex toward the outer cortex resembling an I shape. [89] Then, the zygoma and the zygomatic arch complex are displaced antero-medially.

http://dx.doi.org/10.5772/59088

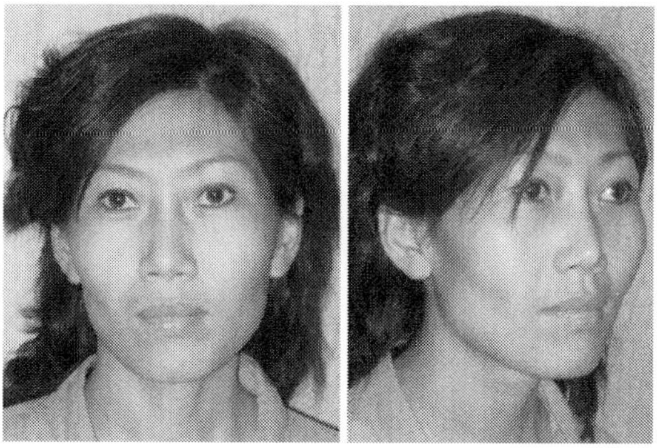

Figure 12. A 38 year-old oriental woman with severe malar prominence. wide faces due to a prominent zygoma are considered unsightly. frontal (left) and oblique (right) views.[from Zou C, et al. midface contour change after reduction malarplasty with modified L-shaped osteotomy: a surgical outcomes study. Aesthetic plast surg.2014]

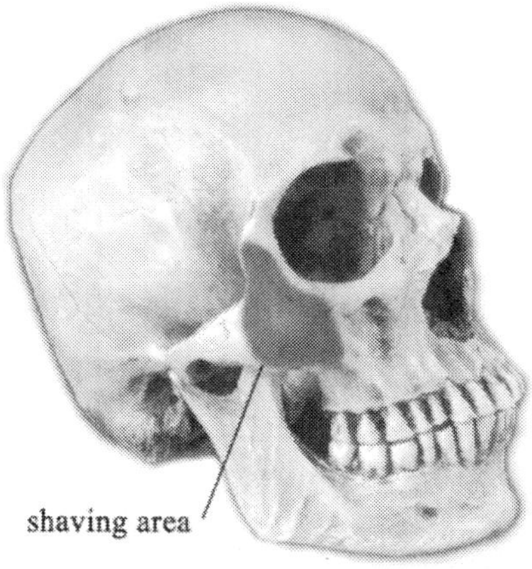

Figure 13. Illustration of zygomatic shaving procedure. Note the shaving area involved the zygoma and the anterior part of zygomatic arch.

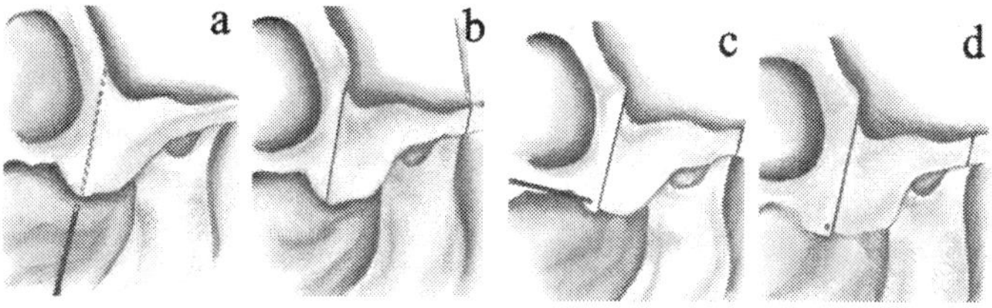

Figure 14. Illustration of I-shaped osteotomy.

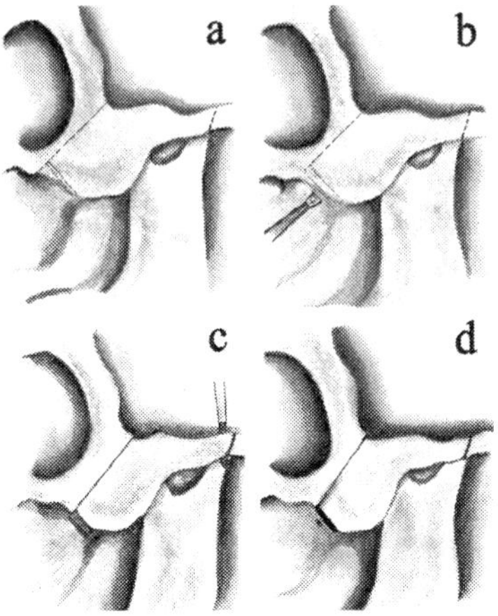

Figure 15. Illustrationof L-shaped osteotomy.

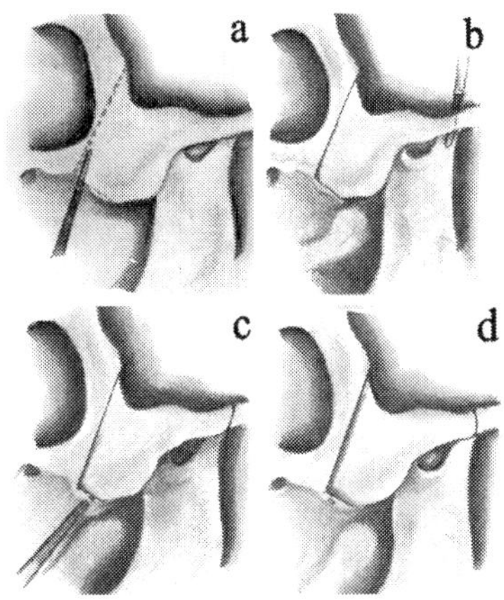

Figure 16. Illustration of C-shaped osteotomy.

L-shaped osteotomy: This technique is similar to I-shaped osteotomy which can be considered in special cases.

C-shaped osteotomy The main difference of this technique with L-shaped osteotomy is in the oblique part of the osteotomy line; the oblique line is moved more toward the external orbital rims in comparison with the L-shaped osteotomy and consists of 2 parallel lines unlike L-shaped osteotomy in which we have only 1 line of osteotomy. [89]

Modified L-shaped Osteotomy: The modified L-shaped osteotomy differed from the original method mainly in that the two parallel osteotomy lines are made vertically so that the zygomatic body and arch can be shifted (Fig. 17).

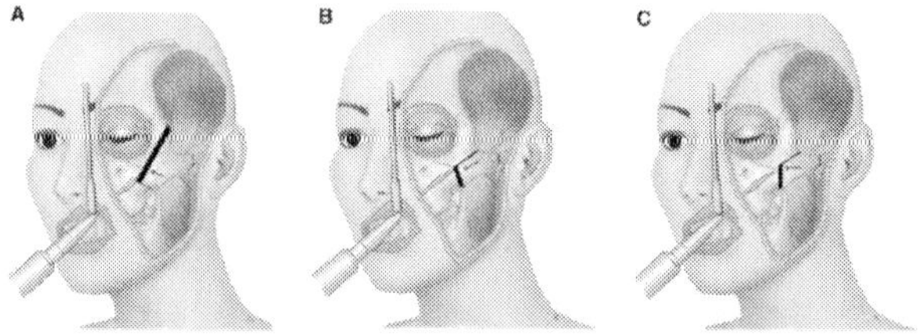

Figure 17. A. Kim's L-shaped osteotomy. **B.** The original L-shaped osteotomy. **C.** The modified L-shaped osteotomy. [fromNakanishi Y, et al. The boomerang osteotomy - A new method of reduction malarplasty. 2012]

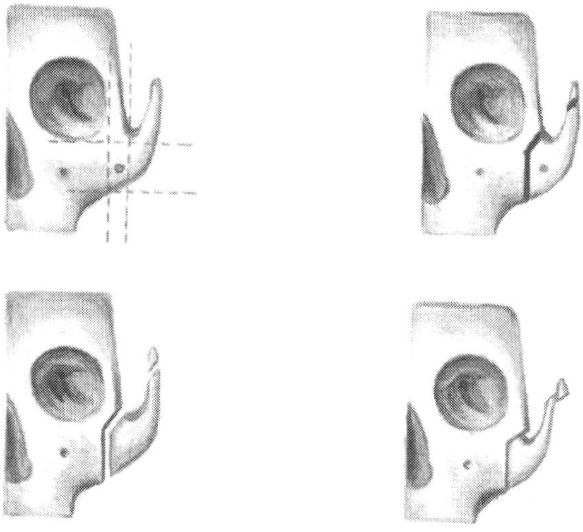

Figure 18. (Left Above) Location of the most prominent part of the zygoma body (red point) (Right Above) Incision of the Boomerang Osteotomy (Left Below) Mobilization of the bone (Right Below) The complex of the zygoma body and zygomatic arch is shifted medially.

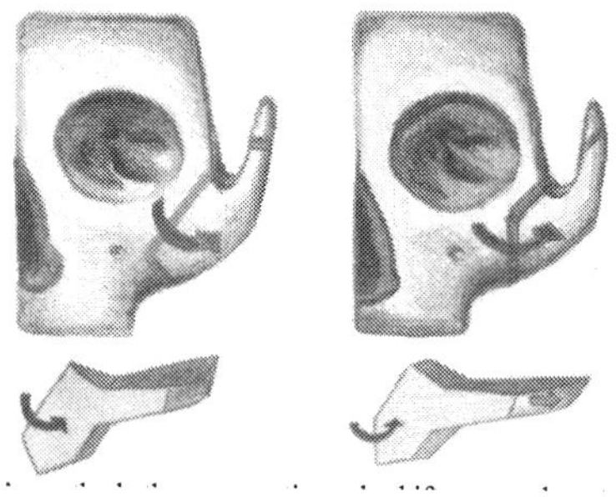

Figure 19. With Kim's method, the zygomatic arch shifts upward as the rotation for subtle adjustment. The vertical height of the zygomatic arch presents no change with boomerang method.

Horizontal v-shaped osteotomy : this technique is similar to L-shaped osteotomy.

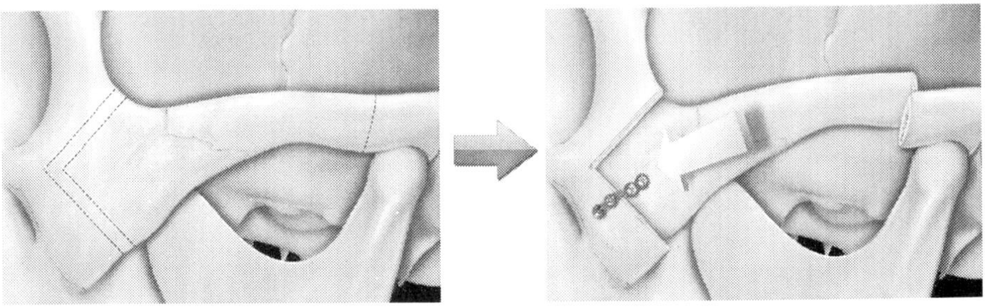

Figure 20. Horizontal V-shaped osteotomy used to correct protrusion of the zygoma and zygomatic arch. Not that the free part of the root of the zygomatic arch was locked into the gap between the rigid part and the temporal bone as a mortice and tenon structure.[fromTang K, et al. New horizontal v-shaped osteotomy for correction of protrusion of the zygoma and the zygomatic arch in East Asiansindication and results. Br J Oral Maxillofac Surg. 2014]

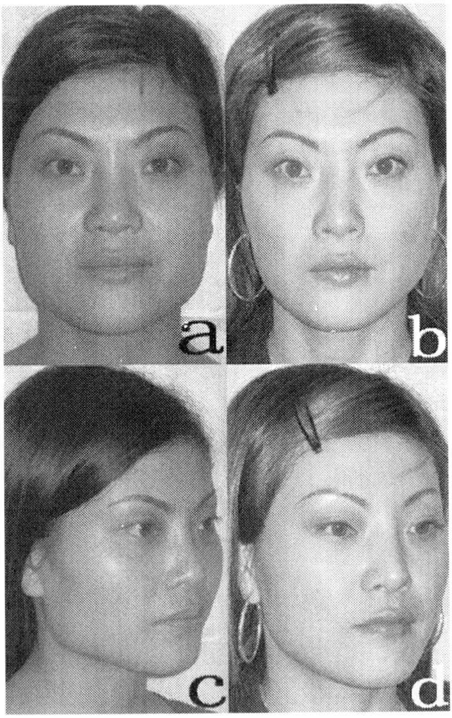

Figure 21. Preoperative views of the same patient **(a, c)**. Postoperative views after an L-shaped malar osteotomy and repositioning and mandibular reduction **(b, d)**.[fromChen T, et al. correction of zygoma and zygomatic arch protrusion in east Asian individuals. Oral Surg Oral Med Oral Pathol Oral Radiol Endod.2011].

4.2. Aumentation malarplasty

Clinical evaluation: Oval shaped face with the key component of malar prominence is considered to be a sign of beauty and youth in Caucasians. [73] Many tricks using artificial highlighting and darkening are developed by makeup artists to accentuate the malar prominence. [73] Flattened cheeks and narrow face makes people look sad and prematurely aged. [73] This transverse midface deficiency can be addressed by widening the bimalar width.[73]

Hinderer[100]	From the frontal view, draw a line from the lateral commissure of the lip to the lateral canthus of the ipsilateral eye and another line from the tragus to the inferior edge of the nasal ala. The area posterior and superior to the junction of these two projections should be the most prominent area of the malar eminence. (Fig. 12a) [100]
Powell et al[77]	Draw a vertical line through the middle of the face, then bisect the segment between the nasion and the nasal tip with a line that curves gently upward to the tragus on both sides. Draw a line from the inferior ala to the lateral canthus and another one, parallel to this one, from the lateral oral commissure toward the ear. The intersection of the curvilinear horizontal line and the line from the oral commissure marks the point where the malar area should be most prominent. (Fig. 12b) [77]
Silver and Guilden[101]	If the malar prominence in the true lateral projection is >5 mm posterior to the nasolabial groove, then a deficiency in the malar area exists. Silver describes the malar prominence triangle. [101] To create this triangle, draw a Frankfort horizontal line across the face in frontal projection and a parallel line that bisects the upper lip. Then draw a perpendicular line through both of these lines and through the lateral canthus. The intersection of the vertical line and the line through the upper lip defines point A.[101] Create a line from point A though the medial canthus and then a second line from point A toward the temporal area-but at the same angle from the vertical that was created by the projection from point A through the medial canthus. This creates the malar prominence triangle with the base being the Frankfort horizontal and the apex being point A. Silver advises that the implant should be placed several millimeters below the Frankfort line. (Fig. 12c)[101]
Wilkinson[102]	The ideal high points as he has suggested is at or just lateral to the outer canthus of the eye on a point a distant of approximately one-third from the lateral canthus to the inferior border of the mandible. (Fig.12d)[102]
Schoenrock[103]	On an oblique view (27 to 35 degrees of rotation from the frontal view) in natural head position,A line from themost lateral point of the malar complex intersected at 90° the commissure-canthus line at 66% of its lengthand The length of thisline was 17% the length of the commissure-canthus line. (Fig. 13)[103]

Table 1. Analyses of malar projection

Malar recontouring involves not only the zygomatic region, but also the infraorbital,paranasal, and buccal regions. Furthermore, imperfections of other facial areas may reflect negatively on the malar region. The buccal region should be slightly concave or flat in adults,within the

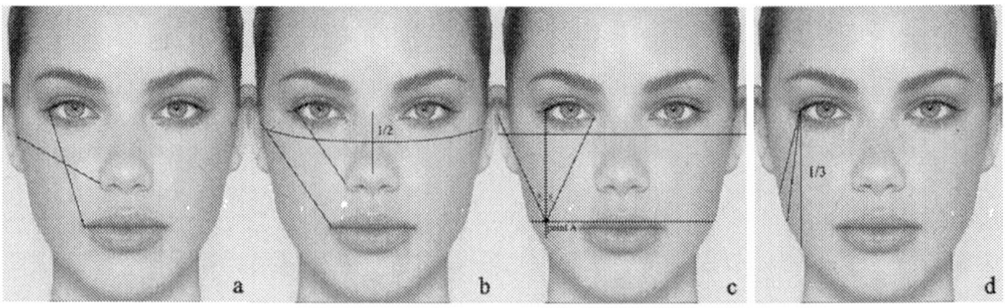

Figure 22. Analyses of malar projection. a, hinderer analysis. b, pwell et al analysis. c, Silver and Guilden. d, Wilkinson analysis.

confines of a tangent from the cheekbone to the mandibular angle. Fullness in the buccal region can give the illusion of a poorly developed malar eminence. In these patients, partial excision of the buccal fat pad may be indicated.[104] Shadowing in the concavity of the buccal area highlights the malar eminence, giving it a sculptured, well-defined look. Caucasian women tend to accentuate this effect by using makeup, whereas Asians prefer much softer contours. But excessive buccal hollowness results in an emaciated, gaunt appearance with exaggerated malar definition. Excessive width and prominence of the mandibular angle and masseter muscles make the malar eminence look small and give the face a square or triangular shape. Reduction of the mandibular angle and masseter muscles might be more adequate than malar augmentation. The malar eminence is also examined relative to the periorbital region. A high and prominent mala eminence enhances the appearance of the beautiful eye. Fullness of the area 10 mm lateral and 15–20 mm inferior to the lateral canthus should be obvious. (Fig. 21)[105]

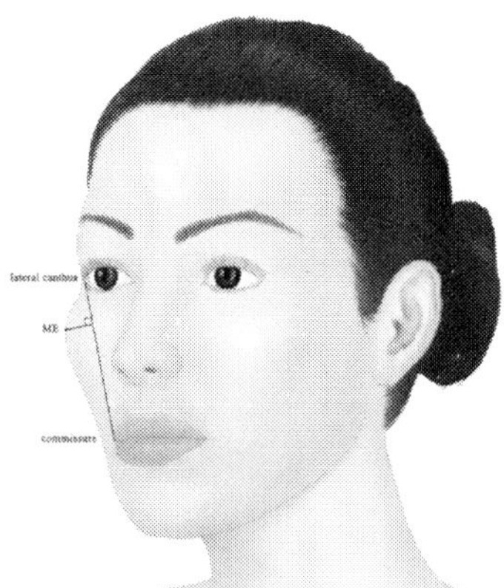

Figure 23. Schoenrock analysis of malar projection in oblique view. (ME): malar eminence.

Surgical thechniques:

Zygomatic arch osteotomy: A subperiosteal flap is raised to expose the ascending malar buttress and the zygomaticomaxillary suture. The position of an oblique sagittal cut is selected

http://dx.doi.org/10.5772/59088

by deciding whether augmentation should include any of the anterior buttress or whether it should be totally lateral to zygomaticomaxillary suture line. The cut is then made with a sagittal reciprocating saw starting from the inferior portion of the zygomaticomaxilary suture to the notch of both lateral orbital rim and malar zygomatic process. A previously selected graft may now be placed between the two segments. The result is an increase in interarch width (zygion-zygion).(Fig 22)

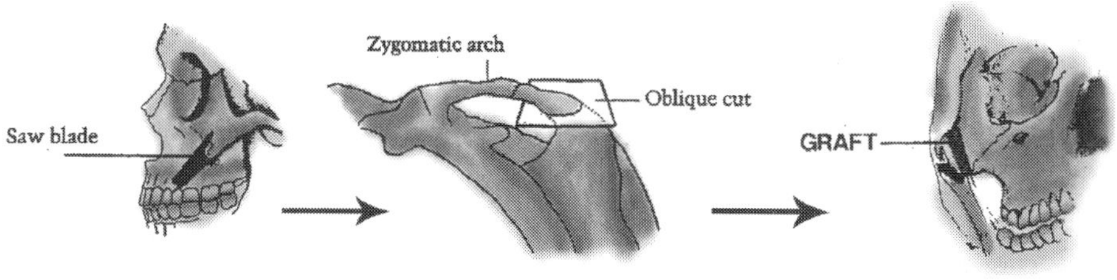

Figure 24. Surgical steps of zygomaticarch osteotomy.

Zygomatic sandwich osteotomy (ZSO): To solve some problems, modifications of zygomatic arch osteotomy technique have been presented. Mommaerts et al [81]modified Powell's technique by connecting a vertical with a semihorizontal osteotomy which both transect the maxillary sinus, thereby maximizing anterior as well as lateral augmentation.

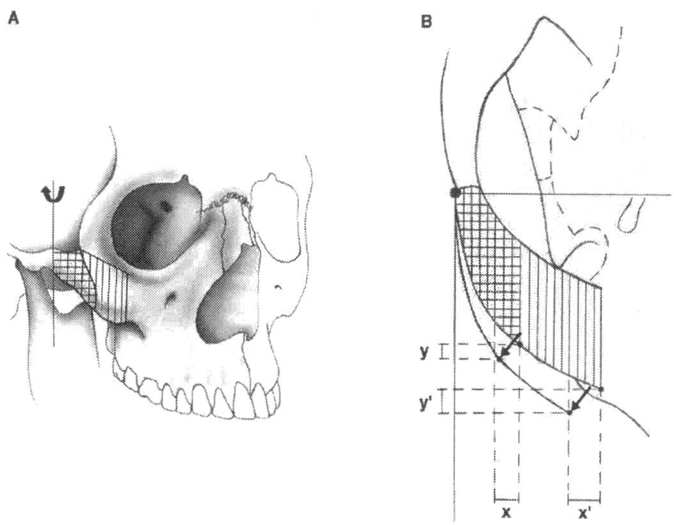

Figure 25. Comparison of zygomatic arch osteotomy (Powell et al) and zygomatic sandwich osteotomy (Mommaerts et al).(A) difference in design (zygomatic arch osteotomy [ZAO] = horizontal lines; zygomatic sandwich osteotomy [ZSO] = verticallines). (B) amount of augmentation, caudal view (x = lateral displacement with ZAO; x′ = lateral displacement with ZSO; y =anterior displacement with ZAO; y′ = anterior displacement with ZSO).

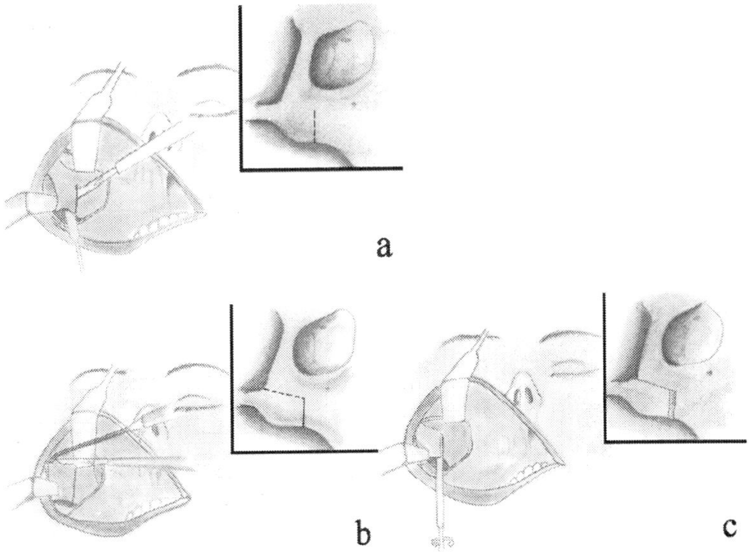

Figure 26. a. vertical osteotomy, **b.** semihorizontal osteotomy,**c.** Opening of the vertical osteotomy and insertion of spacer material.

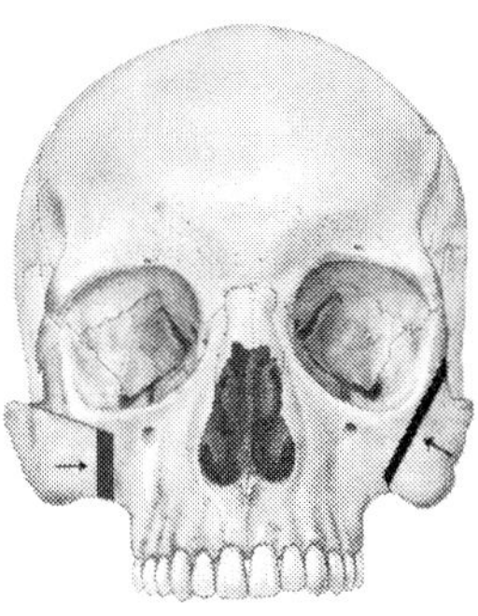

Figure 27. Malar augmentation, differences in osteotomy design: Mommaerts et al (left) compared with Kim and Seul (right).

Zygomatic Sagittal Split Osteotomy (ZSSO):in this technique the zygomatic arch is isolated from its temporal origin to its zygomatic insertion both on its lateral and medial surfaces Using a waver sewer, a sagittal full thickness osteotomy of the zygomatic arch is performed (Fig. 26).Later, 2 separate partial thickness osteotomies: one on the arch's osteotomies are connected with the previously released sagittal osteotomy. After correction of the zygomatic arch according to presurgical programs. Stabilization is achieved using bicortical titanium screws (Fig. 26).

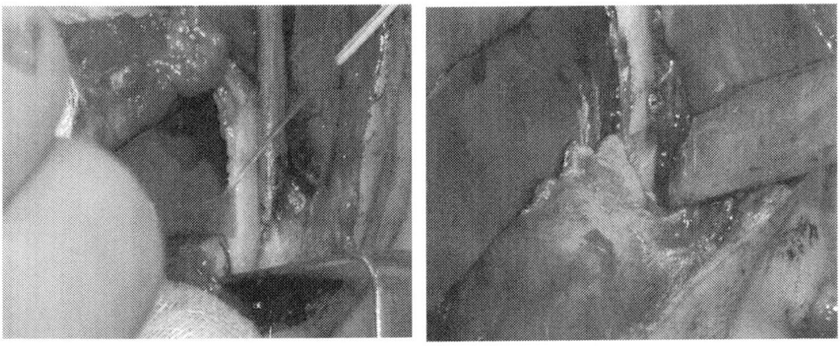

Figure 28. Two vertical partial-thickness osteotomy are performed: one on the posterolateral surface of the zygomatic arch and the other on its anteromedial surface. **left)** Sagittal full-thickness osteotomy of the zygomaticarch, performed with a waver sewer.**right)** Stabilization of the osteotomy with bicortical titanium screws.[fromGasparini G et al. Zygomatic Sagittal Split Osteotomy: A Novel and Simple Surgical Technique for Use in Midface Corrections. J Craniofac Surg.2010]

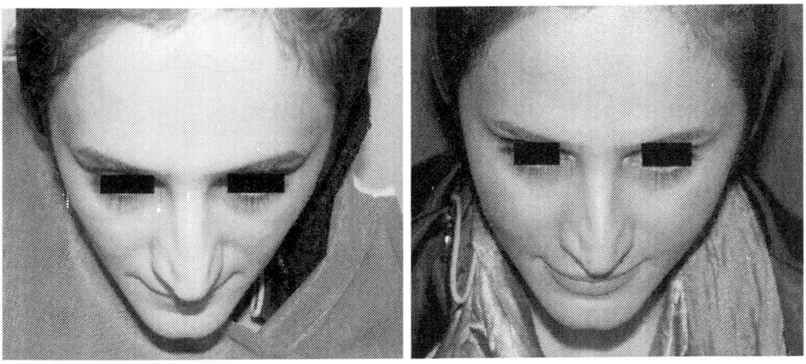

Figure 29. A 32 years woman with malar deficiency, No orthognathic surgery was performed in this case. The patient desired definition of the cheekbones with zygomatic sandwich osteotomy (ZSO) (left) preoperative view, note the triangular shape of she's face; (right) 18 month postoperative view.

5. Frontal modification

Frontal bossing reduction: Frontal Bossing known as a prominent supraorbital region and considers as a masculine characteristic. Generally men have more prominent frontal bossing than women which tends to have a smooth transition from brow area into a forehead. Frontal Bossing patients range from those with craniofacial anomaly such as thalassemias, Crouzon/

apert syndrome, Hurler syndrome to those without any underlying medical problem(figure 28,29). [112]

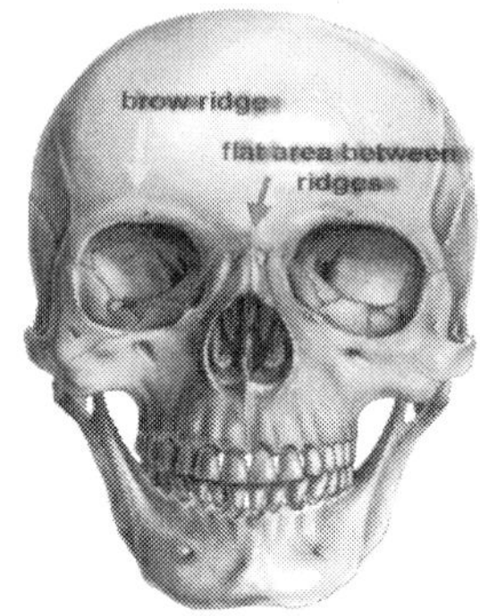

Figure 30. The main difference between male and female foreheads is that males often have a ridge of bone around the upper edge of the eye sockets called the "brow ridge" or "brow bossing". Female foreheads tend to have little or no bossing.Between the ridges of the two eye sockets a flat area can be visible. As women don't have the ridges, also the flat area between them is not present. [from facialfeminization.eu]

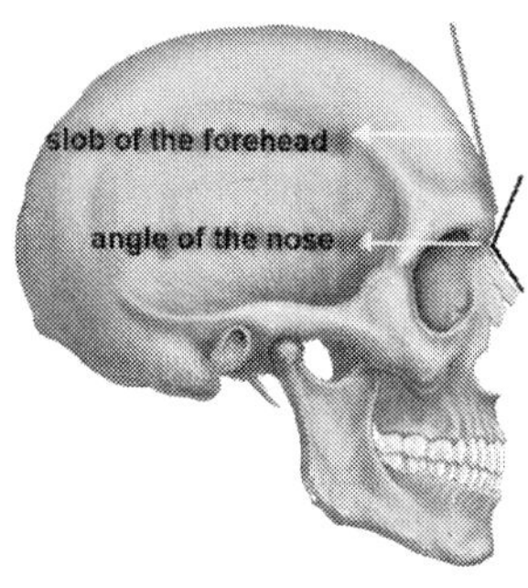

Figure 31. Schematic view of the slob of the forehead. Because of the brow ridge the general angle of the forehead in males (below-right) is steeper and the angle between the forehead and nose is sharper in lateral view. Women,(below-left) because they don't have the brow ridge, have a more vertical appearance of the forehead in lateral view. The angle between nose and forehead is more open. [from facialfeminization.eu]

The most common method of brow bone reduction is an open approach using a bi-coronal flap with either a burring reduction, an infracture technique or osteotomies and reshaping. Simple burring can be effective if the outer table of the brow bone is thick enough.

In the course of normal skull growth, satisfactory reduction of anterior bossing without direct surgical correction of the shape of the forehead can be achieved through sagittal suturectomy along with biparietal barrel stave cuts[113]. More correction of biparietal width and the occipital deformity, on the other hand, may also result in a gradual correction of the frontal

http://dx.doi.org/10.5772/59088

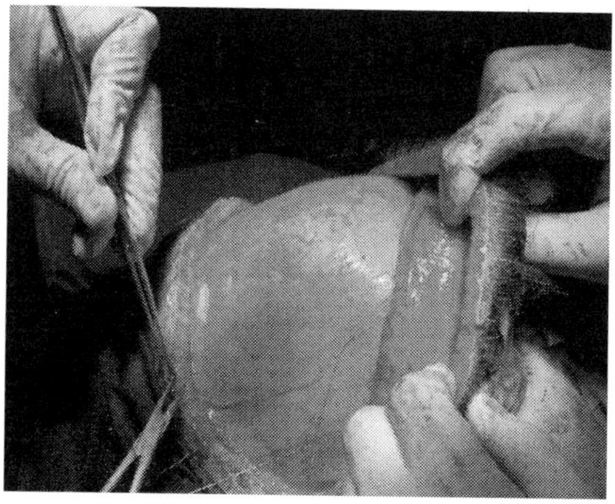

Figure 32. bi-coronal flap.

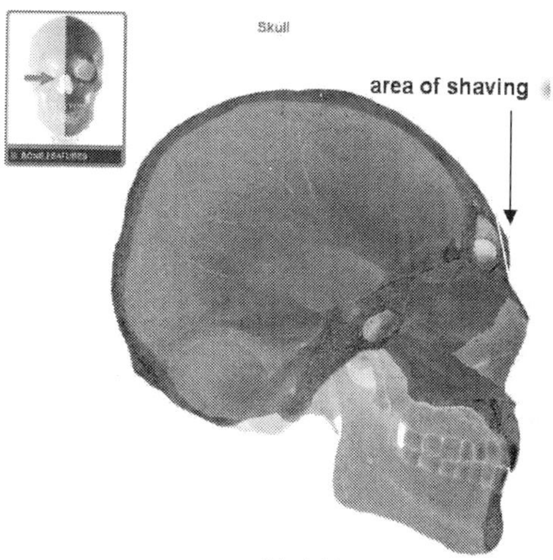

Figure 33. Frontal bossing re-shaping.With the thick bone, the surgeon only has to grind down the bone to the desired level and there will still be plenty of bone left to cover the frontal sinus as you can see.With the thin bone sutgeons can't grind it down to the ideal line or very much at all without breaking through into the sinus. In this case, most FFS surgeons will perform a forehead reconstruction so after grinding down what they can, they actually take the wall of bone apart, re-shape it and move it backwards to the desired position. [from www.virtualffs.co.uk]

deformity to satisfactory. In severe cases, however, the natural development of the calvarial shape with physiological skull growth following the described technique will not suffice as a cosmetically compromising frontal bossing will be most likely to persist. In such cases, a direct surgical correction, including radial osteotomies, rotation of bone flaps, "frontal to occipital switch", π-procedure, morcellation, use of distraction or contraction devices, total cranial vault reconstruction, and other techniques have been suggested in the craniofacial literature.[114] The general approach in these techniques includes excision, remodeling, transposition, and re-insertion of free bone flaps. The direct approach will then require complex bone fixations using wires or plates and screws. More advanced modifications of these techniques to avoid free bone flaps have been discussed where the shortened and re-approximated bone tongues stay attached at their normal calvarial position at the base or the apex of the calvaria. For example, in the technique described by Wagner and Wiewrodt[113] in 2008, following sagittal suturectomy and parietalbarrel stave incisions, four or five lanceolate pieces of thefrontal bone are excised resulting in three or four vertical bone bridges. These osteotomies are designed to extend radially from thecranial base towards the fontanel. Small strips rectangular to the apico-basal axis are then cut out from these bridges, leaving basal and apical bone tongues. [113] The tabula externa at the base of the basal tongues is drilled off and the tongues are bent inward to correct the inferior aspect of the frontal bossing. [113]

Corresponding basal and apical bone tongues arethen re-approached and fixated with sutures.

The gold standard procedure for correction of severe frontal bossing is still open approach with osteotomy of the anterior table of the frontal sinus which provides excellent outcome. Complications such as long coronal scars, alopecia, blood loss, forehead paresthesia, neuromas and traction palsy of the facial nerve makes this operation invasive, with increased chance of morbidity and less desirable for mild to moderate frontal bossing correction. [112]

Despite the widespread use of endoscopic frontal bone operations such as remodeling of bony defects and removal of osteomas of the frontal bone, only recently has "endoscopic frontal bossing correction" been introduced.[112] This emerging method seems to have rendered frontal bossing correction much simpler, significantly safer, and minimally invasive.

Moreover, the introduction of the endoscope revolutionized the surgical approach to the forehead, as it allowed for smaller incisions, magnified visualization, decreased risk of bleeding, faster recovery, and decreased chance of neuropathy by preserving cutaneous nerves. Endoscopic contouring of the forehead was first described by Song et al. on a Korean woman with frontal bone deformities.[115] Since then, most published endoscopic manipulation of the frontal bone and supraorbital ridge has involved osteoma mass excision or frontal sinus fracture repair. Retrospective reviews of patients receiving endoscopic correction of frontal bossing have shown promising aesthetic results with minimal postoperative morbidity. This method of improving forehead contour, however, should be carried out on properly selected groups of patients. Mild deformities of frontal bossing and adequate bone thickness over the frontal sinus makes patients a great choice for endoscopic frontal bossing correction. [112] Some complications such as neurosensory damage, vascular injury, and extended operative time. [112]. Similarities like incision line and dissection planes for this technique with standard endoscopic forehead lift allows easy access to the frontal bone for contouring in patients with frontal bossing and undergoing concurrent forehead rejuvenation.[112]

6. Summary

The major architectural promontories of the facial skeleton, including the malar-midface region, nose, chin,angle of the mandible and frontal buttress provide the base upon which the soft tissues of the face drape. By altering these promontories, dramatic changes can be made in the estheticappearance of the face—much more so than by changing soft tissue and skin alone.Since many years ago numerous surgical and office based techniques have been introduce to augment, reduce or refine the most projected points of the face such as cheek,chin,nose, Para-nasal area, angle of the jaw.When reduction of these esthetic points is planed not only we don't have multiple choices but also without using these methods the precise and predictable correction is almost impossible. In case of augmentation although we have the more options such as soft tissue office based procedures or facial prostheses[110, 111] a precise pre-surgical evaluation in according to patient complaints, social and economic conditions, soft or hard tissue deficiency, amount of augmentation,the past similar procedure, ect. should be considered and the best method for each patient should be selected.Aesthetic adjunct facial osteotomy techniques have proved to be expedient techniques, with low morbidity, producing a controllable and predictable increase or decrease of the facial prominences and stable short and long-term morphological results.The most common complication of esthetic adjunct osteotomy techniques are under- correction and over-correction; pre-surgical evaluation and precise estimation of amount of excess or deficiency is a best method to reduce these complications the relation between hard and soft tissue change is also important,for example the hard tissue to soft tissue ratio in case of advancement genioplasty is almost 1:1 but in case of reduction genioplasty or chin narrowing is almost 1:0.5.Another complication is bad split ; although it is a rare complication and often is simple to manage but in cases in whom correction is impossible the best way is internat fixation,close the incision and set an another appointment with patient. Other complications such as nerve injury, relapse or sever bleeding is very rare. The more surgeon experience the less incidence of complications.

Acknowledgements

Special thanks to MS. Shahrzad Zojaji and Marjan Golpashafor illustrations.

Author details

Seied Omid Keyhan[1,2*], Seifollah Hemmat[3], Peyman Mehriar[4], Arash Khojasteh[5] and Mohammad Ali Asayesh[5]

*Address all correspondence to: keyhanomid@ymail.com

1 Department of Oral and Maxillofacial Surgery, Shahid Sadooghi University of Medical Sciences, Yazd, Iran

2 Department of Oral and Maxillofacial Surgery, Isfahan University of Medical Sciences, Isfahan, Iran

3 Department of Oral and Maxillofacial Surgery, Bandar Abbas University of Medical Sciences, Bandar Abbas, Iran

4 Advanced Education in General Dentistry,Florida Institute, Miami, Florida, USA

5 Department of Oral and Maxillofacial Surgery,Shahis Beheshti University of Medical Sciences,Tehran, Iran

References

[1] Keyhan SO,Khiabani K,Raeisian SH et.al.Zigzag genioplasty;patients evaluation,technique modifications and review of the literature.Am J Cosmetic surg,2013; 30(2):80-88.

[2] Chang E, Lam S, Karen M, Donlevy JL. Sliding genioplasty for correction of chin abnormalities. *ArchFacial Plast Surg.* 2001;3:8–15.

[3] Troulis MJ, Kearns GJ, Perrott DH, Kaban LB. Extended genioplasty: long-term cephalometric, morphometric and sensory results. *Int J Oral Maxillofac Surg.* 2000;29:167–175.

[4] Farifia R, Valladares S, Aguilar L, Pastrian J, Rojas F. M-shaped genioplasty: a new surgical technique for sagittal and vertical chin augmentation: three case reports. *J Oral Maxillofac Surg.* 2012;70:1177–118

[5] Satoh K, Onizuka T. A new osteotomy for genioplasty—stepped osteotomy: preliminary report. *Ann Plast Surg.* 1993;31:186–190.

[6] Thomson ER. Sagittal genioplasty: a new technique of genioplasty. *Br J Plast Surg.* 1985;38:70–74.

[7] Wang J, Gui L, Xu Q, Cai J. The sagittal curving osteotomy: a modified technique for advancementgenioplasty. *J Plast Reconstr Aesthet Surg.*2007;60:119–124.

[8] Celik M, Tuncer S, Buyukcayir I. Splitting advancement genioplasty: a new genioplasty technique. *AnnPlast Surg.* 1999;43:148–153.

[9] Triaca A, Minoretti R, Merz B. Treatment of mandibular retrusion by distraction osteogenesis: a new technique. *Br J Oral Maxillofac Surg.* 2004;42:89–95.

[10] Grime PD, Blenkinsopp PT. Horizontal T genioplasty: a modified technique for the broad or asymmetrical chin. *Br J Oral Maxillofac Surg.* 1990;28:215–221.

[11] Li KK, Riley RW, Powell NB, Troell RJ. Obstructive sleep apnea surgery: genioglossus advancement revisited. *JOral Maxillofac Surg.* 2001;59:1181–118

[12] Zide BM, Mccarthy J. The mentalis muscle: an essential component of chin and lower lip position. Plast Reconstr Surg 1989: 83: 413-20.

[13] Danahey DG, Dayan SH, Benson AG, et al: Importance of chin evaluation and treatment to optimizing neck rejuvenation surgery. Facial Plast Surg,2001;17:91-97,

[14] Frodel JL: Evaluation and treatment of deformities of the chin. Facial Plast Surg Clin North Am,2005; 13:73-84,

[15] Frodel JL, Sykes JM, Jones JL: Evaluation and treatment of vertical microgenia. Arch Facial Plast Surg,2004; 6:111-119,

[16] Hofer O. Operation der Prognathic und Mikrogenie. Dtsch Zahn Mund Kieferheilkd 1942: 9: 81.

[17] Gillies HD, Millard DR. The principles and art of plastic surgery. Boston: Little Brown, 1957.

[18] Trauner R, Obwegeser H. The surgical correction of mandibular prognathism and retrognathia with consideration of genioplasty. Part I. Surgical procedures to correct mandibular prognathism and reshaping of the chin. Oral Surg 1957: 10: 677-89.

[19] Hinds EC, Kent JN. Genioplasty: the versatility of horizontal osteotomy. J Oral Surg 1969: 27: 690-700.

[20] Schendel SA. Genioplasty: a physiological approach. Ann Plast Surg 1985: 14: 506-14.

[21] Bell WH, Gallagher DM. The versatility of genioplasty using a broad pedicle. J Oral Maxillofac Surg 1983: 41: 763-9.

[22] Wolfe S. Chin advancement as an aid in correction of deformities of the mental and submental regions. Plast Reconstr Surg 1981: 6: 624-9.

[23] Tessier E Chin advancement as an aid in correction of deformities of the mental and submental regions: discussion. Plast Reconstr Surg 1981: 67: 630.

[24] Behrman S J, Complications associated with orthognathic surgery. In: IRBY WB, ed.: Current advances in oral surgery. St Louis: CV Mosby, 1974: 137.

[25] Mercuri LG, Laskin DM. Avascular necrosis after anterior horizontal augmentation genioplasty. J Oral Surg 1977: 35: 296-8.

[26] Ellis E, Dechow PC, Mcnamara JA,etal. Advancement genioplasty with and without soft tissue pedicle. J Oral Maxillofac Surg 1984: 42: 637-45.

[27] Storum KA, Bell WH, Nagura H. Microangiographic and histologic evaluation of revascularization and healing after genioplasty by osteotomy of the inferior border of the mandible. J Oral Maxillofac Surg 1988: 48: 210-6.

[28] Posnick JC, Al-qattan MM, Sterner NM. Alteration in facial sensibility in adolescents following sagittal split and chin osteotomies of the mandible. Plast Reconstr Surg 1996: 97: 920-7.

[29] Spear SL, Kassan M. Genioplasty. Clin Plast Surg 1989: 16:695 706.

[30] Lindquist CC, Obeid G. Complications of genioplasty done alone or in combination with sagittal split ramus osteotomy. Oral Surg 1988: 6: 13-6.

[31] Conwrse JM, Wood-Smith D. Horizontal osteotomy of the mandible. Hast Reconstr Surg 1964: 34: 464-71.

[32] Precious DS. A retrospective study of advancement genioplasty using a special bone plate: discussion. J Oral Maxillofac Surg 1992: 50: 347.

[33] Trimble LD, West RA. Steinman pin stabilization after horizontal mandibular osteotomy. J Oral Maxillofac Surg 1982: 40: 461-3.

[34] Turvey AT, Childers DA, Ntynn DR. Kirshner wire stabilization of the horizontal ostectomy of the inferior border of the mandible. Oral Surg 1982: 54: 513-6.

[35] Schow SR, Stein aM, Cardenas L. Intraoperative control and stabilization of the distal osseous segment in genioplasty. J Oral Maxillofac Surg 1995: 53: 481-2.

[36] Defreitas CE, Ellis E, Sindde A.retrospective study of advancement genioplasty using a special bone plate. J Oral Maxillofac Surg 1992: 50: 340-6.

[37] Polido WN, Declairfont RL, Bell WH. Bone resorption, stability and soft tissue changes following large chin advancements. J Oral Maxillofac Surg 1991: 49: 251-6.

[38] Precious DS, Armstrong JE, Morals D. Anatomic placement of fixation devices in genioplasty. Oral Surg 1992: 73: 2-8.

[39] Edwards RC, Kiely KD, Eppley BL: Resorbable fixation techniques for genioplasty. J Oral Maxillofac Surg 58:269-272, 2000

[40] Dolce C, Hatch JP, Van Sickels JE, et al: Five-year outcome and predictability of soft tissue profiles when wire or rigid fixation is used in mandibular advancement surgery. Am J Orthod Dentofacial Orthop124:249-256, 2003

[41] Proffit WR, Turvey T, Moriarty J. Augmentation genioplasty as an adjunct to conservative orthodontic treatment. Am J Orthod 1991: 79: 473-91.

[42] Wider TM, Spiro SA, Wolfe SA. Simultaneous osseous genioplasty and melo plasty. Plast Reconstr Surg 1997: 99: 1274-81.

[43] Wolford LM, Bates JD. Surgical modification for the correction of chin deformities. Oral Surg.1988: 66: 279-86.

[44] Uckan S, Soydan S, Veziroglu F, Arman A. Transverse reduction genioplasty to reduce width of the chin: indications, technique, and results. *JOral MaxillofacSurg.* 2010:68:1432–1437.

[45] Park S, Noh JH. Importance of the chin in lower facial contour: narrowing genioplasty to achieve a feminine and slim lower face. *Plast Reconstr Surg.* 2008;122:261

[46] Putnam J, Donovan M.modified reduction genioplasty.*J Oral Maxillofac Surg.* 1989:47:203-205

[47] Keyhan SO, Khiabani K, Hemmat S, Varedi P. Zigzag genioplasty: a new technique for 3-dimensional reduction genioplasty. *Br J Oral Maxillofac Surg.*2013:51(8):e317-e318

[48] Khiabani KH,Keyhan SO et al.Buccal fat pad lifting;an alternative open technique for malar augmentation.*J Oral Maxillofac Surg.*2014:72(2):e1-e15

[49] Badri AA,Keyhan SO,Surgical correction of facial skeletal deformity of patients with thalassemia.Am J Cosmetic surg.2014:31(2):107-115

[50] Herna´ndez-Alfaro F, Garcıa E, Martı C, Porta A. U-shaped osteotomy in management of paranasal deficiency.Int. J. Oral Maxillofac. Surg. 2006; 35: 1145–1148

[51] Epker BN. Correction of the skeletalnasal base in rhinoplasty. J Oral Maxillofac Surg 1991: 49: 938–946.

[52] Reyneke JP, Widgerow AD. Nasomaxillaryosteotomy for the correction of Binder's syndrome. Int J Adult OrthodonOrthognath Surg 1996: 11: 117–126

[53] Adams JR, Kawamoto HK. Late infectionfollowing aesthetic malar augmentation with proplast implants. PlastReconstr Surg 1995: 95: 382–384.

[54] Berghaus A. Porous polyethylene inreconstructive head and neck surgery.Arch Otolaryngol 1985: 11: 154–160.

[55] Bikhazi HB, Van Antwerp R. The useof Medpor in cosmetic and reconstructive surgery: Experimental and clinical evidence.In: Stucker FJ, ed: Plastic and Reconstructive Surgery of the Head andNeck. St. Louis: Mosby 1990: 271–273

[56] Cohen SR, Kawamoto HK. Infection ofproplast malar implants following dental injections. Plast Reconstr Surg 1992: 89:1148–1151.

[57] Constantino PD, Friedman CD, LaneA. Synthetic biomaterials in facial plastic and reconstructive surgery. Facial PlastSurg 1993: 9: 1–15.

[58] Davis PKB, Jones SM. The complicationsof silastic implants: Experience with 137 consecutive cases. Br J Oral MaxillofacSurg 1971: 24: 405–411

[59] Frodel JL, Lee S. The use of high densitypolyethylene implants in facial deformities. Arch Otolaryngol Head Neck Surg1998: 124: 1219–1223

[60] Morehead JM, Holt GR. Soft tissueresponse to synthetic biomaterials. Otolaryngol Clin North Am 1994: 27: 195–201

[61] Rubin JP, Yaremchuk MJ. Complicationsand toxicity of implantable materials used in facial reconstructive andaesthetic surgery: A comprehensivereview of the literature. Plast ReconstrSurg 1997: 100: 1336–1353.

[62] Whear NM, Cousley RR, Liew G,Henderson D. Postoperative infectionof proplast facial implants. Br J OralMaxillofac Surg 1993: 31: 292–295.

[63] Yaremchuk MJ, Israeli D. Paranasalimplants for correction of midface concavity. Plast Reconstr Surg 1998: 102:1676–1684

[64] Chow TK, Yu CN, Fung SC. Pyriformrim sandwich osteotomy: A new regional osteotomy for correction of para-alar deficiency.J Oral Maxillofac Surg 2004: 62: 256–260

[65] Haffner CL, Pessa JE, Zadoo VP, et al: A technique for threedimensional cephalometric analysis as an aid in evaluating changes in the crainofacial skeleton. Angle Orthod 1999: 69:345,

[66] Hirohi T, Yoshimura K.Lower face reduction with full-thickness marginal ostectomy of mandibular corpus-angle followed bycorticectomy. JPlast Reconstr Aesth Surg. 2010: 63, 1251-1259

[67] Baek SM, Kim SS, Bindiger A. The prominent mandibular angle: Preoperative management, operative technique, and results in 42 patients. Plast Reconstr Surg 1989;83: 272-8

[68] Yang DB, Park CG. Mandibular contouring surgery for purely aesthetic reseons.Aesthetic Plast Surg.1991;15:53-6

[69] Honda T, Sasaki K, Takeuchi M, et al. Endoscope-assistedintraoral approach for masseteric hypertrophy. Ann Plast Surg 1997;38:9-14

[70] Kim SK, Han JJ, Kim JT.Classification and Treatment of Prominent Mandibular Angle.Aesth. Plast. Surg.2001; 25:382–387

[71] Han K, Kim J. Reduction mandibuloplasty: ostectomy of the lateral cortex around the mandibular angle. J Craniofac Surg 2001;12:314-25

[72] Yamanouchi S, Ishihara K, Shirato Y, et al. Facial pattern of the present day Japanese associated with normal occlusion. J Jpn Orthod Soc 1995;54:93-101

[73] Layoun W, Guyot L, Richard O, Gola R.Augmentation of cheek bone contour using malar osteotomy. Aesthetic Plast Surg. 2003;27(4):269-74.

[74] Choi JY, Lee SH, Baek SH: Effects of facial hard tissue surgery on facial aesthetics: Changes in facial content and frames. J Craniofac Surg. 2012;23:1683.

[75] Jones RH, Ching M. Intraoral zygomatic osteotomy for correction of malar deficiency. J Oral Maxillofac Surg. 1995 Apr;53(4):483-5.

[76] Powell NB, Riley RW: Cranial bone grafting in facial aesthetics and reconstructive contouring. Arch Otolaryngol Head Neck Surg. 1987; 113:713.

[77] Powell N, Riley RW, Laub DR: A new approach to evaluation of the malar complex. Ann Plast Surg. 1988;30:206.

[78] Donovan MG: Augmentation of the malar prominence by sagittal osteotomy of the zygoma and interpositional bone grafting, in Bell WH (ed): Modern Practice in Orthognathic and Reconstructive Surgery, vol 3. Philadelphia, PA, Saunders, 1992, pp 2298-2304.

[79] Walji S: Letter to the Editor: Mommaerts MY, Abeloos JVS, De Clercq CAS, et al: The sandwich zygomatic osteotomy. J Craniomaxillofac Surg. 1996;24:131.

[80] Gimenez EJ: Osteotomia de1 hueso malar. Revista Assoc Odont Argent. 1973;61:303.

[81] Mommaerts MY, Abeloos JVS, De Clercq CAS, et al: The "sandwich" zygomatic osteotomy: Technique, indications and clinical results. J Craniomaxillofac Surg. 1995;23:12.

[82] Onizuka T, Watanabe K, Takasu K, et al. Reduction malarplasty.Aesthetic Plast Surg 1983;7:121–125.

[83] Baek SM, Chung YD, Kim SS. Reduction malarplasty. Plast Reconstr Surg 1991;88:53–61.

[84] Sumiya N, Kondo S, Ito Y, Ozumi K, Otani K, Wako M. Reduction malarplasty. Plast Reconstr Surg 1997;100:461–7.

[85] Baek RM, Kim J, Lee SW. Revision reduction malarplasty with coronal approach. J Plast Reconstr Aesthet Surg 2010;63:2018–24.

[86] Kim YH, Seul JH. Reduction malarplasty through an intraoral incision:a new method. Plast Reconstr Surg 2000;106:1514–9.

[87] Lee JG, Park YW. Intraoral approach for reduction malarplasty: a simple method. Plast Reconstr Surg 2003;111:453–60.

[88] Zou C, Niu F, Liu J, Chen Y, Wang M, Su R, et al. midface contour change after reduction malarplasty with modified L-shaped osteotomy: a surgical outcomes study. Aesthetic plast surg.2014;38(1):177-83.

[89] Chen T, Hsu Y, Li J, Hu J, Khadka A, Wang Q, et al. correction of zygoma and zygomatic arch protrusion in east Asian individuals. Oral Surg Oral Med Oral Pathol Oral Radiol Endod.2011;112(3):307-14.

[90] Tang K, Hsu Y, Hu J, Zhao Y, Wang Q, Li J. New horizontal v-shaped osteotomy for correction of protrusion of the zygoma and the zygomatic arch in East Asians: indica-

tion and results. Br J Oral Maxillofac Surg. 2014; http://dx.doi.org/10.1016/j.bjoms. 2014.04.016.

[91] Nakanishi Y, Nagasao T, Shimizu Y, Miyamoto j, kishi K, Fukuta K. The boomerang osteotomy - A new method of reduction malarplasty J Plast Reconstr Aesthet Surg 2012;65(5):111-20.

[92] Song WC, Choi HG, Kim SH, et al. Topographic anatomy of the zygomatic arch and temporal fossa: a cadaveric study. J Plast Reconstr Aesthet Surg 2009;62:1375-8.

[93] Uhm KI, Lew JM. Prominent zygoma in Orientals: classification and treatment. Ann Plast Surg 1991;26:164-70.

[94] Hwang YJ, Jeon JY, Lee MS. A simple method of reduction malarplasty. Plast Reconstr Surg 1997;99:348-55.

[95] Kim T, Baek SH, Choi JY. ReductionMalarplasty According to Esthetic Facial Unit Analysis: Retrospective Clinical Study of 23 Cases. J Oral Maxillofac Surg. 2014;72(8): 1565-78.

[96] Jung H, Lee Y, Doo JH, et al. Prevention of complication and management of unfavorable results in reduction malarplasty. J Korean Soc Plast Reconstr Surg. 2008;35:465–470.

[97] Hong SE, Liu SY, Kim JT, Lee JH. Intraoral Zygoma Reduction Using L-shaped Osteotomy. J Craniofac Surg. 2014;25(3):758-61.

[98] Morris DE, Moaveni Z, Lo LJ. Aesthetic facial skeletal contouring in the Asian patient. Clin Plast Surg 2007;34:547-56.

[99] Whitaker LA. Temporal and malar-zygomatic reduction and augmentation. Clin Plast Surg 1991;18:1-4.

[100] Hinderer UT. Malar implants for improvement of facial appearance. Plast Reconstr Surg.1975;56(2):157-65.

[101] Blyer SM. Facial ilants in cosmetic surgery. In: Fonseca RJ, Turvey TA (editors). Oral and maxillofacial surgery. Second ed.Missouri: ELSEVIER SAUNDERS;2009.690.

[102] Wilkinson TS. Complications in esthetic malar augmentation.Plast Reconstr Surg. 1983;71:643.

[103] Prendergast M, Shoenrock LD. Malar augmentation. Patient classification and placement. Arch Otolaryngol Head Neck Surg. 1989;115(8):964-9.

[104] Stuzin JM, Wagstrom L, Kawamoto HK, et al. The anatomy and clinical applications of the buccal fatpad. Plast Reconstr Surg 1990;85(1):29– 37.

[105] Bettens RMA, Mommaerts MY, Sykes JM. Aesthetic malar recontouring: the zygomatic sandwich osteotomy. Facial Plast Surg Clin N Am. 2002;10: 265–277.

[106] Li KK. Discussion, six years' experience with the zygomatic "sandwich" osteotomy for correction of malar deficiency. J Oral Maxillofac Surg. 1999;57:14 – 5.

[107] Lorenz HP, Schendel SA. Facial bone sculpturing. In: Ward-Booth P, Hausamen JE, Schendel SA, editors.Maxillofacial surgery, vol 2. London: Churchill Livingstone; 1999. pp. 1441– 56.

[108] Mommaerts MY, Nadjmi N, Abeloos JVS, et al. Six years experience with the zygomatic sandwich osteotomy for correction of malar deficiency. J Oral Maxillofac Surg. 1999;57:8–13.

[109] Gasparini G, Saponaro G, Moro A, Boniello R, Cervelli D, Pelo S. Zygomatic Sagittal Split Osteotomy: A Novel and Simple Surgical Technique for Use in Midface Corrections. J Craniofac Surg.2010;21(6):1872-5.

[110] Keyhan SO,Badri AA,Hemmat S ET AL.Use of platelet-rich fibrin and platelet-rich plasma in combination with fat graft: which is more effective during facial lipostructure? J Oral Maxillofac Surg. 2013:71 (3), 610-621

[111] Khiabani K,Keyhan SO,Hemmat S.Buccal Fat Pad Lifting: An Alternative Open Technique for Malar Augmentation.J Oral Maxillofac Surg.2014:72 (2), 403. e1-403. e15

[112] Guyuron B, Lee M, Larson K, Amirlak B. Endoscopic correction of frontal bossing. Plastic and reconstructive surgery. 2013 Mar;131(3):388e-93e.

[113] Wagner W, Wiewrodt D. A simple technique for the correction of frontal bossing in synostotic scaphocephaly. Child's nervous system : ChNS : official journal of the International Society for Pediatric Neurosurgery. 2008 Mar;24(3):373-7.

[114] Alvarez-Garijo JA, Cavadas PC, Vila MM, Alvarez-Llanas A. Sagittal synostosis: results of surgical treatment in 210 patients. Child's nervous system : ChNS : official journal of the International Society for Pediatric Neurosurgery. 2001 Jan;17(1-2):64-8.

[115] Song IC, Pozner JN, Sadeh AE, Shin MS. Endoscopic-assisted recontouring of the facial skeleton: the forehead. Annals of plastic surgery. 1995 Mar;34(3):323-5

Chapter 11

Surgical Techniques to Improve the Smile

Mazen Almasri

Additional information is available at the end of the chapter

http://dx.doi.org/10.5772/59213

1. Introduction

A smile has always been an important key in our social life, not to mention if it is an attractive one. The type, degree, tone, at static or a dynamic figure concerns facial beauty as well as the internal mood, or what might be called " the internal smile." The society in the current century is turning towards social media, gadgets, electronics and advertisements mainly based on pictures. Those corporates seeking to recruit applicants for job positions assess the persons photograph in addition to their CV because a photo can tell a lot about an applicant. Hence, there is a growing trend towards enhancement of facial esthetics.

Among the medical professions, many specialties are dealing with smiles; however, the approach to management can vary considerably due to improper diagnosis and lack of knowledge toward the variable treatment options. Specialists such as restorative dentist, prosthodontist, orthodontist, periodontist, maxillofacial surgeon, plastic surgeon, and dermatologist are working around the "smile complex"; however, no clear inter-specialty communication exists to provide the best intervention for patients. This might be a reason for variable management to smile imperfections via different specialties.

In this chapter, the "unattractive smile", is being discussed from different angles and in a totally different manner. The objective is to collect the expertise of variable cosmetic specialties in a single chapter to help practitioners in future decision-making processes in "smile management." Hence, the concepts are presented along with multiple challenging cases with different interventions. Interventions such as restorative veneers in the maxillary anterior teeth can be the answer to all patients' troubles if used in the right cases; while crown lengthening as a sole procedure or in combination with veneers can be the ultimate solution for others [1].

Maxillary surgical procedures such as LeFort 1 may be the only solution in others. Laser therapy for lip irregularities can provide more convenient results in case of fine wrinkles, while Botox and fillers may provide better outcomes for some gummy smiles. The case can be a little bit more challenging if the patient is known to have a repaired cleft lip, previous lip trauma, or secondary facial deformity [2].

Other situations where patients visit clinics with a clear demand of what can make them feel happier, such as piercing or cheek dimples can be linked to the patient's own personal satisfaction. On other occasions, clients may be confused, and complain of resenting their profile pictures without clear understanding of their problem needing correction. It is well known, that in the current era of cosmetic revolution and subspecialty care and techniques, continuous evaluation and research regarding the principles of "smile management" are evolving. Therefore, practitioners should keep in mind that proper training in the field, careful case selection, and inter-specialty communication can provide the best results with the least possible complications.

2. Definition of smile

A smile is expressed as a form of one's feature reflecting pleasure and happiness usually shown by upturning the corners of the mouth [1]. It can be presented in a static state mostly during taking pictures, or can be as part of a dynamic state during articulation. However, the personal self-evaluation can be more complicated due to the era of advanced social networking. Hence, it is not surprising that critics of smiles and perfectionism are increasing [2].

3. Components of the smile

Medical practitioners may describe the smile as a status of the orofacial complex where muscles of the facial expression are harmonized. Muscles such as the frontalis, orbicularis oculi, orbicularis oris, zygomaticus major, risorius, platysma and depressor anguli oris are working in harmony to provide various facial expressions [3]. A common mistake is considering the oral complex as the only item composing the smile, though midfacial muscles such as the zygomaticus major and minor originate from the midface and hence affect the general character and smile. The muscles around the orbital complex are critical to facial expression as a reflection of youth and beauty when lacking heavy wrinkles [4]. Hence, the components of a smile can be evaluated according to different factors namely:

a. Anatomical components

b. Smile lip line

c. Dental smile lines

d. Facial character

Anatomical components: The smile is composed of the upper lip, the maxillary bone, the maxillary teeth, and the gingival tissue envelope [5, 6].

The upper lip represents the area from the point subnasal to the upper lip stomion which varies between 18-22mm (Figure 1) [5]. The width of the lip is composed of mucosa, orbicularis muscle, fat, and skin, which varies between individuals in height and thickness. However, the extension of muscles into the surrounding structures such as the nose can affect the nasal shape when smiling. A lot of patients have their nasal tips turned downward when they smile, or have the alae of the nose extremely widen or flare, which can be unsightly [7].

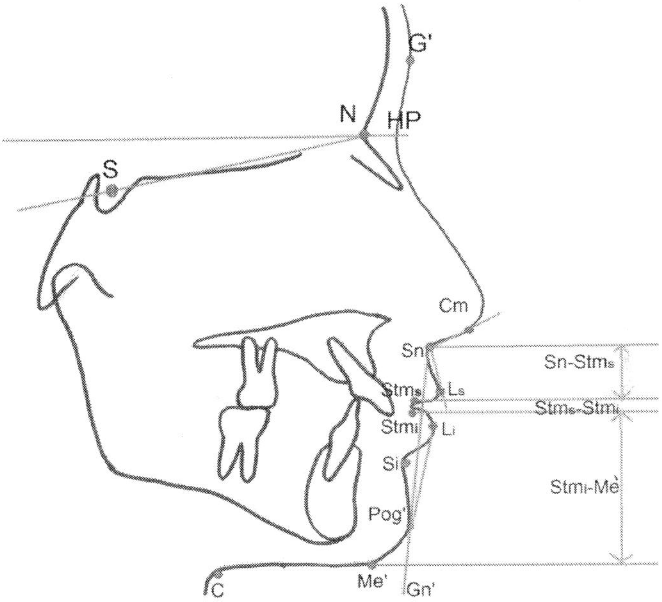

Figure 1. Lateral cephalometric analysis showing the lip form and position. Nasolabial angle (Cm-Sn-Ls), mentolabial sulcus depth (Si to Li-Pog'), maxillary incisor exposure (Stms-1). Upper lip protrusion (Ls to Sn-Pog'), lower lip protrusion (Li to Sn-Pog'), vertical lip-chin ratio (Sn-Stms/Stmi-Me'), interlabial gap (Stms- Stmi). [5]

The maxillary bone and teeth constitute the second and third parts. The maxilla extends from the subnasal down to the alveolar component housing the teeth. The width of the smile is correlated with the width of the maxilla, as transverse deficiency will lead to narrow V-shaped maxillary arch and a wide buccal corridor which is not pleasant, and vice versa. While in the vertical dimension, maxillary excessive growth will lead to over expression of gum and teeth during smiling or a gummy smile; while extreme maxillary bone vertical deficiency will lead to absence of teeth and gingival show at static or dynamic orofacial states reflecting an unpleasant aging character. Evaluation of the maxillomandibular complex is accomplished via clinical and radiographic modalities clarified later in this chapter [5].

The gingival architecture is the fourth factor. Gingival recession exposing more tooth structure and roots is as unpleasant as gingival overgrowth -leading to short clinical crowns. As the crown shape, including height, width, curvature, and alignment have an important role [3], once the dental smile arc line is upturned posteriorly it will reflect better cosmetic results compared to a flat or downturned arc line. [6] Hence, a defect in a single component or inappropriate harmony between each can provide patients with unpleasant smiles. Therefore it is very critical to diagnose the major contributor to the disharmony and formulate the best management plan accordingly.

Smile lip line: This is divided into high, moderate or low horizontal smile lines according to the magnitude of upper lip coverage of the maxillary anterior teeth when static and smiling. [6] A high lip line refers to a smile showing the maxillary anterior teeth and part of the gingival tissue, while a low lip line shows 0-2mm of the anterior teeth. A high smile line is considered to be a challenging factor when rehabilitating the anterior maxilla. As any defect in the crown or gingival tissue can be disclosed; unlike patients with moderate or low smile lines (Figure 2).

Dental smile line (smile arc): This pertains to maxillary teeth from the incisor going along to the 1st molar and describes the best cosmetic relation as evaluated by an expert restorative dentist.[4,6] A smooth transition of dental lines, alignment, shape, and color can provide pleasant smiles. The dental smile line is an imaginary line drawn from the incisal edges of the maxillary anterior teeth and following the upper lip inferior border curvature. It can be flat, upturned, or downturned. These lines do have more fine details that a specialist restorative dentist can analyze. [3, 4, 6] The fine dental line details are beyond the scope of the chapter.

4. Case

A young female patient referred complaining that she does not like her smile. On examination the patient was presented an option of orthodontic treatment to adjust the spaces and dental relation before any final restorative esthetic procedures. However, the patient did not prefer any orthodontic intervention. Hence, the cosmetic restorative team evaluated the patient for possible prosthetic rehabilitation of the smile and anterior teeth via dental veneers. Proper examination, impression and lab simulation using wax up models was performed and showed a favorable outcome. Therefore, the team elected to proceed with the treatment. Although the team advised the patient to receive restorative therapy of the premolar teeth, the patient refused, as she was mainly interested in betterment of the anterior tooth show (Figure 2).

Facial character: The overall shape, color, and harmony of the face and maxillomandibular relationship should be evaluated clinically as well as radiologically. Clinical pictures of the frontal and profile views from different angles are necessary for documentation. Static evaluation as well as dynamic evaluation of the facial expression is important and any facial asymmetry should not go unforeseen. [2, 7, 8]

Beside the clinical examination of the head and neck region, radiographic evaluation is important to investigate the maxillomandibular complex, temporomandibular joint, and dentition using panoramic radiography and cephalometrics. [5, 7, 8]

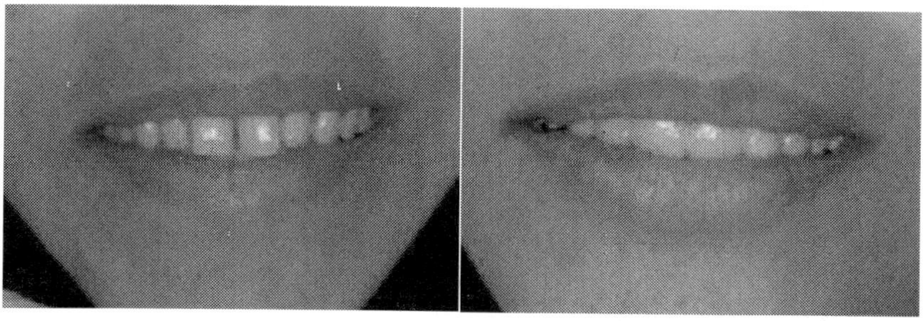

Figure 2. (Left) a moderate smile lip line, with unfavorable dento-gingival relationship and dental esthetics. (Right) Postoperative results after treatment with restorative veneers (Courtesy of Professor Motaz Ghulman, King Abdulaziz University).

4.1. Principles of managing an unpleasant smile

Unpleasant smiles can be due to clear defect in one or more of the major smile components, lack of harmony of the smile pillars, or loss of self-satisfaction, which can be due either to a specific demand the patient is requesting (such as cheek dimples) or pure personal psychological dissatisfaction. The most important principle in managing such patients is to diagnose the etiology to see if it is actually an organic anatomical issue or is it an issue of self-concept. The answer is usually explored via careful teamwork consultation that will help guide the patient to the proper treatment channels.

4.1.1. The use of botox and fillers for smiles: [9, 10]

Botox (Botulinum toxin) is a neurotoxin that is derived from the bacterium Clostridium Botulinum that has several serologically distinct subtypes, A, B, C, D, E, and G. It acts by blocking acetylcholine release at the neuromuscular junction, and hence preventing muscular contraction leading to smoothening of the hyperkinetic unpleasant looking facial rhytids or skin lines. The most common one is Botulinum A, Botox. [9, 10]

Botox has many applications in medical fields such as:

1. Treating facial rhytids: forehead, periorbital, and paranasal area
2. Treating neck vertical platysmal bands
3. Myofacial pain of the head and neck
4. Migraines
5. Muscle palsy
6. Muscle hypertrophy, commonly masseter and temporalis muscle hypertrophy.

For smiles with hyperactive muscular complex of the upper lip, Botox can be carefully deposited in the main hyperactive areas to reduce the action and hence to allow better draping of the upper lip complex on the maxillary teeth. [11]

The advantages are: easier application, less invasive, quick procedure, reasonable price, reasonably fast onset, and duration of about 6 months.

Disadvantages are: the action may start with fine dropping of the upper lip that patients may perceive as unpleasant, it takes from days to weeks to stabilize, asymmetric smile, uncomfortable injections, requiring re-injection after 6 months to stabilize results. [9, 11]

4.1.2. Case presentation

A 29-year-old woman complained that she was unsatisfied with her smile and that she had to use her hand to cover her mouth while laughing. On examination it was noticed that she had a hyperactive upper lip muscles, orbicularis oris and elevator labii alaeque nasi. She agreed to start management with a simple non-invasive method such as Botox therapy of the hyperactive areas (Figure 3, 4).

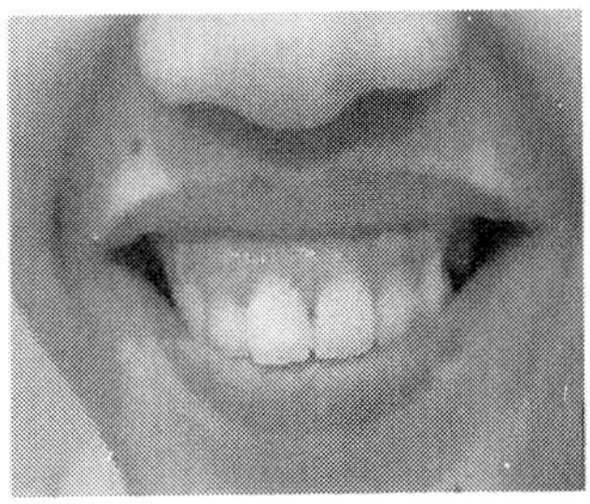

Figure 3. A 29-year-old woman with a gummy smile.

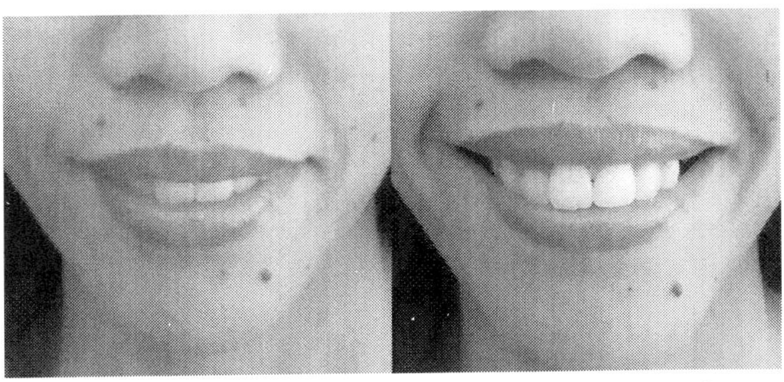

Figure 4. The patient after treatment with selective Botox therapy at the hyperactive muscular areas. The pictures showing two pleasant smile poses, as compared to the preoperative smile in Figure 3.

4.2. Lefort 1 maxillary surgery

A LeFort 1 maxillary procedure is a surgical intervention where the maxillary bone is osteotomized in the semi-horizontal plane to disengage it from the cephalic end and allow moving the disengaged part into a more favorable position as dictated in relation to the opposing jaw and thus, improving the general facial harmony. The movement can be accomplished in three dimensions as needed. A maxillofacial surgeon trained in the field of orthognathics and facial reconstruction usually performs the procedure [5, 12]. Preoperative evaluation and consultation with an orthodontist trained in the field is necessary to estimate the defect and treatment planning including a thorough preoperative work up. This usually includes the following: Facial clinical photographs, intraoral photographs, panoramic radiograph, lateral cephalometric radiograph, anteroposterior cephalometric radiograph, impressions to develop study casts, mounting casts and a face bow transfer to aid in the cast mounting (Figure 5) [5,12]. Once this is accomplished, a proper data analysis is required for each aspect to develop a preoperative documented record, a diagnosis, and a provisional plan.

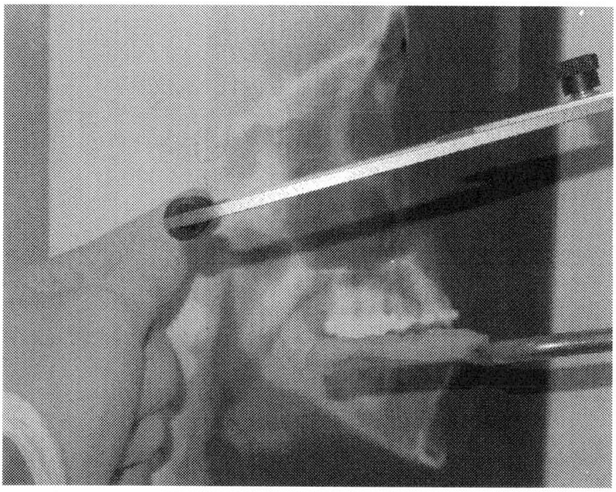

Figure 5. Lateral cephalometric radiograph with superimposing face bow transfer is a method to insure proper dentoskeletal relation before sending the face bow and impressions to the laboratory.

One of the most common indications is in gummy smile cases due to maxillary vertical excess. The procedure can be more challenging in cases with a short upper lip that contributes to the unpleasant smile complex. The procedure is mainly directed toward reducing the maxillary excess by moving the maxilla in the superior direction, and hence, it improves the smile.

The advantages of such a procedure are that it provides a major improvement in the shape of the face and smile.

The disadvantages are that it is done under general anesthesia, requires hospitalization, requires prolonged recovery time that can be up to a month (hence usually done during a prolonged vacation), postoperative expectations include swelling, pain, midface paresthesia, difficulty eating, minor changes in nasal shape, and general discomfort. [12, 13]

4.2.1. Case presentation

A 27-year-old patient with an unpleasant smile and difficulty eating. Clinical and radiographic evaluation revealed vertical maxillary excess and mandible deviation. The patient underwent multi-team comprehensive consultation and found it best to be treated via orthognathic surgery. LeFort 1 maxillary osteotomy was done to position the maxilla in upward position and correct the rotation, while the mandible underwent bilateral sagittal split osteotomy to optimize symmetry and occlusion. The patient still requires final orthodontic treatment (Figure 6).

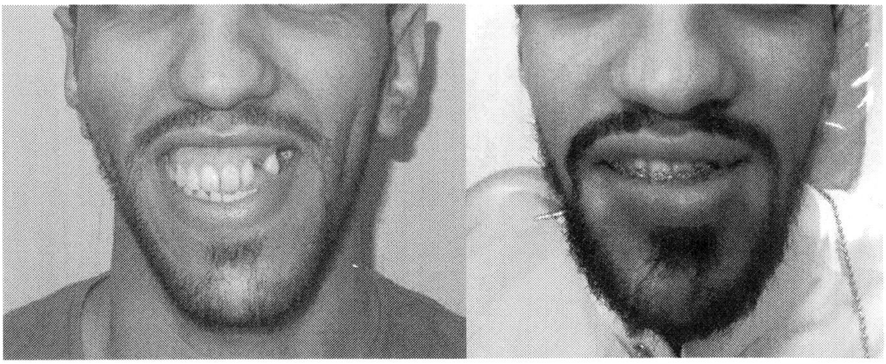

Figure 6. Maxillary vertical excess that required orthognathic surgery intervention to correct the deformity seen on the left. The right picture shows the postoperative favorable results.

4.3. Upper lip enhancement procedures

Facial aging is a continuous process that can be accelerated by smoking, sun exposure, or personal genetic predisposition. The loss of elastic fibers and replacement with collagen fibers leads to reduction in skin elasticity and sagging of the skin complex. Hence, cosmetic procedures such as facial fillers, lipofillers, chemical peeling, surgical lifting procedures, and laser treatment can optimize the general results. [10-14]

Other surgical procedures are not as common such as upper lip elongation or shortening that can treat cases of short upper lip that require some elongation to redrape the maxillary teeth. The upper lip is measured from the subnasal point to upper lip stomion, and has an average of 18-22mm length. [8]

A subnasal upper lip-lift is a procedure used to shorten a long upper lip and to evert it outward. This will allow more maxillary teeth show, upper lip outward eversion, and hence, a more pleasant youthful smile. It can be designed in a W-lift direction to provide better enhancement of the cupid bow area. The W arms can be designed in asymmetric fashion to manage upper lip asymmetric deformities. [2]

The lips can be in inverted, everted, hypoplastic, or with fine mucosal irregularities [13]. Such lip irregularities can be managed using laser therapy to eliminate superficial folds, or even cut and plan the rotation movements needed (Figure 7). [13, 14]

4.3.1. Case presentation

A 23-year-old female referred complaining of unesthetic upper lip and unpleasant smile. The patient had had multiple cleft lip and palate repair procedures in the past. The patient was presented an option of asymmetric upper lip lift and fat transfer to the upper lip. The procedure took place under general anesthesia and the results were immediately noticed (Figure 7, 8).

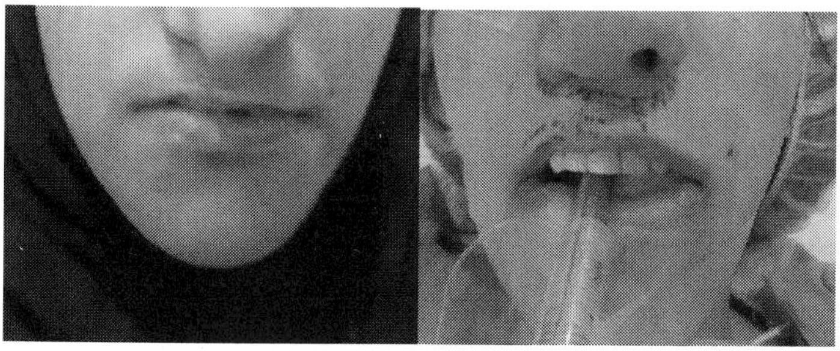

Figure 7. The patient at the preoperative stage (left); the upper lip is thin, inverted and flat. The plan surgically was to lift up the upper lip, evert it outward, and augment it using fat transfer. The picture on the right shows the preoperative W-lift marking. [2]

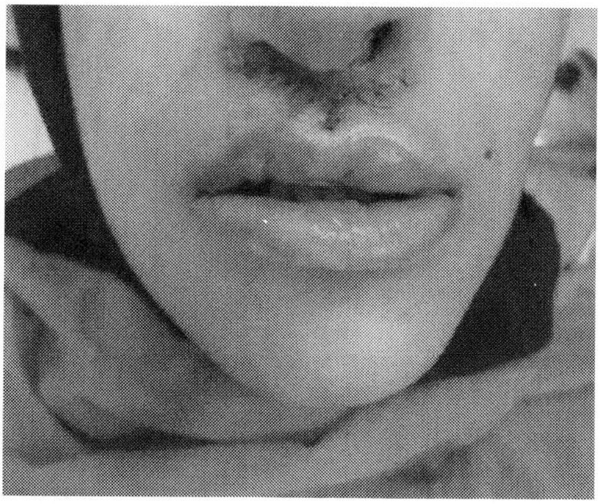

Figure 8. One-week postoperatively showing the upper lip volume, lip lift, and outward eversion of the patient in Figure 7.

Upper lip volume enhancement can be accomplished using autogenous grafts such as fascia, muscle, and periosteum especially if more volume is needed in compromised sites such as repaired cleft lip with notching or whistle deformity (Figure 9). Synthetic fillers are a common option now days to achieve lip volume enhancement or final border definition [7-9, 13].

4.3.2. Case presentation

A 34-year-old male patient referred complaining of extramucosal fold of his upper lip that shows more during smiling. The patient was presented an option of Erbium-Yag laser therapy to remove the mucosal folds under local anesthesia (Figure 9).

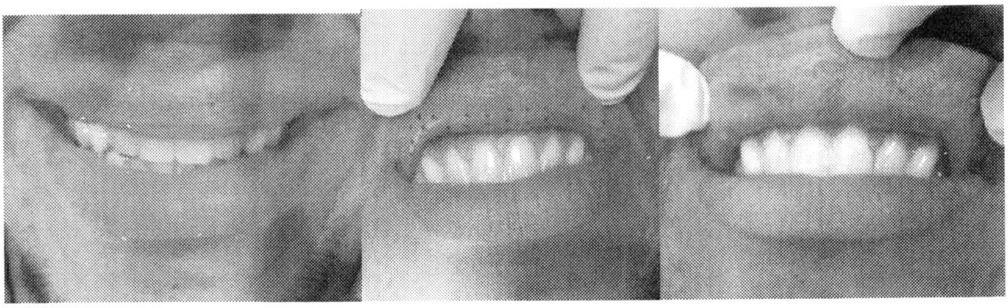

Figure 9. The left picture presents a smile of a 34-year-old male patient complaining of extramucosal fold of his upper lip that shows more during smiling. The patient was presented an option of Erbium-Yag laser therapy to remove the mucosal folds under local anesthesia. The picture on the right showing the result immediately after laser therapy, indicating the dry field and a potential of favorable secondary intentional healing.

4.3.3. Case presentation

A 23-year-old female presented with severe whistle deformity and notching of the upper lip secondary to repaired cleft lip 6 years ago. She was presented an option of upper lip revision; however, she was not keen to do so. Hence, she was presented the option of periosteum-muscular graft augmentation harvest from the lower lip / chin mass and transfer to the upper lip (Figure 10).

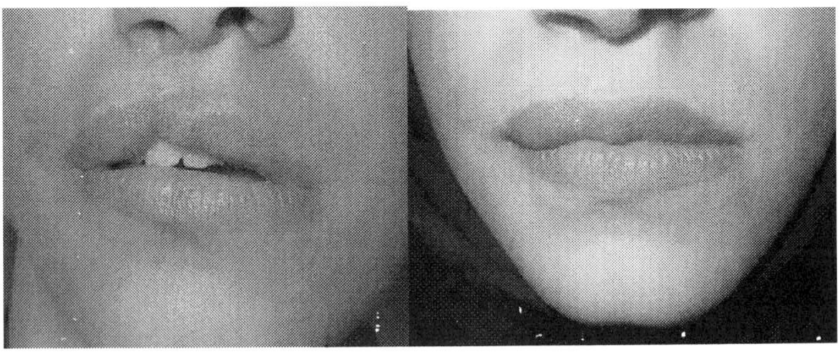

Figure 10. Reconstruction of an upper lip with severe notch deformity on the left picture using autologous muscular graft. The photograph on the right is three months postoperative. Final fine-tuning of lip boundaries can be achieved using synthetic fillers.

4.4. Crown lengthening

Crown lengthening is defined as a procedure used to increase the height of the clinical crowns by removing part of the gingival tissue with or without the crestal alveolar bone [14]. The procedure is usually designed according to the demand of the clinical crown height or the planned prosthetic crown or veneer. The tissue ablation is performed using blades, lasers, or less favorably, electrocautery, which has the tendency to damage the soft tissue cuff when compared to laser-based precise cutting capabilities. However, Laser treatment will require a set up to be ready, such as machine position, extensions, wires plastic covers, goggle's for the team and patient, surgical sites protections, and proper infection control protocol (Figure 11). [14]

The dental gingival relation describes the maxillary teeth height, width, shape, and alignment status in relation to the gingival envelope. This can never be satisfying unless it was reflected in a beautiful smile [1, 2]. Therefore, a specialized restorative dentist should evaluate the case to verify the needed consultation and intervention, which can vary from simple odontoplasty, placing veneers, crowns, orthodontic treatment, or even extraction, alveolar bone reconstruction and implant-based rehabilitation (Figure 12).[15-17] Hence, teamwork is always the key to reach the best dento-gingival relation to provide a satisfying smile. This can be clarified through two examples, the first one illustrating the role of the oral and maxillofacial surgeon to evaluate a poor alveolar bone supporting the gingival tissue that requires alveolar reconstruction in horizontal and/ or vertical dimensions before prosthetic rehabilitation. [17] The second example illustrates the role to manage patients with short lip and vertical maxillary excess that will never be managed properly if crown-lengthening procedure was only performed. Such a case will require a LeFort 1 surgical procedure to reposition the maxilla superiorly first. [5, 12]

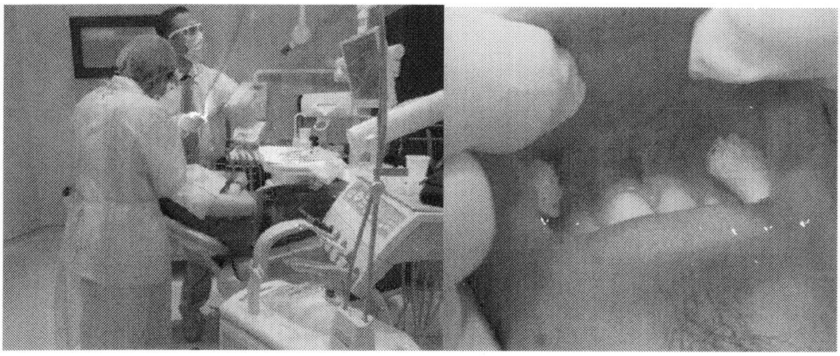

Figure 11. Showing the laser setup in the dental office as well as surgical site preparation for laser assisted labial frenoplasty.

The indication for crown lengthening is: cases of satisfying harmony of the upper lip height and maxillary bone relation, healthy dentition and periodontium but with poor dentogingival relation such as gingival overgrowth or poor architecture. It is used as well to optimize the restorability of the coronal portion of teeth. [14, 15]

The advantages: done under office local anesthesia, can be done using a laser for less bleeding and better postoperative recovery.

The disadvantages: Asymmetry, might require re-treatment to remove more gingival tissue or/ and bone, gingival recession, discomfort that lasts for few days. [14, 15]

4.4.1. *Case presentation*

A young male patient referred complaining of unesthetic anterior maxillary teeth. On clinical and radiographic evaluation, the patient had a poor dentogingival relation of the anterior maxillary teeth, poor crown shape, color and texture. The patient was presented to the team which advised a multi-step intervention starting from proper planning to restore the eight anterior teeth after a crown lengthening procedure using laser therapy (Figure 12).

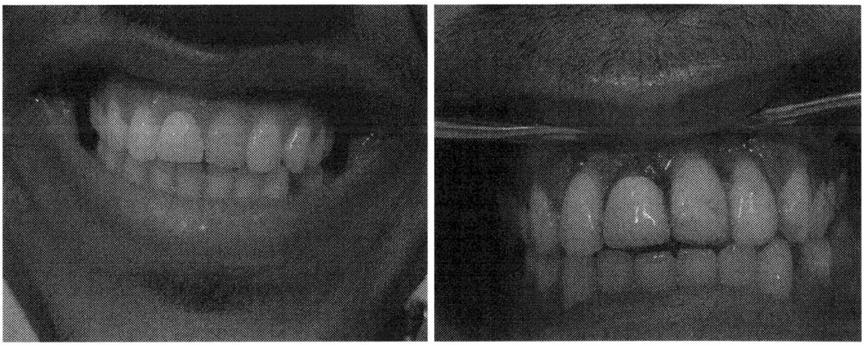

Figure 12. The picture on the left showing poor dentogingival relation of the anterior maxillary teeth. The right figure is showing the poor alveolar crestal bone relation to the first maxillary right crowned incisor, which looks short and misshapen. Those poor relations lead to esthetically non-balanced anterior maxillary teeth.

4.5. Internal smile procedures (patient's personal satisfaction)

Some patients can be unsatisfied with their smiles regardless of the type of treatment planned. Unless the operator figures out the exact factor contributing to the problem treatment will not really work. To provide examples, patients might be looking for cheek, lip, or chin piercing as the major key factors to their internal satisfaction while others, regardless of the procedures performed on their teeth, a single cheek dimple may be the change that the patient desires. And once that left cheek dimple procedure is performed, self-satisfaction is reflected positively on the actual smile (Figure 13). [18]

http://dx.doi.org/10.5772/59213

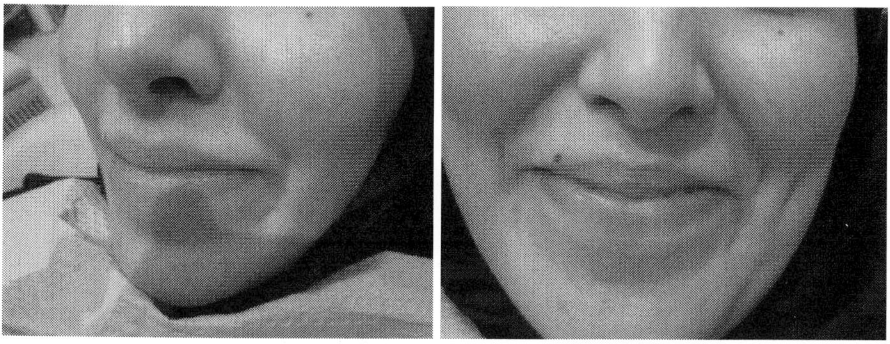

Figure 13. The patient had the desire to get a dimple on the left cheek that made her satisfied with her smile. The post-operative picture on the right side indicates a more pleasant smile.

Another situation, is where patients can have acceptable jaw skeletal relations, however, microgenia (small chin bone) or macrogenia (large chin bone) reduces their self-satisfaction of their smiles (Figure 14). Such chin deformities can be treated with genioplasty, chin augmentation or chin reduction procedures [2, 5, 7, 9, and 13].

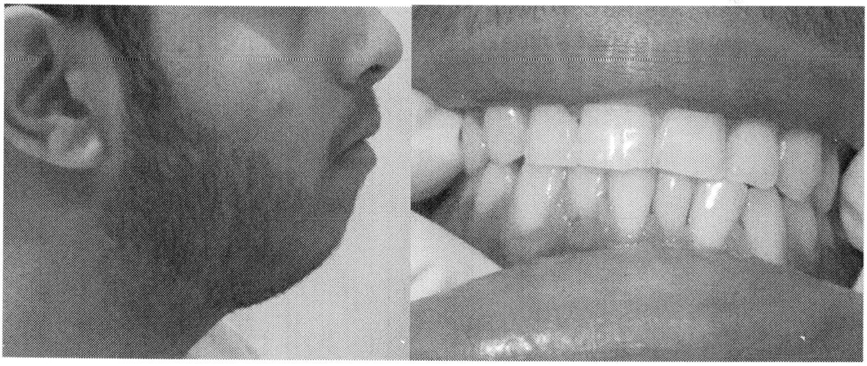

Figure 14. Although the patient presented with what looks like a retruded lower jaw (left), his occlusion is in an acceptable relation, that clarifies that the defect is mainly at the chin level, microgenia (right).

5. Conclusion

In conclusion, this chapter presents the major components of a "smile" from the anatomical aspect as well as the evaluation methodology. A multi team approach can provide the best evaluation and management plan. Hence, the term "Smile Team" is appropriate to be embraced in the medical and dental professions.

The trick is always the proper diagnosis, treatment plan, and best implementation of one or more of the treatment modalities.

6. Recommendations

It is recommended that dental students, medical students, general practitioners, and residents dealing with the facial complex consider applying training rotations at the involved specialty departments in order to get a clear exposure to the capabilities of each specialty. Such will help expanding their skills in treatment planning and seeking interspecialty care. As well, it should be noted that dealing with smiles is considered to be a very challenging task at every step of treatment, hence, managing teeth in the anterior maxillary zone with veneers, placing dental implants, or lips enhancement procedures should always be approached with caution and perhaps under the supervision of specialized providers.

Acknowledgements

The author would like to thank:

The administration of Umm Alqura University for the research support.

My colleagues and friends; Professor Motaz Ghulman (Vice dean of the faculty of dentistry at King Abdulaziz University) for his continuous support of the "smile team" patient management. As well as special gratitude to Dr Khalid Zawawi, Dr Ibrahim Yamani, Dr Mohammad Khalil, and Dr Ahmad Halawani for their interspecialty patient care.

My dear colleagues; the resident at the Saudi Board of Oral Maxillofacial Surgery, the dental students in Umm Alqura University and King Abdulaziz University whom have always been of continuous help in research and case documentation.

Author details

Mazen Almasri*

Address all correspondence to: mazen_ajm@yahoo.com

Oral and Maxillofacial Surgeon, Umm Alqura University, Saudi Arabia

References

[1] Manne P1, Zakkula S, Atla J, Muvva SB, Sampath A. Redefining smile-a multidisciplinary approach. J Clin Diagn Res. 2013 Jul;7(7):1527-9

[2] Mazen Almasri. Cosmetic considerations in facial defect reconstruction, A text book of advanced oral maxillofacial surgery, volume I. InTech Pub, 2013;573-592

[3] Nold SL, Horvath SD, Stampf S, Blatz MB. Analysis of Select Facial and Dental Esthetic Parameters. Int J Periodontics Restorative Dent. 2014 Sep;34(5):623-629.

[4] Karen L. Schmidt, Jeffrey F. Cohn. Human Facial Expressions as Adaptations: Evolutionary Questions in Facial Expression Research. Am J Phys Anthropol. 2001; Suppl 33: 3–24.

[5] Mazen Almasri, Sara Bukhari. Considerations to planning orthognathic surgery in different regions of Saudi and the Middle East. American Journal of Public Health Research, 2014, Vol. 2, No. 1, 6-9

[6] Kourkouta S., Implant therapy in the esthetic zone: smile line assessment. Int J perio Restorative Dent, 2011:31(2):195-201

[7] Niamtu J. Cosmetic oral and maxillofacial surgery options. Journal of the American Dental Association. 2000;131:756-764. 2.

[8] Al-Gunaid, T., Yamada, K., Yamaki, M., Saitod, I, "Soft-tissue cephalometric norms in Yemeni men." Am. J. Orthod. Dentofacial Orthop. 132, 2007, pp. 576.

[9] Niamtu J. New technologies in cosmetic facial surgery. VaDent J. 2000;77:9-12. 3.

[10] Alster TS, West TB. Human-derived and new synthetic injectable materials for soft-tissue augmentation: current status and role in cosmetic surgery. Plast Reconstr Surg. 2000;105:2515-2528.

[11] Burcu Bas, Bora Özan, Nükhet Çelebi. Treatment of masseteric hypertrophy with botulinum toxin: A report of two cases, Med Oral Patol Oral Cir Bucal. 2010 Jul;15 (4):649-52.

[12] Liu X, Zhu S, Hu J. Modified versus classic alar base sutures after LeFort I osteotomy: a systematic review. Oral Surg Oral Med Oral Pathol Oral Radiol. 2014 Jan;117(1): 37-44.

[13] John McLurdy, Sameul Lam. Cosmetic surgery of the Asian face. Thieme 2005.

[14] Flax H. Soft and hard tissue management using lasers in esthetic restoration Dent Clin North Am. 2011 Apr;55(2):383-402, x. doi: 10.1016/j.cden.2011.01.008

[15] Ribeiro FV1, Hirata DY, Reis AF, Santos VR, Miranda TS, Faveri M, Duarte PM. Open-flap versus flapless esthetic crown lengthening: 12-month clinical outcomes of a randomized controlled clinical trial. J Periodontol. 2014 Apr;85(4):536-44

[16] Mazen Almasri. Does Immediate Reconstruction of Postextraction Lost Buccal Plate Reduce the Chances of Implant Surface Exposure after Crown Placement? Surgical Science, 2013, 4, 110-113

[17] Mazen Almasri, Bone graft for future dental implants, the truthful reality. Lambert publishing 2013.

[18] Bao S, Zhou C, Li S, Zhao M. A new simple technique for making facial dimples. Aesthetic Plast Surg. 2007 Jul-Aug;31(4):380-3.

Section 3

Surgical Management of Periapical Lesions, Cysts of the Maxillary Sinus and Benign Tumors of the Jaws in Children

Chapter 12

Surgical Treatment of Odontogenic Periapical Lesions

Onur Gonul, Kamil Göker, Sertac Aktop and
Hasan Garip

Additional information is available at the end of the chapter

http://dx.doi.org/10.5772/59270

1. Introduction

Periradicular surgical practise is done for the treatment or prevention of periradicular pathologies. Abscess drainage, periapical surgery, corrective surgery, intentional replantation, and root removal are the most commonly performed types of periradicular surgery. Conventional endodontic treatment is generally a successful procedure; however, in 10% to 15% of cases the symptoms can persist or spontaneously recur. Findings such as a draining fistula, pain on mastication, or the incidental noting of a radiolucency increasing in size indicate problems with the initial endodontic procedure. Surgery then becomes a an important part of treatment in such cases. A decision on whether to approach the case surgically or to consider orthograde (through the coronal portion of the tooth) endodontic retreatment is dictated by various clinical and anatomic situations. Apicoectomy, apical surgery, endodontic surgery, root resection, root amputation are the terms which are used for surgery involving the root apex to treat the apical infection. It is the cutting off of the apical portion of the root and curettage of periapical necrotic, granulomatous, inflammatory or cystic lesions. In spite of adequate endodontic treatment, if periapical lesions are not resolved, then apical surgery is taken to consideration.

2. Indications

- Apical anomaly of root that blocks appropriate root canal theraphy
- Presence of lateral/accessory canal/apical region perforations
- Roots with broken instruments/overfillings

- Fracture of apical third of the root
- Formation of periapical granuloma or odontogenic cyst related with apex
- Draining sinus tract/nonresponsive to RCT
- Extension of root canal sealant cement/filling beyond the apex

3. Contraindications

- Presence of systemic diseases—leukaemia, uncontrolled diabetes, anaemia, thyrotoxicosis, etc.
- Teeth damaged beyond restoration
- Teeth with deep periodontal pockets and grade III mobility
- Traumatic occlusion
- Poor root crown ratio
- Acute infection which is nonresponsive to the treatment
- Anatomic structures (e.g., adjacent nerves and vessels)
- Structures interfere with access and visibility

4. Assessment for surgical procedures

The basic purpose of periapical surgery can be determined as follows:

- Elimination of disease
- Prevention of disease
- Removal of damaged or redundant tissue
- Improvement of function and esthetics.

In order to achieve these goals, following principles have to be estimated:

Preoperatively;

- Developing a surgical diagnosis

Intraoperatively;

- Aseptic technique
- Flap design
- Tissue handling

- Haemostasis
- Dead space management
- Decontamination and debridement
- Suturing

Post operatively;

- Oedema control
- İnfection control
- Patient's general health and nutrition
- Follow-up.

5. Incision and flap design

Surgical access is a compromise between the need for visibility of the surgical site and the potential damage to adjacent structures. A properly designed and carefully reflected flap results in good access and uncomplicated healing. Although several possibilities exist, the three most common incisions are

- Submarginal curved (i.e., semilunar) (fig:1)
- Submarginal, and full mucoperiosteal (i. e., sulcular) (fig:2)
- Submarginal and full mucoperiosteal incision has a three-corner (i.e., triangular, trapezoidal, rectangular).(fig:3)

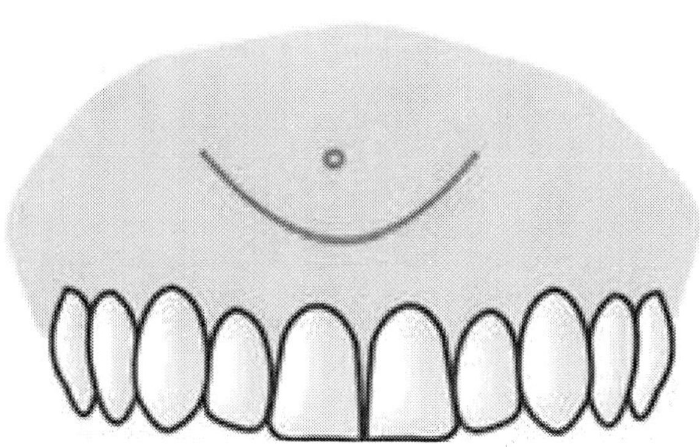

Figure 1. Semilunar incision

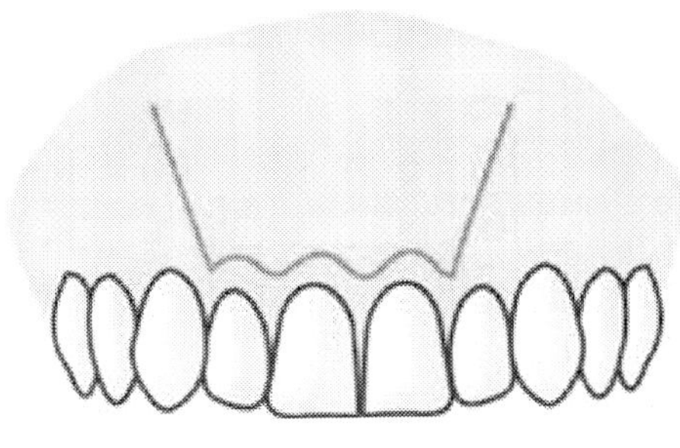

Figure 2. Submarginal incision

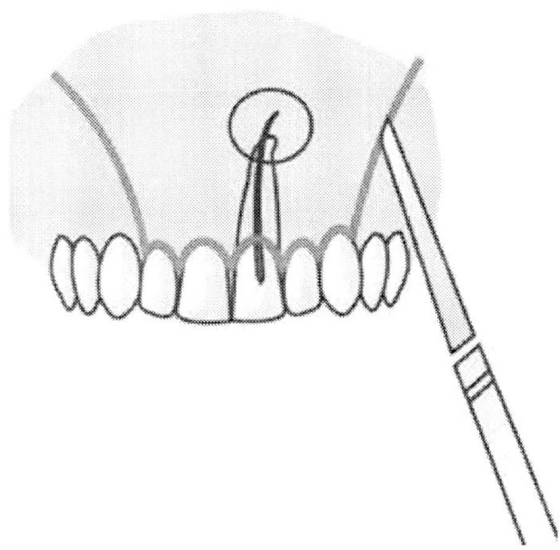

Figure 3. Full mucoperiosteal incision

6. Semilunar incision

Despite the commonly use of semilunar incision among practitioners, it's limitations and potential complications should be considered deply before surgery. Semilunar incision

is a slightly curved half-moon horizontal incision in the alveolar mucosa. Although the location allows easy reflection and quick access to the periradicular structures, it limits the clinician in providing full evaluation of the root surface. The incision is based primarily in the unattached or alveolar mucosa, which heal more slowly with a greater chance of dehiscence than a flap based primarily in attached or keratinized tissue. In addition, the flap design carries the flap over the inflamed surgical site, and this inflamed mucosa is at a high risk of breakdown. Other disadvantages to this incision include excessive hemorrhage, delayed healing, and scarring; this design is therefore contraindicated for most endodontic surgery.

7. Submarginal incision

The horizontal component of the submarginal incision is in attached gingiva with one or two accompanying vertical incisions. Generally, the incision is scalloped in the horizontal line, with obtuse angles at the corners. The incision is used most successfully in the maxillary anterior region or, occasionally, with maxillary premolars with crowns. Because of the design, prerequisites are at least 4 mm of attached gingiva and good periodontal health. The major advantage is esthetics. Leaving the gingiva intact around the margins of crowns is less likely to result in bone resorption with tissue recession and crown margin exposure. Compared with the semilunar incision, the submarginal provides less risk of incising over a bony defect and provides better access and visibility. Disadvantages include hemorrhage along the cut margins into the surgical site and occasional healing by scarring, compared with the full mucoperiosteal sulcular incision.

8. Full mucoperiosteal incision

The full mucoperiosteal incision is made into the gingival sulcus, extending to the gingival crest. This procedure includes elevation of interdental papilla, free gingival margin, attached gingiva, and alveolar mucosa. One or two vertical relaxing incisions may be used, creating a triangular or rectangular design.

The full mucoperiosteal design is preferred over the other two techniques. The advantages include maximum access and visibility, not incising over the lesion or bony defect, fewer tendencies for hemorrhage, complete visibility of the root, allowance of root planing and bone contouring, and reduced likelihood of healing with scar formation. The disadvantages are that the flap is more difficult to replace and to suture; also, gingival recession can develop if the flap is not reapproximated well, exposing crown margins or cervical root surfaces.

9. Periapical exposure

Periapical exposure must be achievedafter full thickness flap elevation by using a sterile round surgical burr. Mostly the cortical bone overlying the apex has been resorbed due to underlying apical pathosis, exposing a soft tissue lesion. If the opening is small, it is enlarged, until approximately half the root and the lesion are visible. With a limited bony opening, radiographs are used in conjunction with root and bone topography to locate the apex. Regardless of the handpiece used, there should be copious irrigation with a syringe or through the handpiece with sterile saline solution. Enough overlying bone should be removed to expose the area around the apex and at least half the length of the root. Good access and visibility are important; the bony window must be adequate. The clinician should not be concerned about the bone removal because once the infection resolves, the bone will reform. The exposure of the root is done before resecting the root to avoid the potential of blending the root in with the bone and losing surgical orientation. This is especially critical in the mandible where the bone is dense. Lower incisor roots are carefully exposed because the proximity with adjacent teeth could lead to treatment of the wrong apex. Fig:4

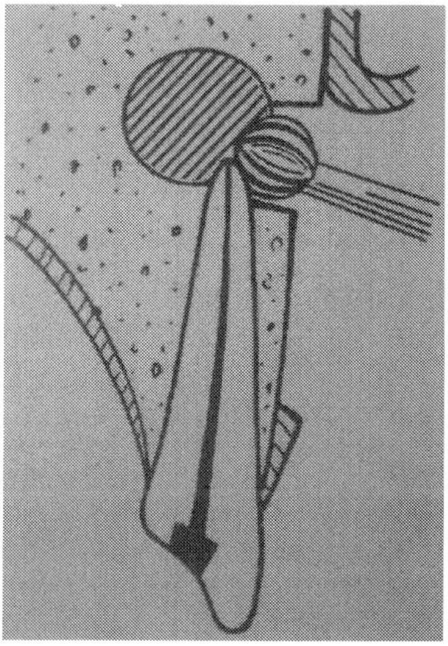

Figure 4. Periapical exposure

10. Curettage

Granulomatous, inflamed tissue around the periradicular area should be removed to gain access and visibility of the apex, to obtain a biopsy for histologic examination (when indicated), and to minimize hemorrhage. If possible, the tissue should be enucleated with a suitably sized sharp curette. Fig:5

11. Root end resection/prepertion/restoration

Apical third of the root is most likely the most difficult part to obturate properly. Presence of accessory canals increases at the apex as well, which may have not been initially cleaned and debrided, thereby leaving a source of continued infection. In general, approximately 2 to 3 mm of the root is resected more if necessary for apical access or if an instrument is lodged in the apical region; less if too much removal would further compromise stability of an already short root.Fig:5

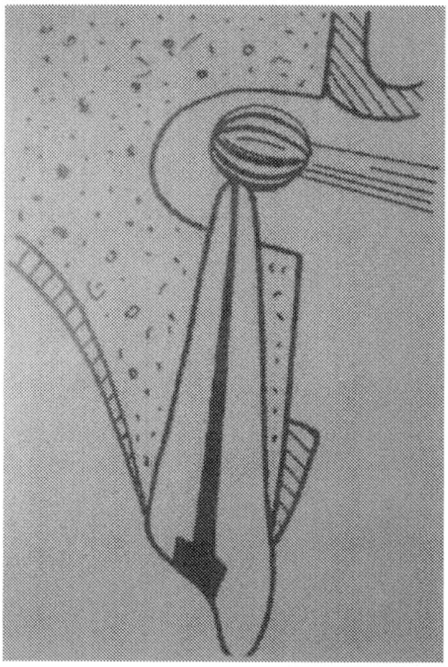

Figure 5. Root resection

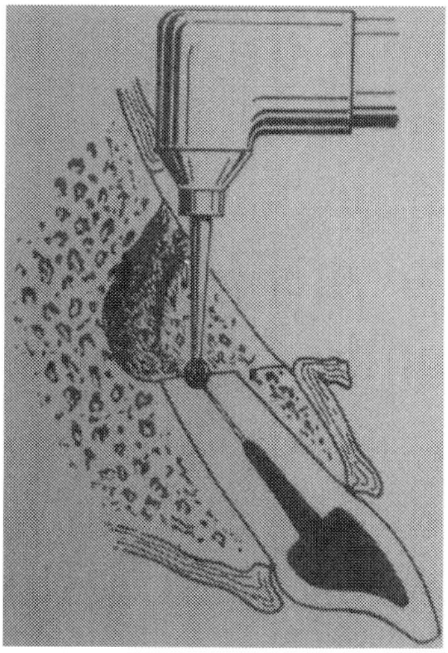

Figure 6. Root preperation for retrograd filling

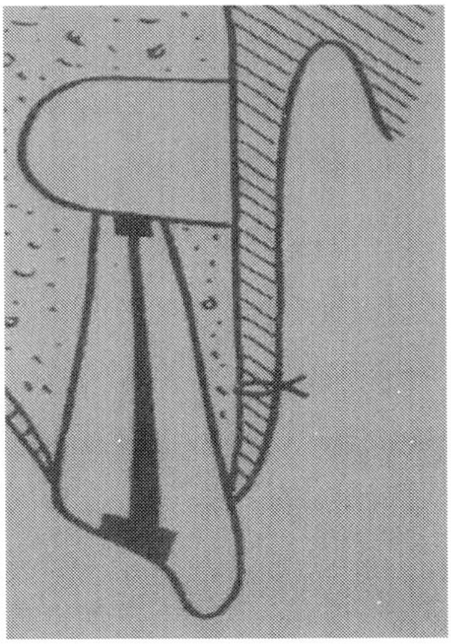

Figure 7. Suturing after retrograd filling

An angled micro handpiece and micro round bur or ultrasonic tip can be used for retropreparation. The bur or tip is placed at the apical opening of the canal and guided gently deeper into the canal as it cuts. Once the retropreparation is completed the prepared cavity is inspected. The gutta-percha at the base is recondensedwith small 0.5 mm microplugger (Fig:6). After that orot end filling material can be applied. The aim of placing root end filling material is to establish an apical seal that inhibits the leakage of residual irritants from the root canal into the surrounding tissues (Fig:7).

12. Flap replacement and suturing

After finishing surgical procedures the flap is returned to its original position and is held with moderate digital pressure and moistened gauze. Primary closure of the elevated flap is gained by basic or interrupted sutures. Absorbable monoflament or sling suture material is commonly used. After suturing, the flap should again be compressed digitally with moistened gauze for several minutes to express more hemorrhage. This limits postoperative swelling and promotes more rapid healing and adequate positioning of the flap.

13. Postoperative care

Oral and written information should be supplied in simple, straightforward language. Patient should be informed about the procedure and what is coming next. A chart like the one below can be prepared and given to patient.

- Do not raise the lip to look at the suture.
- Place an icepack on the outside of the face 20 min. out of every 1½ hour for the first

day of surgery

- Instruct to do salt wateror clorhexidine rinsing 3 times daily preferably after meal.
- Do not chew any hard food with the tooth for 1 week.
- Do not brush in the area of surgery for 1 week.
- Maintain good oral hygiene.
- Soft diet is suggested for the first 4 days.

14. Complications

Damage to the anatomic structures, bleeding, splattering of retrograd filling material at the operation site, incomplete root resection and curettage process, inadequate flap closure, healing problems of soft tissue, scar formation are the most common complications that may occur should be considered during and after the surgical procedure.

15. Prognosis

Healing capacity of involved tissues after periapical surgery is considered as good. Under the conditions that the diagnosis and treatment planning is held carefully and the intraoperative procedures achieved successfully most of the cases reveals long term uneventful follow up.

16. Sample cases

16.1. Case 1

The patient applied to our our clinic with the complaint of swelling at right maxillar buccal area. Via radiographic and clinical examination, an intrabony lesion was observed between right maxillary lateral and first molar tooth apices about 5x2 cm in size. All teeth related to lesion were devital. An aspiration biopsy performed and characteristic yellowish fluid which has kollesterin crystals in it was gained which lead us to define the lesion as a radicular cyst due to necrose pulp tissues.

Treatment plan was to have endodontic treatment after that to enucleate the cyst totally, achieve apicoectomies to all related teeth apexes and reconstruct the intrabony defect by cancellous-bone grafts and membranes. We receipt postoperative antibiotic theraupy per os (amoxicillin 875 mg+clavulanate 125 mg 2x1) for ten days. Defect area started to filled with healing tissue from the base of the cavity and the complaints of the patient disappeared considerably.

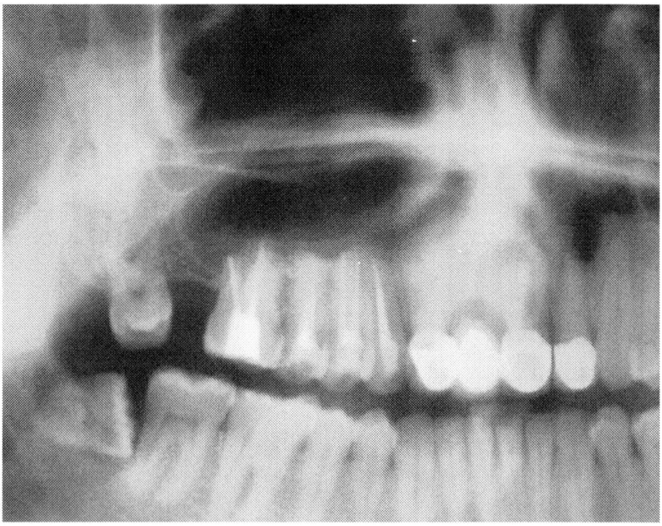

Figure 8. OPTG view before surgery

http://dx.doi.org/10.5772/59270

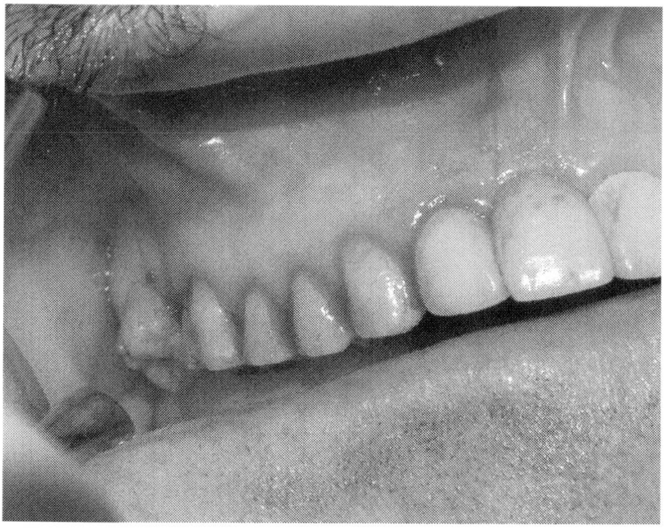

Figure 9. Incision

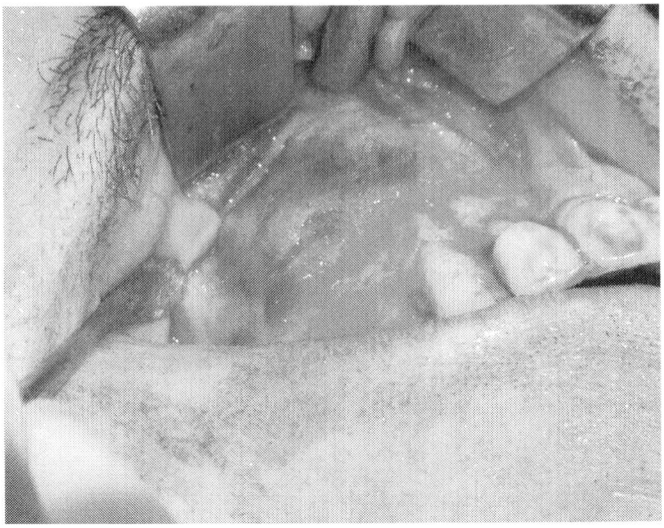

Figure 10. Exposure of Cystic Lesion

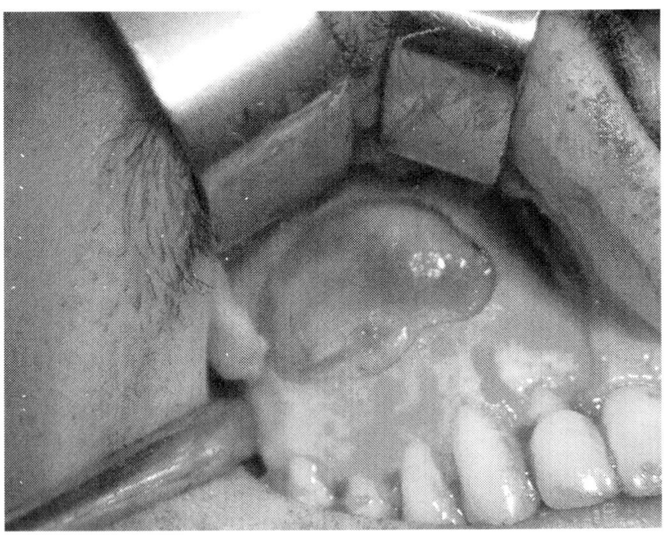

Figure 11. Elevation of Cyst Epithelium

16.2. Case 2

A 43-year-old female patient referred to our clinic with incidental OPTG examination finding of a homogenous radiolucent, sharply lined lesion located between canine teeth in anterior maxilla. On clinical examination, oral mucosa was intact and there was no evidence of bony expansion on both buccal and palatal sides. Pulp vitality testing was performed for all maxillary anterior teeth, 12 and 22 were found to be non-vital. With an inital diagnosis of inflammatory dentigerous cyst, enucleation of the lesion was planned. Prior to surgery, endodontic treatment of all involved teeth were completed. On surgical exploration, there was no expansed buccal bone was observed. After reaching the cyst capsule and performing resection of the involved roots, two seperate cystic cavities extending palatally behind the roots that have been seperated on the midline with a bony septa were encountered. Lesions were totally enucleated and submitted to histopathological examination. Result of histopathological examination was fibrotic capsule with medium degree of mononuclear cell infiltration, hyperplastic stratified squamous epithelium. In the postoperative period, healing was uneventful.

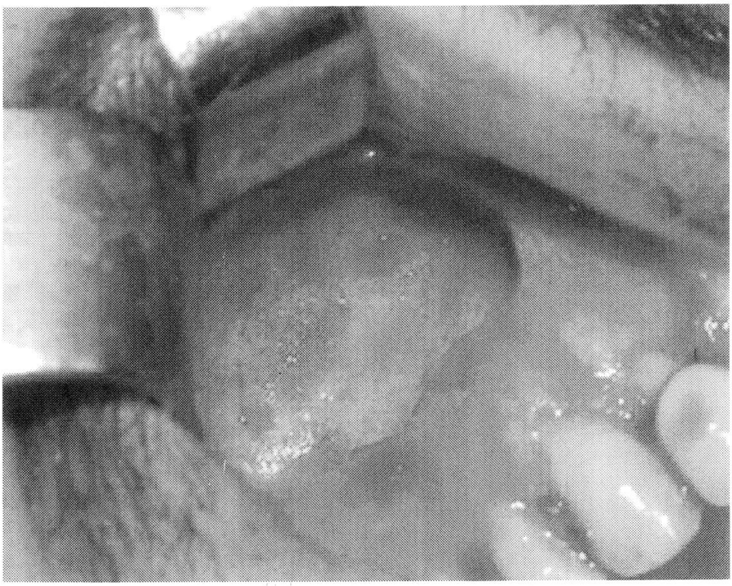

Figure 12. Cystic cavity

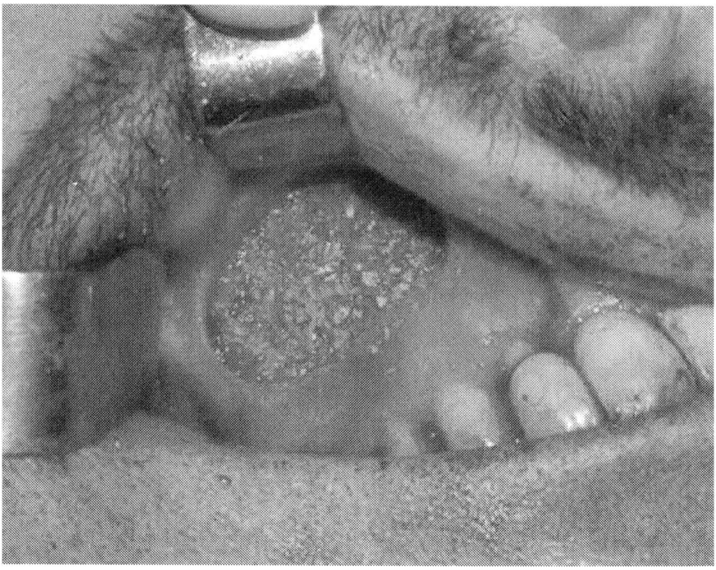

Figure 13. Graft material

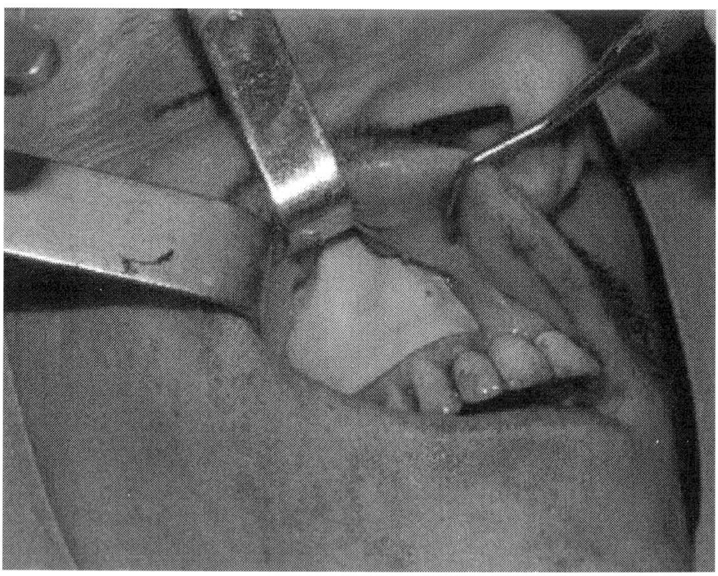

Figure 14. Application of collagen membrane

http://dx.doi.org/10.5772/59270

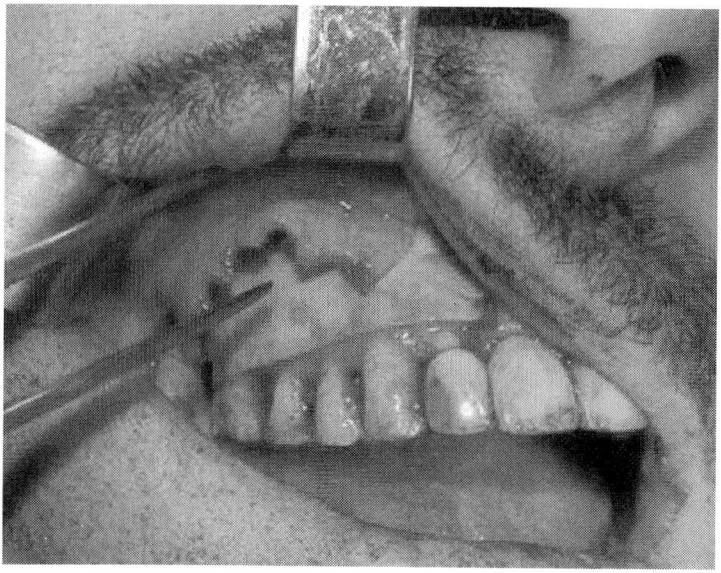

Figure 15. Adaptation of flap

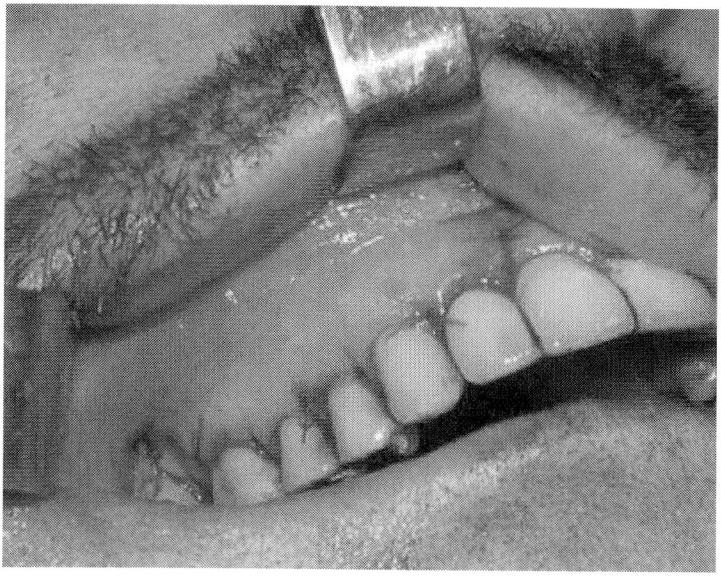

Figure 16. Primary closure of area

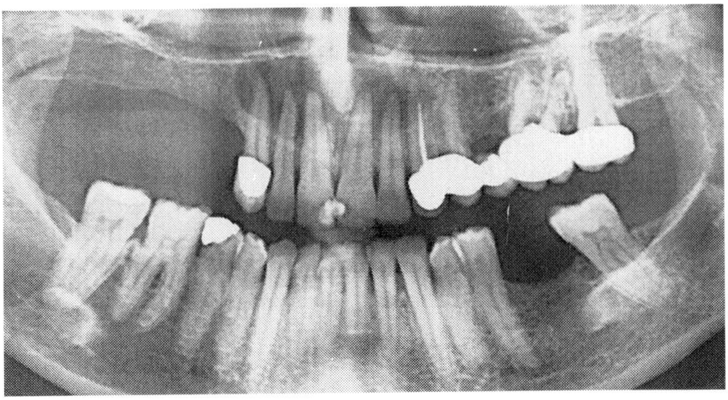

Figure 17. OPTG view

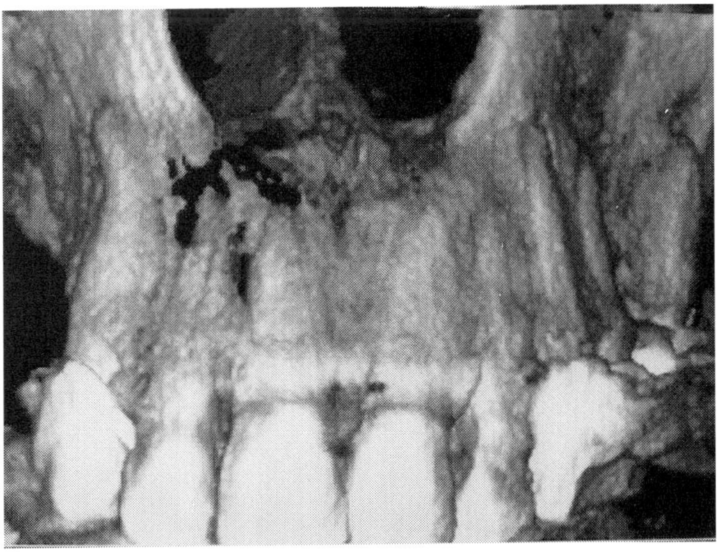

Figure 18. CT image

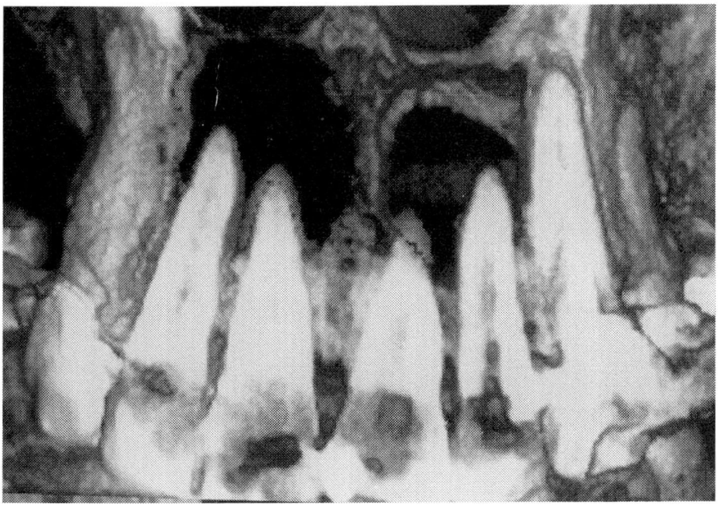

Figure 19. CT image

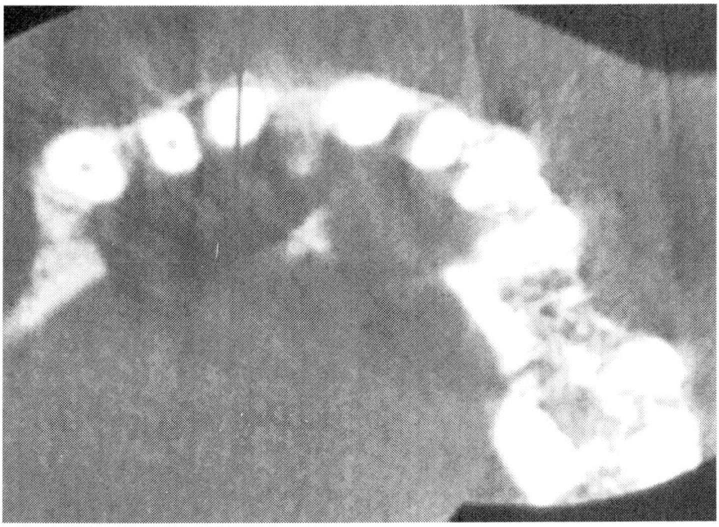

Figure 20. CT image

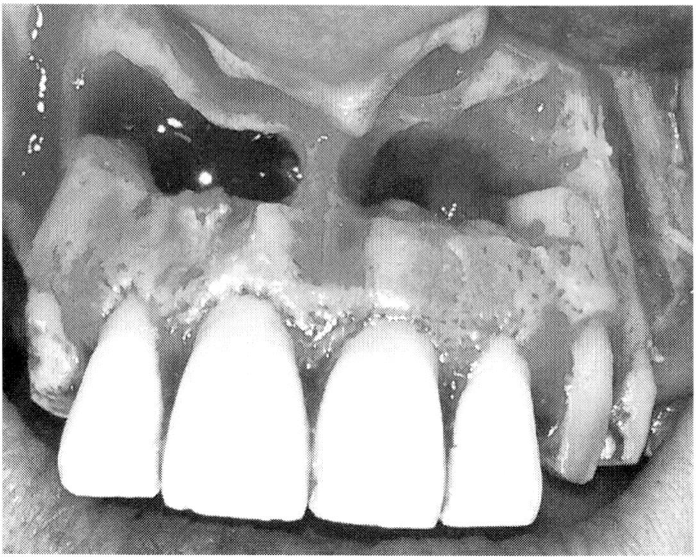

Figure 21. Cystic cavity

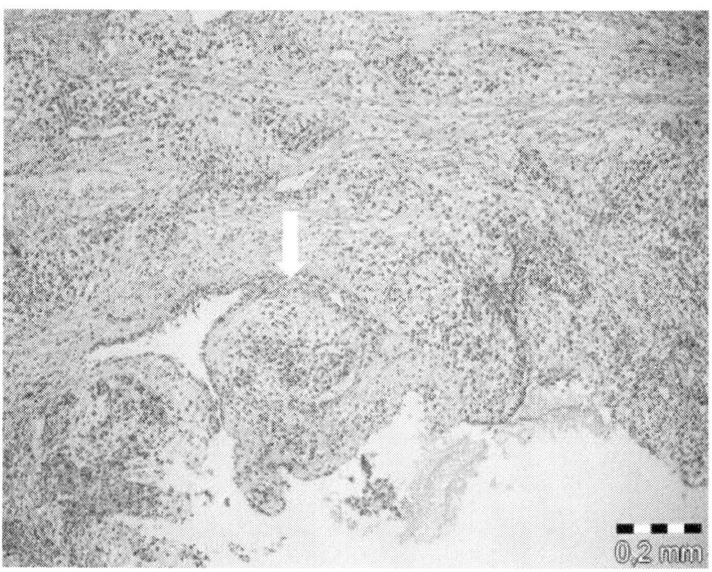

Figure 22. Histopathologic evaluation

16.3. Case 3

36-year-old female patient admitted to our clinic with complaints of pain.Clinical and radiographic examination revealed a demarcated radiolucent leson at the the apexes of the teeth no: 25,26,27. An electrical vitality test examination related to the teeth 24, 25and 27 was performed which found that teeth are non-vital, and these findings suggest that lesion was caused by non vital pulp tissues of related teeth. CT results showed that maxillary sinus bone compact and buccal cortex were perforated elevated and sinus floor was elevated by the lesion. After completion of endodontic treatment of related teeth patient have been operated under intravenous conscious sedation. During the operation, primarily by aspiration of cyst fluid pressure is reduced and the 2,3x2x1 cm sized radicular cyst was enucleated. Apical resections of relevant teeth were performed an operation region was primarily closed by 3.0 silk suture. Enucleated lesionwas sent to histopathologic examination for definitive diagnosis sent for and diagnosis was confirmed as periradicular cyst epithelium.

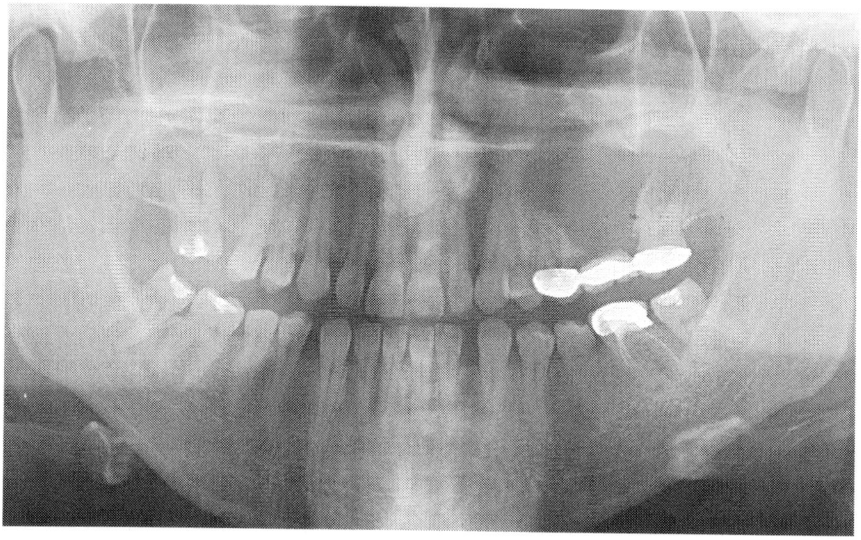

Figure 23. OPTG view

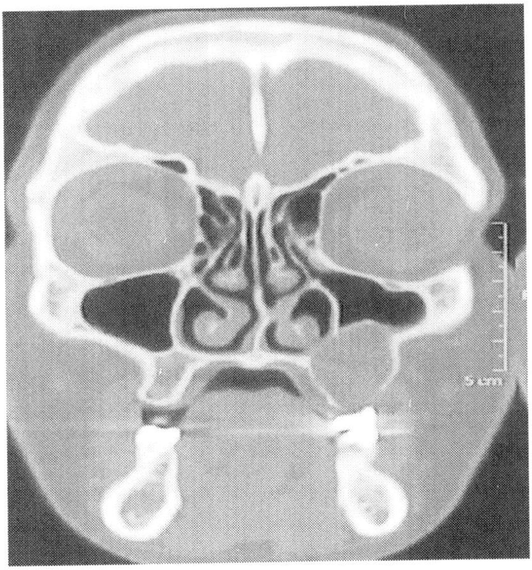

Figure 24. CT image

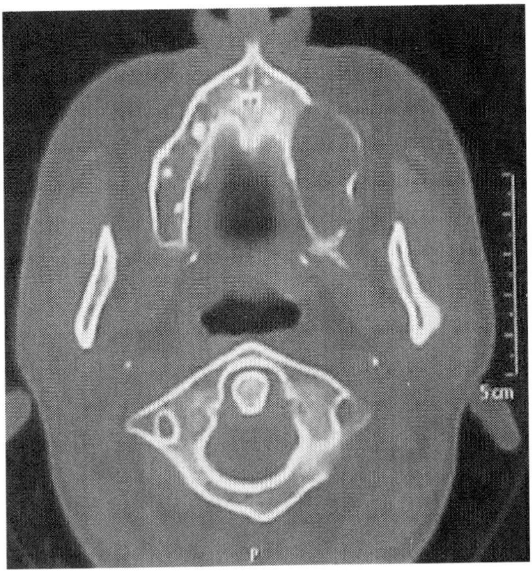

Figure 25. CT image

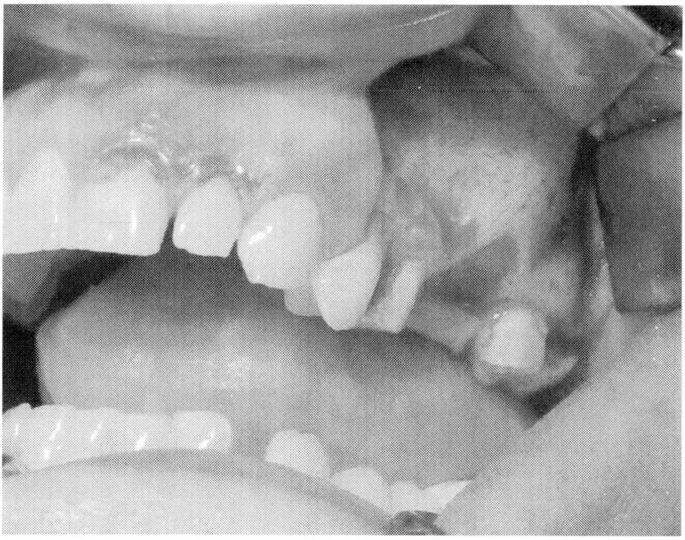

Figure 26. Exposure of lesion area

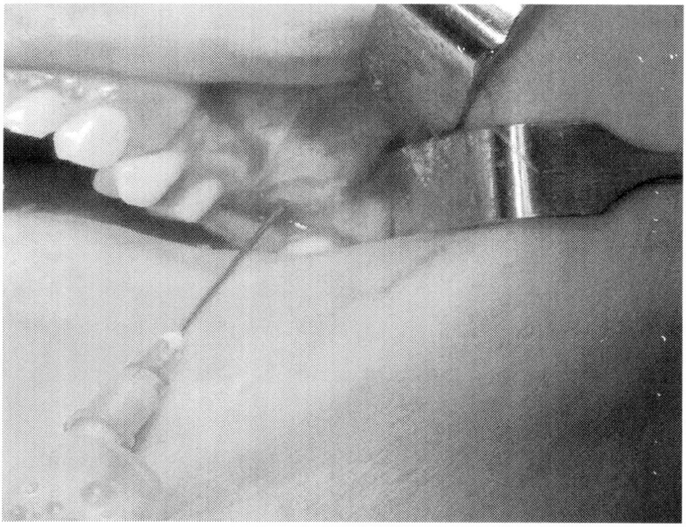

Figure 27. Aspiration of cystic liquid

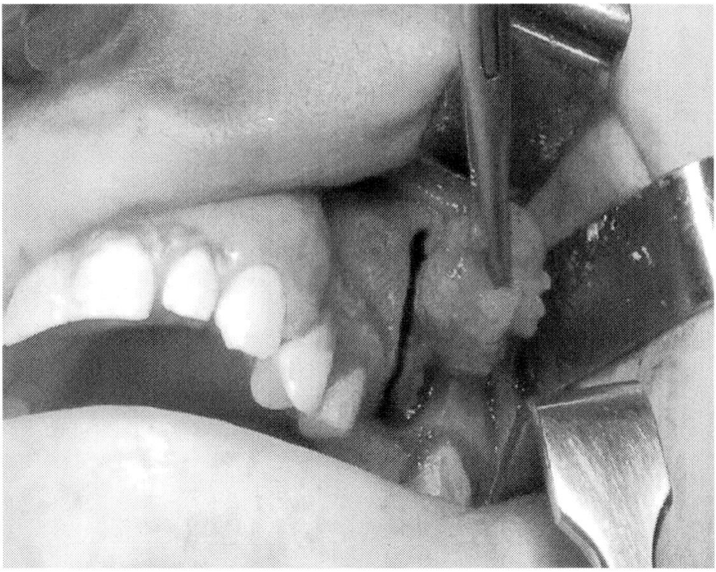

Figure 28. Enucleation of cyst epithelium

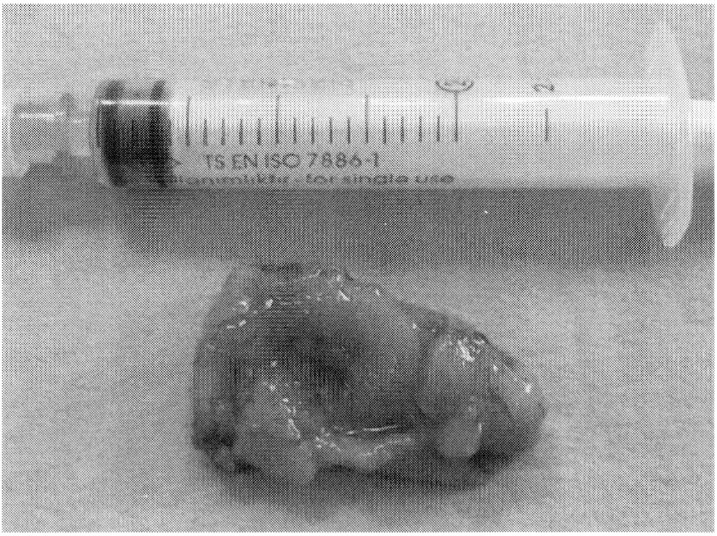

Figure 29. Cyst epithelium

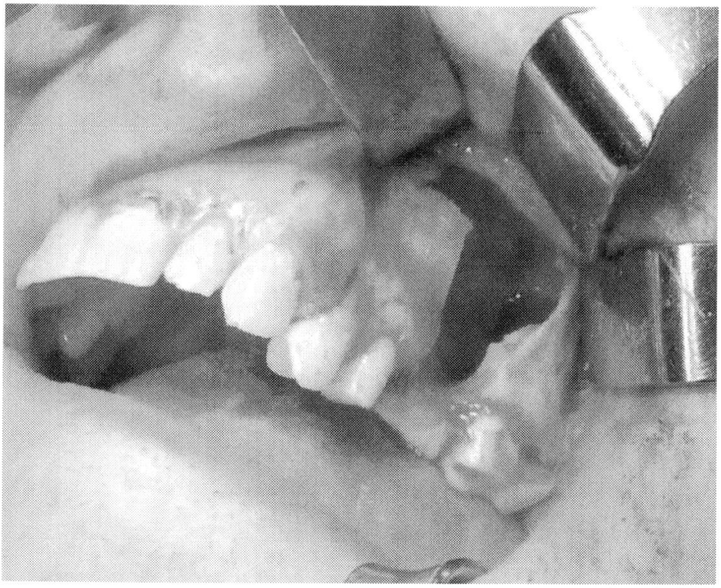

Figure 30. Cystic cavity

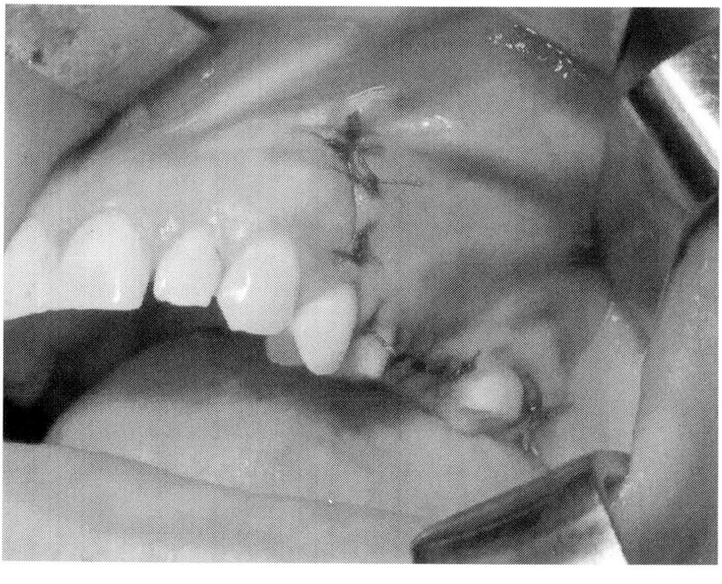

Figure 31. Primary closure of lesion area

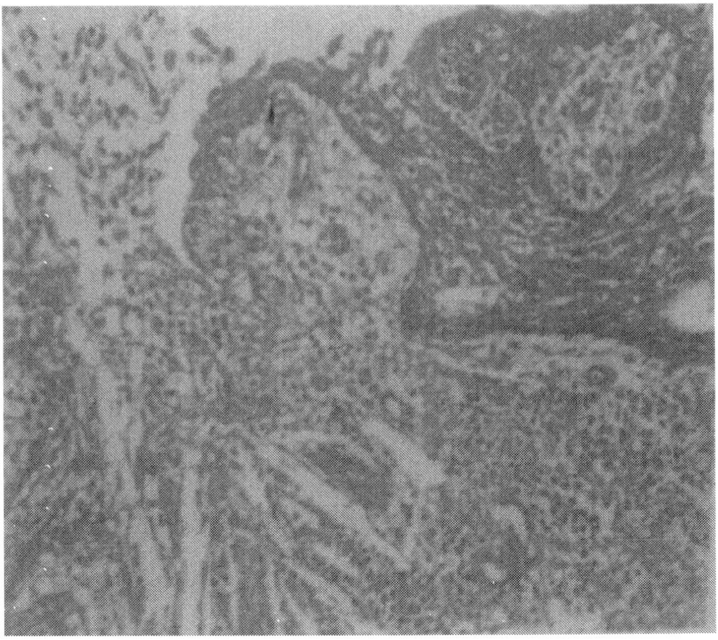

Figure 32. Histopathologic evaluation

Author details

Onur Gonul*, Kamil Göker, Sertac Aktop and Hasan Garip

*Address all correspondence to: onurgonul@yahoo.com

Marmara University, Faculty of Dentistry, Department of Oral and Maxillofacial Surgery, Istanbul, Turkey

References

[1] Sanghai S., Chatterjee P. A Concise Textbook of Oral and Maxillofacial Surgery, Jaypee Brothers Medical Publishers (P) Ltd, New Delhi, 2009

[2] Archer WH. Oral and Maxillofacial Surgery.5th Edition, WB Saunders Co. Philadelphia 1975.

[3] Baumann L, Rossman SR. Clinical Roentgenologic and Histopathologic Findings in Teeth with Apical Radiolucent Areas. Oral Surg 1956;9:1330.

[4] Shafer WG, Hine MK, Levy BM. Textbook of Oral Pathology. 4th Edition, WB Saunders Co. Philadelphia, 1983.

[5] Textbook of Oral and Maxillofacial Surgery 2008, Neelima Anil Malik Gutmann JL, Jaypee Brothers Medical Publishers (P) Ltd, New Delhi, 2008

[6] Harrison JW: Logical endodontics, Boston, 1994, Blackwell Scientific

[7] Zuolo ML, Ferreira MOF, Gutmann JL: Prognosis in periradicular surgery: a clinical prospective study, lnl Enclad J 33:9 1, 2000.

[8] Contemprary Oral and Maxillofacial Surgery Fifth Edition James R. Hupp Edward Ellis III Myron R. Tucker. Mosby, Inc., an affiliate of Elsevier Inc. 2008

[9] Illustrated Manual of Oral and Maxillofacial Surgery. Geeti Vajdi Mitra, Jaypee Brothers Medical Publishers, New Delhi; 2009

[10] Oral Surgery. Fragiskos D. Fragiskos (Ed.), Springer-Verlag Berlin Heidelberg 2007

[11] Practical lessons in Endodontic surgery Donald. E. Arens. Quintessence Publishing co,İnc 1998

[12] Barnes IE (1981) Surgical endodontics – introduction, principles,and indications. Dent Update 8:89–92, 95–99

[13] Bellizzi R, Loushine R. A Clinical Atlas for Endodontic Surgery. Quintessence, Chicago, Ill.1991

[14] Ferreira FB, Ferreira AL, Gomes BP, Souza-Filho FJ (2004) Resolution of persistent periapical infection by endodonticsurgery. Int Endod J 37(1):61–69

[15] Harrison JW(1992) Surgicalmanagement of endodontically treated teeth. Curr Opin Dent 2:115–121

[16] Taylor GN, Bump R (1984) Endodontic considerations associated with periapical surgery. Oral Surg 58:450–455

[17] Danin J, Linder LE, Lundqvist G et al: Outcomes o[periradicular surgery in cases with apical pathosis and u ntreated canals, Oral Surg Oral Med Oral Pat/101 Oral Radial Endad 87:227, 1999.

[18] Lubow RM, Wayman BE, Cooley RL: Endodontic flap design: analysis and recommendation for current usage, Oral 5urg Oral Med Oral Pathol 58:207, 1984.

[19] McDonald N, Torabinejad M : Surgical endodontics. I n Walton R, Torabinejad M, editors: Principles and practice of endodontics, ed 3, Philadelphia, WB Saunders 2002.

[20] Zuolo ML, Ferreira MOF, Gutmann JL: Prognosis in periradicular surgery: a clinical prospective study, lnl Enclad J 33:9 1, 2000

[21] Sauveur G, Roth F; Sobel M et al: The control of haemorrhage at the operative site during peri radicular surgery, lilt Endod) 32:225, 1999.

Chapter 13

Treatment Approaches for Odontogenic Cysts of the Maxillary Sinus

Hasan Garip, Sertac Aktop, Onur Gonul and
Kamil Göker

Additional information is available at the end of the chapter

http://dx.doi.org/10.5772/59087

1. Introduction

Cysts of the maxillary sinus are detected primarily as incidental findings on radiographs. These cysts often appear as rounded, dome-shaped, soft tissue masses, which are usually located on the floor of the maxillary sinus. Ectopic teeth in the maxillary sinus are readily diagnosed radiographically because they are radiopaque. Water's view, panoramic radiography and plain skull radiography are simple and inexpensive methods that can be used in daily practice. The shape and extent of the cysts can vary widely, and the position of ectopic teeth may be found very close to the eye; in such situations, conventional radiographs may not be sufficient for determining their dimensions or relationship with anatomical structures. Thus, computed tomography (CT) should be used, and patient observation should be initiated using a multidisciplinary team that includes specialists from radiology, dentistry, and surgery departments.

Multidisciplinary treatment planning is an important key component in the long-term success and quality of treatment. In some cases, endodontic treatment should be performed by a dentist or endodontist before the operation, and the vitality of the teeth should be observed closely after the operation. Generally, treatment includes enucleation of the cyst and/or surgical excision, including endoscopic observation in some cases. Long-term multidisciplinary postoperative patient observation should be performed, especially in cases with high recurrence. The aim of this section is to shed new light on treatment approaches for cysts localized in the maxillary sinus.

2. Anatomy of the maxilla

The maxillae are the largest bones of the face, after the mandible. Each assists in forming the boundaries of three cavities: the roof of the mouth, the floor and lateral wall of the nose, and the floor of the orbit. They also enter into the formation of the fossae infratemporal and fossae pterygopalatine, and two fissures, the inferior orbital and pterygomaxillary. [1] The body of the maxilla is somewhat pyramidal in shape, and contains a large cavity, the maxillary sinus (antrum of Highmore). [1]

2.1. Blood supply and venous drainage of the maxillary teeth

The arteria (a.) maxillaris arises from the a. carotis externa, which supplies the maxillary teeth. The maxillary arch is supplied by a plexus of three arterial branches: the a. alveolares superiores anteriores, a. alveolares superiores medialis, and a. alveolares superiores posteriores. The a. alveolares superiores posteriores arises from the third division of the a. maxillaris before the a. maxillaris enters the fossa pterygopalatine (Figure 1). It continues on and enters the infratemporal surface of the maxilla to supply the maxillary sinus, the premolars, and the molars (Figure 1).

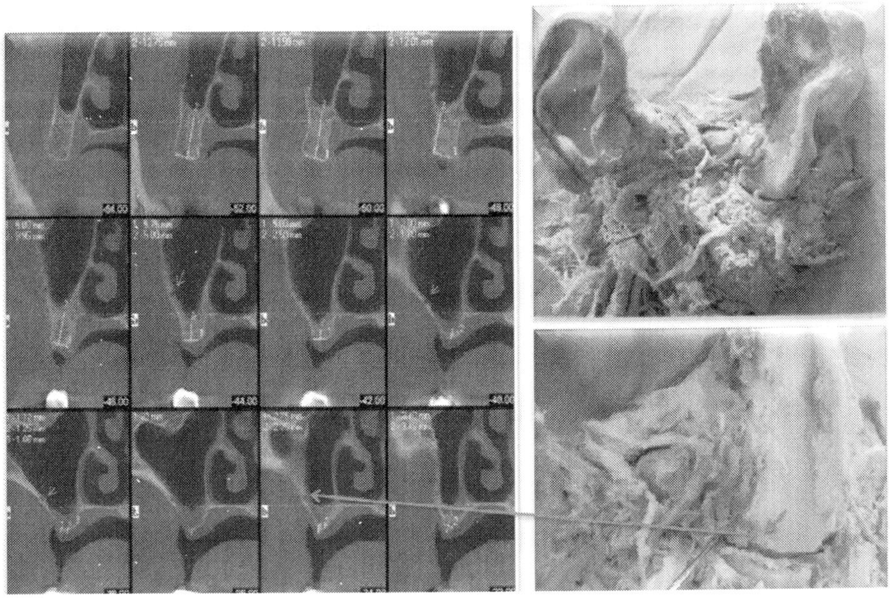

Figure 1. A. maxillaries and a. alveolares superiores posteriores.

During operations performed in this area there may be spontaneous bleeding from these vessels during surgery and sometimes serious bleeding in the postoperative period after local anesthetics lose activity. This situation may put the patient in a dangerous situation at two time points: immediately after the operation, because of bleeding, and later, after the operation, because of infection of formed clots. Careful CT examinations before the operation and appropriate surgical management will help to avoid all intraoperative and post-operative bleeding complications.

The a. alveolares superiores medialis arises from the a. infraorbitalis as does the a. alveolares superiores anteriores. It arises within the infraorbital canal where it descends to supply the maxillary sinus and plexus at the level of the canine. The a. alveolares superiores anteriores also arises at the level of the middle superior alveolar artery and runs with it to supply the anterior portion of the maxillary arch, maxillary sinus, and anterior teeth.

The venous (v.) drainage of v. alveolares superiores posteriores, v. alveolares superiores medialis, and v. alveolares superiores anteriores drain into the plexus venosus pterygoideus. [3] Some of the most important points during operations in the maxillary part of the body are first, during the design of the flap, to protect the plexus venosus pterygoideus and lymphatic drainage and, second, to be gentle during the retraction of soft tissues.

2.2. Innervation of the maxilla and of the maxillary teeth

The nervus trigeminus (the fifth cranial nerve) is a mixed nerve (n.) responsible for sensation in the face and certain motor functions, such as biting and chewing. It has three major branches: the n. ophthalmicus, n. maxillaris, and the n. mandibularis. The n. ophthalmicus and n. maxillaris are purely sensory. The n. mandibularis has both sensory and motor functions (Figure 2). [1]

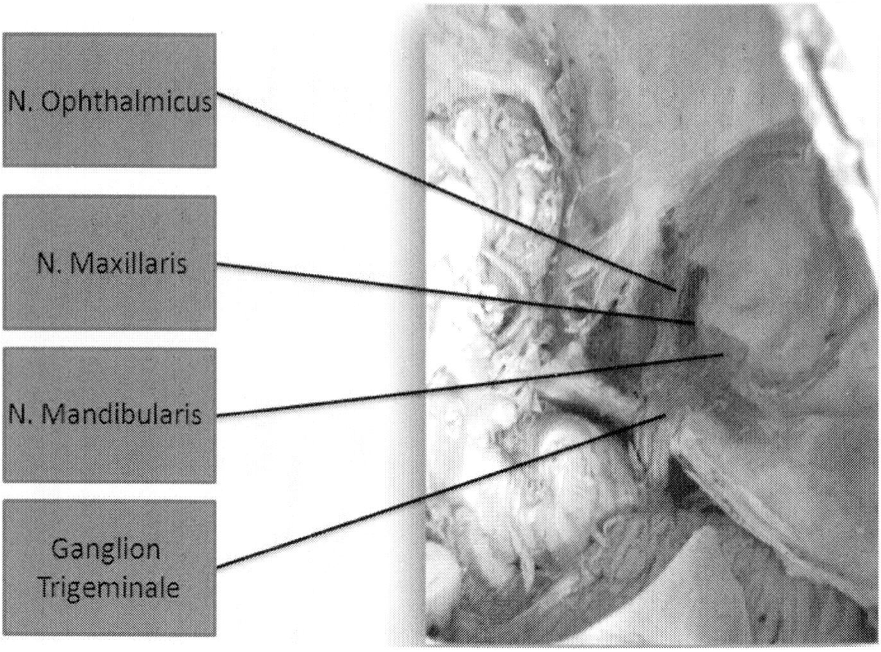

Figure 2. The nervus trigeminus

- The n. ophthalmicus carries sensory information from the scalp and forehead, the upper eyelid, the conjunctiva and cornea of the eye, the nose, the nasal mucosa, the frontal sinuses, and parts of the meninges.
- The n. maxillaris carries sensory information from the lower eyelid and cheek, the nares and upper lip, the upper teeth and gums, the nasal mucosa, the palate and the roof of the pharynx, the maxillary, ethmoid and sphenoid sinuses, and parts of the meninges. It leaves the ganglion trigeminale between the n. ophthalmicus and the n. mandibularis lateral to the sinus cavernosus. The nerve leaves the cranium forward, through the foramen rotundum and enters the fossa pterygopalatina where it divides into three main branches: the n. zygomaticus, n. infraorbitalis, and truncus pterygopalatinus.
- The n. infraorbitalis is a direct extension of the n. maxillaris. It leaves the fossa pterygopalatina and enters the orbit through the fissura orbitalis inferior, together with a. infraorbitalis. The nerve runs forward on the floor of the orbita in one fulcrum, which turns anteriorly to the canalis infraorbitalis. Going forward it leaves the maxilla through the foramen infraorbitale (Figure 3), positioned on the anterior wall of the maxilla under the sutura zygomaticomaxillaris, and gives rise to terminal branches.

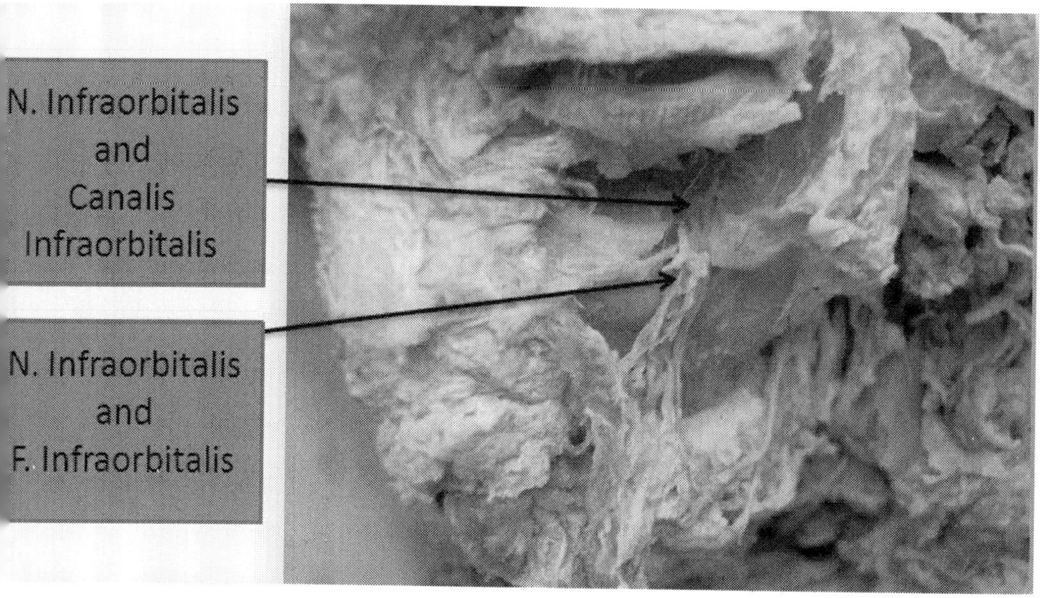

Figure 3. N.infraorbitalis, c. infraorbitalis and f.infraorbitalis

The n. alveolares superiores arises from the n. maxillaris in the fossa pterygopalatina just before n. infraorbitalis enters the orbita or arises from the n. infraorbitalis in the sulcus infraorbitalis. The upper alveolar nerves are divided in three groups: the n. alveolaris superior posterior, the n. alveolaris superior medius, and the n. alveolaris superior anterior. [4] Working 5 mm above the roots of the teeth in the maxilla will avoid damage to the neurovascular plexus. [5] This is one of the most important points during surgical procedures performed in the maxillary sinuses when the teeth are vital (Figure 4). A second important point is to avoid damage to the n. infraorbitalis, which is commonly damaged during elevation and retraction of mucoperiosteal flaps.

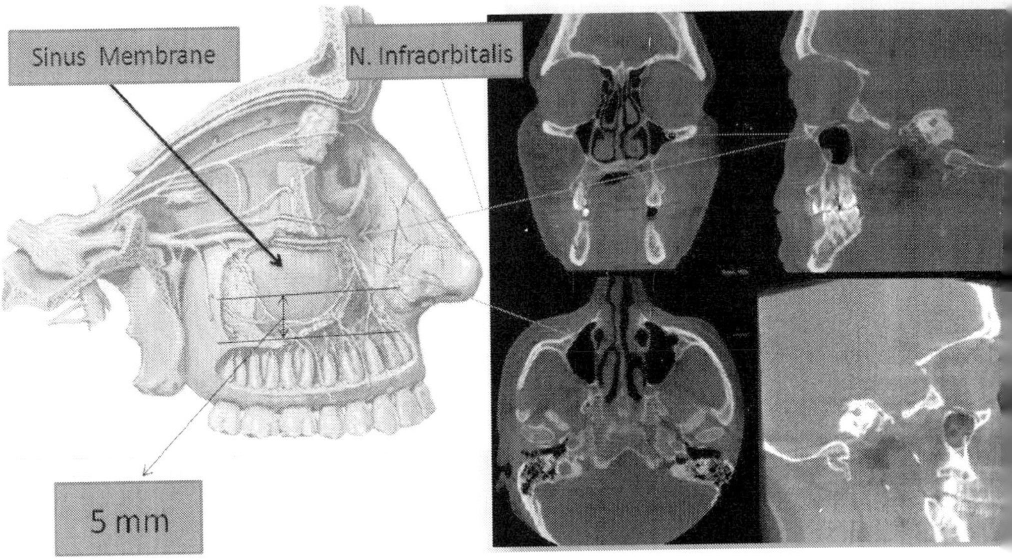

Figure 4. N. infraorbitalis, c. infraorbitalis and f. infraorbitalis (part of figure adapted from Netter).

The n. mandibularis carries sensory information from the lower lip, the lower teeth and gums, the chin and jaw, parts of the external ear, and parts of the meninges. The mandibular nerve carries touch/position and pain/temperature sensation from the mouth. It does not carry the taste sensation; the chorda tympani is responsible for taste. However, one of its branches, the lingual nerve, carries somatic sensation from the tongue.

3. History and anatomy of the maxillary sinus

The maxillary sinus was first discovered and illustrated by Leonardo da Vinci (1452-1519), but the earliest scientific description is attributed to the British surgeon Nathaniel Highmore (1613-1685). [2] The sinus maxillaris is located behind the anterior wall of the os. maxillaris, under the orbital cavities and above the alveolar bone of the teeth. It has the shape of a pyramid, with a volume of ~15 cc, inferosuperior length of 33 mm, a mediolateral length of 23 mm, and anteroposterior length of 34 mm (Figure 5). The deepest point of the maxillary sinus is normally located in the area of the molar roots; the next deepest area is at the premolar roots. Thus, the risk of exposing the maxillary sinus intraoperatively is greatest when molar teeth are extracted (Figure 6). [6-10]

Kiliç et al. [8] evaluated the maxillary sinus regions from 92 patients, using dental cone-beam CT. This study showed that ~10.5% of molar roots were located in the maxillary sinus. Jung and Cho [9] in their study showed that 28.1% of molar roots were located in the maxillary sinus. Hirata et al. [10] investigated 1337 patients after 2038 molar extractions and found 3.8% maxillary sinus perforations. In addition to the relationship between the roots and the maxillary sinus floor, exposing the maxillary sinus intraoperatively when molar teeth are extracted depends on the shape and distance of the roots from each other, extraction technique, skill and experience. Knowledge of the anatomical shape of the maxillary sinus and the relationship between the sinus floor and tooth apices, careful planning, and good extraction technique will avoid maxillary sinus perforations.

The paranasal sinuses and the majority of the nasal cavity itself are lined with pseudostratified columnar ciliated epithelium (respiratory type). The cilia suspend a mucous blanket, which is secreted by goblet cells in the mucous membrane. [11] The sinus maxillaris has an opening for drainage, the ostium, located on the medial wall into the hiatus semilunaris. The position of the ostium does not help draining of sinus contents when the head is in an upright position. Before operation, this opening should be checked in CT scans for any obstruction. Ordinarily, it has a diameter of 5-7 mm and a length of 1-2 mm.

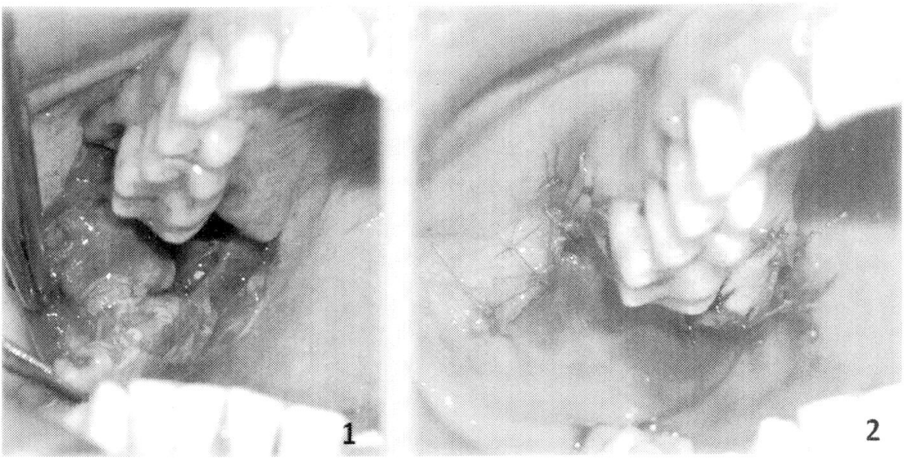

Figure 6. Maxillary sinus exposed after second molar tooth extraction.

Janner et al. [12] reported that the thickness of the Schneiderian membrane showed a wide range, with a minimum value of 0.16 mm and a maximum value of 3.461 mm. The highest mean values, ranging from 2.16 to 3.11 mm, were found for the mucosa located in the mid-sagittal regions of the maxillary sinus. Dagassan-Berndt et al. [13] stated that in the molar regions with periodontal destruction, Schneiderian membrane thickening occurred, particularly in combination with small bone layers above the root tips or periapical lesions.

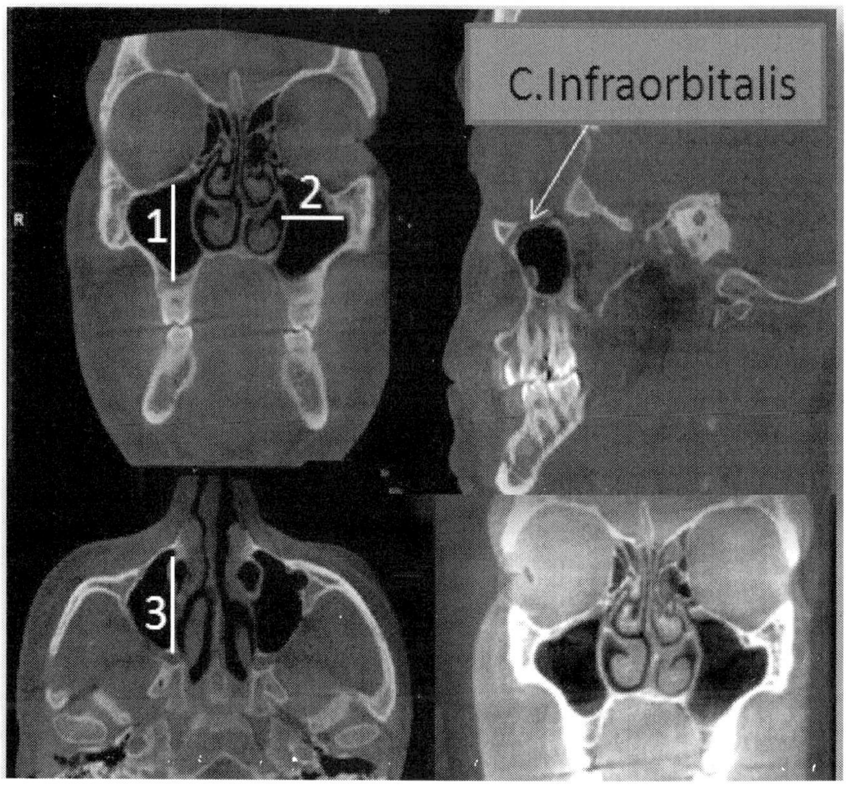

Figure 5. The sinus maxillaries. Volume ~15 cc and pyramidal shape. 1. inferosuperior length 33 mm, 2. Mediolateral length 23 mm, 3. Anteroposterior length 34 mm.

4. Etiology of cysts localized in the maxillary sinus

A cyst is a lesion consisting of an epithelial sac, filled with fluid or semisolid material, and is surrounded by a connective tissue capsule. Cysts are more commonly seen in the maxilla than the mandible. The most common causes of cysts localized in the maxillary sinus are chronic infection, allergic sinonasal disease, trauma, previous surgery, obstruction of the sinus ostium, accumulations of secretions, ectopic teeth, foreign bodies (e.g., dental implant, tooth roots, graft materials), dental infections, incomplete sealing of all communications between the root canal system and periradicular tissues during endodontic treatment, mechanical obstruction of mucociliary flow, defects in ciliary capabilities to propel the mucous blanket and genetic factors. Pathologically, a cyst can develop and grow in the sinus until it reaches a large size with no serious complaint by the patient because of the anatomy of the sinus. [14-16]

5. Cyst treatment options

Marsupialization (Partsch I) procedure is a technique for making a surgical incision in the cyst capsule, minimizing intracystic pressure, and evacuating its contents, then suturing the edges of the cyst to the healthy surface of the oral mucosa to establish a large permanent opening (Figure 7).[17]

Decompression is a technique that relieves the pressure within the cyst by making a small opening in the cyst and keeping it open. This can be achieved with a drain or obturator. Each day the obturator should be removed and the cyst cavity should be irrigated. The cyst size will decrease and any damage to important structures upon enucleation will be diminished (Figures 8, 9). [18]

The decompression and marsupialization of cysts were first suggested by Partsch in the German literature in the late 19th century. [18] Indications for such marsupialization and decompression are large cysts with thin bony walls that may cause spontaneous fracture, cysts that are very close to structures such as the n. alveolaris inferior or nasal floor, and infected cysts. [17, 18, 19]

Enucleation (Partsch II procedure) is a procedure in which all pathological tissue is removed and wound edges are closed (Figure 10). [18]

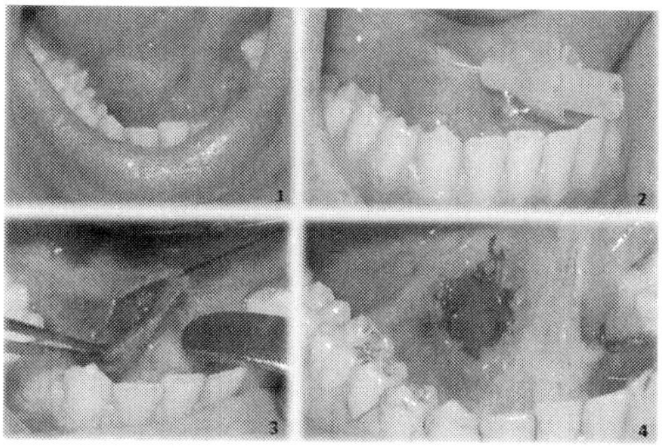

Figure 7. Marsupialization (Partsch I) procedure of a ranula.

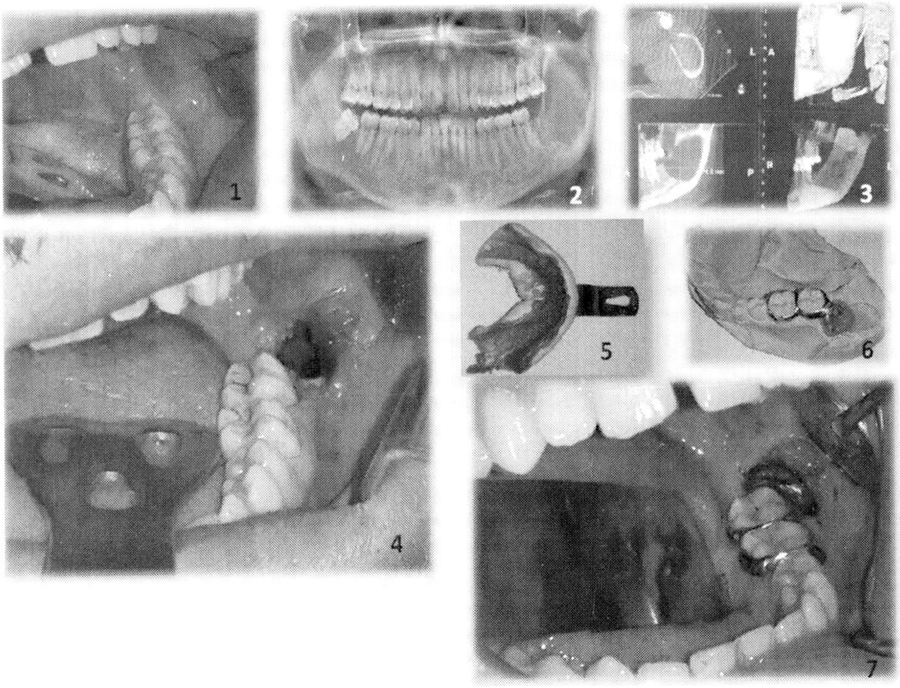

Figure 8. Decompression technique for a dentigerous cyst.

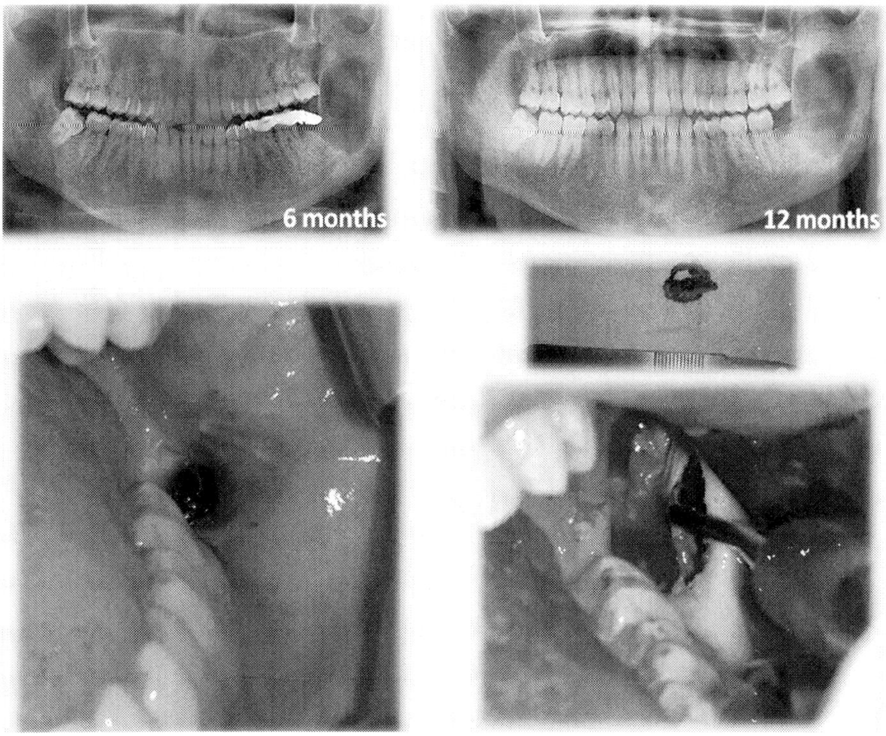

Figure 9. Enucleation after 12 months of decompression.

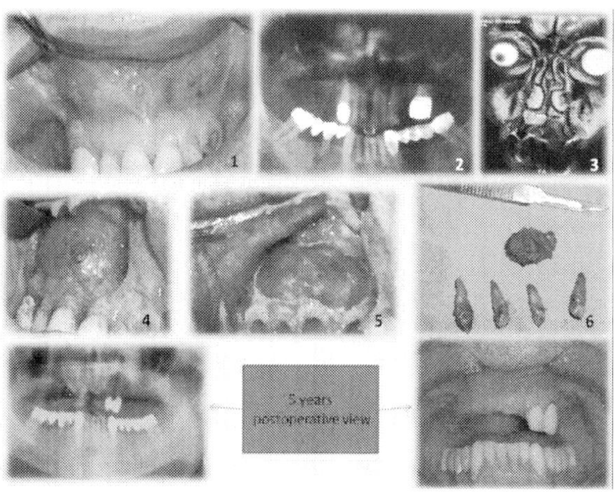

Figure 10. Enucleation (Partsch II procedure) of an odontogenic keratocyst.

6. Cases

6.1. Case 1

A 19-year-old male was referred to our department of oral and maxillofacial surgery with a 3-week history of swelling on the right side of the face. There was no history of trauma, pain, paresis, paresthesia, or lymphadenopathy. There was slight but obvious facial asymmetry caused by the swelling over the right maxillary region. The mass was firm and non-tender on palpation and not adherent to the overlying skin. Intra-oral examination showed little expansion of the upper right third molar region.

A panoramic radiograph and CT showed a well-defined unilocular radiolucency involving the right maxillary sinus along with the impacted third molar in the top part of the maxillary sinus in conjunction with the orbital floor. A vitality test was performed; all the teeth were vital.

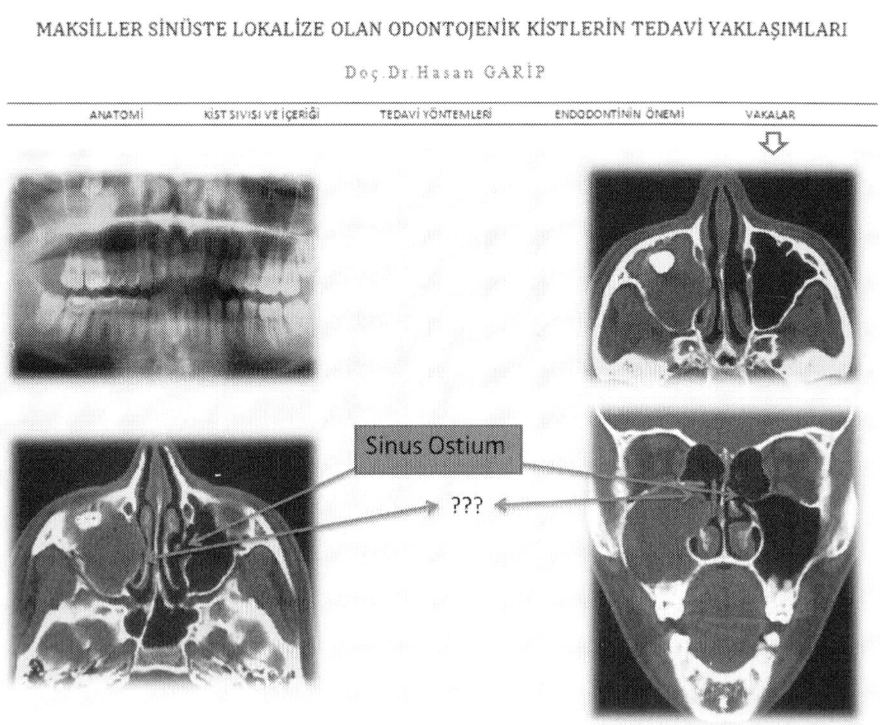

Figure 11. Panoramic radiograph and CT views.

In cases like this, careful examination is important. Points that should be checked include possible obstruction of the sinus ostium (Figures11, 12), the need for an antrostomy procedure, the route of the canalis nasolacrimalis, resorption of the posterior bony wall of the sinus, continuity of the orbital floor, and eye examinations before and after the operation. In such operations where visualization is a problem, an endoscopic-assisted approach is mandatory. [20] Endoscopic sinus surgery has been performed for various indications in maxillofacial surgical practice. It has been used for the assessment of antral pathologies, removal of foreign bodies, orthognathic procedures, and the treatment of facial fractures. [21, 22] Especially after finishing the removal of a cyst and tooth in operations like this using endoscopy, the surgeon should check any remaining pathology of the cyst, continuity of the orbital floor, to assess the possibility of a blow-out fracture [23], root tips of the teeth and any possible damage, check the aperture of sulcus nasolacrimalis, and perform an antrostomy using endoscopic assistance as needed. [24]

The operation was performed under general anesthesia, combined with local anesthesia. A mucoperiosteal flap was opened in two layers (Figure 13). Through a modified Caldwell-Luc approach, the cyst was exposed (Figure 14). At this stage in the operation, saving teeth vitality is the most important point, so it is important to work at least 5 mm away from the teeth apices. After the pus was removed from the cyst, the tooth was carefully extracted under endoscopic assistance and the remaining part of the cyst was then enucleated (Figure 15, 16). Using endoscopy, the cavity was checked (Figure 17) and packing of the sinus (Figure 18) was performed; this was removed 3 days later. Vitality of the teeth were checked for the last time at 3 months after the operation and all teeth were vital.

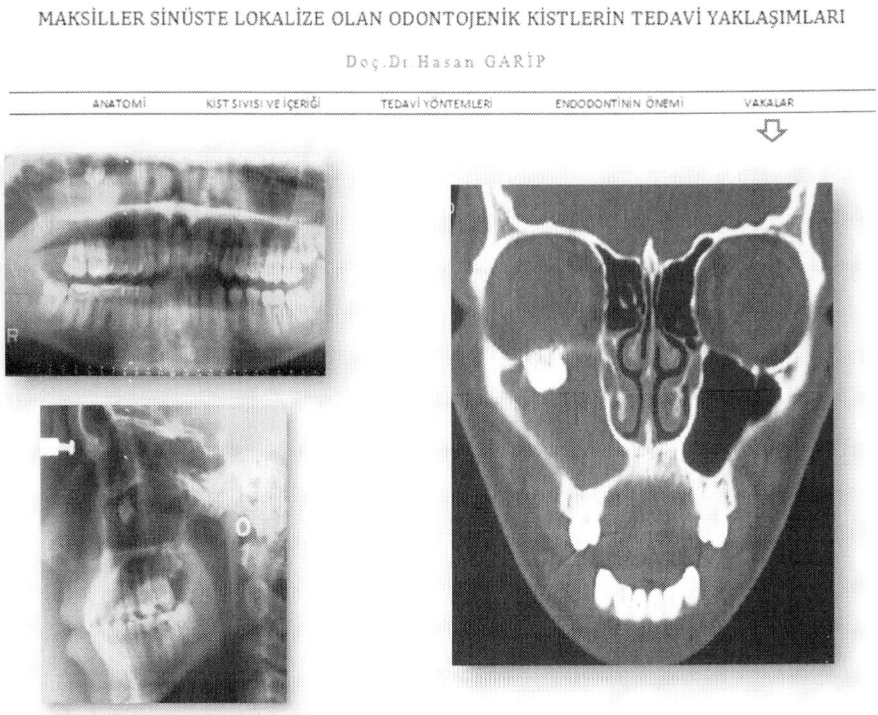

Figure 12. Panoramic radiograph, lateral cephalometric and CT views showing tooth in the right maxillary sinus.

http://dx.doi.org/10.5772/59087

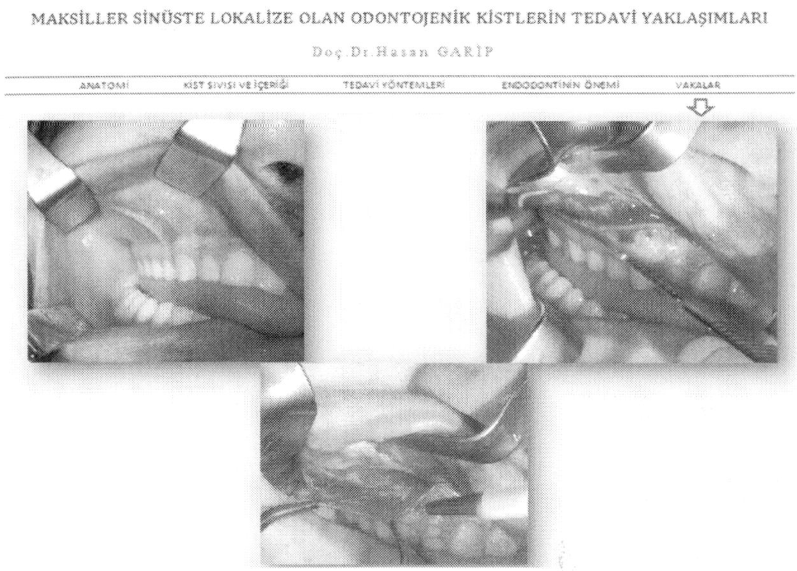

Figure 13. Mucoperiosteal flap preparation.

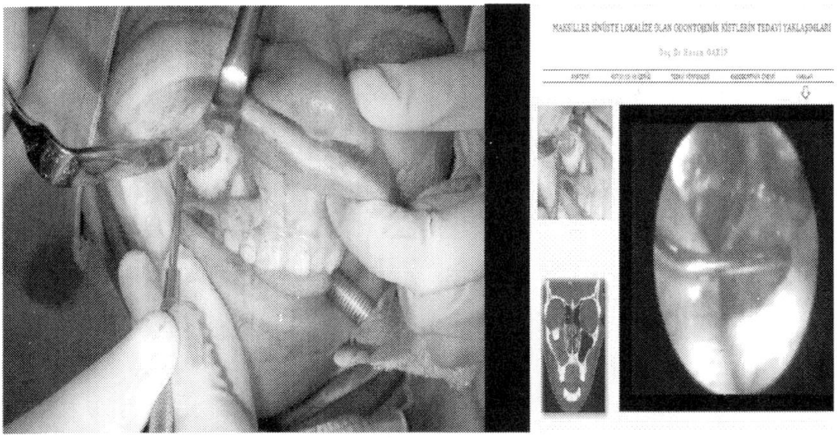

Figure 14. Exposure of the cyst. Endoscopic view (right).

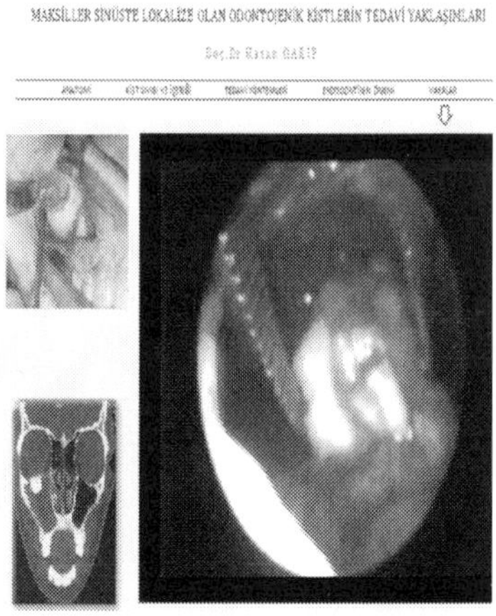

Figure 15. Enucleation of the cyst.

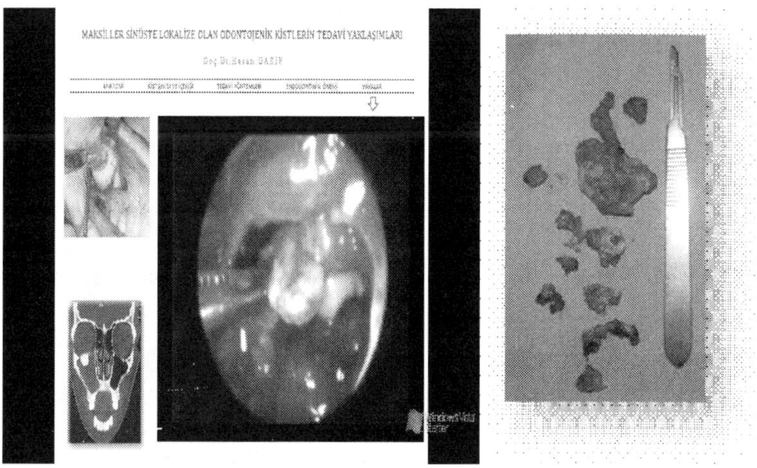

Figure 16. Extraction of the tooth.

http://dx.doi.org/10.5772/59087

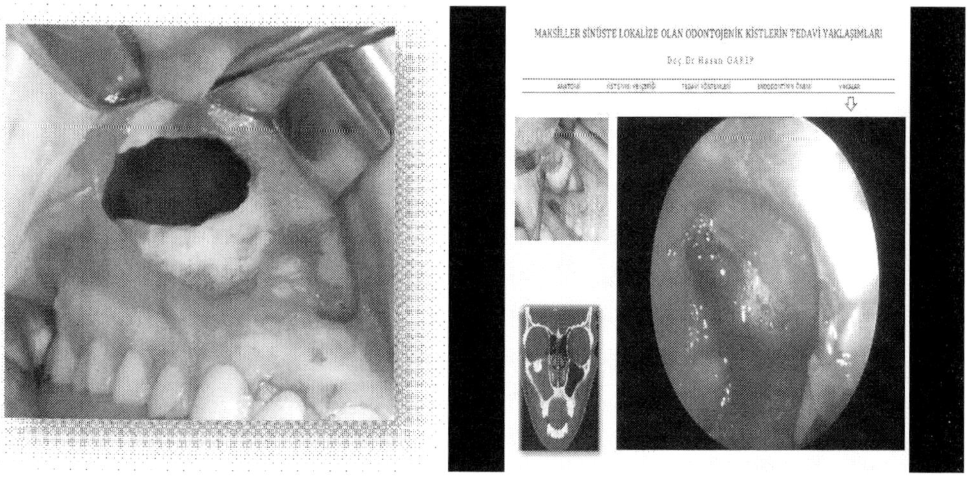

Figure 17. Postoperative cavity checking.

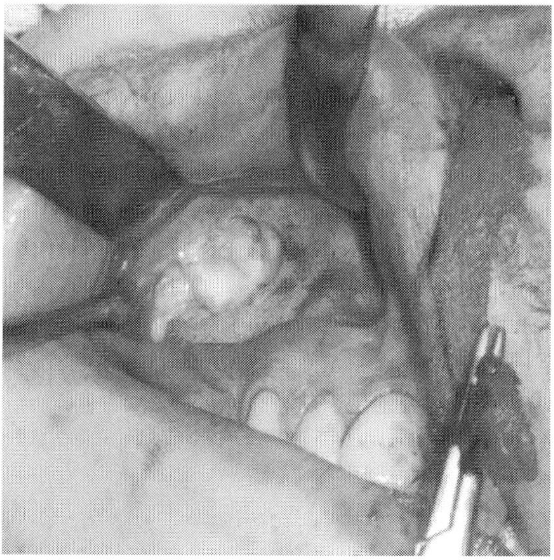

Figure 18. Packing of the sinus after antrostomy.

6.1.1. Intranasal inferior meatal antrostomy technique

An intranasal inferior meatal antrostomy is a process of making an opening in the nasoantral wall of the inferior meatus by an intranasal route. The nasoantral wall of the inferior meatus is perforated with a curved hemostat and then this opening is enlarged. The opening should be 1.5-2 cm in diameter and as close to the floor of nose as possible (Figure 19). Intrasinus pus/ debris should be removed by suction. Packing into the sinus is achieved from the posterior, packing layer-by-layer upwards and forwards (to facilitate removal through the antrostomy) and nose packing may also be required if there is severe bleeding (Figure 20). [25]

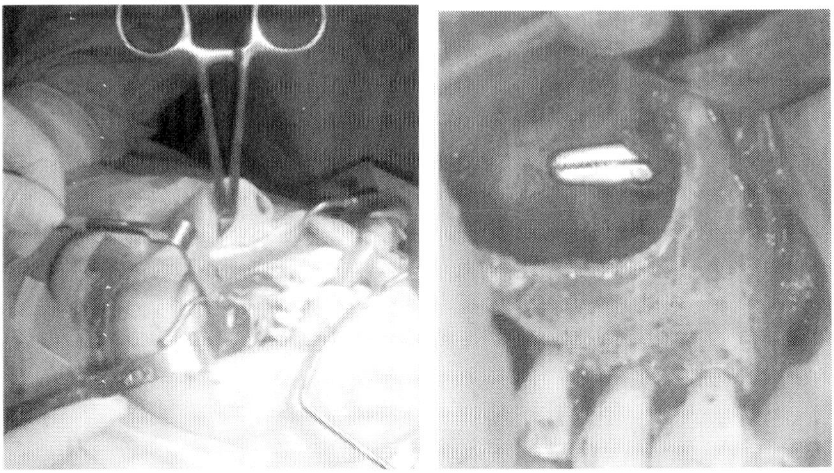

Figure 19. Intranasal inferior meatal antrostomy technique.

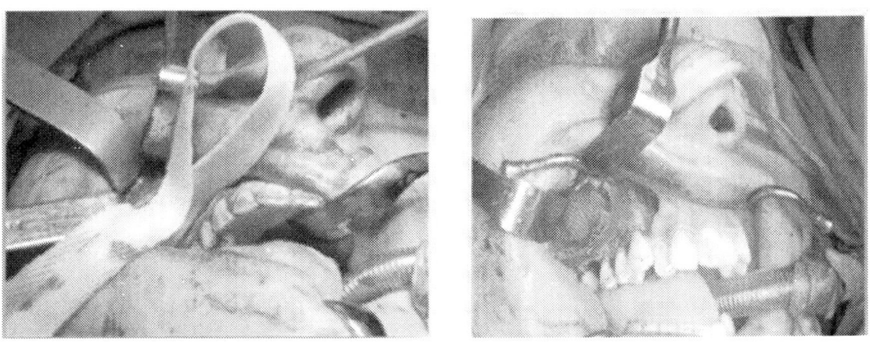

Figure 20. Packing of the sinus maxillaris.

6.2. Case 2

During an incidental radiological exam (orthopantomograph, OPG, Figure 21 at our department of radiology, a 51-year-old male with no complaints and no history of any trauma, pain, paresis, paresthesia, or lymphadenopathy, was discovered to have an ectopic tooth in the right maxillary antrum. A CT scan (Figure 21) was performed and all important points were checked. An operation was performed under general anesthesia with combined local anesthesia. Using a crestal incision, a trapezoid mucoperiosteal flap was designed and carefully elevated. The tooth was extracted under endoscopic assistance (Figures 22, 23) and a dentigerous cyst was enucleated (Figure 24). Using endoscopy, all cavities were checked and packing of the sinus was performed; this was then removed 3 days later.

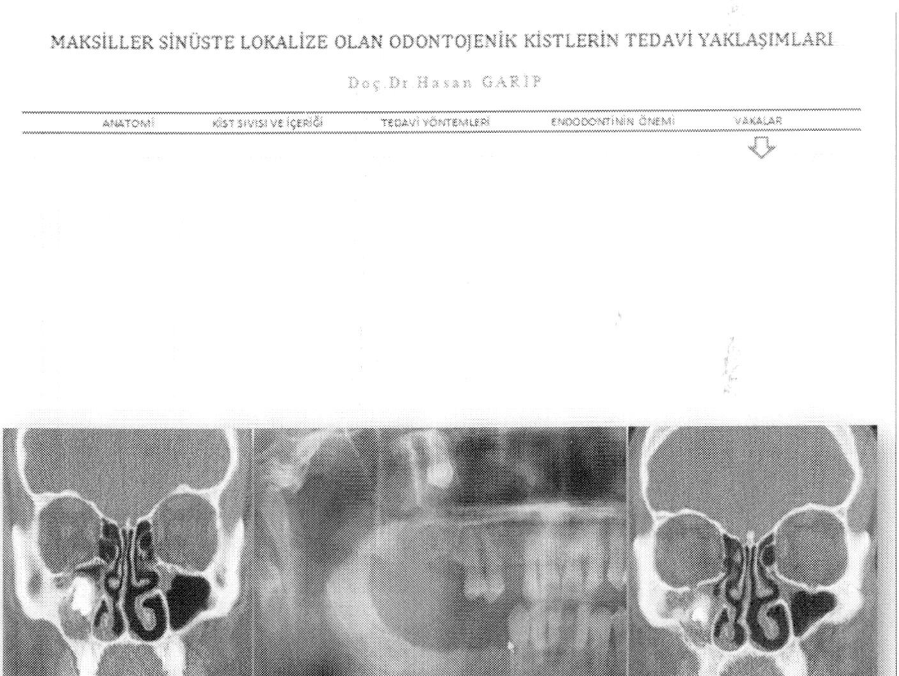

Figure 21. OPG and CT views.

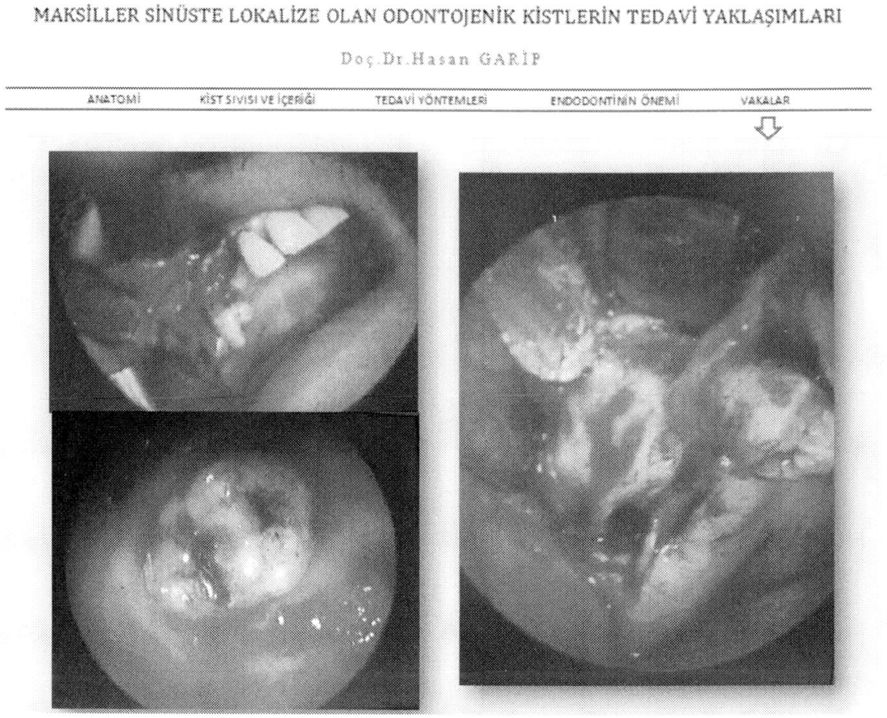

Figure 22. Extraction under endoscopic assistance.

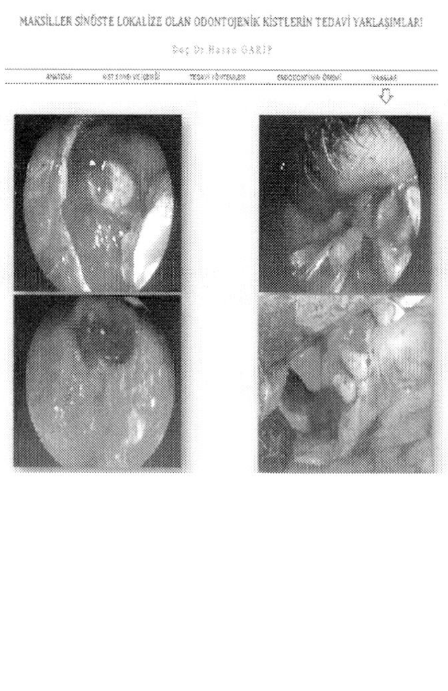

Figure 23. Extraction under endoscopic assistance.

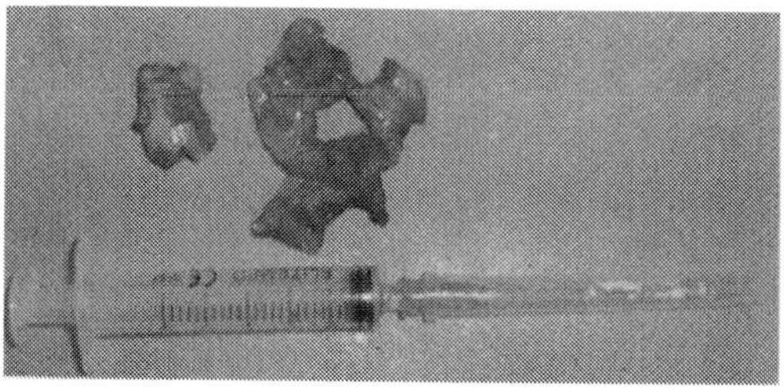

Figure 24. Enucleated dentigerous cyst.

6.3. Case 3

A 23-year-old female was referred to our department of oral and maxillofacial surgery with headache, fatigue, and difficulty in nasal breathing. After a radiological examination (figure 25), it was seen that there was an ectopic third molar in the left sinus and a wisdom lower left third molar in conjunction with a cyst. A CT scan (Figure 26) was performed and all important points were checked and it was seen that the third molar in the maxillary sinus was associated with a cyst that had occupied over two-thirds of the left maxillary sinus.

An operation was performed under general anesthesia with combined local anesthesia. A trapezoid mucoperiosteal flap was designed and carefully elevated (Figure 27). The tooth was extracted (Figure 28) and the cyst was enucleated (Figure 29). An intranasal inferior meatal antrostomy was performed with packing of the sinus (Figure 30); this was removed 3 days later. After the operation, all symptoms of headache, fatigue, and difficulty in nasal breathing resolved. Pathological specimens were sent for examination and the report showed that the cyst was an orthokeratotic odontogenic cyst.

During the operation, using envelope incision, the lower-left-third molar was also extracted and its cyst was enucleated (Figure 31). The pathological report for the lower cyst showed it to be dentigerous. The patient remains under observation (Figure 32).

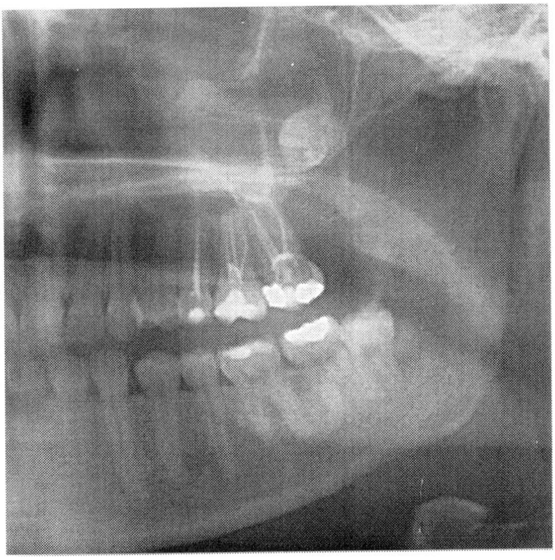

Figure 25. OPG view.

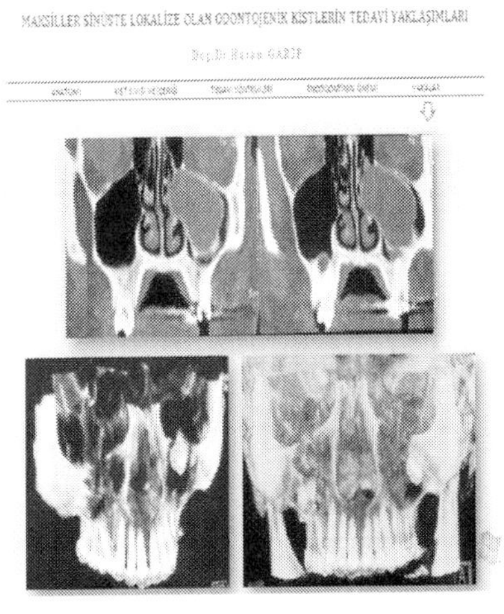

Figure 26. CT views.

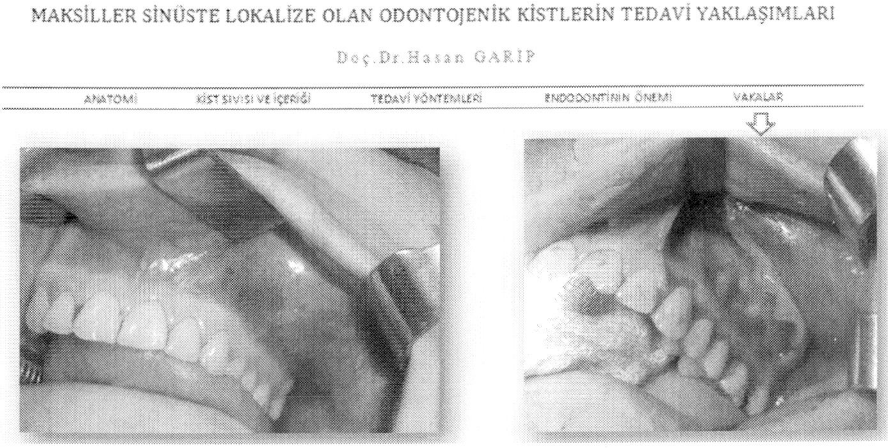

Figure 27. Mucoperiosteal flap preparation.

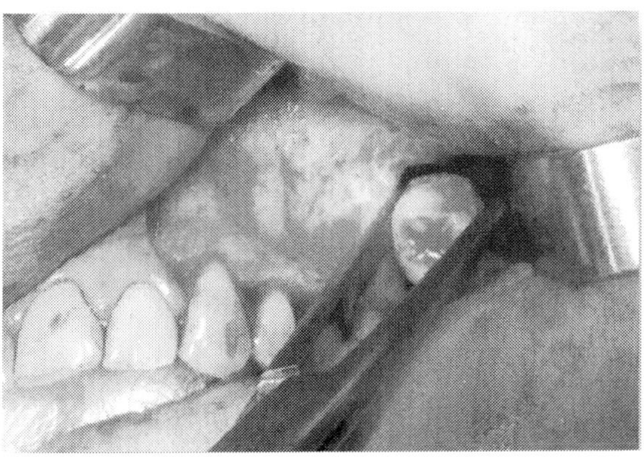

Figure 28. Tooth extraction.

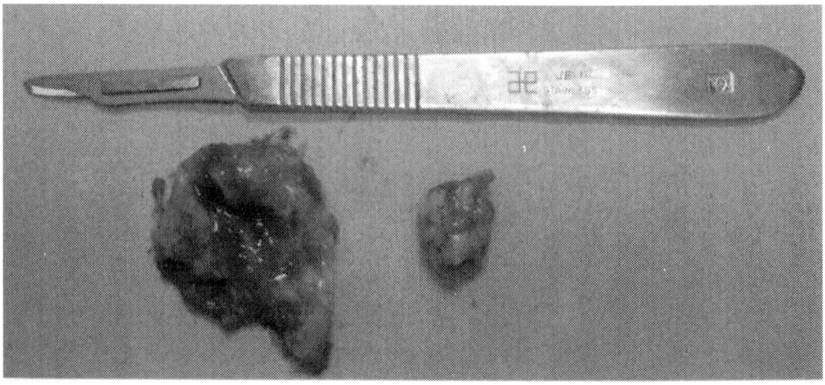

Figure 29. Enucleated cyst and extracted tooth.

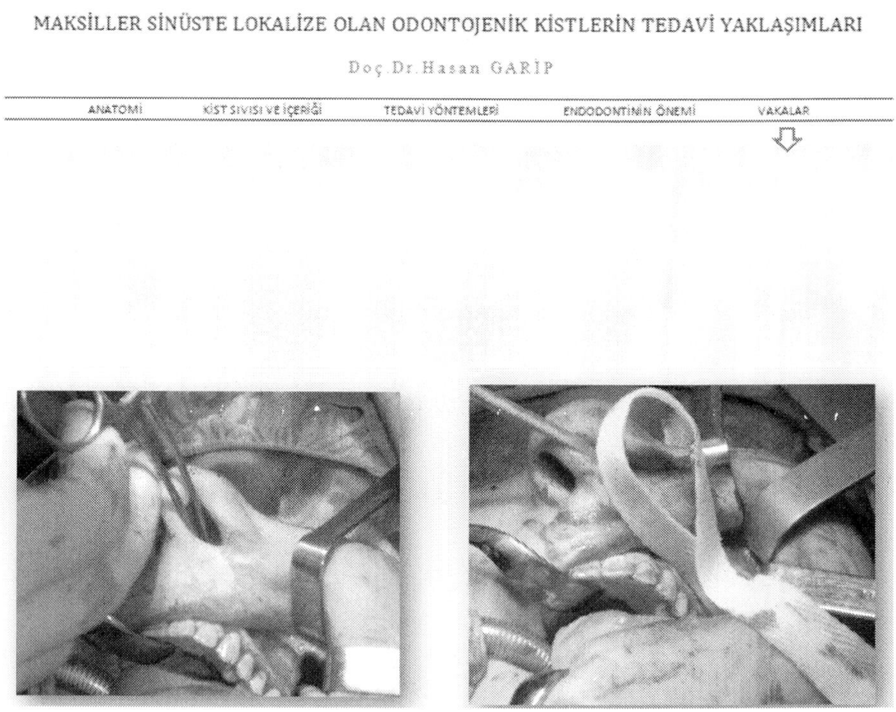

Figure 30. Intranasal inferior meatal antrostomy and packing of the sinus maxillaris.

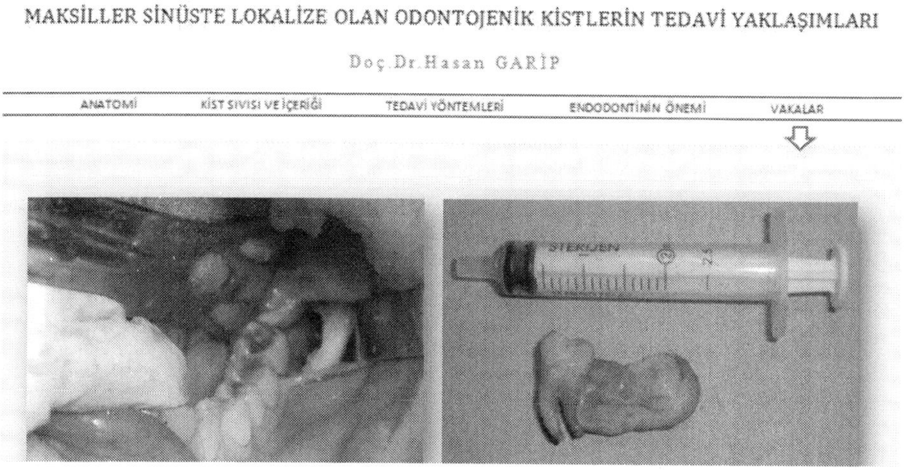

Figure 31. Extracted lower tooth.

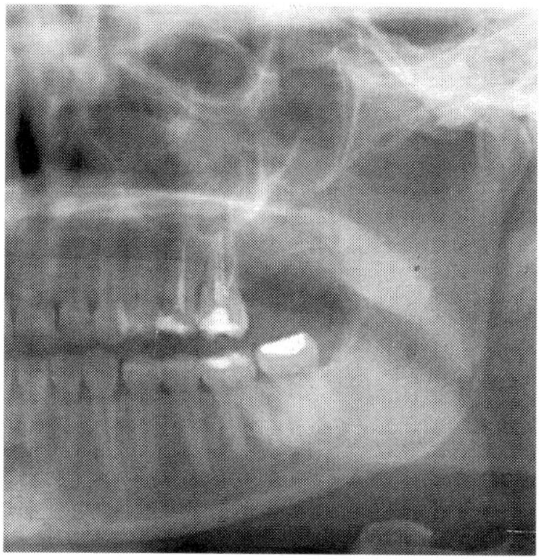

Figure 32. 5 year postoperative OPG.

6.4. Case 4

A 26-year-old female was referred to our department with severe headache, fatigue, difficulty in nasal breathing, halitosis, and a slowly growing facial deformity on the right site of the face. After radiological assessment (OPG and CT) and clinical examination (Figure 33), it was seen that there was a cyst that almost completely filled the right maxillary sinus and there was slight, but obvious, facial asymmetry caused by the swelling over the right maxillary region. The mass was firm and non-tender on palpation and not adherent to the overlying skin. Intra-oral examination showed expansion of the upper right molar region.

Endodontic treatment was performed for the upper right first and second premolars and for the second molar tooth. It was decided that the first molar roots and third molars would be extracted. All important anatomical points were carefully checked on CT scans.

An operation was performed under general anesthesia, with combined local anesthesia. A trapezoid mucoperiosteal flap was designed and carefully elevated (Figure 34). The teeth were extracted and the cyst was enucleated (Figure 35); and apical resection was performed (Figure 36). An intranasal inferior meatal antrostomy was performed as was packing of the sinus (Figures 37, 38); this was removed 3 days later. Endoscopic assistance was not used because of good visualization. Pathological specimens were sent for examination and report confirmed a radicular cyst (Figure 39).

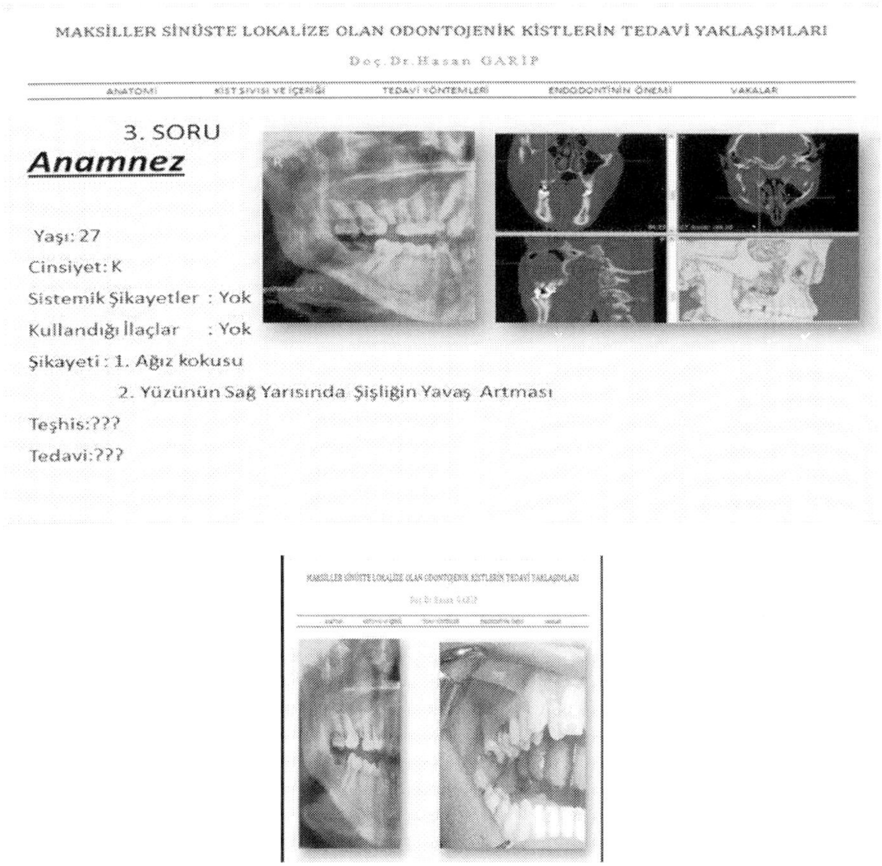

Figure 33. Radiological (OPG and CT) and intraoral clinical views.

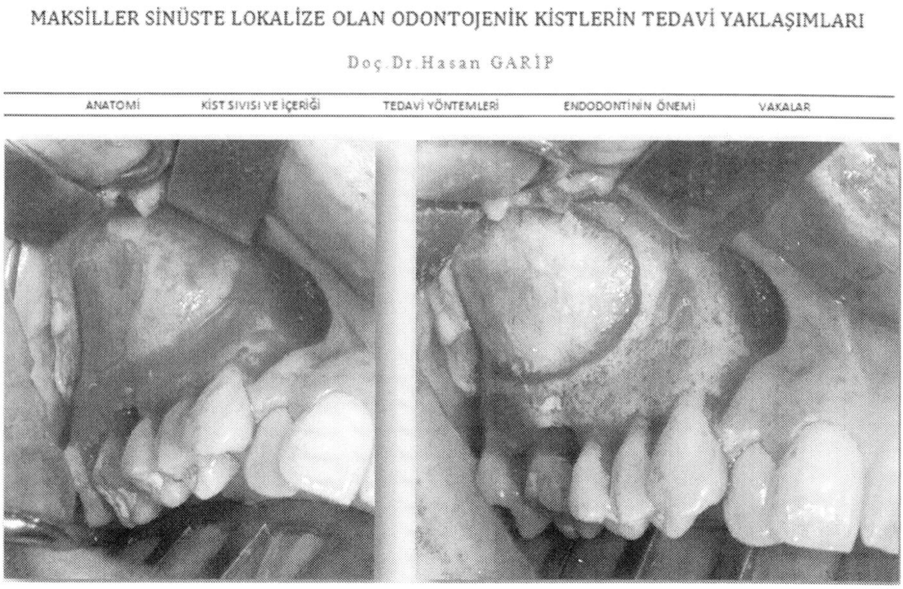

Figure 34. Mucoperiosteal elevation and cyst exposure.

http://dx.doi.org/10.5772/59087

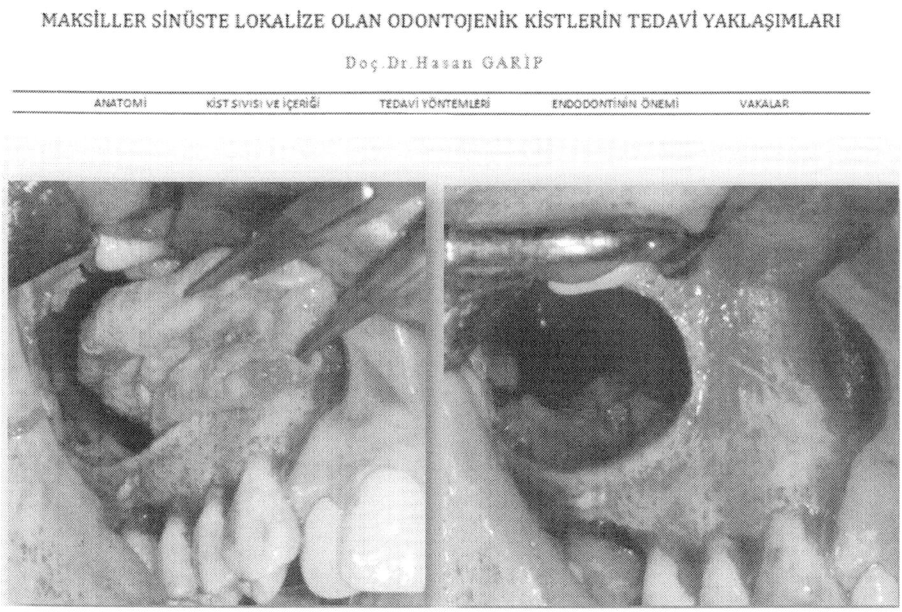

Figure 35. Cyst enucleation.

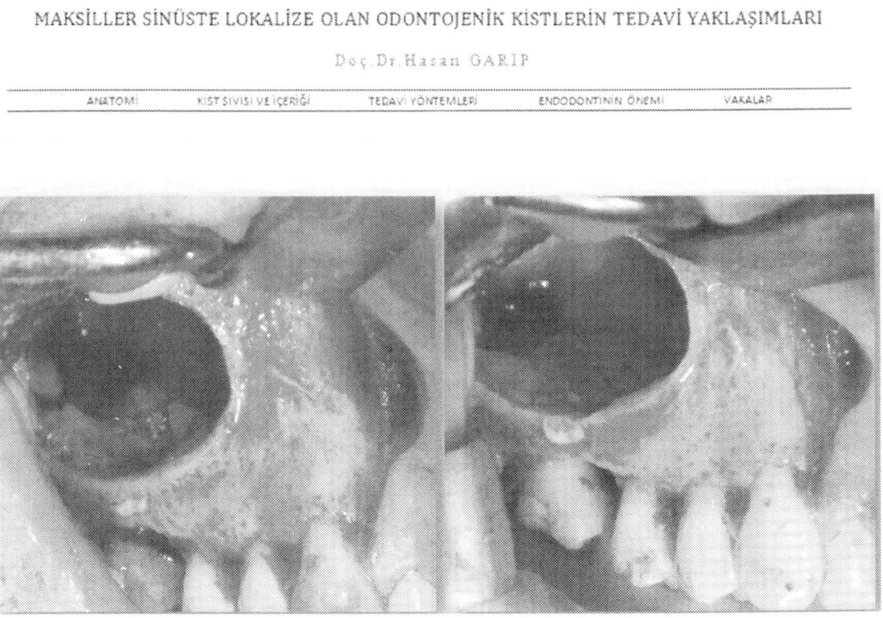

Figure 36. Apical resection.

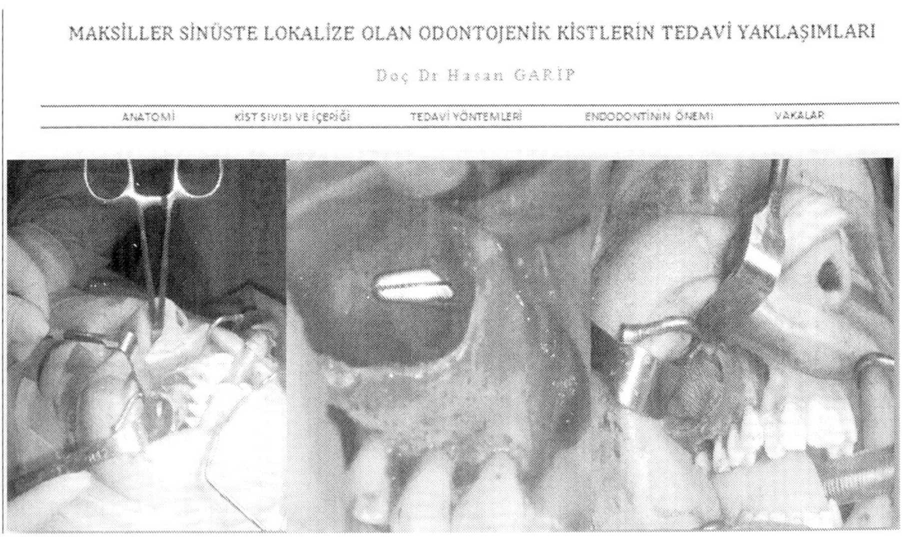

Figure 37. Intranasal inferior meatal antrostomy and packing of the sinus maxillaris.

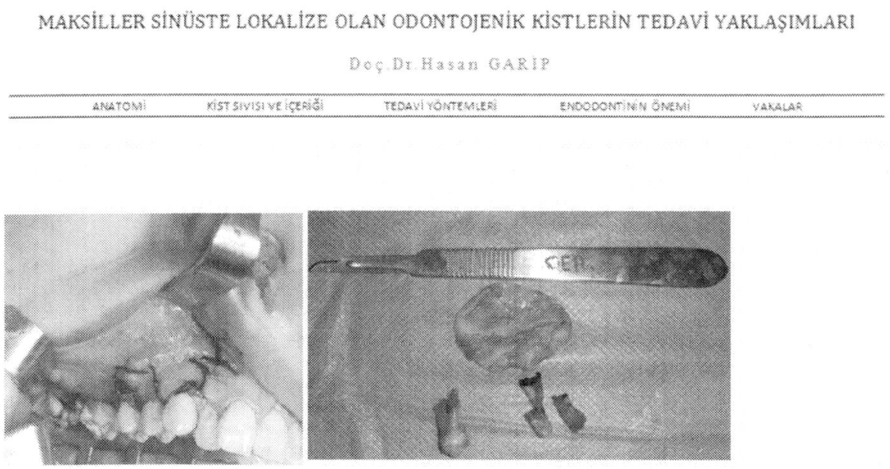

Figure 38. Closed mucoperiosteal flap and enucleated cyst.

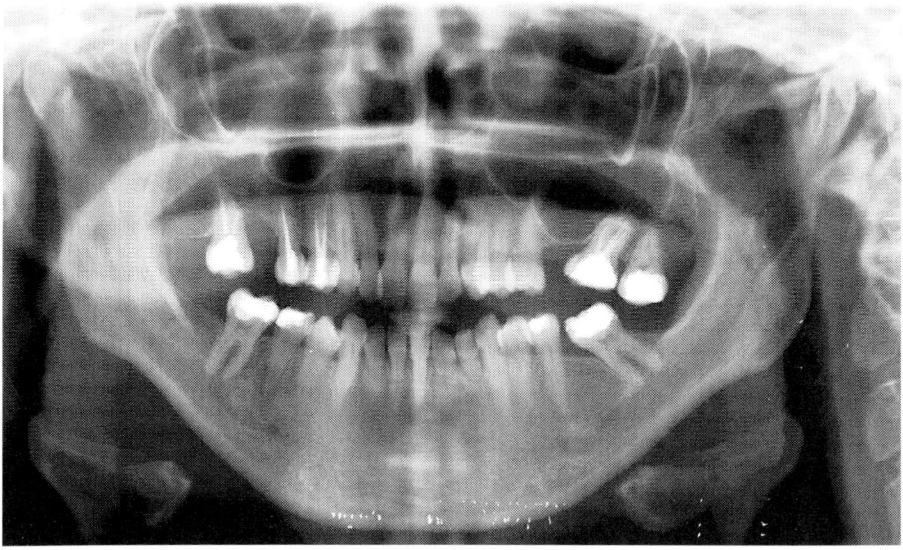

Figure 39. 5 year postoperative OPG

6.5. Case 5

A 33-year-old male was referred to our department with difficulty in nasal breathing, halitosis, and a slowly growing facial deformity on the left side of the face. From radiological (OPG and CT) and clinical examinations (Figure 42), it was seen that there was a cyst, which was related to the left maxillary teeth and nasal floor, uplifting the sinus floor, although it did not obliterate the sinus ostium and the sinus mucosa was not infected. This information was important for the decision as to whether to perform an intranasal inferior meatal antrostomy or not. In this case, because the parameters for maxillary sinus ventilation were ideal, we did not perform an antrostomy. Before the operation all teeth on the left site underwent endodontic treatment (Figure 41).

An operation was performed under general anesthesia combined with local anesthesia. A trapezoid mucoperiosteal flap was designed and carefully elevated (Figure 42). The buccal cortex was decorticated using a round bur without damaging the cyst wall (Figure 43). Intracystic liquid was aspirated with a 20-cc syringe (Figure 44). During aspiration, cholesterol crystals were observed clearly in the cyst fluid. After enucleation of cyst (Figure 45), apical resection plus MTA retrograde filling was performed and the mucoperiosteal flap was sutured. Pathological specimens were sent for examination and the report was a radicular cyst.

Endodontic surgery involves a combination of curettage of infected tissue and removal of an infected or damaged root apex. Among the causes of failure in endodontic surgery, the most frequent is the incomplete sealing of all communications between the root canal system and periradicular tissues. Many studies have shown that bacteria that remain in the root canal system have access to the periradicular tissues after resection [26, 27] The main purpose of the root-end filling material is to provide an apical seal that prevents the movement of bacteria from the root canal system into the periapical tissues. Recently, an experimental substance, MTA, was suggested as a potential root-end filling material. In a series of *in vitro* studies, the sealing ability of MTA was evaluated, compared with commonly used root-end-filling materials. It was shown that MTA had significantly less dye and bacterial leakage. [26, 28, 29] Some studies have shown that when the root canal is confined hermetically and an adequate retrograde cavity depth is prepared, then variation in the root-end cutting angle does not necessarily cause any difference in microleakage. [26]

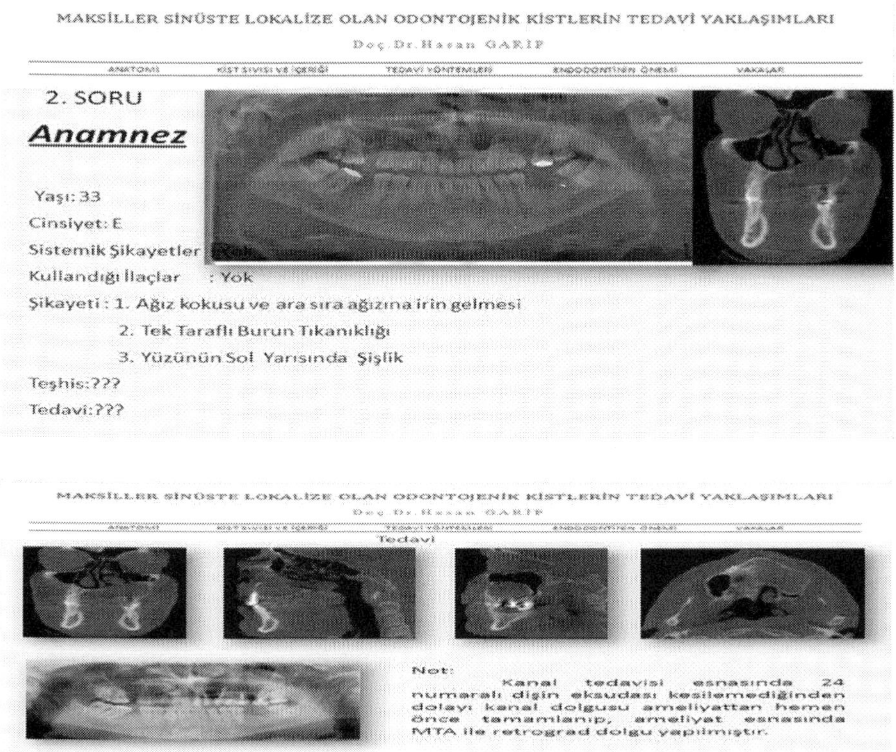

Figure 40. Radiological (OPG and CT) examination.

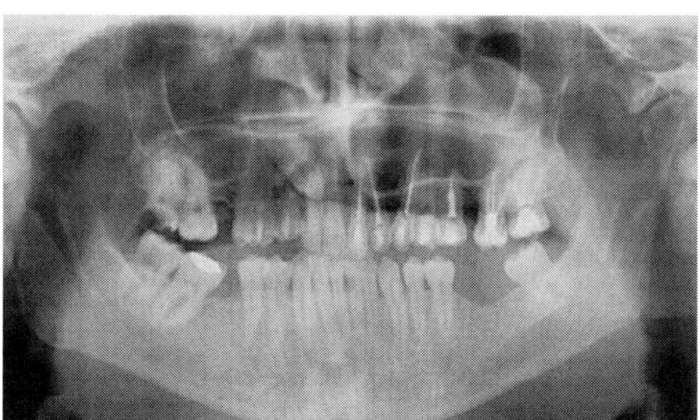

Figure 41. Endodontic treatment of the teeth.

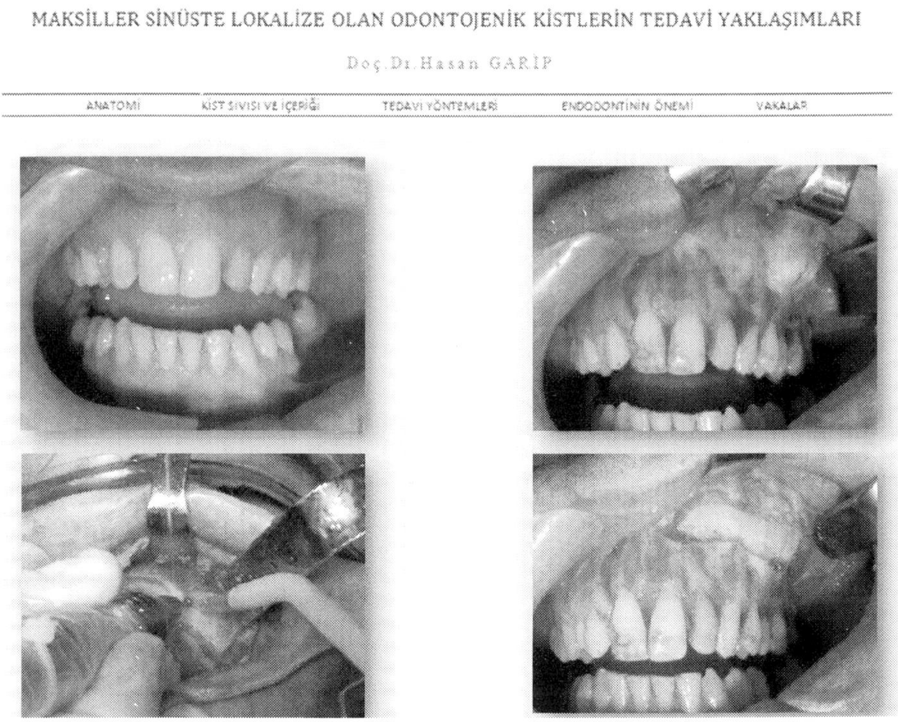

Figure 42. Preparation and elevation of the mucoperiosteal flap.

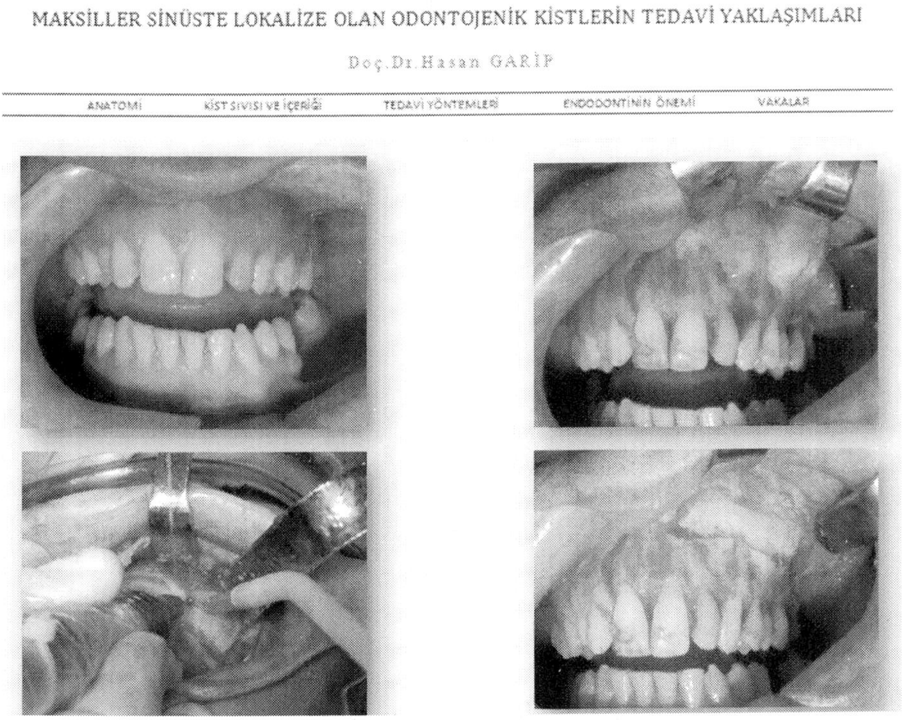

Figure 43. Buccal cortex decortication.

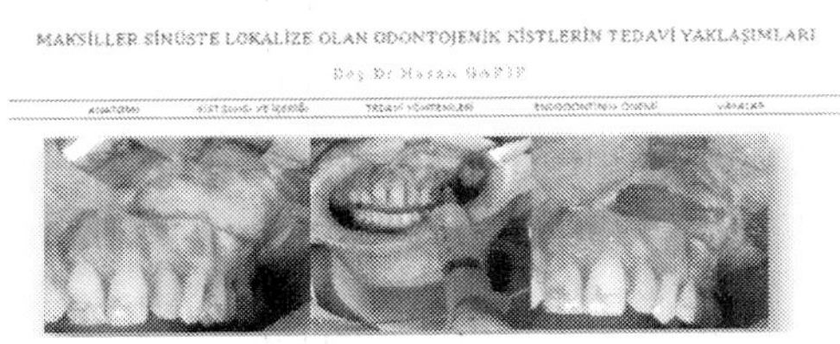

Figure 44. Intracystic liquid aspiration with a 20-cc syringe and view of cholesterol crystals.

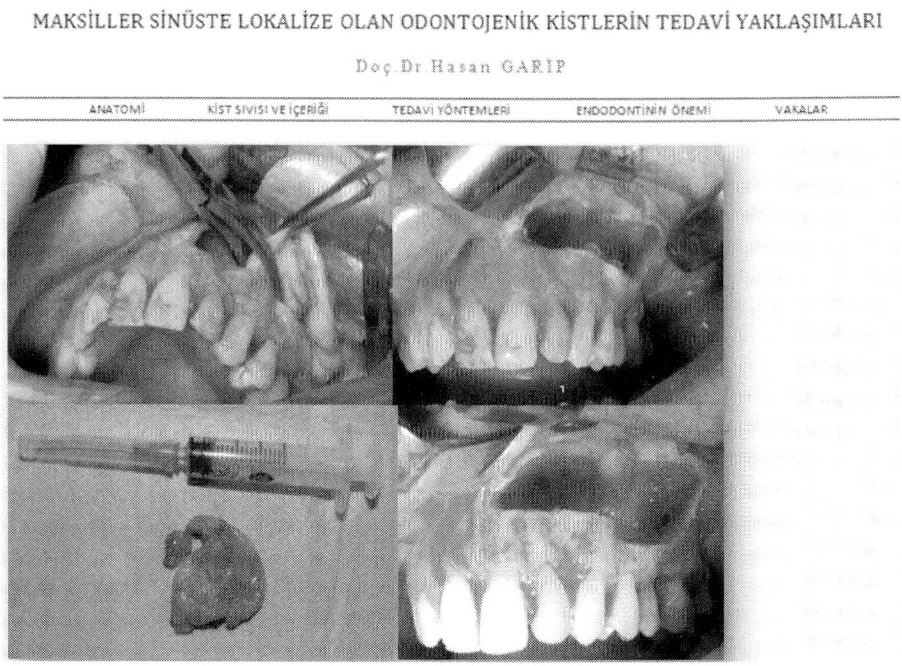

Figure 45. Enucleation of the cyst.

7. Conclusions

Because of the anatomy of the maxillary sinus, pathological structures that develop and grow in the sinus can reach a large size without any serious complaint by the patient, making early diagnosis unlikely and treatment is important to address morbidity.

OPG and CT scans aid in the diagnosis of cysts localized in the sinus and CT scans are indispensable in surgical strategy planning. Good visualization during the operation provides a better opportunity for good cleaning of pathologies, better bleeding control, and minimal trauma. For better visualization, the use of endoscopy during the operation can simplify and enhance the procedure. Also, close observation of patients in the early postoperative period and regular follow-up in the later postoperative period are important.

Author details

Hasan Garip*, Sertac Aktop, Onur Gonul and Kamil Göker

http://dx.doi.org/10.5772/59087

*Address all correspondence to: hasangarip@yahoo.com

Dear Authors, Add Your Respected Institutions, Town, Country

References

[1] Gray's anatomy.

[2] http://en.wikipedia.org/wiki/Maxillary_sinus

[3] www.kenhub.com/en/library/anatomy/innervation-and-blood-supply-of-the-teeth

[4] Sarachev E, Uzunov H. Klinichna I Topographska Anatomoya na Litsevo-Chelusnata Oblast. ISBN 9549806-14-6, 2001 Plovdiv, 449-495.

[5] Miloro M. Peterson's Principle of Oral and Maxillofacial Surgery. Second Edition.. In Miloro M., Ghali G. E., Larsen P. E., Waite P. Editors. BC Decker Inc. 2004 p. 1179-1205

[6] Aydinlioğlu A, Diyarbakirli S, Şakul U B, Keleş P, Arslan H, Kiriş M. Surgical Anatomy Of The Paranasal Sinuses: Cadaver And Ct Study I-Sinus Maxillaris And Frontalis.Turkiye Klinikleri J Dental Sci 1997;3(1):6-11

[7] Jensen, Ole T. The Sinus Bone Graft, Quintessence Publishing Co, Inc, 1999 p. 31-48

[8] Kılıc C, Kamburoğlu K, Yüksel SP, Özen T. An Assessment of the Relationship between the Maxillary Sinus Floor and the Maxillary Posterior Teeth Root Tips Using Dental Cone-beam Computerized. Tomography. Eur J Dent. 2010 Oct;4(4):462-7.

[9] Jung YH, Cho BH. Assessment of the relationship between the maxillary molars and adjacent structures using cone beam computed tomography. Imaging Sci Dent. 2012 Dec;42(4):219-24.

[10] Hirata Y, Kino K, Nagaoka S, Miyamoto R, Yoshimasu H, Amagasa T. A clinical investigation of oro-maxillary sinus-perforation due to tooth extraction. Kokubyo Gakkai Zasshi. 2001 Sep;68(3):249-53

[11] Miloro M. Peterson's Principle of Oral and Maxillofacial Surgery. Second Edition.. In Miloro M., Ghali G. E., Larsen P. E., Waite P. Editors. BC Decker Inc. 2004 p.295-312

[12] Janner SF, Caversaccio MD, Dubach P, Sendi P, Buser D, Bornstein MM. Characteristics and dimensions of the Schneiderian membrane: a radiographic analysis using cone beam computed tomography in patients referred for dental implant surgery in the posterior maxilla. Clin Oral Implants Res. 2011 Dec;22(12):1446-53.

[13] Dagassan-Berndt DC, Zitzmann NU, Lambrecht JT, Weiger R, Walter C. Is the Schneiderian membrane thickness affected by periodontal disease? A cone beam computed tomography-based extended case series. J Int Acad Periodontol. 2013 Jul; 15(3):75-82.

[14] Han MH, Chang KH, Lee CH, Na DG, Yeon KM, Han MC. Cystic expansile masses of the maxilla: differential diagnosis with CT and MR. AJNR Am J Neuroradiol. 1995 Feb;16(2):333-8.

[15] Caylakli F, Yavuz H, Cagici AC, Ozluoglu LN. Endoscopic sinus surgery for maxillary sinus mucoceles. Head Face Med. 2006 Sep 6;2:29.

[16] Buyukkurt MC, Omezli MM, Miloglu O. Dentigerous cyst associated with an ectopic tooth in the maxillary sinus: a report of 3 cases and review of the literature. Oral Surg Oral Med Oral Pathol Oral Radiol Endod. 2010 Jan;109(1):67-71.

[17] Scott A. Martin. Conventional Endodontic Therapy of Upper Central Incisor Combined with Cyst Decompression: A Case Report. JOE 33(6), 2007, 753-757

[18] Pogrel M A. Treatment of Keratocysts: The Case for Decompression and Marsupialization. J Oral Maxillofac Surg 63:1667-1673, 2005

[19] Miloro M. Peterson's Principle of Oral and Maxillofacial Surgery. Second Edition.. In Miloro M., Ghali G. E., Larsen P. E., Waite P. Editors. BC Decker Inc. 2004 p.575-596

[20] Bello SA, Oketade IO, Osunde OD. Ectopic 3rd molar tooth in the maxillary antrum. Case Rep Dent. 2014;2014:620741.

[21] Varol A, Türker N, Göker K, Basa S. Endoscopic retrieval of dental implants from the maxillary sinus. Int J Oral Maxillofac Implants. 2006 ;21(5):801-4

[22] Kim JW, Lee CH, Kwon TK, Kim DK. Endoscopic removal of a dental implant through a middle meatal antrostomy. Br J Oral Maxillofac Surg. 2007, 45(5):408-9.

[23] Chen CT, Chen YR. Endoscopically assisted repair of orbital floor fractures. Plast Reconstr Surg. 2001 Dec;108(7):2011-8

[24] Nour YA. Variable extent of nasoantral window for resection of antrochoanal polyp: selection of the optimum endoscopic approach. Eur Arch Otorhinolaryngol. 2014 Jul 11.

[25] Dhingra PL, Dhingra S. Diseases of Ear, Nose and Throat. Chapter 82 5th edition, Elsevier 2010

[26] Garip H, Garip Y, Oruçoğlu H, Hatipoğlu S. Effect of the angle of apical resection on apical leakage, measured with a computerized fluid filtration device. Oral Surg Oral Med Oral Pathol Oral Radiol Endod. 2011 Mar;111(3):e50-5.

[27] Lin LM, Pascon EA, Skribner J, Langleland K. Clinical, radiographic, and histologic study of endodontic treatment failures. Oral Surg Oral Med Oral Pathol 1991;71:603-11.

[28] Torabinejad M, Watson TF, Pitt FTR. Sealing ability of a mineral trioxide aggregate when used as a root end filling material. J Endod 1993;19:591-5.

[29] Torabinejad M, Higa RK, McKendry DJ, Pitt FTR. Dye leakage of four root end filling materials: effects of blood contamination.J Endod 1994;20:159-63.

Chapter 14

Multidisciplinary Management of Benign Jaw Tumors in Children

Mehmet Cemal Akay, Mert Zeytinoğlu,
Birant Şimşek and Işıl Aras

Additional information is available at the end of the chapter

http://dx.doi.org/10.5772/59341

1. Introduction

A tumor is defined, in brief, as abnormal growth of tissue; tumoral formations are classified under two main headings, benign and malignant. The oro-facial region including the jaw bones, maxilla and mandible, is a site for a multitude of neoplastic conditions. Odontogenic tumors (OTs) constitute a wide range and diverse kind of lesions derived from tooth forming apparatus and its remnants. OTs originate from epithelium or ectomesenchyme or from both, showing varying degrees of inductive interaction between these embryonic components of the developing tooth germ. [1]. The majority of these tumors occur intraosseously within the maxillofacial skeleton, while extraosseous odontogenic tumors occur nearly always in the tooth-bearing mucosa. Due to their specific structure and location they have been identified and classified by pathologists into a separate group, differing in histogenesis, biology, clinical findings and radiological signs from other tumors developing in the oral cavity and facial bones (Figure 1).

The aim of the chapter is to review multidisciplinary treatment approaches to pediatric patients with benign jaw tumors from a radiological and clinical point of view and assess advantages and disadvantages of the current treatment techniques, possible complications and their prevention in the light of the recent literature.

1.1. Etiology of odontogenic tumors

According to current literatures, it is known that the potential sources for development of an odontogenic tumor are varied, and these include:

1. **The pre-functional dental lamina** (odontogenic epithelium with ability to produce a tooth), which is more abundant distal to the lower third molars.

2. **The post-functional dental lamina**, a concept that covers those epithelial remnants such as Serre´s epithelial rests, located within the fibrous gingival tissue; the epithelial cell rests of Malassez in the periodontal ligament and the reduced enamel organ epithelium, which covers the enamel surface until tooth eruption.

3. **The basal cell layer of the gingival epithelium**, which originally gave rise to the dental lamina.

4. **The dental papilla**, origin of the dental pulp, which has the potential to be induced to produce odontoblasts and synthesize dentin and/or dentinoid material.

5. **The dental follicle.**

6. **The periodontal ligament**, which has the potential to induce the production of fibrous and cemento-osseous mineralized material [2].

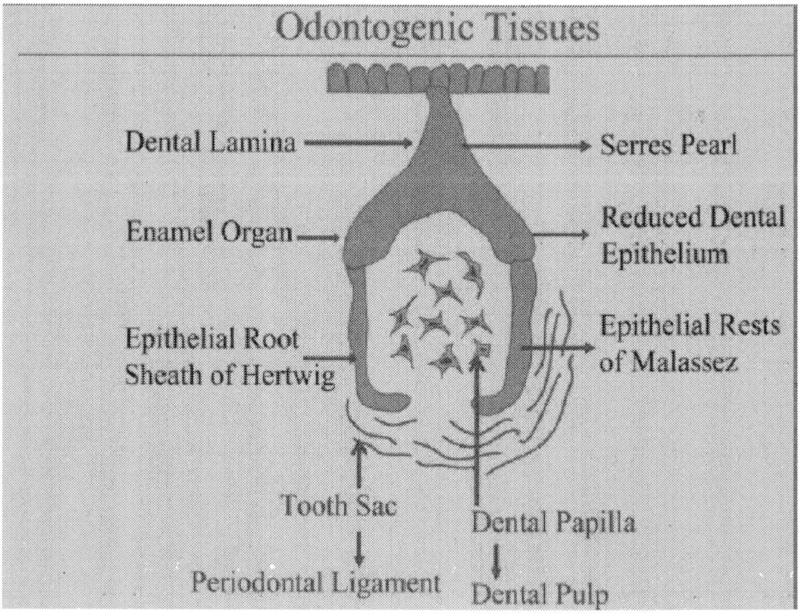

Figure 1. Odontogenic tumors arising from odontogenic tissues

From a biological point of view, some of these lesions represent hamartomas with varying degrees of differentiation, while the rest are benign or malignant neoplasms with variable aggressiveness and potential to develop metastases. These tumors constitute a heterogeneous group of diseases with diverse clinical and histopathological features [3]. The relative frequency of OTs obtained from studies from different parts of the world, have varied widely. Some authors have reported that OTs are rare with a relative frequency of 1%, while others have reported OTs constitute up to 32% of jaw lesions [4-6]. These disparities have been suggested to be due to the differences in terminology and classification and also, possibly due to racial and or genetic differences in the occurrence of the various types of OTs. OTs comprise a large heterogeneous group of lesions originating from the epithelium and/or odontogenic ectomesenchyme and remnants. OTs include entities of a hamartomatous nature, such as odontoma, benign neoplasms, some of which are aggressive as is the case of ameloblastoma and myxoma and malignant neoplasms capable of metastasis [2, 7].

Primary jaw tumors are broadly classified into odontogenic and nonodontogenic groups. The World Health Organization (WHO) classified this group of lesions in 1971 and 1992. In 2005, the WHO published the latest updated edition of the classification of OTs. There were 6 major changes in this schema from the previous versions namely:

1. parakeratinized variant of odontogenic keratocyst is now classified as a benign tumor and termed KCOT
2. adenomatoid odontogenic tumor (AOT) originates from the odontogenic epithelium with mature fibrous stroma and without ectomesenchyme
3. calcifying odontogenic cyst (COC) is divided into 2 benign and 1 malignant groups
4. clear cell odontogenic tumor is a malignant lesion and termed clear cell odontogenic carcinoma (CCOC)
5. odontogenic carcinosarcoma is not included due to the lack of evidence for the existence of this type and
6. some changes were made regarding terminology and subtypings [5-7].

The latest WHO classification has been used as a global standard for the last 10 years but our knowledge of odontogenic tumors continues to evolve.

The latest WHO classification of odontogenic tumors

1. Malignant odontogenic tumors

Odontogenic carcinomas

Metastasizing (malignant) ameloblastoma

Ameloblastic carcinoma - primary type

Ameloblastic carcinoma - secondary type (dedifferentiated), intraosseous

Ameloblastic carcinoma - secondary type (dedifferentiated), peripheral

Primary intraosseous squamous cell carcinoma solid type

Primary intraosseous squamous cell carcinoma derived from keratocystic odontogenic tumor

Primary intraosseous squamous cell carcinoma derived from odontogenic cysts

Clear cell odontogenic carcinoma

Ghost cell odontogenic carcinoma

Odontogenic sarcomas

Ameloblastoma fibrosarcoma

Ameloblastic fibrodentino-and fibro-odontosarcoma

2. Benign odontogenic tumors

Odontogenic epithelium with mature, fibrous stroma without odontogenic ectomesenchyme

Ameloblastoma, solid/multicystic type

Ameloblastoma, extraosseous/peripheral type

Ameloblastoma, desmoplastic type

Ameloblastoma, unicystic type

Squamous odontogenic tumor

Calcifying epithelial odontogenic tumor

Adenomatoid odontogenic tumor and Keratocystic odontogenic tumor

Odontogenic epithelium with odontogenic ectomesenchyme, with or without hard tissue formation

Ameloblastic fibroma

Ameloblastic fibrodentinoma

Ameloblastic fibro-odontoma

Odontoma

- Odontoma, complex type

- Odontoma, compound type

Odontoameloblastoma

Calcifying cystic odontogenic tumor

Dentinogenic ghost cell tumor

Mesenchyme and/or odontogenic ectomesenchyme with or without odontogenic epithelium

Odontogenic fibroma

Odontogenic myxoma and myxofibroma

Cementoblastoma

Bone-related (Fibro-osseous) lesions

Ossifying fibroma

Fibrous dysplasia

Osseous dysplasia

Periapical Osseous Dysplasia

Focal Osseous Dysplasia

http://dx.doi.org/10.5772/59341

Florid Osseous Dysplasia

Central giant cell granuloma

Cherubism

Aneurysmal bone cyst

Solitary (Simple) bone cyst

Other tumors

Melanotic neuroectodermal tumor of infancy

Classification of the Latest Benign Fibro-Osseous Lesions of the Craniofacial Complex: [8]

1. Bone dysplasias

a. Fibrous dyspla

i. Monostotic

ii. Polyostotic

iii. Polyostotic with endocrinopathy (McCune-Albright)

iv Osteofibrous dysplasia

b. Osteitis deformans

c. Pagetoid heritable bone dysplasias of childhood

d. Segmental odontomaxillary dysplasia

2. Cemento-osseous dysplasia

a. Focal cemento-osseous dysplasia

b. Florid cemento-osseous dysplasia

3. Inflammatory/reactive processes

a. Focal sclerosing osteomyelitis

b. Diffuse sclerosing osteomyelitis

c. Proliferative periostitis

4. Metabolic Disease: hyperparathyroidism

5. Neoplastic lesions (Ossifying fibromas)

a. Ossifying fibroma

b. Hyperparathyroidism jaw lesion syndrome

c. Juvenile ossifying fibroma

i. Trabecular type

ii. Psammomatoid type

d. Gigantiform cementomas

In pace with new findings of new genetic and molecular changes, classification of odontogenic tumors will necessitate further modification and subsequent changes in the classification system. Hence a new and revised version of the classification will always be dynamic. Characteristics and epidemiology of jaw tumors have been described mostly in adults. Compared with their adult counterparts, jaw tumors in childhood show considerable differences. Tumors of the head and neck represent only 2% to 5% of all pediatric tumors. OTs in children constitute approximately 3% of all tumor like growths in the oral cavity, jaws and salivary glands in all age groups [9]. In general, OTs in the pediatric population are rare and considerably more so than in the adult population. There are differences in the spectrum of diseases seen in this group and in adults. When the diseases are similar, there are sometimes differences in their clinical behavior. There are additional management concerns when working with children. Treatment burden is given relatively greater consideration in children since they are growing and developing and treatment may exert untoward influences therein. It is important for the clinicians involved in the diagnosis and treatment of pediatric head and neck tumors to understand certain patterns that follow the development of these lesions, so that misdiagnosis and delays in treatment can be avoided. Because of their relative rarity, this broad spectrum of lesions require careful attention and close collaboration between pediatricians, medical oncologists, radiotherapists, pathologists and surgeons working in the head and neck area. Pathology is uncommon among the pediatric age group, its incidence and prevalence has been increasing in recent years, and it remains a significant cause of morbidity and mortality in this population. Recently, Jones and Franklin performed a retrospective investigation of oral and maxillofacial pathologies within a 30-year period. Those authors verified that biopsies in patients aged between 10 and 16 years represented 8.2% of all cases reported.[10]

Classification of pediatric jaw tumors

The various classifications systems proposed by authors are enumerated as below:

1. Jaw Tumors in Children (11)

1.Classification of non-odontogenic jaw tumors in children

I. Benign mesenchymal tumors

- a) Giant cell lesions
- b) Fibro-osseous lesions
- c) Myxoma

II. Hematopoietic and reticuloendothelial tumors

- a) Langerhans cell histiocytosis
- b) Burkitt's lymphoma
- c)Lymphoma

III. Neurogenic tumors

- a) Neurofibroma
- b) Neurilemmoma
- c) Neuroma
- d)Ganglioneuroma
- e) Neuroblastoma

f)Melanotic neuroectodermal tumor

IV. Vascular lesions

a)Vascular malformation (capillary, lymphatic, venous, arterial, combined)

b)Hemangioma

c)Aneurysmal bone cyst

V. Malignant mesenchymal tumors

a) Osteogenic sarcoma

b) Chondrosarcoma

c) Fibrosarcoma

d) Ewing's sarcoma

VI. Malignant epithelial tumors

a)Squamous cell carcinoma

b)Mucoepidermoid carcinoma

c)Adenoid cystic carcinoma

d)Adenocarcinoma

2. **Classification of odontogenic jaw tumors in children**

I. Epithelial tumors

a) Ameloblastoma (Peripheral, Unicystic, Solid, Multicystic)

b) Adenomatoid odontogenic tumor

c) Calcifying epithelial odontogenic tumor

II. Mesodermal tumors

a)Cementoma

b)Periapical cemental dysplasia

c)Cementifying fibroma

d)Cementoblastoma

e)Odontogenic fibroma

III. Mixed tumors

a)Ameloblastic fibroma

b) Odontoma

3. Classification of Small Round Cell Tumors in children

1. Soft tissue Rhabdomyosarcoma

Soft tissue (extraosseous) Ewing's sarcoma

Hemangiopericytoma

2. Osseous Ewing's sarcoma

Small cell osteosarcoma

Mesenchymal chondrosarcoma

Hemangiopericytoma of bone

3. Neural

Neuroblastoma

Peripheral neuroectodermal tumors

- Askin's tumor

- Neuroepithelioma

Pheochromocytoma

4. **International classification of childhood cancer (12)**

Malignant Bone tumors

a) Osteosarcomas

b) Chondrosarcomas

c) Ewing tumor and related sarcomas of bone

d) Other specified malignant bone tumors

e) Unspecified malignant bone tumors

Soft tissue and other extraosseous sarcomas

a) Rhabdomyosarcomas

b) Fibrosarcomas, peripheral nerve sheath tumors and other fibrous neoplasms

c) Kaposi's sarcoma

d) Other specified soft tissue sarcomas

e) Unspecified soft tissue sarcomas

2. Clinical sign and symptoms of pediatric jaw tumors

Pediatric patients encompass a very interesting study group, as several long term physiological changes take place in the maxillofacial area. During the mixed dentition period, children can refer with a complaint of swelling in the maxillofacial area, which may or may not be associated with pain. These mostly include both hard and soft tissue pathologies. When involving bone, only odontogenic cysts or odontogenic tumors as a category have been considered. Intra-osseous pediatric jaw lesions can present in diverse clinical patterns and their diagnoses can vary from odontogenic to non-odontogenic pathogeneses, which can rarely include connective tissue pathology. The great majority of pediatric jaw tumors are non-odontogenic [13,14].

OTs can be observed casually or after the appearance of nonspecific symptoms. Because of their slow-growth tendency, usually they do not cause pain. The odontogenic tumors grow in the jaw, through the haversian system, without metastases but with a high probability of relapse. In the majority of cases, tumors of the head and neck in children are first seen by general practitioners or pediatricians with subsequent delays in investigations and diagnosis. Some of these tumors may disappear spontaneously without any treatment. During the mixed dentition period, children can report with complaint of swelling in the maxillofacial area, which may or may not be associated with pain. A history of trauma also needs to be elicited, because they are prone to falling down during playing, which can affect the jaws. Because of the complex anatomy and development of the head and neck, neoplasms during infancy and childhood arising at this site represent the most difficult challenges in clinical practice. [15]

3. Diagnosis of pediatric jaw tumors

The odontogenic cysts and tumors are a diverse group of lesions that represent deviation from normal odontogenesis. The physical signs and symptoms of odontogenic cysts and tumors will depend to a certain extent on the dimensions of the lesion. A small lesion is unlikely to be diagnosed on a routine examination of the mouth because signs will not be demonstrable. Such lesions are only likely to be detected at an early stage as the result of routine radiographic examination. Exceptions are some early lesions that may present in conjunction with a devitalized tooth, which is detectable on clinical examination. Some cystic lesions may become secondarily infected, leading to their diagnosis. Clinical absence of one or more teeth without the history of extraction may also be a clinical indicator of an undiagnosed odontogenic cyst or tumor because many of these lesions are associated with impacted or congenitally missing teeth. As the lesion grows, other indirect changes may occur. An enlarging lesion between two teeth can cause the crowns to converge and the roots to diverge. Growth that is nearly undetectable visually may lead to difficulty with denture retention. As the lesion enlarges even further, expansion of the bone may be seen directly. This is usually toward the buccal surface of the alveolar bone because this is the thinnest area and expansion occurs here most easily. Clinically evident expansion is often a late finding, especially in lesions developing within the ramus or angle of the mandible or within the maxillary sinus. Lesions in these areas may become extremely large before expansion is observed clinically. Masses in the neck confront the pediatrician with greater opportunities for evaluation before a decision regarding biopsy or excision is reached. Signs of systemic involvement must also be determined.

3.1. Radiographic and imaging studies

- The primary goals of radiographic assessment are to more precisely define the primary lesion and to detect metastatic disease for clinical staging
- Chest radiographs are useful screens for mediastinal lymphadenopathy
- Ultrasound is able to differentiate a solid from a cystic mass, and give general relationships of the mass to adjacent structures
- Axial and coronal computerized tomography (CT) allows documentation of bone erosion and invasion of adjacent structures
- Magnetic resonance imaging (MRI) offers improved tissue contrast and definition
- Angiography delineates the blood supply to a lesion, and offers the ability to embolize specific factors to decrease blood loss associated with excision of vascular lesions
- Bone scans and liver spleen scans offer modalities to detect systemic disease. [9, 16]

A tissue diagnosis becomes necessary in order to diagnose and initiate proper therapy.

3.2. Biopsy

- Biopsy of OTs allows histologic evaluation of the mass
- Excisional biopsy is often therapeutic as well as diagnostic
- Incisional biopsy is required in cases where the lesion is large, or the lesion is relatively inaccessible

- Fine needle aspiration for cytologic study is useful in salivary gland and thyroid gland lesions. However, its generalized use for all pediatric head and neck masses is limited due to the rarity of squamous or glandular neoplasms developing in children
- Large bore needle biopsy has no established role in the evaluation of head and neck malignancies in children and has been reported to cause seeding along the needle tract in children. [9, 16]

OTs have a specific histological structure reflecting various stages of odontogenesis and are located mainly in the jaws, rarely in other parts of the skeletal system. Due to their specific structure and location they have been identified and classified by pathologists into a separate group of neoplasms differing from other lesions developing in the oral cavity and facial bones [17]. Odontogenic tissue is programmed to produce dentin and enamel due to active interactions between odontogenic mesenchyme and epithelium. Tooth formation is achieved via odontogenic mesenchyme and epithelium stage- and spatial-specific differentiation from early tooth development to late maturation [18]. Therefore, when odontogenic tissue becomes undifferentiated and undergoes tumoral changes, it has the potential to produce abnormal calcifications with enameloid, dentinoid, and cementum-like material histologic features. For this reason, these odontogenic calcifications are important odontogenic tumor characteristics and occasionally are accompanied by odontogenic epithelium ghost cell change and amorphous odontogenic mesenchyme hyalinization [19].

Aspiration cytology, a well established diagnostic tool in adult oncology, is recently gaining acceptance in pediatric population, as clinicians add this technique to their diagnostic armamentarium. Fine-needle aspiration cytology is a useful and reliable tool in the diagnosis of head and neck OTs with no contraindications and minimal complications even in children [20].

More than 95% of all OT reported in large series are benign and around 75% are represented by odontomas, ameloblastomas and myxomas (which could be considered as "relatively frequent OT"). Due to the inclusion of the odontogenic keratocyst as a tumor, these figures will be modified significantly, as this lesion is more frequently diagnosed than the other three entities. Some studies have shown epidemiological data that demonstrate that there is a second group of OT, which, although rare in terms of general pathology, are of "intermediate frequency" with respect to other OT, which have to be considered in the differential diagnosis of tumors of the oral and maxillofacial regions; therefore they have to be included within the contents of pathology of the graduate and post-graduate courses of oral and general pathology. The lack of specific markers to confirm the odontogenic origin of all the lesions included in the current WHO classification makes diagnoses mainly on anatomic considerations, or on the histomorphological similarities among some tumors with the above mentioned odontogenic structures. However, as most OT contain variable amounts of epithelium, and the fact that such tissue may express several of the more than 20 cytokeratin markers (intermediate filaments of the epithelial cells) known to date, there are some studies that have demonstrated that cytokeratins 14 and 19 are the more frequently expressed by OT, and that these are also expressed in the different epithelial structures of the developing tooth [21, 22], leading to promote their use as a diagnostic tool to support the odontogenic nature of these entities. Additionally, the expression of amelogenin, a representative protein of the enamel matrix, which is produced by secretory ameloblasts and that seem to actively participate in the process of production and mineralization of enamel, has been consistently demonstrated within the enamel matrix and the cytoplasm of the cells of the reduced enamel epithelium, stratum intermedium and stellate reticulum of the enamel organ, as well as in some epithelial OT, particularly at the basal endings of the cuboidal or columnar cells of ameloblastomas and in cells of calcifying epithelial odontogenic tumor, malignant ameloblastoma and ameloblastic carcinoma [22]. Therefore, the use of these markers is a valuable tool to discard other types of epithelial lesions that may develop within the oral and maxillofacial regions. More recently, calretinin, a 29-kDa calcium-binding protein has been shown to be expressed in both unicystic and solid ameloblastomas but not in other types of odontogenic cysts, and this finding led some authors to propose it may be considered a specific immunohistochemical marker for neoplasitic ameloblastic epithelium [23] and an important diagnostic aid in the differential diagnosis of cystic odontogenic lesions, particularly the keratocystic odontogenic tumor [24]. In the same way, the expression of cytodifferentiation of neoplastic epithelium via epithelial-mesenchymal interactions and mineralization markers, such as bone morphogenetic protein (BMP) is of great value to study those lesions that are characterized by the production of hard dental tissues [25, 26].

4. Treatment of pediatric jaw tumors

The majority of tumors of the mouth and jaw in children are benign. Tanaka et al. reported that only 3% of their cases were malignant in nature. In another study, benign tumors composed 93% of the cases (13, 14, 27).

Treatment consists of a range of surgical methods, from surgical curettage to hemimandibulectomy and reconstruction with bone graft. Generally, surgical excision, curettage, cryosurgery or en bloc resection are adequate for treatment of these tumors. However, some patients need multiple treatment because of its specific criterias such as the clinical behavior and extent of the lesion. Odontogenic lesions encompasses a wide spectrum of lesions and their variants, which either can be a cyst or a tumor. Odontogenic cysts are derived from the epithelium associated with the development of the dental apparatus while a tumor forms through some aberration from the normal pattern of odontogenesis. But the fact, that these lesions can mimic each other can complicate the diagnosis. The Adenomatoid Odontogenic Tumor is a benign, nonaggressive odontogenic tumor which has been known by a number of descriptive names since it was first reported. In almost all instances, the lesion may be removed by surgical enucleation. Unicystic Ameloblastoma is another tumor of the odontogenic series which has been described as benign but locally invasive. The Dentigerous Cyst, a cyst of odontogenic origin, has the potential of transforming into an Ameloblastoma. The Odontogenic Keratocyst, is characterized by aggressive behavior has debatable treatment options. All OTs can have a similar clinical and radiographic features which can mislead the dentist and a biopsy is needed to make a final diagnosis. Of all odontogenic tumors, ameloblastomas are the most controversial in terms of treatment. Treatments range from surgical curettage to bloc excision or resection [28]. Surgical excision in the infant or child is sometimes met with resistance by both parents and physicians, yet with many tumors surgery is clearly the best treatment. A wide resection for some tumors may pose psychological and cosmetic difficulties that parents can learn to accept if these difficulties are discussed in an open and helpful manner. When parents accept their children disabilities, the children in turn, can adjust very well functionally and psychologically following operations [29]. Cryosurgery is relatively new to the management of head and neck tumors in children. Local freezing has the ability to destroy tumor cells. A wide variety of probe tips are available to treat lesions of the skin, nose, mouth, nasopharynx, oropharynx, hypopharynx and larynx. Unlike surgical excision or radiation therapy, cryosurgery has the capability of destroying the tumor and only minimally affecting the surrounding normal tissue; also unlike radiation therapy,cryosurgery can be repeatedly administered to a specific area should the tumor persist or recur. The role of cryosurgery is still being assessed, but the potential is both great and exciting [29]. In planning treatment for pediatric tumors, authors stress the importance of the growth development of the jaw, and of esthetics and functional concerns in later periods of life [30].

5. Benign odontogenic tumors

5.1. Odontogenic epithelium with mature, fibrous stroma without odontogenic ectomesenchyme

5.1.1. Ameloblastomas have been classified as follows (WHO 2005 classification)

- Ameloblastoma, solid/multicystic type
- Ameloblastoma, extraosseous/peripheral type
- Ameloblastoma, desmoplastic type
- Ameloblastoma, unicystic type

Ameloblastoma is a tumor of the odontogenic epithelium, first described by Cusick in 1827. Ameloblastoma is perhaps the most perplexing of all odontogenic neoplasms due to its unexplainable clinical and histopathological behavior [31] It accounts for less than 1% of all odontogenic cysts and tumors. Although all ameloblastomas have the same cell of origin, there are several biologically distinct forms. The differences are especially important in pediatric cases. Central ameloblastomas occur as unicystic, multicystic or solid lesions. Ameloblastoma is non-encapsulated and infiltrates surrounding bone marrow. Even though they are locally infiltrative, they can rarely metastasize. They may occur in any part of both jaws but most are in the middle and posterior regions of the mandible. Ameloblastomas are always purely radiolucent and may be unilocular but frequently become multilocular as they increase in size. If not found and treated early, they will expand the jaws. Despite being categorized as benign tumors, ameloblastomas have a high rate of recurrence, and there is a risk of malignant transformation when treated inadequately. Clinically, ameloblastoma frequently manifests as a painless swelling, which can be accompanied by facial deformity, malocclusion, and loss of dentition, ulceration and periodontal disease. Sometimes pain occurs with varying intensities, but often quite low. It is not known whether the cause of the pain is pressure from the tumor on peripheral nerves or secondary infection [32].

The unicystic ameloblastoma resembles a dentigerous or primordial cyst clinically and radiographically and often occurs in teenage patients. Multicystic or solid ameloblastomas occur most commonly in patients 30 to 50 years of age and are extremely rare in childhood. Choung and Kaban in review of pediatric jaw tumors found only one case in 10 years. In the pediatric population, ameloblastoma must be considered in the differential diagnosis of radiolucent lesions of the jaws. In the vast majority of pediatric cases, however, these turn out to be either odcontogenic or non-odontogenic cysts or non-odontogenic primary jaw tumors. The two ameloblastic lesions that are found in childhood are the ameloblastic fibroma and the unicystic ameloblastoma.The ameloblastic fibroma appears as an asymptomatic radiolucent lesion, often associated with an impacted tooth and indistinguishable from an odontogenic cyst. The patients are usually under 12 years of age. The unicystic ameloblastoma occurs in teenagers, most commonly in the mandible. The patient exhibits a painless facial swelling or radiolucency, usually associated with an impacted third molar. The lesion is most commonly unilocular and may produce cortical expansion or perforation. Roots of adjacent teeth may be displaced or resorbed. Aspiration reveals clear serous fluid from a cystic mass [33].

There has been some debate regarding the most appropriate method for surgical removal of ameloblastomas. These range from conservative to radical modes of treatment. The conservative modalities include curettage, enucleation and cryosurgery; while the radical modalities are marginal, segmental and composite resections. The recommended treatment for ameloblastoma in children should be radical resection, 0.5 to 1 cm past what appears to be normal bone [34]. Treatment of both unicystic ameloblastomas and ameloblastic fibromas consists of enucleation [33] Simple curettage is usually met with recurrence. It has been reported that pediatric ameloblastomas are generally unicystic and do not extend beyond the cystic wall of the tumor cell. [30] This type of tumor has a much better prognosis (Figure 2).

Early diagnosis is the most important component of therapy for this odontogenic tumor, which does not have specific radiographic features in the early stages. In particular, unilocular ameloblastoma may be difficult to diagnosis for the surgeon. Surgical enucleation with bony curettage and intra-operatory cryostat examination of the lesion allows preservative treatment and reduction of the risk of relapse [35]. The loss of permanent teeth, removed during the surgical treatment, will require orthodontic-prosthetic rehabilitation when the patient reaches adult age. Peripheral ameloblastoma occurs in soft tissue outside and overlying the alveolar bone. This neoplasm arises from the basal layer of the surface epithelium or remnants of the dental lamina. It occurs most frequently in the fourth to sixth decade and has a slight male predilection. The mandible is affected twice as frequently as the maxilla. Seldom does this neoplasm exhibit any radiographic findings. Superficial erosion in the alveolar region is occasionally observed. The microscopic pattern of peripheral ameloblastoma is similar to that of central ameloblastoma; however, it lacks the invasiveness of its central counterpart. Most peripheral ameloblastomas are acanthomatous. This lesion can be confused with peripheral odontogenic fibroma because features of both lesions may be present. However, in the hands of an experienced oral pathologist the

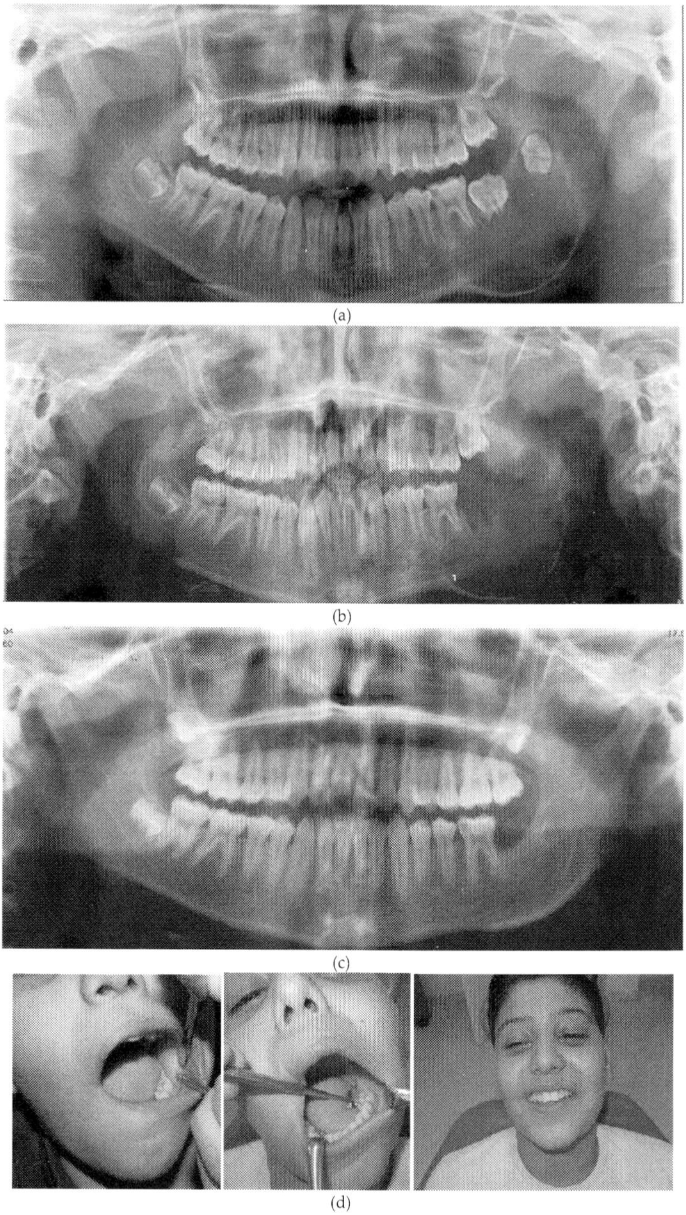

Figure 2. (a): Ameloblastoma: Orthopantomograph of a 12-year-old boy who had a painless bony- hard swelling of the left mandible associated with cortical expansion. (b): Radiological appearance after surgical treatment. (c): Radiological appearance taken 24 months post-operatively. (d): Presurgery photographs showing the left mandible associated with cortical expansion and postoperative clinical control at 12 and 24 months

diagnosis is generally not difficult. Because this lesion is relatively innocuous, noninvasive, and displays little tendency for recurrence, it is treated by local excision. Despite its behavior, 1-year follow-up examinations are recommended [36, 37].

5.1.2. *Squamous odontogenic tumor*

The squamous odontogenic tumor (SOT) is a rare and benign neoplasm frequently located within the jaws. In 1975, Pullon et al. identified this entity and reported it for the first time in a series of 6 cases. This benign tumor has a slow and gradual growth that might invade the trabecular bone, destroying the cortical bone and infiltrating adjacent structures. Its aetiology remains unknown although it could be originated from the epithelial remnants of the Malassez. It usually appears over the lateral radicular surface of an erupted tooth and diminishes the height of alveolar bone causing tooth mobility. There is a similar entity that is characterized by squamous odontogenic tumor like proliferations (SOTLP) with a very similar histological pattern than the SOT. This lesion commonly is located in the wall of an odontogenic cyst and has a non-neoplastic character like in the SOT, representing probably, an hamartomatous lesion. [38]

5.1.3. *Calcifying epithelial odontogenic tumor*

The calcifying epithelial odontogenic tumor (CEOT) is a rare tumor. It was first described as a separate pathologic entity by a Dutch pathologist Jens Jorgen Pindborg in 1955. The term "Pindborg's tumor" was first used by Shafer and colleagues in 1963. CEOT is a rare benign odontogenic epithelial neoplasm representing about 0.4-3% of all odontogenic tumors. This tumor more frequently affects adults in the age range of 20-60 years, with a peak incidence in the 5th decade of life with equal sex predisposition. CEOT is a rarely seen odontogenic tumor in pediatric patients. It is a benign, but locally aggressive tumor; of all the odontogenic tumors, CEOT accounts for 1% of the cases. Approximately 200 cases have been reported to date. Although the tumor is clearly of odontogenic origin, its histogenesis is still uncertain. It usually involves the premolar-molar area of the mandible with about 50% cases associated with unerupted or embedded teeth. Etiology of this lesion is not clear. In the 113 cases reviewed by Franklin and Pindborg, patients ranged from 8 to 92 years with a mean age of 40 years. Radiographically, this tumor is often mistaken for a dentigerous cyst or ameloblastoma [39]. The diagnosis of CEOT is based on histological examination, revealing polyhedral neoplastic cells which have abundant eosinophilic, finely granular cytoplasm with nuclear pleomorphism and prominent nucleoli. Most of the cells are arranged in broad ramifying and anastomosing sheet-like masses with little intervening stroma. An extracellular eosinophilic homogenous material staining like amyloid is characteristic of this tumor with concentric calcified deposits, resembling psammoma bodies called "Liesegang rings. A painless, slow-growing swelling is the most common presenting sign. The differential diagnosis includes adenomatoid odontogenic tumor, calcifying odontogenic cyst, dentigerous cyst, ameloblastic fibro-odontoma and odontoma. It is an infiltrative neoplasm and causes destruction with local expansion. Definitive resection of the entire mass with tumor-free surgical margins (en bloc resection) is the preferred treatment as tumor will recur if not completely removed. Long-term follow ups are recommended (Figure 3). Local recurrence rates of 10-15% have been reported [40]

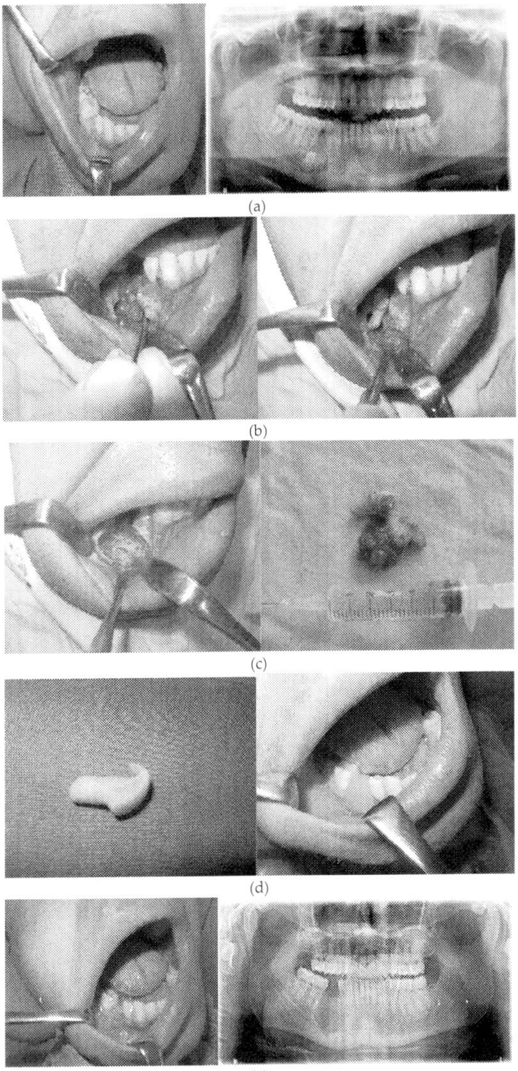

(a)

(b)

(c)

(d)

(e)

Figure 3. (a): Pindborg (CEOT) tumor associated with impacted premolar. Preoperative clinical (left) and radiological appearance of CEOT (right). (b): Clinical appearance of CEOT and impacted premolar tooth. (c): Postoperative operation site and macroscopic appearance of the mass. (d): Application of surgical obturator. (e): Postoperative clinical (left) and radiological control (right) at 12 months.

5.1.4. Adenomatoid Odontogenic Tumor (AOT)

This is a tumor mostly of teenagers. It occurs in the middle and anterior portions of the jaws in contrast to ameloblastoma which is found mostly in the posterior segment. Two-thirds occur in the maxilla and it is more common in females. The tumor may be partially cystic, and in some cases solid lesion may be present as masses in the wall of a large cyst. It is believed that lesion is not a neoplasm" Philipsen et al. subdivided this condition into three groups referred to as follicular, extrafollicular, and peripheral. These variants have common histologic characteristics that indicate a common origin as derived from the complex system of dental lamina or its remnant [41].The follicular and extrafollicular variants account for 96% of all AOT and of these 71% are follicular variants.The peripheral variant is the rarest with only 18 cases reported so far [42]. The follicular variant is predominantly associated with the crown and often part of the root of an impacted (unerupted) tooth (Figure 4). The most frequently associated tooth is the maxillary canine rarely the permanent molars. Based on the clinical and radiographic examination the follicular variant is often initially mistaken as dentigerous cyst. This tumor is encapsulated and is treated by curettage with a recurrence rate approaching zero. The radiographic appearance is a unilocular radiolucency, often around the crown of an unerupted tooth in which case they resemble a dentigeous cyst.. A homogeneous, eosinophilic and amorphous material may occasionally be found in AOT [43]. If they are present in sufficient size and number, they may show on the radiograph as a "snow-flake" pattern

5.1.5. Keratocystic odontogenic tumor

The Keratocystic Odontogenic Tumor (KCOT) has been defined by the World Health Organization In 2005, as a benign intraosseous neoplasm of odontogenic origin with characteristic lining of parakeratinized squamous epithelium. It represents approximately 10 percent of all jaw cysts and may occur in a wide age range of patients. About 70 percent or more cases involve the mandible, especially in the molar, angle and ramus regions. The clinical features associated with the keratocystic odontogenic tumor show it to be a unilocular or multilocular radiolucency. It is generally believed that these lesions originate from remnants of the dental lamina in the same way as the primordial cyst. However, a tooth is generally not missing and, therefore, they are believed to originate from additional remnants of the lamina not involved in tooth formation. Alternatively, in some cases they may arise from the oral mucosa, particularly in the retromolar region, because daughter cysts are found between the oral mucosa and the cyst in the retromolar region [44].

Symptoms such as pain, swelling and drainage may be present, especially with larger lesions. However, at least half of all lesions are discovered as incidental radiographic findings. Due to the propensity of KCOTs to grow within the medullary bone, they have the potential to become extremely large without causing any clinical signs or symptoms. Radiographically, the KCOT presents as a well defined radiolucency with thin corticated margins. These tumors are normally diagnosed histologically from a sample of the lining. With simple enucleation, it seems that the recurrence rate may be from 25% to 60%. Approximately 20-40 percent of these tumors are associated with an unerupted tooth and can be identical in appearance to a dentigerous cyst (Figure 5). Root resorption is relatively uncommon. The classic treatment of

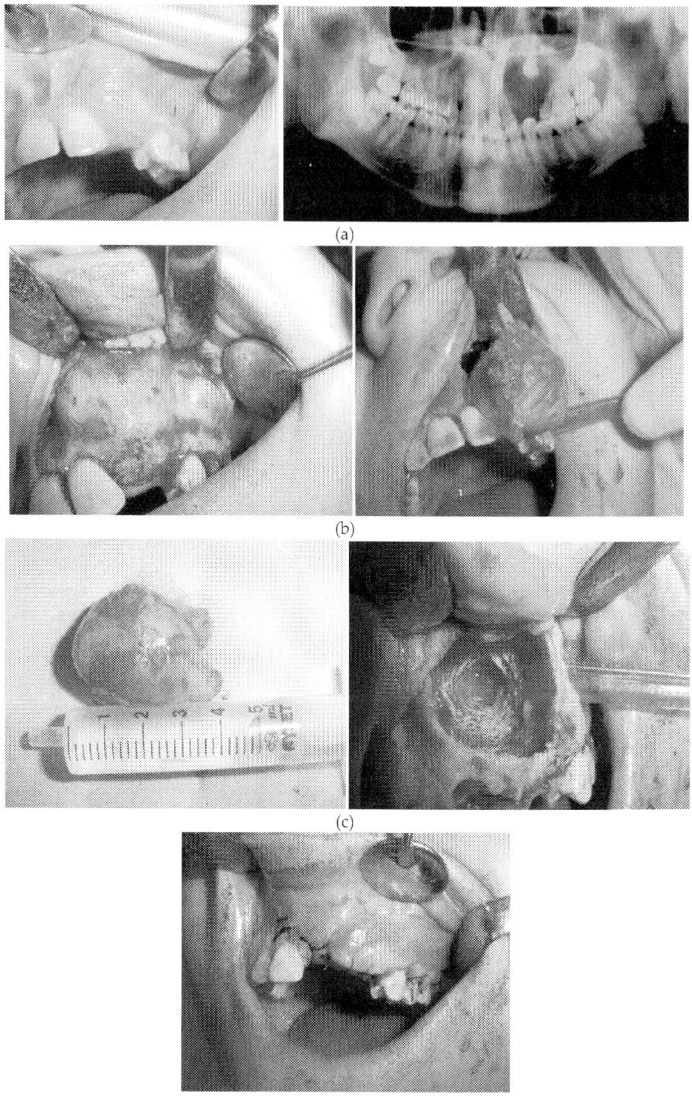

Figure 4. AOT associated with canine tooth. Oral photograph showing an anterior maxillary swelling in a 16-year-old girl. Preoperative radiological appearance of AOT. (b): Oral photograph showing large buccal anterior exspansion. Clinical appearance of the mass being removed. (c): Clinical appearance of the encapsulated mass and the operation site after enucleation. (d): Postoperative appearance of the operation site

this lesion is surgical marsupialization, enucleation and curettage being performed through an intraoral approach. KCOTs have a high recurrence rate and develop more aggressively than

http://dx.doi.org/10.5772/59341

any other jaw cyst. Based on the high rate of recurrence, most authors advocate radical enucleation for small unilocular keratocysts and suggest resection and bone grafting for very large lesions. But there is a general agreement that complete removal of large multilocular KCOTs of the mandible ramus may be difficult because of the possibility that remnants of cystic tissue or that satellite microcysts may be left behind. Most authors have shown the successful treatment of large KCOTs using the technique of decompression and irrigation. The benefits of this protocol over more conventional approaches (enucleation, en bloc resection) lie in the minimal surgical morbidity. In addition, the associated structures such as the inferior alveolar nerve and developing teeth are less vulnerable to damage. Morgan et al. reported that treatment with Carnoy's solution did not show a significant association with recurrence. Most reports point out that recurrence will appear within the 5 to 7 years [45, 45].

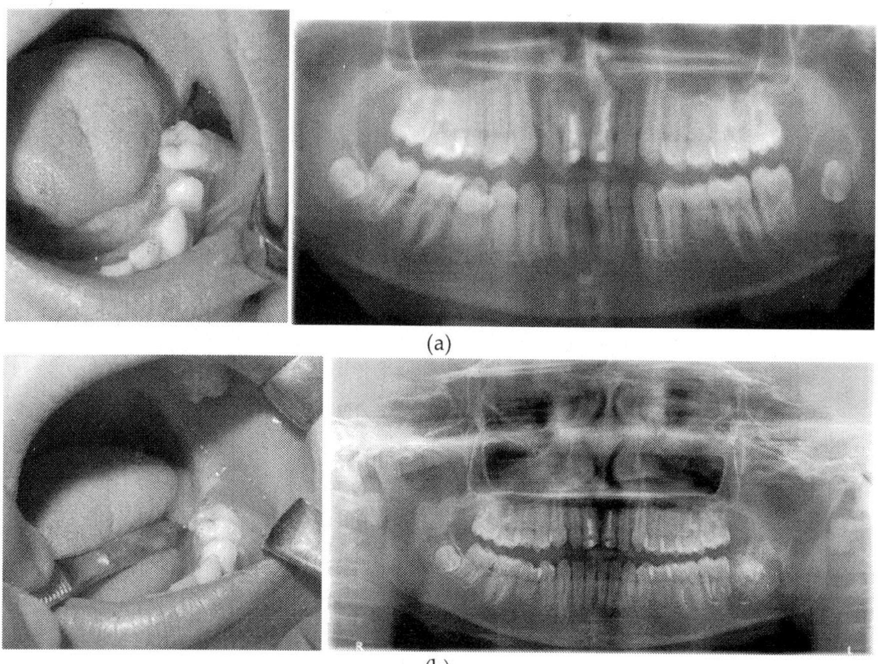

Figure 5. (a): KCOT. Frontal photograph and radiograph showing a 14-year-old boy presenting a posterior mandibular radiolucency associated with impacted left third molar. (b): Oral and radiographic appearance of the operated area with gauze tamponade after cystostomy and application of the surgical obturator.

5.2. Odontogenic epithelium with odontogenic ectomesenchyme, with or without hard tissue formation

5.2.1. *Ameloblastic fibroma*

This tumor, at least conceptually, is a compound odontoma and which includes the ameloblastic fibradentinoma, ameloblastic odontoma and complex odontoma [46]. All show evidence of inductive interaction between odontogenic epithelial and ectomesenchymal components, but only the ameloblastic fibroma lacks hard tissue formation. The ameloblastic fibroma presents as a jaw swelling and multilocular radiolucency in the lower premolar or molar region or, less commonly, in the maxilla. This is a tumor of childhood, the typical patient is about 12 –14 years old, seldom is it seen beyond age 20 yrs. The posterior segment of the mandible is the most common location. Local swelling or failure of teeth to erupt on time or in proper alignment may call attention to the tumor. Ameloblastic fibromas are purely radiolucent. Small lesions may be unilocular but larger lesions are ordinarily multilocular. Both odontogenic epithelium and odontogenic ectomesenchyme contribute to this tumor (an odontogenic mixed tumor not to be confused with the mixed tumor of the salivary gland). The epithelium grows in small islands and cords. This tumor is clearly benign and is ordinarily treated by vigorous curettement. The recurrence rate is placed at about 15 %. Even though this tumor is comprised of both odontogenic epithelium and odontogenic ectomesenchyme, it does not secrete either enamel matrix or dentin. Its microscopic structure like its radiographic appearance, is reminiscent of that of the ameloblastoma, but with two major differences: the connective tissue component resembles dental papilla; and the stellate reticulum zone of the epithelium is poorly developed. The ameloblastic fibroma poses two further problems: for the histopathologist, it must be distinguished from a developing complex odontoma; and for the surgeon, the requirement for complete excision must be weighed against the need to preserve the developing jaw bones and dentition [40].

5.2.2. *Ameloblastic fibrodentinoma and Ameloblastic fibro-odontoma*

Ameloblastic fibrodentinoma (AFD) and ameloblastic fibroodontoma represent, at least for didactic purposes, intermediate stages between the ameloblastic fibroma and the complex odontoma. They also represent the interface between hamartomas and neoplasms, and occur in late adolescence or in early adulthood. A classic site for the formation of an ameloblastic fibrodentinoma is within, or adjacent to, the follicle of an unerupted tooth, typically a lower third molar, in its path of eruption. Most often it presents as a symptomless radio-opacity and may not be the cause of the failure of the underlying tooth to erupt (Figure 6). The ameloblastic fibro-odontoma is a more variable entity and, as already noted, may be hard to distinguish, clinically, radiographically and histopathologically, from a developing complex odontoma or ameloblastic fibroma. The majority of ameloblastic fibro-odontomas are small, mixed radio-opaque / radiolucent lesions that occur across a similar age-range to the ameloblastic fibro-dentinoma, and most are small and unilocular with limited growth potential after completion of tooth formation. They show features that suggest the formation of tooth-like structures, complete with tubular dentine and varying degrees of enamel matrix calcification. That this is not a developing odontoma is suggested by its perceived continued growth potential (hence the belief that at least some are true neoplasms) and its presentation at an age when odontomes have normally "matured" and become quiescent, as well as incorporating an extensive soft tissue (radiolucent) component that somewhat resembles ameloblastic fibroma [40, 46]. A regular follow-up protocol should be established to rule out any evidence of recurrence and malignant transformation. A detailed study is required in order to understand the relationship of AFD and related lesions, their biological behavior and management strategies [47].

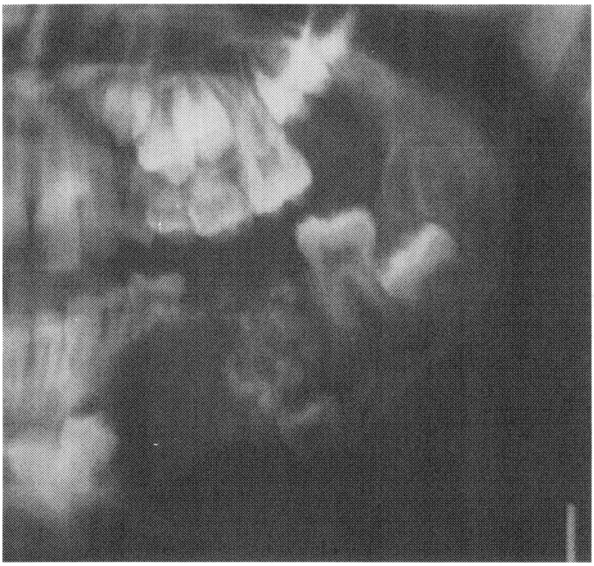

Figure 6. Ameloblastic fibro-odontoma. This combines the radio-opaque component that resembles a complex odontoma with radiolucent soft tissue that histologically combines the features of ameloblastic fibroma with the early stages of tooth germ development.

5.2.3. Odontoma

- **Odontoma, complex type**
- **Odontoma, compound type**

Odontomas are hamartomas of aberrant tooth formation, which occur due to budding of extra-odontogenic epithelial cells or detachment of odontogenic cells from the dental lamina [48]. These odontogenic cells may in turn differentiate and deposit enamel, dentine, cementum or pulp in the form of multiple teeth like structures (compound odontoma), amorphous calcified masses (complex odontoma) or a combination of both (composite odontoma and compound-complex odontoma). Trauma to the tooth bud during its early developmental stages has been proposed as a possible predisposing factor for the origin of odontoma. [49,50].

As a result, these tumors are mostly radiodense. In the compound odontoma, multiple small and malformed tooth-like structures are formed creating a "bag of marbles" radiographic appearance. In the complex odontoma, there is little or no tendency to form tooth-like structures. The dentin and enamel are entwined in a mass that bears no resemblance to teeth. Both types of odontoma are found in the early years, usually in the teens or early twenties. Compound odontoma is more common in the anterior jaw segment whereas the complex type is found more commonly in the posterior jaws (Figure 7). Many are associated with an unerupted tooth. Odontomas behave more like developmental abnormalities (hamartomas) than true neoplasms. Although they may reach a large size, they do eventually cease growing in contrast to true neoplasms which show continuous growth. Treatment is elective surgery. They have a limited growth potential and cause no pain or cosmetic deformity [46].

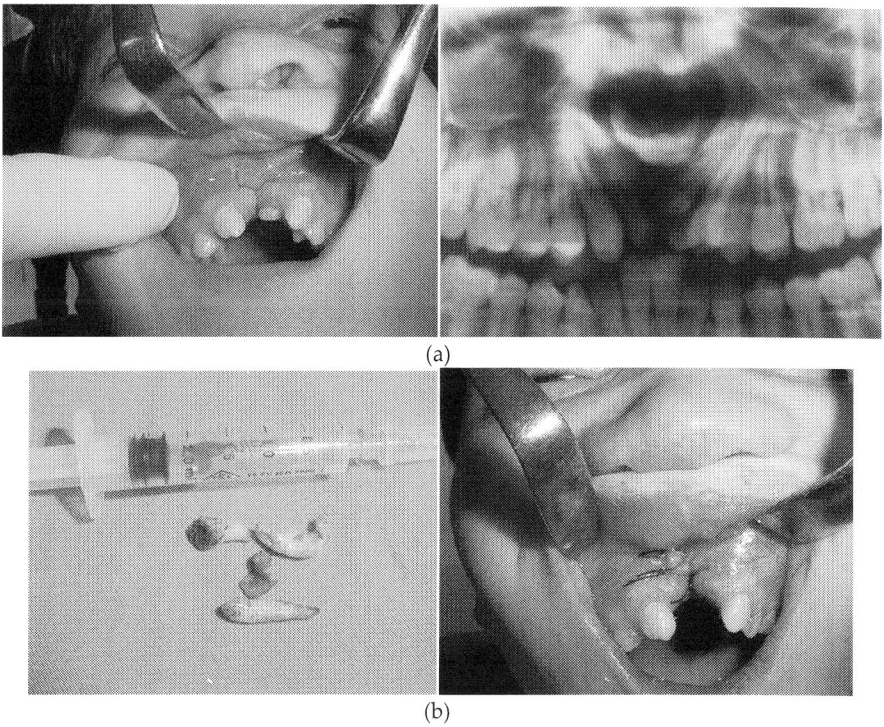

NOTE: We have skipped odontoameloblastoma, calcifying cystic odontogenic tumor, dentinogenic ghost cell tumor, malignant ameloblastoma,ameloblastic carcinoma, clear cell odontogenic carcinoma because they are exceedingly rare.

Figure 7. a): Compound odontoma associated with two mesiodens. Photograph and radiograph showing a 11-year-old boy presenting an anterior maxillary radiolucency with impacted supernumerary teeth and radio-opaque mass. (b): Macroscopic appearance of the supernumerary teeth and postoperative operation site

5.3. Mesenchyme and/or odontogenic ectomesenchyme with or without odontogenic epithelium

5.3.1. *Odontogenic fibroma*

Central odontogenic fibromas are encountered as unilocular radiolucencies that turn out to be solid, rather than cystic, following enucleation. They are rare, far rarer for example than ameloblastomas, and arise usually anterior to the molars, more commonly in the maxilla and mainly in women, as a small, well-circumscribed radiolucency that may cause resorption and/or displacement of adjacent vital teeth (Figure 8). A wide age-range is noted among the relatively few reported cases, and a scalloped radiographic margin may denote a more aggressive behavior pattern. Following enucleation, most odontogenic fibromas do not recur, although there have been occasional reports of some following a more aggressive course; however, there seems to be little correlation with the histological pattern [40, 46]

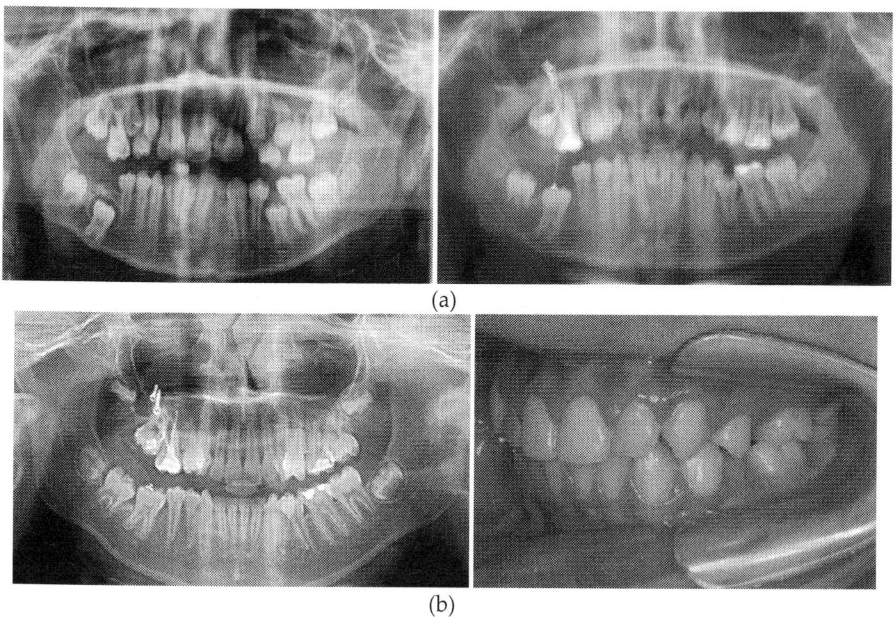

Figure 8. (a): Odontogenic fibroma. Radiograph showing a 12-year-old boy presenting with a posterior mandibular mass associated with an impacted left first molar tooth. (b): Orthodontic extrusion of the impacted first molar using the zygomatic bone anchor and clinical appearance after the right first molar extrusion

5.3.2. *Odontogenic myxoma/myxofibroma*

Despite the name similarity, the odontogenic myxoma is quite a different entity from the odontogenic fibroma in almost all respects. Odontogenic myxoma (OM) of the jaws, first described by Thoma and Goldman in 1947, is believed to arise from odontogenic ectomesenchyme [51, 52]. It is a rare benign tumor characterized grossly by mucoid or gelatinous grayish-white tissue that replaces the cancellous bone and expands the cortex. OMs are locally invasive, non-metastasizing neoplasms of the jaws, almost exclusively seen in tooth-bearing areas. It accounts for 0.2-17.7% of odontogenic tumors. It predominantly involves the mandible and maxillary tumors are known to be more aggressive than tumors involving the mandible [53]. Most frequently, OMs occur in the 2 nd and 3 rd decades of life. Cortical expansion and perforation are common findings; however, maxillary myxomas often extend into the sinus [54]. Radiographically, the tumor presents as a unilocular or multilocular radiolucent lesion with fine, bony trabeculae within its interior structure expressing a honeycombed, soap bubble, or tennis racket appearance [55]. A histologic characteristic of this tumor resembles the mesenchymal portion of a tooth in development. The lesion is not encapsulated being characterized by the proliferation of a few rounded cells, fusiforms and star cells, being included in abundant myxomatous stroma with a few collagen fibers [56]. They are uncommon. Extragnathic skeletal lesions are a rarity. Since it does not produce a calcified matrix material, it is purely radiolucent. If allowed to reach a large size, it takes a big operation to remove it [40].

5.3.3. Cementoblastoma

Cementoblastoma in the current World Health Organization classification of odontogenic tumors, is in the category of tumors of mesenchyme and/or odontogenic ectomesenchyme with or without odontogenic epithelium [57]. The lesion was first recognized by Noeberg in 1930 [58]. The lesion is considered as the only true neoplasm of cementum origin. It generally occurs in young persons, comprises <1-6.2% of all odontogenic tumors and is characterized as being attached to the roots, most frequently associated with first permanent molars [59]. The differential diagnosis for a periapical radiopacity include cementoma, osteoblastoma, periapical cemental dysplasia, condensing osteitis and hypercementosis. The majority of these tumors are radiopaque, but a radiolucent tumor may occur in rare instances. Histologically, it presents as a well-circumscribed tumor composed of cementum like tissue surrounded by a fibrous capsule. Surgical enucleation of the cementoblastoma with the associated tooth is usually curative, although recurrences have been reported following incomplete excision. The recurrence rate is 21.7-37.1% [60, 61].

5.4. Bone-related (Fibro-osseous) lesions

5.4.1. Juvenile ossifying fibroma

Benign fibro-osseous lesions of the head and neck region are uncommon and constitute a wide range of tumors sharing some histopathological features. This group includes developmental, reactive or dysplastic lesions as well as neoplasm such as fibrous dysplasia (FD), ossifying fibroma (OF), and cemento-osseous dysplasia (COD) [62]. Ossifying fibromas are rare benign, neoplasms arising from undifferentiated cells of the periodontal ligament tissues (63). These have been described as demarcated or rarely encapsulated neoplasms consisting of fibrous tissue containing varying amounts of mineralized material resembling bone and/or cementum which is one of its principal characteristics [64]. In 1872, Menzel first described ossifying fibroma, but in 1972, Montgomery assigned terminology to it. It accounts for 3.1% of all oral tumors and for 9.6% of all gingival lesions. There are two types of ossifying fibroma, central and peripheral. The central type arises from the endosteum or periodontal ligament adjacent to the root apex and expands from the medullary cavity of the bone. The peripheral type occurs solely on the soft tissue overlying the alveolar process. Trauma or local irritants are known to precipitate the development of this lesion [65]. It is common in young adults (especially, 2nd and 3rd decades) with a female predominance and is generally asymptomatic until the growth produces a noticeable swelling most often found in interdental gingiva, located anterior to molars and in the maxilla [66]. The suggested etiology although unknown has been associated with inflammatory hyperplasia of the periodontal ligament [67]. When ossifying fibroma is diagnosed in young people the term "juvenile" is used. The accurate nature and classification of JOF has undergone considerable debate among pathologists, resulting in a confusing evolution of competing nomenclatures [68] According to the WHO classification of odontogenic tumors 2005, JOF is further subdivided into two distinct clinic-pathological variant i.e., juvenile psammornatoid ossifying fibroma (JPOF) and juvenile trabecular ossifying fibroma (JTOF) [69]. Juvenile psammornatoid ossifying fibroma (JPOF) is a rare fibro-osseous neoplasm that arises within the craniofacial bones in individuals under 15 years of age, and these lesions are usually benign and tend to grow slowly. JPOF is rare fibro-osseous neoplasm. Probability of malignancy makes this lesion worrysome. The lesion is nonencapsulated but well demarcated from surrounding bone. JPOF mainly involves the bones of the orbit and paranasal sinuses, whereas the trabecular type commonly involves the jaws. JPOFs are rare, benign, potentially aggressive fibro-osseous tumors of the craniofacial bones characterized by the presence of numerous calcified spherules within an actively proliferating connective tissue stroma. They are mainly seen in the sino-naso-orbital region of young individuals. Males and females are equally affected. The maxilla and the mandible are the dominant sites of incidence. Occurrence in the maxilla is slightly more frequent than in the mandible (Figure 9) The incidence of JPOF is still unknown because of relatively few cases reported till date. The pathogenesis of JPOF jaw lesions are related to the maldevelopment of basal generative mechanism that is essential for root formation. The developing tooth can either be displaced, missing or remain unerupted. It tends to occur at younger age group and is locally aggressive and these characteristics make them different from conventional ossifying fibroma and other fibro-osseous lesions. Moreover, this lesion may clinically manifest with rapid painless expansion of the affected bone as an aggressive lesion mimicking malignancy such as osteosarcoma. JPOF can be easily excluded from malignant bone tumors on the routine histological examination. Additionally, it may be difficult to distinguish JPOF from other fibro-osseous lesions because of the overlapping features. It is important to accurately recognize JPOF for reaching the diagnosis and treatment planning. Because of this lesion's aggressive nature and high recurrence rate, early detection and complete surgical excision are essential [40, 46].

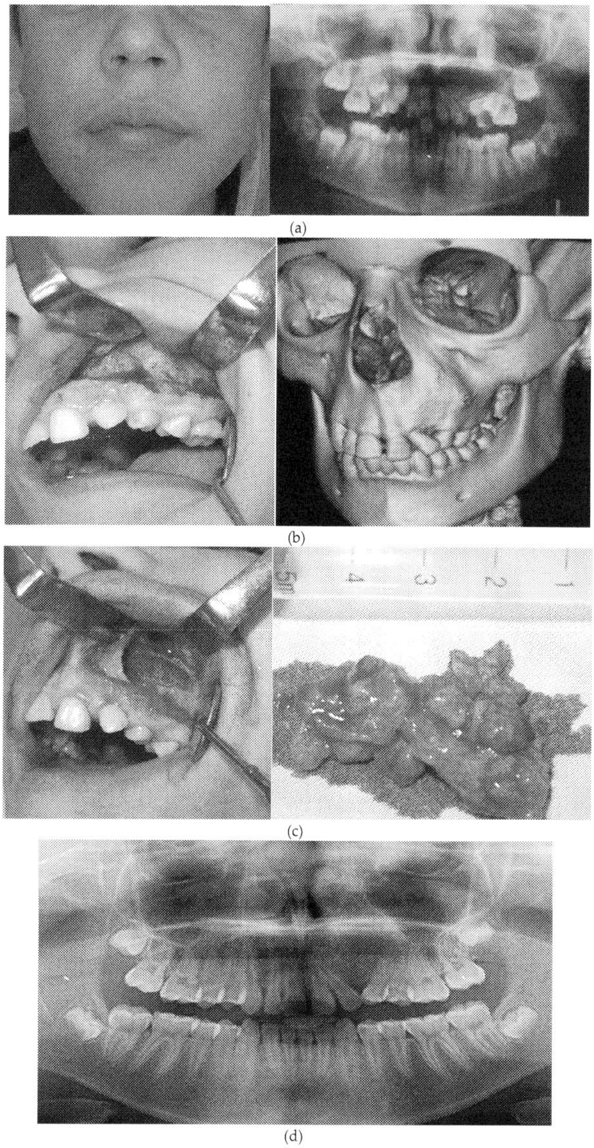

Figure 9. (a): JPOF. Photograph showing a 14-year-old boy presenting an anterior maxillary expansion associated with impacted left canine tooth ; Preoperative facial view showing asymmetry of face (left); Preoperative radiograph showing large radiolucency, well-defined sclerotic border around the upper left impacted canine tooth (right). (b): Clinical and radiographical appearance of buccal cortical expansion. (c): Clinical appearance after enucleation and the mass. (d): Postoperative panoramic radiograph showing normal bone pattern

5.4.2. Central giant cell granuloma

There are a number of lesions that occur in the jaws that contain giant cells within them. They include cherubism, giant cell granuloma of the jaws, giant cell tumor, aneurysmal bone cyst, traumatic bone cyst and brown tumor of hyperparathyroidism. Their relationship to each other, however, is ill defined. The histological similarities with the finding of multinucleated giant cells of osteoclastic origin and the lesions themselves greatly differ in their genetic origin, etiopathogenesis and clinical behaviour. Central giant cell granuloma (CGCG) is fairly common in the jaws and it is a nonneoplastic bone disease, probably reactive to some unknown stimulus. CGCG constitutes approximately 7% of the benign jaw tumors. Usually, it occurs in patients 30 years of age or younger with painless swelling and an asymmetry in facial appearance. The clinical behavior of CGCG ranges from a slowly growing asymptomatic lesion to an aggressive lesion manifesting with pain, local bone destruction, root resorption, or displacement of teeth. The highest rate of occurrence is the mandible, and most mandibular lesions occur anterior to the first molars.

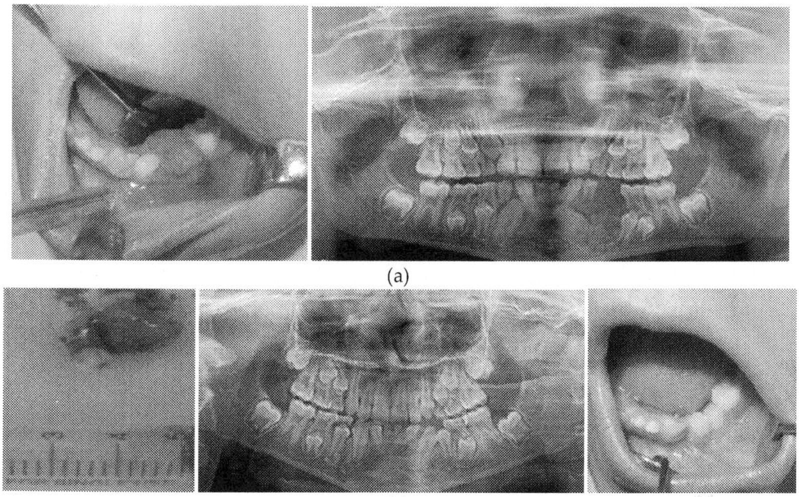

(a)

(b)

Figure 10. (a). CGCG: Photograph showing a 13-year-old boy presenting a posterior mandibular lesion at premolar region (a): Preoperative facial view showing ulcerative mass (left): Preoperative radiograph showing the lesion. (b): Excised pathologic mass associated with tooth ; Postoperative panoramic radiograph showing normal bone pattern. Clinical view taken 13 months post-operatively

Its etiology is still unknown and its biological behavior is poorly understood. This lesion occurs almost exclusively within the jaw bones. It usually presents as a painless swelling of the jawbone. Radiographically, CGCG presents as radiolucent defect, which may be unilocular or multilocular. The defect usually is well-circumscribed and, in some cases, displacement of teeth can be found (Figure 10). Conventional treatment for the CGCG has been local curettage and this has been associated with a high success rate and low recurrence rate. The conservative surgical treatment of CGCG usually involves curettage alone or along with peripheral ostectomy with no evidence of disease in a 2 year follow up perior. The margins of the CGCG may also be thermally sterilized with a laser or a cryoprobes. Radical surgical techniques of resection without continuity defect, peripheral ostectomy and en-bloc resection have sometimes been justified for aggressive CGCG. Pediatric patients necessitate conservative management to prevent long term developmental defects. Steroids and calcitonin have been advocated recently for inhibition of osteoclastic activity. Equal parts of triamcinolone acetonide (10mg/ml) and 0.5% bupivacaine injected into the lesion for a period of 11 weeks has been shown to be effective in a child patient. Relative contraindications do exist in certain medical conditions, such as diabetes mellitus, peptic ulcer and generalized immunocompromised states. Calcitonin nasal spray 200 U/spray once or twice daily was reported to be safe and effective for the treatment of CGCG [40,46].

6. Conclusion

Literature reveals very few reported studies involving pediatric pathologies and there are different treatment modalities for pediatric jaw tumors in the recent literatures. Many surgeons find it difficult to decide which technique offers better results, and are also uncertain about the factors which might influence their techniques of choice. The rapid growth and development process in childhood and adolescence affects the growth potential of tumors and tumor like lesions and occasionally results in considerable morbidity. There are many rare odontogenic tumors that may involve the head and neck in the pediatric population. Each of them deserves careful attention by a multidisciplinary tumor board that includes pediatric oncologists, radiation oncologists, dentists, and surgeons. Clinicians need to keep abreast of the various intraosseous lesions with their presenting signs and symptoms, so that the patient can be treated without any delay and avoiding unnecessary administration of antibiotics. Subsequent to an unresponsive antibiotic therapy radiographs are taken to reveal a radiolucent or radiodense lesion in the jaws. As a consequence the contribution of pathological examination remains imperative in odontogenic cyst or tumor diagnosis. It is very important to consider surgical and permanent dental concerns during jaw tumor treatment planning. Facial growth and aesthetic results should be considered in the surgical planning.

Author details

Mehmet Cemal Akay[1*], Mert Zeytinoğlu[1], Birant Şimşek[1] and Işıl Aras[2]

*Address all correspondence to: cemalakay@yahoo.com

1 Ege University, Faculty of Dentistry, Department of Oral and Maxillofacial Surgery, Bornova, Izmir, Turkey

2 Ege University, Faculty of Dentistry, Department of Orthodontics, Izmir, Turkey

References

[1] Pindborg, JJ. & Kramer, IRH. (1971) Histological typing of odontogenic tumours, jaw cysts, and allied lesions (International Histological Classification of Tumours No. 5). Geneva World Health Organization

[2] Taylor, AM. (2008) New findings and controversies in odontogenic tumors. Med Oral Patol Oral Cir Bucal. Sep1; 13(9): E555-8.

[3] Slootweg, PJ., Van den Bos, T.& Straks, W. (1985) Glycosaminoglycans in myxoma of the jaw: a biochemical study. J Oral Pathol. Apr;14(4):299-306.

[4] Ulmansky, M., Lustmann, J.& Balkin, N. (1999) Tumors and tumor-like lesions of the oral cavity and related structures in Israeli children, Int J Oral Maxillofac Surg. Aug; 28(4):291-4.

[5] Barnes, L., Eveson, JW., Reichart, P.& Sidransky, D. (2005) (editors). World Health Organisation classification of tumours. Pathology and genetics of head and neck tumours. Lyon: IARC Press, p. 283-328.

[6] Philipsen, HP. & Reichart, PA. (2006) Classification of odontogenic tumours. A historical review, Oct;35(9):525-9.

[7] Tawfik, MA. & Zyada, MM. (2010) Odontogenic tumors in Dakahia, Egypt: analysis of 82 cases. Oral Surg Oral Med Oral Pathol Oral Radiol Endod 109: e67–e73.

[8] Eversole, R., Su, L.& ElMofty,S. (2008) Benign fibro-osseous lesions of the craniofacial complex. A review. Head Neck Pathol. Sep;2(3):177-202.

[9] Cunningham, MJ., Myers,EN.& Bluestone, CD. (1987) Malignant tumors of the head and neck in children: a twenty-year review. Int J Pediatr Otorhinolaryngol. Oct;13(3): 279-92.

[10] Jones, AV.& Franklin, CD. (2006) An analysis of oral and maxillofacial pathology found in children over 30-year period. International Journal of Paediatr Dent. 16:19-30.

[11] Choung, R.& Kaban, LB. (1985) Diagnosis and treatment of jaw tumours in children. J Oral Maxillofac Surg. 43: 323-332.

[12] Steliarova-Foucher, E., Stiller, C., Lacour, B.& Kaatsch, P. (2005) International Classification of Childhood Cancer, third edition. Apr 1;103(7):1457-67.

[13] Tanaka, N., Murata, A., Yamaguchi, A.& Kohama, G. (1999) Clinical features and management of oral and maxillofacial tumors in children. Oral Surg Oral Med Oral Pathol. Jul;88(1):11-5.

[14] Tanrikulu, R., Erol, B.& Haspolat, K. (2004) Tumors of the maxillofacial region in children: retrospective analysis and long-term follow-up outcomes of 90 patients. Turk J Pediatr. Jan-Mar;46(1):60-6.

[15] Rapidis, AD., Economidis, J., Goumas, PD., Langdon, JD., Skordalakis, A., Tzortzatou, F., Anagnostopoulos, D.& Matsaniotis, N. (1988) Tumours of the head and neck in children. A clinico-pathological analysis of 1,007 cases. J Craniomaxillofac Surg. Aug;16(6):279-86.

[16] Willging JP. (2000) Head and Neck Masses in Children. American Academy of Otolaryngolgy Annual Meeting, Washington, D.C. September.

[17] Mullapudi, SV., Putcha, UK.& Boindala S. (2011) Odontogenic tumors and giant cell lesions of jaws--a nine year study. World Journal of Surgical Oncology. Jul 5;9:68.

[18] Slavkin, HC., Cummings, E., Bringas, P. & Honig, LS. (1982) Epithelial-derived basal lamina regulation of mesenchymal cell differentiation. Prog Clin Biol Res. 1982;85 pp: 249-59.

[19] Badger, KV.& Gardner, DG. (1997) The relationship of adamantinomatous craniopharyngioma to ghost cell ameloblastoma of the jaws: a histopathologic and immunohistochemical study. J Oral Pathol Med. Sep;26(8):349-55.

[20] Alam, K.,, Khan, R., Jain, A., Maheshwari, V., Agrawal, S., Chana, RS.& Harris, SH. (2009) The value of fine-needle aspiration cytology in the evaluation of pediatric head and neck tumors. International Journal of Pediatric Otorhinolaryngology Jul; 73(7):923-7.

[21] Crivelini, MM., de Araújo, VC., de Sousa, SO. & de Araújo, NS. (2003) Cytokeratins in epithelia of odontogenic neoplasms. Oral Dis. Jan;9(1):1-6.

[22] Kumamoto, H., Kimi, K. & Ooya, K. (2001) Detection of cell cycle-related factors in ameloblastomas. J Oral Pathol Med. May;30(5):309-15.

[23] Coleman, H., Altini, M., Ali, H., Doglioni, C., Favia, G.& Maiorano, E. (2001) Use of calretinin in the differential diagnosis of unicystic ameloblastomas. Histopathology. Apr;38(4):312-7.

[24] DeVilliers, P., Liu, H., Suggs, C., Simmons, D., Daly, B., Zhang, S., Raubenheimer, E., Larsson, A. & Wright T. (2008) Calretinin expression in the differential diagnosis of human ameloblastoma and keratocystic odontogenic tumor. Am J Surg Pathol. Feb; 32(2):256-60.

[25] Gao, YH., Yang, LJ.& Yamaguchi, A. (1997) Immunohistochemical demonstrationof bone morphogenetic protein in odontogenic tumors. J Oral Pathol Med. Jul;26(6) : 273-7.

[26] Kumamoto, H. & Ooya K. (2006) Expression of bone morphogenetic proteins and their associated molecules in ameloblastomas and adenomatoid odontogenic tumors. Oral Dis. Mar;12(2):163-70.

[27] Sato, M., Tanaka, N., Sato, T. & Amagasa, T. (1997) Oral and maxillofacial tumours in children: a review. Br J Oral Maxillofac Surg. 63:92-5.

[28] Regezi, J.& Sciubba, J. (1993) Odontogenic tumors. In: Regezi J, Sciubba J editor. Oral Pathology. ed 2. Philadelphia, PA: Saunders; p. 362–397.

[29] Jaffe, BF. (1973) Pediatric head and neck tumors: a study of 178 cases. Laryngoscope Oct;83(10):1644-51.

[30] Feinberg, SE.& Steinberg, B. (1996) Surgical management of ameloblastoma.Oral Surg Oral Med Oral Pathol Oral Radiol Endod. 81:383-8.

[31] Ramesh, V., Singh, S., Bailwad, SA., Kiran, K., Agarwal, RK. & Singh A. (2014) The Complexity of Stromal Changes in Desmoplastic Ameloblastoma. Ann Med Health Sci Res. Mar-Apr; 4(Suppl 1): S14–S17.

[32] Peter, AR.& Philipsen, HA. (2000) Odontogenic tumors and allied lesions, London: Quintessence, pp.43–58.

[33] Troulis, MJ., Williams, WB.& Kaban, LB. (2004) Staged protocol for resection, skeletal reconstruction, and oral rehabilitation of children with jaw tumors. J Oral Maxillofac Surg. Mar;62(3):335-43.

[34] Vohra, FA., Hussain, M., Mudassir, MF. & Mudassir, MS. (2009) Ameloblastomas and their management: A review Journal of Surgery Pakistan 14(3):136–52.

[35] Asamoa, EA., Ayanlere, AO., Olaitan, AA.& Adekeye, EO. (1990) Paediatric tumours of the jaws in northern Nigeria. Clinical presentation and treatment.Apr;18(3):130-5.

[36] Simpson, HE. (1974) Basal-cell carcinoma and peripheral ameloblastoma.Aug;38(2): 233-40.

[37] Gold, L. (1991) Biologic behavior of ameloblastoma. Oral Maxillofac Surg Clin N Am. 3:21–71.

[38] Sala-Pérez, S., Marco-Molina, V.& Gay-Escoda, C. (2013) Squamous odontogenic tumor-like proliferation in a radicular cyst: A case report. J Clin Exp Dent. Dec 5(5): e298-301.

[39] Lee, SK.& Kim YS.(2014) Current Concepts and Occurrence of Epithelial Odontogenic Tumors: II. Calcifying Epithelial Odontogenic Tumor Versus Ghost Cell Odontogenic Tumors Derived from Calcifying Odontogenic Cyst. The Korean Journal of Pathology 48: 175-187.

[40] Morgan, PR. (2011) Odontogenic tumors: a review. Periodontology 2000, Oct;57(1): 160-76.

[41] Philipsen, HP.& Reichart, PA. (1991) Adenomatoid odontogenic tumour: facts and figures. Oral Oncology, 35(2),pp.125–131.

[42] Philipsen, HP., Reichart, PA., Zhang, KH., Nikai, H.& Yu, QX. (1991) Adenomatoid odontogenic tumor: Biologic profile based on 499 cases. Journal of Oral Pathology and Medicine, 20(4),pp.149–158.

[43] Acharya, S. Goyal, A., Rattan, V., Vaiphei, K.& Bhatia, SK.(2014) Dentigerous Cyst or Adenomatoid Odontogenic Tumor: Clinical Radiological and Histopathological Dilemma. Case Reports in Medicine, Article ID 514720, 5 pages.

[44] Arcuri, F., Grivetto, F., Poglio, G., Brucoli, M.&Benech, A. (2011) Simultaneous palatal pleomorphic adenoma and mandibular keratocystic odontogenic tumor in a pediatric patient. J Craniofac Surg. Nov;22(6):2347-50.

[45] Hyun, HK., Hong, SD.& Kim, JW. (2009) Recurrent keratocystic odontogenic tumor in the mandible: a case report and literature review. Oral Surg Oral Med Oral Pathol Oral Radiol Endod. Aug;108(2):e7-10.

[46] Pogrel, MA. (2013) Clinical Pathology: Odontogenic and Nonodontogenic Tumors of the Jaws. Chapter 23, pp 490-534.

[47] Sankireddy, S., Kaushik, A., Krishna, BA., Reddy, AL., Vinod, VC.& Sridevi, V. (2013) Ameloblastic fibrodentinoma involving anterior maxilla: a rare case report. J Indian Soc Pedod Prev Dent. Oct-Dec;31(4):275-8.

[48] Wood, NK., Goaz, PW.& Lenher, JF. (2006) Mixed radiolucent-radiopaque lesions associated with teeth. In: Wood NK, Goaz PW (eds), Differential diagnosis of oral and maxillofacial lesions, 5th edition, Mosby Co., St. Louis, 423–426.

[49] Glasstone, S.(1952) The development of halved tooth germs; a study in experimental embryology, J Anat, 86(1):12–15.

[50] Levy, BA. (1968) Effects of experimental trauma on developing first molar teeth in rats, J Dent Res, 47(2):323–327.

[51] Neville, BW., Damm, DD., Allen, CM.& Bouquot, JE., (2010) editors. Odontogenic cysts and tumors. In: Oral and Maxillofacial Pathology. 3 rd ed. Philadelphia: WB Saunders; p. 678-740.

[52] Noffke, CE., Raubenheimer, EJ., Chabikuli, NJ.& Bouckaert, MM. (2007) Odontogenic myxoma: Review of the literature and report of 30 cases from South Africa. Oral Surg Oral Med Oral Pathol Oral Radiol Endod 104:101-9.

[53] Jaswal, A., Jana, AK., Biswas, M., Sikder, B.& Nandi, TK.(2008) Recurrent odontogenic myxoma of maxilla: A diagnostic and operative dilemma. Indian J Otolaryngol Head Neck Surg 60:41-4.

[54] Singaraju, S., Wanjari, SP.& Parwani, RN.(2010) Odontogenic myxoma of the Maxilla: A report of a rare case and review of the literature. J Oral Maxillofac Pathol.4:19-23.

[55] Sivakumar, G., Kavitha, B., Saraswathi, TR.& Sivapathasundharam, B. (2008) Odontogenic myxoma of maxilla. Indian J Dent Res ; 19:62-5.

[56] Aquilino, RA., Tuji, FM., Eid, NL., Molina, OF., Joo, HY.& Neto, FH. (2006) Odontogenic myxoma in the maxilla: A case report and characteristics on CT and MR. Oral Oncol Extra 42:133-6.

[57] Huber, AR.& Folk, GS. (2009) Cementoblastoma. Head Neck Pathol. 3:133-5.

[58] Pynn, BR., Sands, TD.& Bradley, G. (2001) Benign cementoblastoma: A case report. J Can Dent Assoc 67:260-2.

[59] Sumer, M., Gunduz, K., Sumer, AP.& Gunhan O. (2006) Benign cementoblastoma: A case report. Med Oral Patol Oral Cir Bucal. 11:E483-5.

[60] Brannon, RB.& Fowler, CB. (2001) Benign fibro-ossoeus lesions: A review of current concepts. Adv Anat Pathol. 8:126-43.

[61] Sharma, N. (2014) Benign cementoblastoma: A rare case report with review of literature. Contemporary Clinical Dentistry Jan-Mar 5(1)pp:92-4.

[62] Sarode, SC., Sarode, GS., Waknis, P., Patil, A.& Jashika M. (2011) Juvenile psammomatoid ossifying fibroma: A review. Oral Oncol. 47:1110-6.

[63] Godhi,, S., Goyal, S., Giraddi, G.& Goyal, S. (2008) Cementifying fibroma of the mandible: A case report. J Oral Health Comm Dent. 2:42-5.

[64] Keleş, B., Duran, M., Uyar, Y., Azimov, A., Demirkan, A., Esen, HH. (2010) Juvenile ossifying fibroma of the mandible: A case report. J Oral Maxillofac Res. 1:e5.

[65] Yadav, A.& Mishra, MB. (2011) Peripheral cemento- ossifying fibroma of mandible: A case report. Indian J Stomatol. 2:193-6.

[66] Shetty, DC., Urs, AB., Ahuja, P., Sahu, A., Manchanda, A.& Sirohi, Y. (2011) Mineralized components and their interpretation in the histogenesis of peripheral ossifying fibroma. Indian J Dent Res. 22:56-61.

[67] Kenney, JN., Kaugars, GE., Abbey, LM. (1989) Comparison between the peripheral ossifying fibroma and peripheral odontogenic fibroma. J Oral Maxillofac Surg. 47:378-82.

[68] Brannon, RB., Fowler, CB., Carpenter, WM.& Corio, RL. (2002) Cementoblastoma: An innocuous neoplasm? A clinicopathologic study of 44 cases and review of the literature with special emphasis on recurrence. Oral Surg Oral Med Oral Pathol Oral Radiol Endod 93:311-20.

[69] Kramer, IRH., Pindborg, JJ.& Shear, M. (1992) Histological typing of odontogenic tumours. 2nd ed. Berlin: Springer-Verlag.

Section 4

Immunohistochemistry in Maxillofacial Lesions

Chapter 15

Tumor Markers in Common Oral and Maxillofacial Lesions

Taghi Azizi

Additional information is available at the end of the chapter

http://dx.doi.org/10.5772/59342

1. Introduction

Immunohistochemical (ihc) stains are widely used for diagnosis of tumors. In this chapter we present modern immunohistochemical stains for diagnosing those tumors that cannot be evaluated via common or routine stains such as hematoxylin and eosin.

2. Epithelial tumors

Squamous cell carcinoma (SCC) and malignant melanoma are common epithelial lesions that require IHC.

2.1. Squamous cell carcinoma

2.1.1. Definition

SCC is a malignant neoplasm arising from the squamous epithelium of the oral cavity most commonly from the lip, then tongue, floor of mouth, gingiva, palate, and buccal mucosa. Premalignant changes present as white (leukoplakia) or red (erythroplakia) mucosal patches.

2.1.2. Immunohistochemical stains

Squamous carcinomas are nearly always positive for CK.

- Common CK expression in squamous carcinomas includes AE1/AE3 and CKs 5, 5/6, 14, and 17.

- Nuclear p63 expression is common in squamous cell carcinomas but is not specific
- Cytokeratin stains may help detect subtle metastatic foci especially in post-treatment lymph nodes (Figure 1).
- Over expression of p53 may be linked to response to radiation and/or chemotherapy
- p16 positive: strong and diffuse nuclear and cytoplasmic expression in oropharyngeal carcinoma (HPV associated). [1-5]

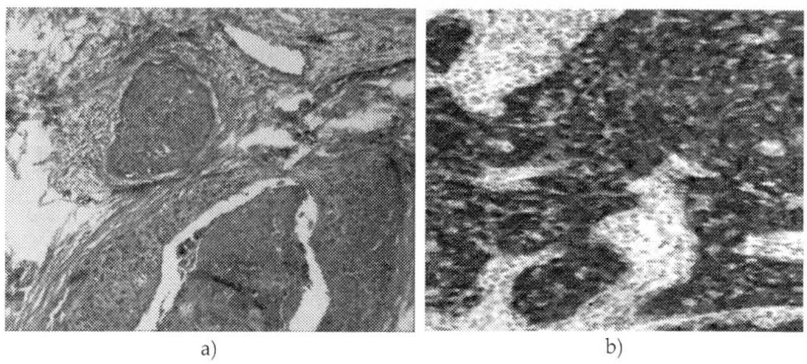

Figure 1. a) Squamous cell carcinoma (H&E). b) Cytokeratin stains in SCC.

2.2. Mucosal melanoma

2.2.1. Definition

Malignant mucosal melanoma (MMM) is a neural crest–derived neoplasm originating from melanocytes and demonstrating melanocytic differentiation.

2.2.2. Immunohistochemical stains

S100 protein, Melan A, HMB45, tyrosinase, vimentin are positive, Keratin and muscle markers are negative (Figure 2). [6-13]

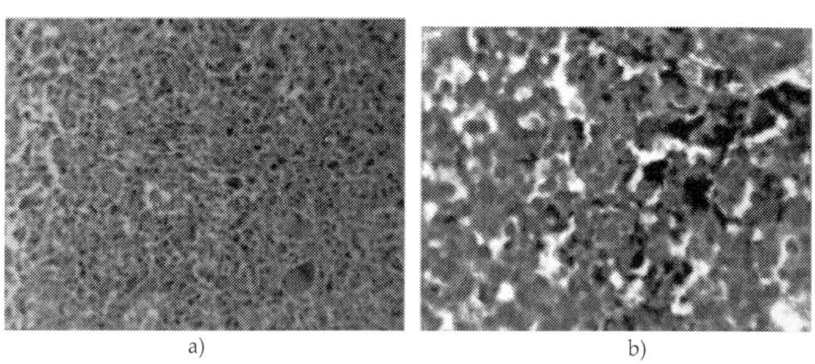

Figure 2. a) Mucosal melanoma (H&E) b) IHC staining for HMB-45

http://dx.doi.org/10.5772/59342

3. Salivary gland tumors

The common salivary gland tumors needing IHC are:

- PLEOMORPHIC ADENOMA
- BASAL CELL ADENOMA
- CANALICULAR ADENOMA
- ONCOCYTOMA
- PAPILLARY CYSTADENOMA LYMPHOMATOSUM (WARTHIN TUMOR(
- SEBACEOUS ADENOMA/LYMPHADENOMA
- MUCOEPIDERMOID CARCINOMA
- ADENOID CYSTIC CARCINOMA
- POLYMORPHOUS LOW-GRADE ADENOCARCINOMA
- EPITHELIAL-MYOEPITHELIAL CARCINOMA
- CLEAR CELL CARCINOMA
- ACINIC CELL CARCINOMA

3.1. Pleomorphic adenoma

3.1.1. Definition

A benign neoplasm composed of ductal epithelial and myoepithelial cells set within a mesenchymal stroma.

3.1.2. Immunohistochemical stains

Cytokeratin cocktail, S100 protein, SMA, p63, calponin, MSA, GFAP, and CD10 reactive the cells are highlighted by a mixture of epithelial and myoepithelial markers that include AE1/AE3, CK5/6, CK7, and CK14; S-100 protein; p63; SMA; calponin; and GFAP. (Figure 3). [14-16]

3.2. Basal cell adenoma

3.2.1. Definition

Basal cell adenoma is a benign salivary gland epithelial neoplasm composed of a proliferation of small basaloid cells in solid, tubular, trabecular, or membranous patterns. (Figure 4).

3.2.2. Immunohistochemical stains

Immunohistochemical Inner luminal cells: cytokeratin cocktail, CK7, and CD117 Peripheral basaloid cellS_100 protein, p63, SMA, and MSA [17 -19]

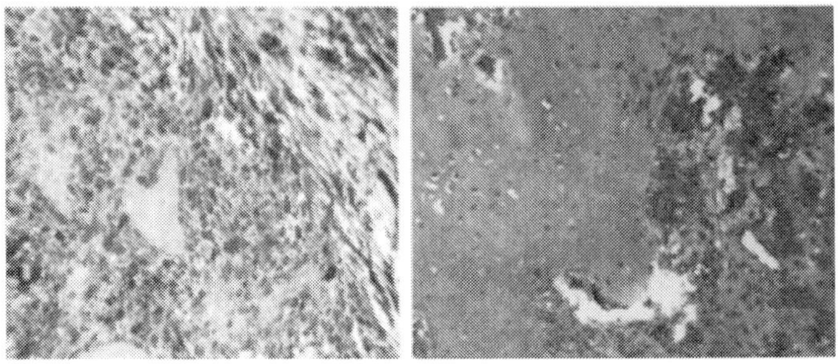

a) b)

Figure 3. a) Pleomorphic adenoma shows a mixture of myoepithelial cells and isolated duct-tubular structures b) S-100 protein in the myoepithelial cells.

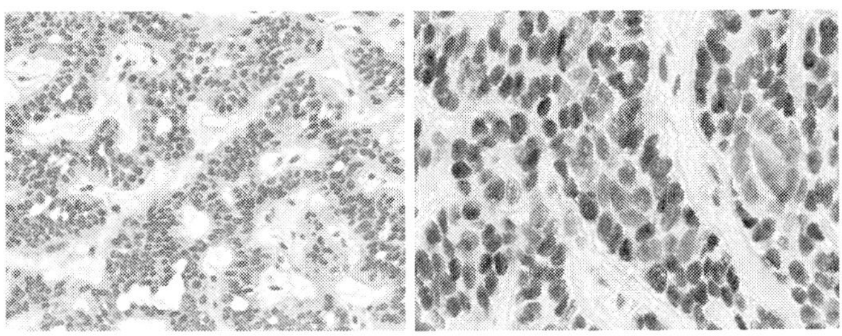

a) b)

Figure 4. a) Basal cell adenoma, trabecular type b) p63 highlights the basal cells

3.3. Canalicular adenoma

3.3.1. Definition

Canalicular adenoma is a benign epithelial salivary gland neoplasm characterized by chains of columnar cells and preference for the minor salivary glands.

3.3.2. Immunohistochemical stains

Cytokeratin and S100 protein reactive GFAP is reactive at the tumor/connective tissue interface (Figure 5.) [17-23].

3.4. Oncocytoma

3.4.1. Definition

Oncocytoma (oncocytic adenoma) is a putative neoplastic proliferation of oncocytically altered cells.

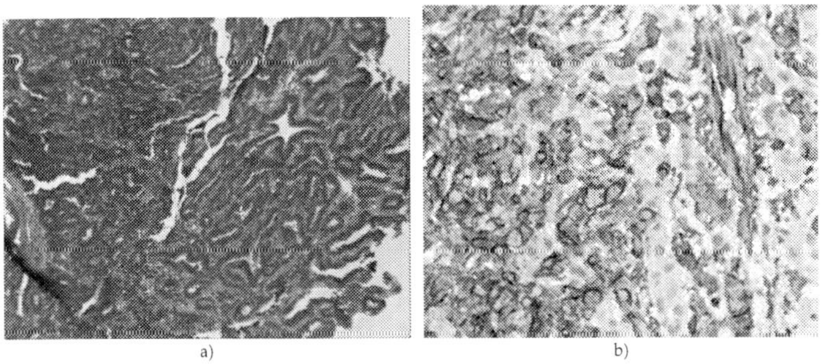

Figure 5. a) Canalicular adenoma, b) GFAP staining is positive

3.4.2. *Immunohistochemical stains)*

Cytokeratin, p63, and PTAH reactive (Figure 6) [17- 19, 21, 22]

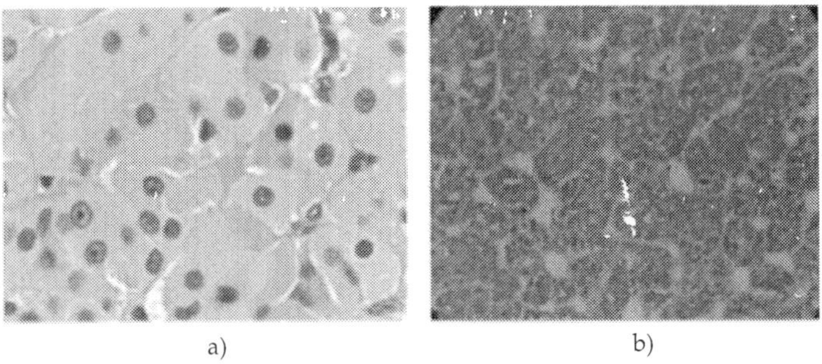

Figure 6. a) Oncocytes are Cytokeratin, highly positive polygonal cells with abundant granular eosinophilic cytoplasm and round, centrally placed nuclei, with or without nucleoli. b) p63 reactive.

3.5. Papillary cystadenoma lymphomatosum (Warthin's tumor)

3.5.1. *Definition*

Warthin's tumor is a relatively common lesion composed of a double layer of oncocytic and cystic architectural pattern cells, and a dense lymphoid epithelium in a papillary stroma. (Figure7)

3.5.2. *Immunohistochemical stains*

Epithelial component keratin reactive Lymphoid component reactive with B- and T-cell markers [17- 19]

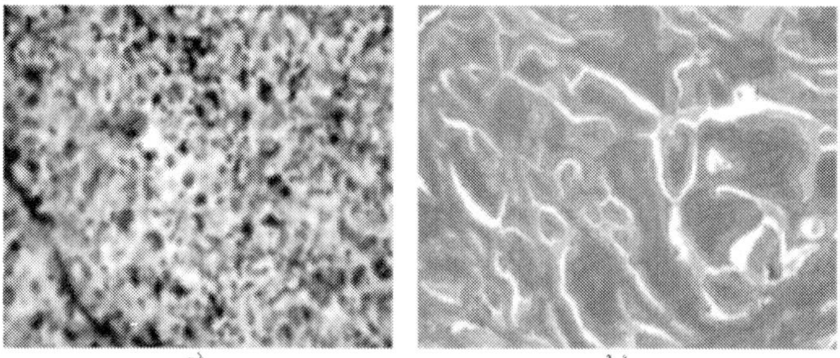

a) b)

Figure 7. a) Papillary-cystic tumor associated with a dense lymphoid stroma. b) KI 67 positive B- cell component.

3.6. Sebaceous adenoma / lymphadenoma

3.6.1. Definition

Sebaceous adenoma is a benign epithelial neoplasm composed of proliferating, incompletely differentiated sebaceous glands. Sebaceous lymph adenoma is a rare variant in which the epithelial proliferation is supported by a dense lymphoid stroma and possibly arises from entrapped salivary gland tissue within intraparotid or periparotid lymph nodes (Figure 8).

3.6.2. Immunohistochemical stains

Immunohistochemistry can be used to confirm the sebaceous differentiation (such as with CD15, androgen receptor, or EMA Epithelial component is cytokeratin and is EMA reactive) [17-19]

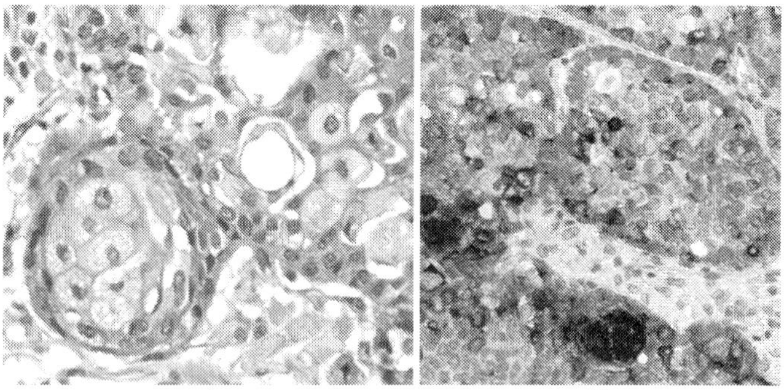

a) b)

Figure 8. a) Sebaceous lymphadenoma b) EMA highlights the sebocytes

3.7. Mucoepidermoid carcinoma

3.7.1. Definition

A malignant glandular epithelial neoplasm characterized by mucus, intermediate, and epidermoid cells. This common salivary gland malignancy represents between 2% and 16% of all salivary gland tumors and up to one third of malignant salivary gland tumors.

3.8. Immunohistochemical stains

Intermediate and epidermoid cells are immunoreactive for cytokeratin and frequently EMA Three cell populations can generally be seen in MEC- epidermoid cells, mucous cells, and intermediate cells— variably set within a cystic background (Figure 9).

CK5/6, Ki-67, and p63 nuclear expression may help in the differential diagnosis. [23, 24]

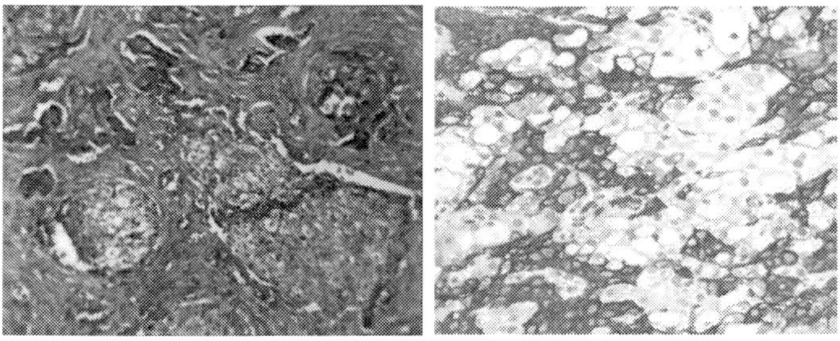

a) b)

Figure 9. a) Mucoepidermoid carcinoma(H&E) and b) CK5/6 highlight the epidermoid and intermediate cells.

3.9. Adenoid cystic carcinoma

3.9.1. Definition

Adenoid cystic carcinoma accounts for 10% of all malignant salivary gland tumors. ACC is cribriform and has two prominent growth patterns: Tubular, and solid, and it is composed of epithelial and myoepithelial cells (Figure 10).

3.9.2. Immunohistochemical stains

Pseudocysts are positive for PAS, Alcian blue, laminin, and type IV collagen Epithelial cells are positive for low-molecular-weight keratins, EMA, and CD117 Myoepithelial cells are positive with calponin, SMA, S100 protein, and p63. [25 – 32].

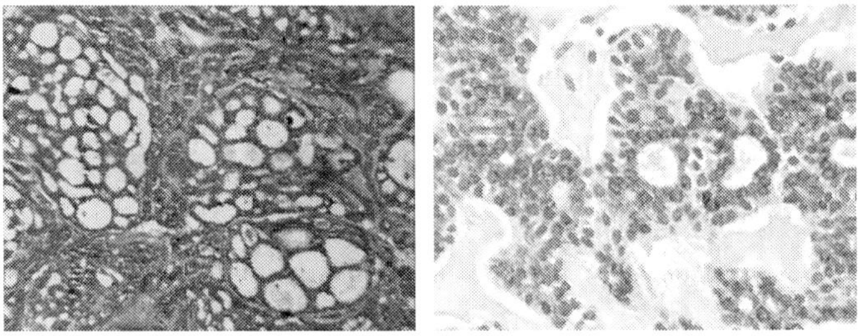

a) b)

Figure 10. a) Adenoid cystic carcinoma showing multiple patterns b) CD117 highlights the epithelial cells.

Polymorphous low-grade adenocarcinoma.

3.9.3. Definition

This is a malignant epithelial tumor characterized by an infiltrative growth of cytologically uniform cells ("low-grade") arranged in architecturally diverse patterns (polymorphous), slowly growing tumor that exclusively affects the minor salivary glands, most often of the palate (Figure 11).

3.9.4. Immunohistochemical stains

Cytokeratin, vimentin, and S100 protein are positive. Variable results are seen with immunohistochemistry and are rarely of diagnostic value. It reacts with EMA, S-100 protein, and Bcl-2; these findings can help differentiate it from PA and ACC. [17-19, 33]

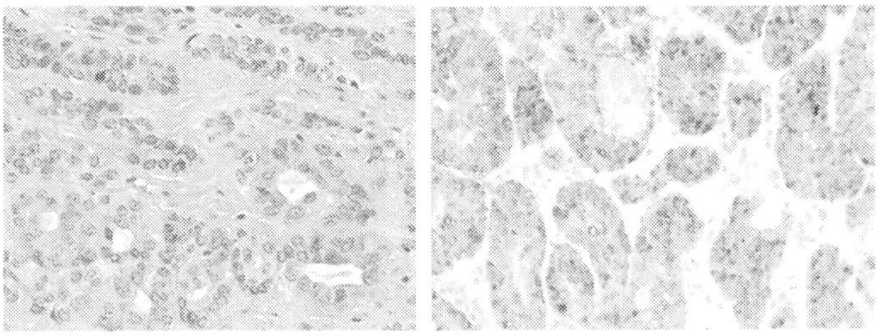

a) b)

Figure 11. a) polymorphous low-grade adenocarcinoma b) S-100 protein

3.10. Epithelial-myoepithelial carcinoma

3.10.1. Definition

Epithelial-myoepithelial carcinoma is a low-grade, malignant, biphasic salivary tumor that comprises 1% to 2% of all salivary neoplasms, the majority of which develop in the parotid gland. It is a malignant neoplasm with biphasic duct-like structures composed of an inner layer of duct lining, epithelium-type cells and an outer layer of clear, myoepithelial-type cells (Figure 12).

3.10.2. Immunohistochemical stains

Inner cells are positive for keratin; outer myoepithelial cells are calponin, SMA, p63, and, less reliably, S100 protein positive; CD117 and bcl-2 are frequently positive. [17- 19, 34

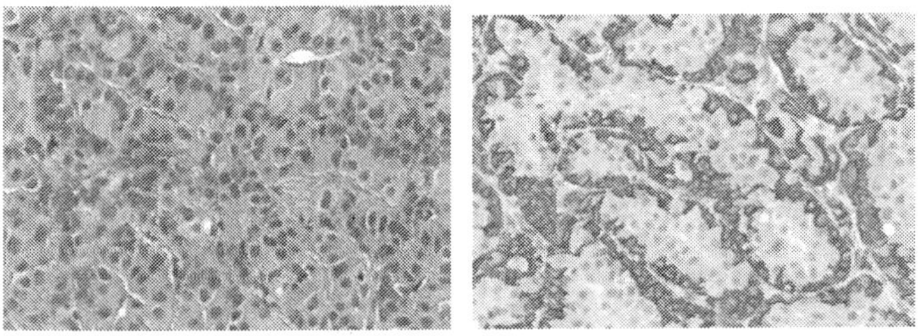

a) b)

Figure 12. a) Epithelial-myoepithelial carcinoma b) smooth muscle actin strongly stains the myoepithelial cells

3.11. Clear cell Carcinoma

3.11.1. Definition

Many salivary and nonsalivary tumors contain clear cells. Among these are mucoepidermoid carcinoma, acinic cell carcinoma, oncocytoma, renal cell carcinoma, myoepithelioma, and clear cell odontogenic carcinoma.

3.11.2. Immunohistochemical stains

The neoplastic cells are positive with AE1/AE3, CAM5. 2, CK7, EMA, and p63; cells are negative with S-100 protein, calponin, actins, and GFAP (Figure 13). They are usually negative for myoepithelial markers that include S-100 protein, MSA, SMA, SMMHC, calponin, and GFAP and are also negative for CD10, CK20, vimentin, desmin, RCC, CA9, and Pax-2 see). [35-37]

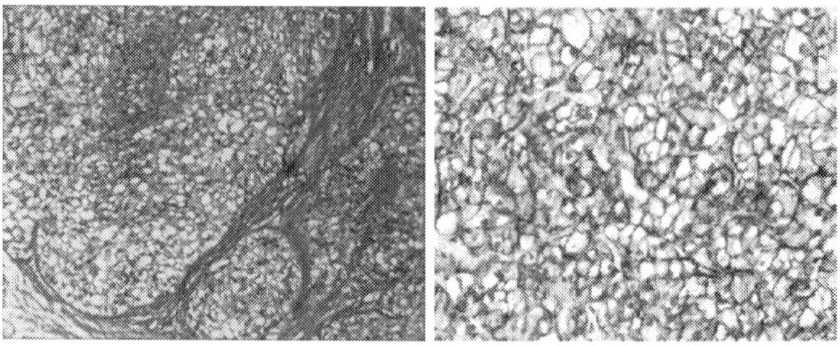

a) b)

Figure 13. a) Clear cell carcinoma b) Highlighted clear cells by S100

3.12. Acinic cell carcinoma

3.12.1. Definition

A malignant epithelial neoplasm demonstrating serous acinar cell differentiation with cytoplasmic zymogen secretory granules (Figure 14).

3.12.2. Immunohistochemical stains

PAS-positive, diastase-resistant zymogen granules. Acinic cells may stain positively for amylase, transferrin, lactoferrin, CEA, VIP, and others. About 10% show some positivity for S100 protein. [38, 39]

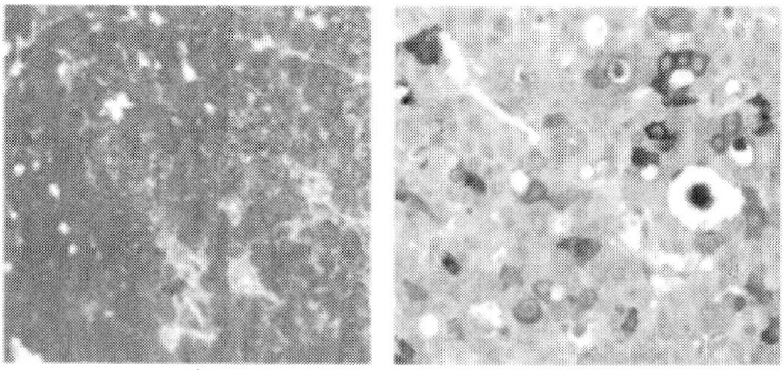

a) b)

Figure 14. a) Serous acinar cells have abundant pale to basophilic, heavily granular cytoplasm (H&E). b) Trypsin is detectable in acinar cells.

4. Soft tissue tumors

The most common soft tissue tumors needing IHC are:

- Lobular capillary hemangioma
- Fibrosarcoma
- Angiosarcoma
- Kaposi Sarcoma
- Leiomyosarcoma
- Synovial Sarcoma
- Rhabdomyosarcoma
- Granular Cell Tumor

4.1. Lobular capillary hemangioma

4.1.1. Definition

Lobular capillary hemangioma previously commonly referred to as "pyogenic granuloma, " is a reactive soft tissue growth with a predilection for the oral cavity that is histologically characterized by a lobular arrangement (Figure15).

4.1.2. Immunohistochemical stains

Positive for endothelial markers including factor VIII–related antigen and CD31 of proliferating small blood vessels. [17-19]

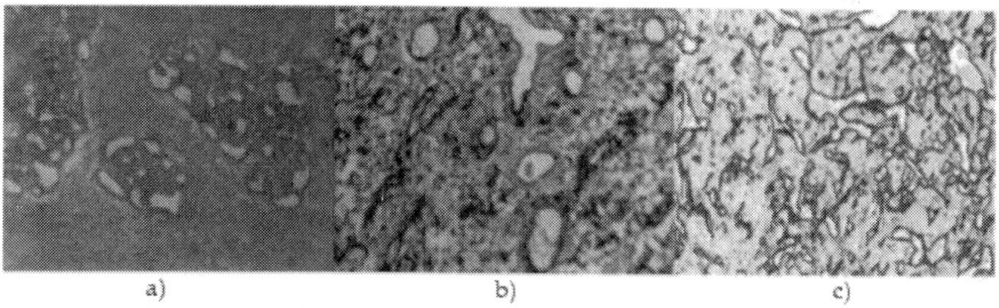

Figure 15. a) H&E capillary hemangioma b) CD31 highlights the endothelial cell C) Factor VIII noted in the endothelial cells.

4.2. Fibrosarcoma

4.2.1. Definition

Malignant neoplasm with only fibroblastic/myofibroblastic differentiation (Figure 16).

4.2.2. Immunohistochemical stains

Vimentin, and rarely, focal actin positivity. [40, 41]

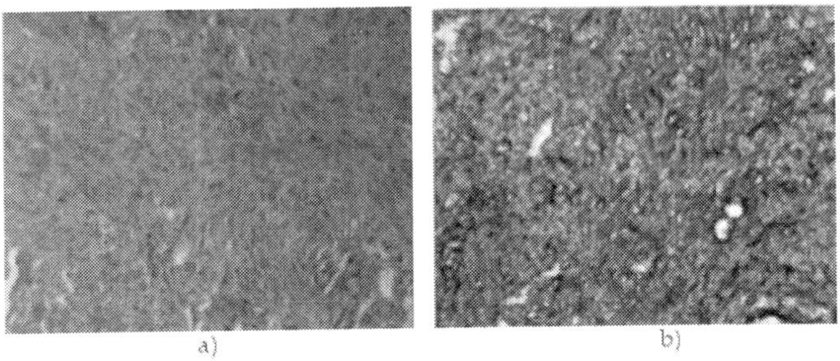

Figure 16. a) Hypercellular tumor, showing spindle cells. b) Vimentin is highly positive

4.3. Angiosarcoma

4.3.1. Definition

Uncommon, high-grade malignant vascular neoplasm, occasionally associated with radiation.

4.3.2. Immunohistochemical stains

Positive with CD34, CD31, factor VIII–RAg, vimentin, podoplanin. ERG shows nuclear positivity in nearly 100% of angiosarcomas. FLI1 expression is found in as many as 100% of angiosarcomas, but utility is limited by poor specificity for vascular lesions. CD31 expression is found in more than 90% of angiosarcomas (Figure 17).

VEGFR3 expression is found in approximately 50% of angiosarcomas, [42-50]

4.4. Kaposis sarcoma

4.4.1. Definition

Kaposi sarcoma is a malignant neoplasm of endothelial cells. Oral lesions are commonly multifocal. Early lesions: are flat, red, and asymptomatic. Older lesions: larger, darker, nodular, and ulcerated. KS is common in patients with AIDS.

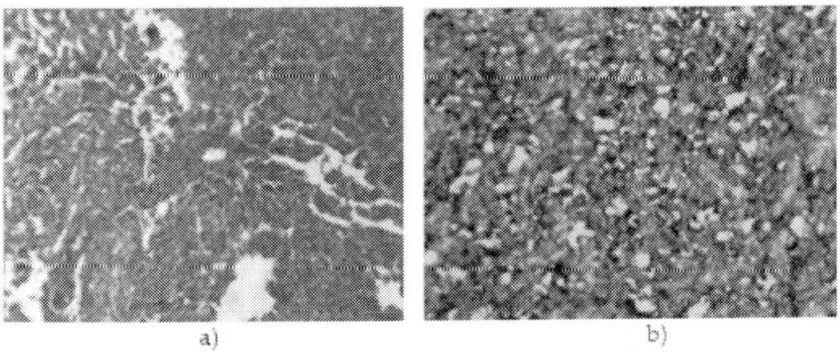

Figure 17. a) Richly vascularized tumor with open vascular channels and mitotic figures b) CD 31 is positive.

4.4.2. Immunohistochemical stains

Human herpes virus 8 has variable expression for endothelial markers (CD31, CD34)[17, 18, 19, 48, 51] (Figure 18).

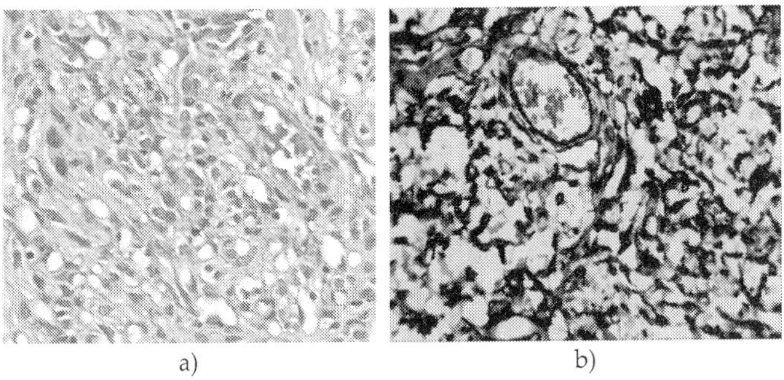

Figure 18. a) Nodular aggregates of spindle cells forming slit-like spaces (H&E). b) CD34 is positive.

4.5. Leiomyosarcoma

4.5.1. Definition

Malignant tumor of smooth muscle

4.5.2. Immunohistochemical stains

Currently, IHC confirmation of smooth muscle differentiation in LMS is based on the demonstration of desmin, α–SMA, muscle actin (HHF-35), and h-Caldesmon PAS with diastase will highlight intracellular glycogen. Tumor cells will be strongly and diffusely reactive with vimentin and actins (smooth muscle, muscle-specific), while variably positive for desmin [49, 50, 51, 52, 53, 54] (Figure 19) [52-57].

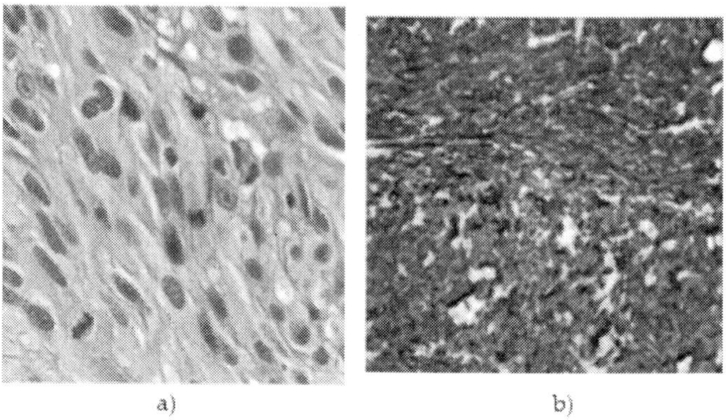

Figure 19. a) Spindle cell population. b) Desmin reactivity.

4.6. Synovial sarcoma

4.6.1. Definition

Synovial sarcoma is a malignant soft tissue tumor that shows epithelial and mesenchymal differentiation and has distinct clinical, genetic, and morphologic features.

Although it was once thought that synovial sarcoma arose in association with synovium, it is now well known that this is not the case and that these tumors may arise at any anatomic location.

4.6.2. Immunohistochemical stains

Morphologically, synovial sarcoma takes three main forms: 1) biphasic, 2) monophasic, and 3) poorly differentiated. Biphasic synovial sarcoma (BSS) consists of a fascicular spindle cell component and an epithelial component that usually shows glandular differentiation, whereas monophasic synovial sarcoma (MSS) lacks the epithelial component. The glandular component of synovial sarcoma expresses cytokeratins, including AE1/AE3. EMA expression is typically observed in both BSS and MSS. however, unlike its biphasic counterpart, MSS tends to be focally and inconsistently reactive for cytokeratins.

In particular, MSS may show reactivity for simple keratins: CK7, CK8, CK18, and CK19. S-100 protein expression is found in approximately 30% of synovial sarcomas. CD99 is commonly observed in MSS, but expression of this marker is also shared by some other spindle cell neoplasms. Strong positivity for BCL2 protein has also been noted in the spindle cell component of synovial sarcoma. [55-58]. TLE1 is positive in synovial sarcoma (Figure 20).

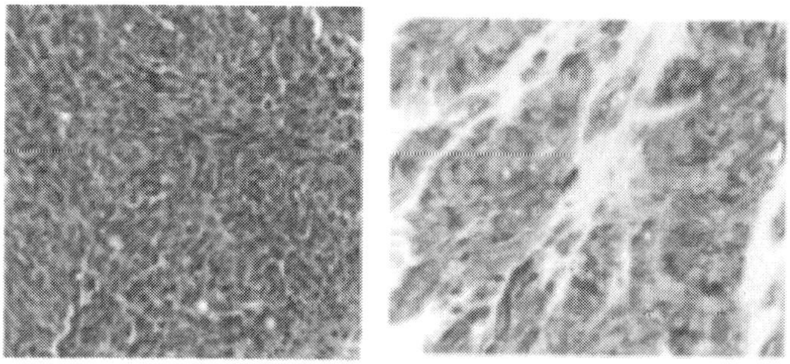

a) b)

Figure 20. a) Spindle or epithelioid cells show a predominantly nested growth pattern. b) TLE1 is positive

4.7. Rhabdomyosarcoma

4.7.1. Definition

A malignant neoplasm with skeletal muscle phenotype: Embryonal type (80%): Alveolar type (20%)

4.7.2. Immunohistochemical stain

MYOD1, SMA positive A variety of myoid markers are positive (desmin, myogenin, MyoD1, myoglobin, actins), but it is important to remember that AE1/AE3, CAM5. 2, and CD56, along with synaptophysin, may be focally positive in some cases. [59, 60, 61] (Figure 21)

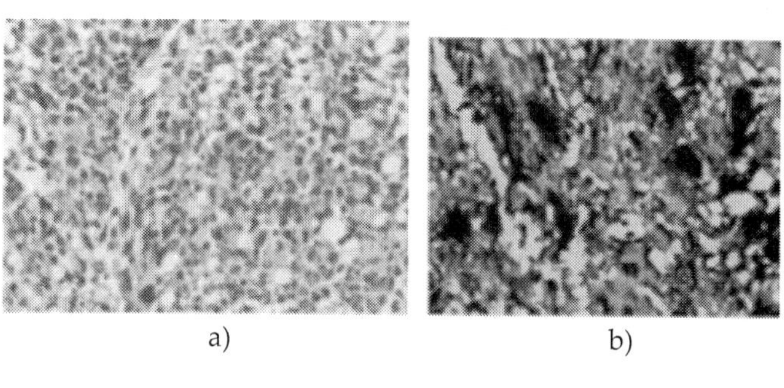

a) b)

Figure 21. a) Mesenchymal cells and rhabdomyoblasts b) Desmin

4.8. Granular cell tumor

4.8.1. Definition

This is an uncommon tumor composed of poorly demarcated granular cells, thought to be Schwann-cell derived, that frequently arise below a mucosa, the latter often showing pseudoepitheliomatous hyperplasia. Granular cell tumor tends to affect the oral cavity (tongue most commonly). Tumors are usually smooth surfaced, poorly demarcated, and are often polypoid, and measure from1 to 2 cm.

4.8.2. Immunohistochemical stains

The neoplastic cells yield a strong and diffuse nuclear and cytoplasmic S-100 protein reaction and are also positive for CD68, NSE, α-1–antitrypsin [17-19, 62] (Figure 22).

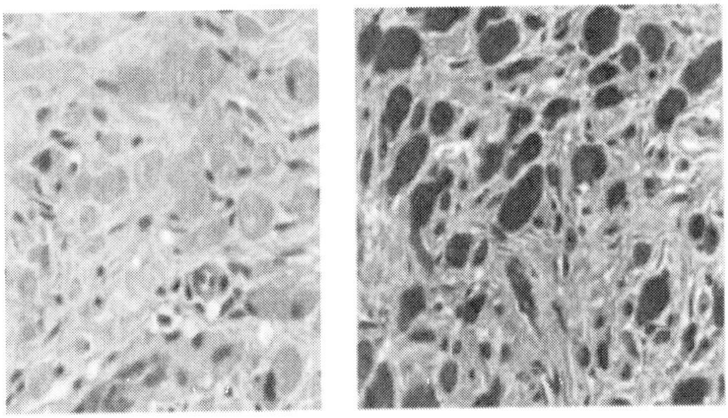

a) b)

Figure 22. a) Polygonal granular cells H&E b) neoplastic ells with s-100

5. Hematologic disorders

The common hematologic disorders that need IHC stains are;

- Hodgkin's lymphoma
- Non – Hodgkin's lymphoma
- Extranodal NK/T-Cell lymphoma, (angiocentric T-cell lymphoma) Midline lethal granuloma
- Burkitt's lymphoma

http://dx.doi.org/10.5772/59342

5.1. Hodgkins lymphoma

This almost always begins in the lymph nodes, and any lymph node group is susceptible.

The most common sites of initial presentation are the cervical and supraclavicular nodes (70% to 75%). Hodgkin's lymphoma is currently classified in the following manner:

- **Lymphocyte-rich**
- **Nodular sclerosis**
- **Mixed cellularity**
- **Lymphocyte depletion**

5.1.1. Immunohistochemical stains

The antibodies most commonly used for diagnosing HL are Ber-H2 (CD30), LeuM1 (CD15), LCA (CD45), L26 (CD20), CD75 (LN1), CD74 (LN2), PAX5, CD3, UCHL1 (CD45RO), ALK, fascin, and EBV-LMP1. EMA and CD57 can be used to recognize NLPHL.

Monoclonal antibody LN1 reacts with H/RSCs in approximately one third of HL cases, most frequently in cases of NLPHL (>75% of cases)(Figure 23). [17-19]

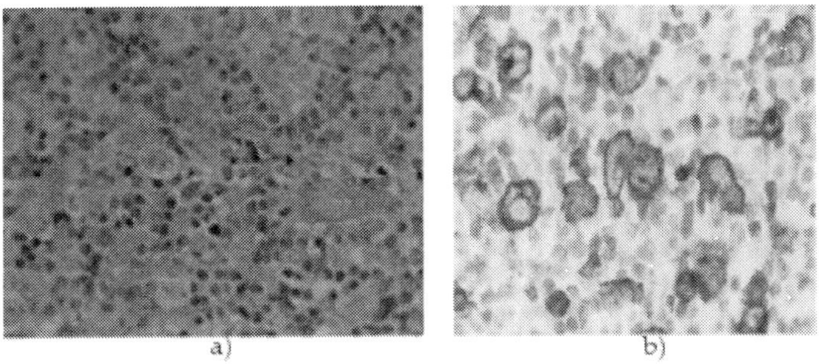

Figure 23. a) Hodgkin/Reed-Sternberg cells b) antigenic Reed-Sternberg cells for CD15

5.2. Non- Hodgkins lymphoma

5.2.1. Definition

Non-Hodgkin's lymphoma most commonly develops in the lymph nodes, In the oral cavity. Lymphoma usually appears as extranodal disease. The malignancy may develop in the oral soft tissues or centrally within the jaws; they most commonly affect the buccal vestibule, posterior hard palate, or gingiva.

5.2.2. Immunohistochemical stains

Small Cell Lymphoid Neoplasms

The lymphoma cells express pan–B-cell antigens (CD19, CD20, CD22, PAX-5). Mantle cell lymphoma (MCL) expresses pan–B-cell antigens (CD19, CD20, CD22), CD5, CD43, Bcl-2, and cyclin D1.

Nodal marginal zone lymphoma (NMZL) will typically express pan–B-cell antigens that include CD19, CD20, PAX5, and CD79a;

Co-expression with Bcl-2 and CD43 is common and occurs in 50%. The vast majority of low-grade follicular lymphoma (FL) are positive for Bcl-2 small lymphocytic lymphoma (CLL/SLL) includes expression of CD5, CD23, CD19, CD43, and Bcl-2 and has a proliferation rate of less than 10%. [17-19] (Figure 24).

Large B-Cell Lymphoid Neoplasms

CD15 expression +

CD30 +

CD45 expression +

PAX5 strong, uniform + CD20 strong, uniform +.

CD79a expression +.

p63 +

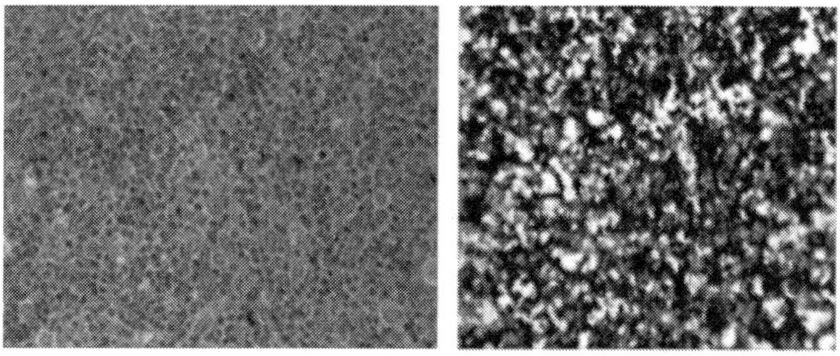

a) b)

Figure 24. a) B-cell lymphoma (H&E) b) CD 20 is positive

T-Cell Lymphoid Neoplasms

Almost all peripheral T-cell lymphomas express pan–T-cell antigens CD3, CD2, and CD43. Anaplastic large-cell lymphoma (ALCL) is positive for CD30, and the expression should be strong and in at least 75% of the cells.

The neoplastic cells of angioimmunoblastic T-cell lymphoma)AITL) are positive for pan–T-cell antigens CD3, CD2, CD5, [17-19]

5.3. Extranodal NK/T-cell lymphoma, (angiocentric T-cell lymphoma) midline lethal granuloma

5.3.1. Definition

NK/T-cell lymphoma is the most common malignant nonepithelial neoplasm found in the upper respiratory tract and most commonly involves the nasal cavity, the maxillary sinus, nasopharynx, and salivary gland. This discussion will be limited to extranodal NK/T-cell lymphoma, nasal type (NK/T LNT), which is more common in the sinonasal region.

5.3.2. Immunohistochemical stains

NK cells express CD2, CD7, CD8, CD56, and CD57. They are positive for cytoplasmic CD3, but not surface CD3, and do not typically express CD5. The neoplastic counterpart, extranodal NK/T-cell lymphomas, express CD2, cytoplasmic CD3, CD56, and, in most cases, EBV. [17-19] (Figure 25, 26).

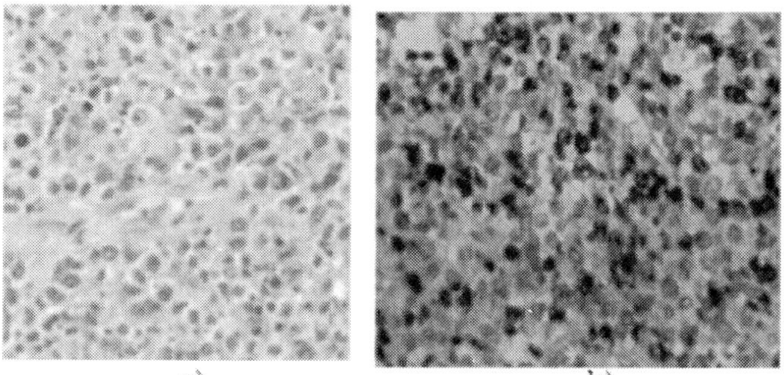

a) b)

Figure 25. a) Extranodal natural killer/T-cell lymphoma b) CD3 staining is positive

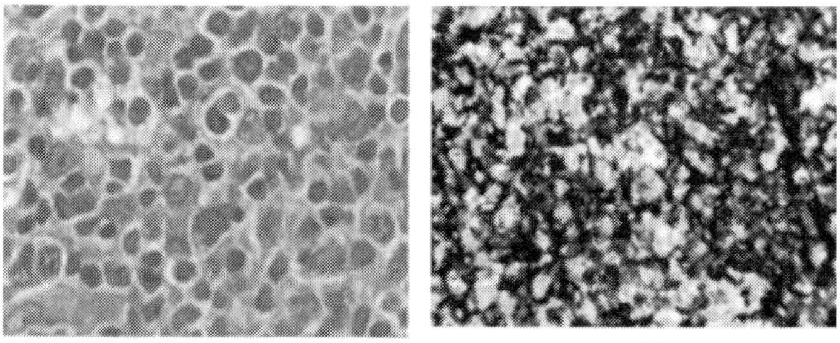

a) b)

Figure 26. a) Atypical lymphoid cells(NK/T-CELL LYMPHOMA) b) Diffusely immunoreactive with CD3C

5.4. Burkitts lymphoma

5.4.1. Definition

Burkitt's lymphoma is a malignancy of B-lvmphocyte origin that represents an undifferentiated lymphoma. The tendency for jaw involvement seems to be age related: nearly 90% of 3-year-old patients have jaw lesions.

5.4.2. Immunohistochemical stains

There were statistically significant differences in the expression of CD10 (28/28 vs. 1/16), bcl-2 (3/28 vs. 11/16), MUM1 (5/28 vs. 15/16), a PI of 95. 0% or more (27/28 vs. 2/16), and combined CD10+/bcl-2-/bcl-6+ (24/28 vs. 1/16) between BLs and DLBCL-HPSSs. Of the BLs, 7 (25%) of 28 and 26 (96%) of 27 were positive for EBER and c-myc rearrangement as compared with 0 of 16 and 1 (7%) of 15 DLBCL-HPSSs, respectively as compared with 0 of 16 and 1 (7%) of 15 DLBCL-HPSSs, respectively. [17-19, 63]

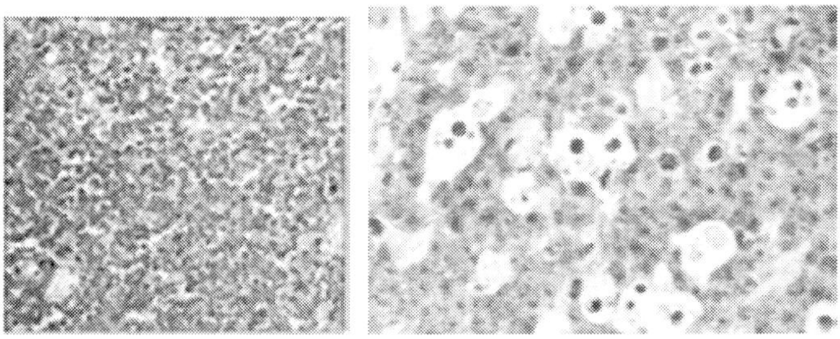

a) b)

Figure 27. a) Burkitt's lymphoma. "starry-sky" appearance b) CD10 staining

6. Bone tumors

The common bone tumors needing IHC are:

- Osteosarcoma
- Chondrosarcoma
- Ewing sarcoma

6.1. Osteosarcoma

6.1.1. Definition

Osteosarcoma is the most common nonhematopoietic primary malignant bone tumor ; it is a malignant mesenchymal tumor producing osteoid from the tumor cells (Figure 28).

6.1.2. Immunohistochemical stains

CD99 positive; rare cytokeratin and smooth muscle actin reaction. Overall, the reported specificity of immunoreactivity for osteonectin and osteocalcin is approximately 40% and 95%, respectively, for the diagnosis of a bone forming tumor. A recent promising marker for identification of osteoblastic differentiation is SATB2, a nuclear matrix protein that plays a role in osteoblast lineage commitment. α-SMA and desmin, which can lead to misdiagnosis. [63-69]

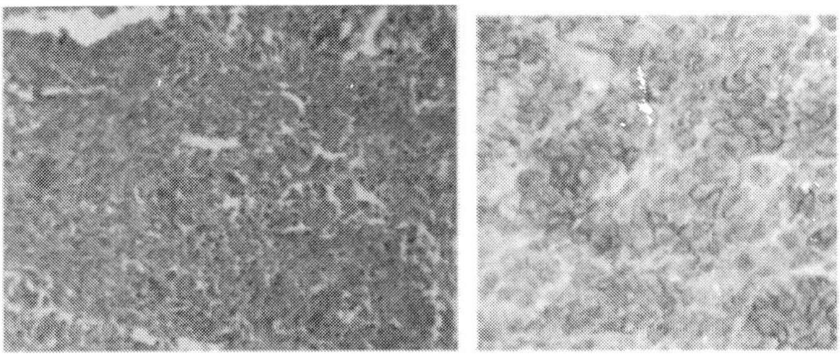

a) b)

Figure 28. a) Osteosarcoma demonstrates irregular trabeculae of tumor osteoid arising from sarcomatous stroma. b) CD99 is positive

6.2. Chondrosarcoma

6.2.1. Definition

Chondrosarcoma is a malignant tumor of bone that shows pure cartilaginous differentiation. Secondary changes that include myxoid features, ossification, and calcification may be present. (Figure 29).

6.2.2. Immunohistochemical stains

Cartilage stains S100 protein positive Mesenchymal chondrosarcoma: Sox9, CD99, and Leu7 positive Although the cartilaginous component of mesenchymal chondrosarcoma is S-100 protein positive, the small-cell component expresses CD99, CD57, and NSE therefore immunohistochemically, there may also be overlap with Ewing sarcoma. However, unlike Ewing sarcoma, MCS is nonreactive for synaptophysin and also typically does not express desmin, actin, cytokeratin, or EMA. In addition, MCS lacks *EWSR1* gene rearrangements. However, a recent study has identified a novel *HEY1-NCOA2* fusion in MCS which appears to be a consistent finding. [70, 71]

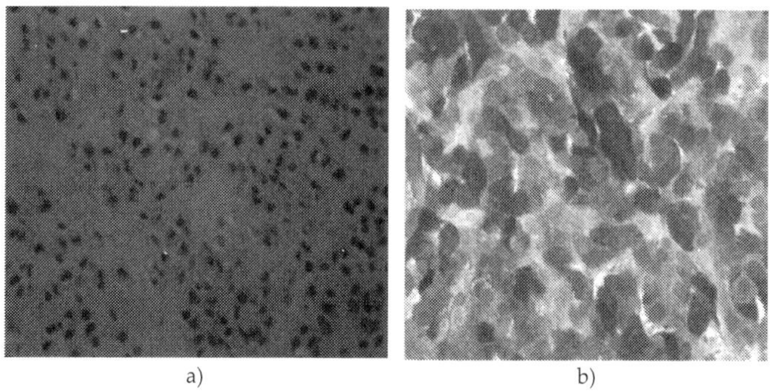

Figure 29. a) High-grade chondrosarcoma b) with marked S100 PROTEN increase in cellularity and myxoid matrix

6.3. Ewing sarcoma

6.3.1. Definition

High-grade, primitive neuroectodermal neoplasm (Figure 30)

6.3.2. Immunohistochemical stains

Positive: FLI1 (nuclear), CD99, vimentin; rarely keratin. May react with other neural markers (NSE, synaptophysin, S100 protein, NFP, GFAP, chromogranin). [72-79]

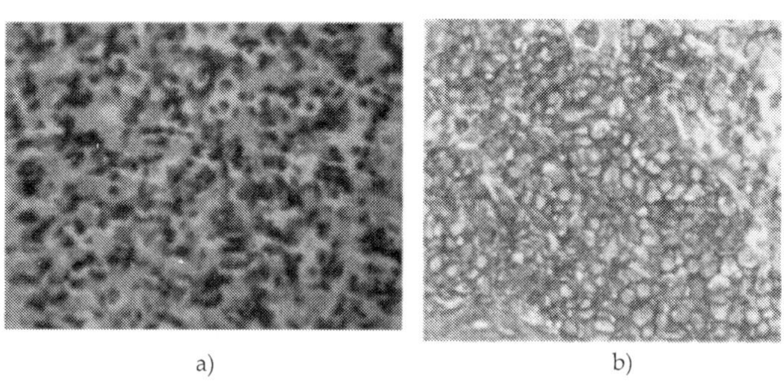

Figure 30. a) Small nucleoli scant cytoplasm with mitosis b) diffuse strong membranous expression of CD99

Author details

Taghi Azizi*

Address all correspondence to: aziziarshia@yahoo.com

Department of Oral and Maxillofacial Pathology, Baqiyatallah University of Medical Sciences Tehran, Iran

References

[1] Lewis JS Jr: p16 Immunohistochemistry As a Standalone Test for Risk Stratification in Oropharyngeal Squamous Cell Carcinoma. *Head Neck Pathol.* 6(Suppl 1):75–82, 2012.

[2] Robinson M, Schache A, Sloan P, et al: HPV Specific Testing: A Requirement for Oropharyngeal Squamous Cell Carcinoma Patients. *Head Neck Pathol.* 6(Suppl 1):83–90, 2012

[3] Lopes V, Murray P, Williams H, et al: Squamous cell carcinoma of the oral cavity rarely harbours oncogenic human papillomavirus. *Oral Oncol.* 47:698–701, 2011.

[4] Cobo F, Talavera P, Concha A: Review article: relationship of human papillomavirus with papillary squamous cell carcinoma of the upper aerodigestive tract: a review. *Int J Surg Pathol.* 16:127–136, 2008.

[5] Lewis JS Jr, Thorstad WL, Chernock RD, et al: p16 positive oropharyngeal squamous cell carcinoma:an entity with a favourable prognosis regardless of tumor HPV status. *Am J Surg Pathol.* 34:1088–1096, 2010.

[6] Frieling G, Al-Zaid T, Prieto V: Placental Alkaline Phosphatase Positivity in Metastatic Melanoma: Report of a Case and Review of the Literature. Annual Meeting of the American Society of Dermatopathology Chicago. 2012

[7] Plaza, JA, et al: Immunohistochemical expression of S100A6 in cellular neurothekeoma: clinicopathologic and immunohistochemical analysis of 31 cases. *Am J Dermatopathol.* 31(5)):419–422, 2009).

[8] Ohsie SJ, Sarantopoulos GP, Cochran AJ, et al: Immunohistochemical Characteristic s of melanoma. *J Cutan Pathol.* 35:433– 444, 2008.

[9] Rao P, Fuller GN, Prieto VG: Expression of Sox-9 in Metastatic Melanoma-A Potential Diagnostic Pitfall. *Am J Dermatopathol.* 32(3):262–266, 2010, 5/2010. e-Pub 1/2010.

[10] Ramos-Herberth FI, Karamchandani J, Kim J, et al: SOX10 immunostaining distinguishes desmoplastic melanoma from excision scar. *J Cutan Pathol.* 37(9):944–952, 2010.

[11] Lee H, Torres FX, McLean SA, et al: Immunophenotypic heterogeneity of primary sinonasal melanoma with aberrant expression of neuroendocrine markers and calponin. Appl Immunohistochem. *Mol Morphol.* 19:48–53, 2011.

[12] Prieto VG: Sentinel lymph nodes in cutaneous melanoma: handling, examination, and clinical repercussion. *Arch Pathol Lab Med.* 134(12):1764–1769, 2010.

[13] Paradela S, Fonseca E, Prieto VG: Melanoma in children. *Arch Pathol Lab Med.* 135:307–316, 2011.

[14] Curran AE, Allen CM, Beck FM, et al: Distinctive pattern of glial fibrillary acidic protein immunoreactivity useful in distinguishing fragmented pleomorphic adenoma, canalicular adenoma and polymorphous low grade adenocarcinoma of minor salivary glands. *Head Neck Pathol.* 1:27–32, 2007.

[15] Shah SS, Chandan VS, Wilbur DC, et al: Glial fibrillary acidic protein and CD57 immunolocalization in cell block preparations is a useful adjunct in the diagnosis of pleomorphic adenoma. *Arch Pathol Lab Med.* 131:1373–1377, 2007.

[16] Antony J, Gopalan V, Smith RA, et al: Carcinoma ex pleomorphic adenoma: a comprehensive review of clinical, pathological and molecular data. *Head Neck Pathol.* 6:1–9, 2012.

[17] David J. Dabbs, Md, Diagnostic Immunohistochemistry, 4th Edition, Saunders, an imprint of Elsevier Inc. (2014)

[18] Lester D. R. Thompson, MD, Head And Neck Pathology, Second Edition, (A Volume In The Foundations In Diagnostic Pathology Series), (2014)

[19] Rosai and Akermans., Surgical Pathology., 10th edition., volume1 Mosby Elsevier. 2011.

[20] Curran AE, Allen CM, Beck FM, et al: Distinctive pattern of glial fibrillary acidic protein immunoreactivity useful in distinguishing fragmented pleomorphic adenoma, canalicular adenoma and polymorphous low grade adenocarcinoma of minor salivary glands. Head Neck Pathol. 1:27–32, 2007.

[21] Liu L, Qian J, Singh H, et al: Immunohistochemical analysis of chromophobe renal cell carcinoma, renal oncocytoma, and clear cell carcinoma: An optimal and practical panel for differential diagnosis. *Arch Pathol Lab Med.* 131:1290–1297, 2007

[22] Paner GP, Lindgren V, Jacobson K, et al: High incidence of chromosome 1 abnormalities in a series of 27 renal oncocytomas: Cytogenetic and fluorescence in situ hybridization studies. *Arch Pathol Lab Med.* 131:81–85, 2007.

[23] Weinreb I, Seethala RR, Perez-Ordonez B, et al: Oncocytic mucoepidermoid carcinoma: clinicopathologic description in a series of 12 cases. *Am J Surg Pathol.* 33:409–416, 2009.

[24] Wolfish EB, Nelson BL, Thompson LD: Sinonasal Tract Mucoepidermoid Carcinoma: A Clinicopathologic and Immunophenotypic Study of 19 Cases Combined with a Comprehensive Review of the Literature. *Head Neck Pathol.* 2011.

[25] Martinez-Rodriguez N, Leco-Berrocal I, Rubio-Alonso L, et al: Epidemiology and treatment of adenoid cystic carcinoma of the minor salivary glands: a meta-analytic study. *Med Oral Patol Oral Cir Bucal.* 16:e884–e889, 2011.

[26] Papaspyrou G, Hoch S, Rinaldo A, et al: Chemotherapy and targeted therapy in adenoid cystic carcinoma of the head and neck: a review. *Head Neck.* 33:905–911, 2011

[27] Mitani Y, Rao PH, Futreal PA, et al: Novel chromosomal rearrangements and break points at the t(6;9) in salivary adenoid cystic carcinoma: association with MYB-NFIB chimeric fusion, MYB expression, and clinical outcome. *Clin Cancer Res.* 17:7003–7014, 2011.

[28] Bell D, Roberts D, Karpowicz M, et al: Clinical significance of Myb protein and downstream target genes in salivary adenoid cystic carcinoma. *Cancer Biol Ther.* 12:569–573, 2011.

[29] Brill LB, Kanner WA, Fehr A, et al: Analysis of MYB expression and MYB-NFIB gene fusions in adenoid cystic carcinoma and other salivary neoplasms. *Mod Pathol.* 24:1169–1176, 2011.

[30] West RB, Kong C, Clarke N, et al: MYB expression and translocation in adenoid cystic carcinomas and other salivary gland tumors with clinicopathologic correlation. Am J Surg Pathol. 35:92–99, 2011

[31] Brown JG, Familiari U, Papotti M, et al: Thymic basaloid carcinoma: a clinicopathologic study of 12 cases, with a general discussion of basaloid carcinoma and its relationship with adenoid cystic carcinoma. Am J Surg Pathol. 33:1113–1124, 2009

[32] Banki F, Khalil K, Kott MM, et al: Adenoid cystic carcinoma of the thymus gland: a rare tumor. Ann Thorac Surg. 90:e56–e58, 2010

[33] Beltran D, Faquin WC, Gallagher G, et al: Selective immunohistochemical comparison of polymorphous low-grade adenocarcinoma and adenoid cystic carcinoma. J Oral Maxillofac Surg. 64:415–423, 2006

[34] Antic T, Venkataraman G, Oshima K: Oncocytic epithelial-myoepithelial carcinoma: an evolving new variant with comparative immunohistochemistry. Pathology. 40:415–418, 2008.

[35] Lai G, Nemolato S, Lecca S, et al: The role of immunohistochemistry in the diagnosis of hyalinizing clear cell carcinoma of the minor salivary gland: a case report. Eur J Histochem. 52:251- 254, 2008

[36] Solar AA, Schmidt BL, Jordan RC: Hyalinizing clear cell carcinoma: case series and comprehensive review of the literature. Cancer. 115:75–83, 2009.

[37] Antonescu CR, Katabi N, Zhang L, et al: EWSR1-ATF1 fusion is a novel and consistent finding in hyalinizing clear-cell carcinoma of salivary gland. Genes Chromosomes Cancer. 50:559– 570, 2011.

[38] Lei Y, Chiosea SI: Re-evaluating historic cohort of salivary acinic cell carcinoma with new diagnostic tools. Head Neck Pathol. 6(2):166–170, 2012.

[39] Griffith C, Seethala R, Chiosea SI: Mammary analogue secretory carcinoma: a new twist to the diagnostic dilemma of zymogen granule poor acinic cell carcinoma. Virchows Arch. 459:117–118, 2011

[40] Doyle LA, Wang WL, Dal Cin P, et al: MUC4 Is a sensitive and extremely useful marker for sclerosing epithelioid fibrosarcoma: association with FUS gene rearrangement. *Am J Surg Pathol*. 36:1444–1451, 2012

[41] Rekhi B, Folpe AL, Deshmukh M, et al: Sclerosing epithelioid Fibrosarcoma—A report of two cases with cytogenetic analysis of FUS gene rearrangement by FISH technique. *Pathol Oncol Res*. 2010.

[42] Kraft S, Fletcher CD: Atypical intradermal smooth muscle neoplasms: clinicopathologic analysis of 84 cases and a reappraisal of cutaneous "leiomyosarcoma". *Am J Surg Pathol*. 35:599–607, 2011

[43] Iwata J, Fletcher CD: Immunohistochemical detection of cytokeratin and epithelial membrane antigen in leiomyosarcoma: a systematic study of 100 cases. *Pathol Int*. 50:7–14, 2000. 2011

[44] Chen E, O'Connell F, Fletcher CD: Dedifferentiated leiomyosarcoma: clinicopathological analysis of 18 cases. *Histopathology*. 59:1135–1143, 2011.

[45] Nicolas MM, Tamboli P, Gomez JA, et al: Pleomorphic and dedifferentiated leiomyosarcoma: clinicopathologic and immunohistochemical study of 41 cases. *Hum Pathol*. 41:663–671, 2010

[46] Shivathirthan N, Kita J, Iso Y, et al: Primary hepatic leiomyosarcoma: Case report and literature review. *World J Gastrointest Oncol*. 3(10):148–152, 2011

[47] Iwata T, Miura T, Inoue K, et al: Primary leiomyosarcoma of the anterior mediastinum encasing the aortic arch, left common carotid and left subclavian arteries. *Ann Thorac Cardiovasc Surg*. 18:140–143, 2012.

[48] Zhang H, Maitta RW, Bhattacharyya PK, et al: γ-Synuclein is a promising new marker for staining reactive follicular dendritic cells, follicular dendritic cell sarcoma, Kaposi sarcoma, and benign and malignant vascular tumors. *Am J Surg Pathol*. 35:1857–1865, 2011.

[49] Kraft S, Fletcher CD: Atypical intradermal smooth muscle neoplasms: clinicopathologic analysis of 84 cases and a reappraisal of cutaneous "leiomyosarcoma". *Am J Surg Pathol*. 35:599–607, 2011

[50] Iwata J, Fletcher CD: Immunohistochemical detection of cytokeratin and epithelial membrane antigen in leiomyosarcoma: a systematic study of 100 cases. *Pathol Int.* 50:7–14, 2000. 2011

[51] Chen E, O'Connell F, Fletcher CD: Dedifferentiated leiomyosarcoma: clinicopathological analysis of 18 cases. *Histopathology.* 59:1135–1143, 2011.

[52] Nicolas MM, Tamboli P, Gomez JA, et al: Pleomorphic and dedifferentiated leiomyosarcoma: clinicopathologic and immunohistochemical study of 41 cases. *Hum Pathol.* 41:663–671, 2010

[53] Iwata T, Miura T, Inoue K, et al: Primary leiomyosarcoma of the anterior mediastinum encasing the aortic arch, left common carotid and left subclavian arteries. *Ann Thorac Cardiovasc Surg.* 18:140–143, 2012.

[54] Shivathirthan N, Kita J, Iso Y, et al: Primary hepatic leiomyosarcoma: Case report and literature review. *World J Gastrointest Oncol.* 3(10):148–152, 2011.

[55] Krskova L, Kalinova M, Brizova H, et al: Molecular and immunohistochemical analyses of BCL2, KI-67, and cyclin D1 expression in synovial sarcoma. *Cancer Genet Cytogenet.* 193:1–8, 2009

[56] Foo WC, Cruise MW, Wick MR, et al: Immunohistochemical staining for TLE1 distinguishes synovial sarcoma from histologic mimics. *Am J Clin Pathol.* 135:839–844, 2011.

[57] Jagdis A, Rubin BP, Tubbs RR, et al: Prospective evaluation of TLE1 as a diagnostic immunohistochemical marker in synovial Sarcoma. *Am J Surg Pathol.* 33:1743–1751, 2009.

[58] Lai JP, Robbins PF, Raffeld M, et al: NY-ESO-1 expression in synovial sarcoma and other mesenchymal tumors: significance for NY-ESO-1-based targeted therapy and differential diagnosis. *Mod Pathol.* 25:854–858, 2012.

[59] Bahrami A, Gown AM, Baird GS, et al: Aberrant expression of epithelial and neuroendocrine markers in alveolar rhabdomyosarcoma: a potentially serious diagnostic pitfall. *Mod Pathol.* 21:795–806, 2008.

[60] van Gaal JC, Flucke UE, Roeffen MH, et al: Anaplastic lymphoma kinase aberrations in rhabdomyosarcoma: clinical and prognostic implications. *J Clin Oncol.* 30:308–315, 2012.

[61] Jo VY, Marino-Enriquez A, Fletcher CD: Epithelioid rhabdomyosarcoma: clinicopathologic analysis of 16 cases of a morphologically distinct variant of rhabdomyosarcoma. *Am J Surg Pathol.* 35:1523–1530, 2011

[62] Thompson LD: Laryngeal granular cell tumor. *Ear Nose Throat J.* 88:824–825, 2009.

[63] Molyneux EM, Rochford R, Griffin B, et al: Burkitt's lymphoma. *Lancet* 379:1234, 2012. *[A review of the pathogenesis and treatment of Burkitt's lymphoma.]*

[64] T Azizi, MHK Motamedi, SM Jafari Gnathic osteosarcoma : A 10- Year multi –center demographic study, Indian Journal of CANCER 46(3) pp;231-233;2009

[65] Lee AF, Hayes MM, Lebrun D, et al: FLI-1 distinguishes Ewing sarcoma from small cell osteosarcoma and mesenchymal chondrosarcoma. *Appl Immunohistochem Mol Morphol.* 19(3):233– 238, 2011.

[66] Gomez-Brouchet A, Mourcin F, Gourraud PA, et al: Galectin-1 is a powerful marker to distinguish chondroblastic osteosarcoma and conventional chondrosarcoma. *Hum Pathol.* 41(9):1220– 1230, 2010.

[67] Yoshida A, Ushiku T, Motoi T, et al: Immunohistochemical analysis of MDM2 and CDK4 distinguishes low-grade osteosarcoma from benign mimics. *Mod Pathol.* 23(9): 1279–1288, 2010.

[68] Yoshida A, Ushiku T, Motoi T, et al: MDM2 and CDK4 immunohistochemical coexpression in high-grade osteosarcoma: correlation with a dedifferentiated subtype. *Am J Surg Pathol.* 36(3):423–431, 2012

[69] Dujardin F, Binh MB, Bouvier C, et al: MDM2 and CDK4 immunohistochemistry is a valuable tool in the differential diagnosis of low-grade osteosarcomas and other primary f ibro-osseous lesions of the bone. *Mod Pathol.* 24(5):624–637, 2011.

[70] de Nigris F, Zanella L, Cacciatore F, et al: YY1 overexpression is associated with poor prognosis and metastasis-free survival in patients suffering osteosarcoma. *BMC Cancer.* 11:472, 2011

[71] Lee AF, Hayes MM, Lebrun D, et al: FLI-1 distinguishes Ewing sarcoma from small cell osteosarcoma and mesenchymal chondrosarcoma. *Appl Immunohistochem Mol Morphol.* 19(3):233– 238, 2011.

[72] Wang L, Motoi T, Khanin R, et al: Identification of a novel, recurrent HEY1-NCOA2 fusion in mesenchymal chondrosarcoma based on a genome-wide screen of exon-level expression data. *Genes Chromosomes Cancer.* 51:127–139, 2012.

[73] Rocchi A, Manara MC, Sciandra M, et al: CD99 inhibits neural differentiation of human Ewing sarcoma cells and thereby contributes to oncogenesis. *J Clin Invest.* 120(3): 668–680, 2010.

[74] Fujiwara T, Fukushi J, Yamamoto S, et al: Macrophage infiltration predicts a poor prognosis for human ewing sarcoma. *Am J Pathol.* 17(3):1157–1170, 2011

[75] van Doorninck JA, Ji L, Schaub B, et al: Current treatment protocols have eliminated the prognostic advantage of type 1 fusions in Ewing sarcoma: a report from the Children's Oncology Group. *J Clin Oncol.* 28(12):1989–1994, 2010.

[76] Lee AF, Hayes MM, Lebrun D, et al: FLI-1 distinguishes Ewing sarcoma from small cell osteosarcoma and mesenchymal chondrosarcoma. *Appl Immunohistochem Mol Morphol.* 19(3):233– 238, 2011.

[77] Wang WL, Patel NR, Caragea M, et al: Expression of ERG, an Ets family transcription factor, identifies ERG-rearranged Ewing sarcoma. *Mod Pathol*. 25:1378–1383, 2012.

[78] Yoshida A, Sekine S, Tsuta K, et al: NKX2. 2 is a useful immunohistochemical marker for Ewing sarcoma. *Am J Surg Pathol*. 36:993–999, 2012.

[79] T Azizi, MHK Motamedi, A textbook of advanced oral and maxillofacial surgery, intechopen, ISBN978-953-51-1146-7, Chapter5, 2013

Section 5

Complex Oral and Maxillofacial Infections

Chapter 16

Considerations for the Spread of Odontogenic Infections — Diagnosis and Treatment

Flaviana Soares Rocha, Jonas Dantas Batista,
Cláudia Jordão Silva, Roberto Bernardino Júnior and
Luis Henrique Araújo Raposo

Additional information is available at the end of the chapter

http://dx.doi.org/10.5772/59161

1. Introduction

The goal of this chapter is to present the basis for correct diagnosis and management of severe odontogenic infections. The knowledge of the anatomy of fascial spaces is essential for the correct diagnosis and treatment of head and neck infections, because both facial and cervical fasciae work as an effective barrier against the spread of infections in this region[1, 2]. Once these infections occur, they are often difficult to assess accurately by clinical examinations and conventional radiographic techniques, and the outcome may be serious and potentially life-threatening[3]

The fasciae of the neck are glossy and divided into two separated layers: the superficial fascia and the deep fascia. The superficial fascia is actually a component of the fatty subcutaneous tissue while the deep cervical fascia is divided into three layers: the superficial layer, the visceral or middle layer, and the pre vertebral or deep layer. The deep cervical fascia plays an important role in determining the location and course of spread of infections within the soft tissues of the neck. The infections that commonly affect head and cervical areas are frequently from odontogenic origin and to a lesser frequency, proceeding from foreign bodies or trauma to this region[4]. An impacted mandibular third molar is one of the most frequent causes of odontogenic infection[5-7]. Moreover, an semi-impacted third molar results in odontogenic infection more commonly than fully erupted or completely impacted molars [7].

Odontogenic infections occasionally spread beyond the barriers of the fascial spaces, which are formed, as seen, by the deep cervical fascia of the suprahyoid regions of the neck[2]. Among various spaces, the submandibular space is one of the first to be involved in odontogenic infections, similar to the masticatory space[2]. As infection may spread along deep cervical facial planes and neck cavities, widespread cellulitis, necrosis, abscess formation, and sepsis may occur in these cases[4]. Therefore, it is important to understand the anatomy, rate of progression and potential for airway compromise of an infection[7].Spontaneous dissemination of an odontogenic infection is however, very rare in immunocompetent patients[8, 9]. In patients with anatomical abnormalities, systemic diseases or immunosuppression, bacteremia caused by dental procedures may lead to generalized or metastatic systemic infection complications leading to hospital care[10, 11]. In particular, patients with poorly controlled diabetes mellitus are more susceptible to bacterial infections[12-14]. However, death from odontogenic infection is quite rare [9, 15, 16].

Despite being rare, facial and neck fasciae spaces involved by infections from odontogenic origin may lead to a very morbid condition. The diagnosis delay and late or wrong therapeutic approachs to deep infections in these areas are the main causes of high mortality rate in this life-threatening situation.[4] Dentistry has made great progress in prevention and early intervention of odontogenic infection. The introduction of antibiotics reduced significantly the mortality and morbidity of these infections, however, even in this contemporary postantibiotic era, serious infections such as a descending necrotizing mediastinitis still have a high mortality rate with a fulminating course, leading frequently to death.[17-20]

2. Facial and cervical space anatomy

The knowledge of the relevant facial and cervical anatomy of the face is essential for todays clinical practice, allowing precise and successful diagnosis. Figure 1 describes the principal anatomic structures and spaces of the face.

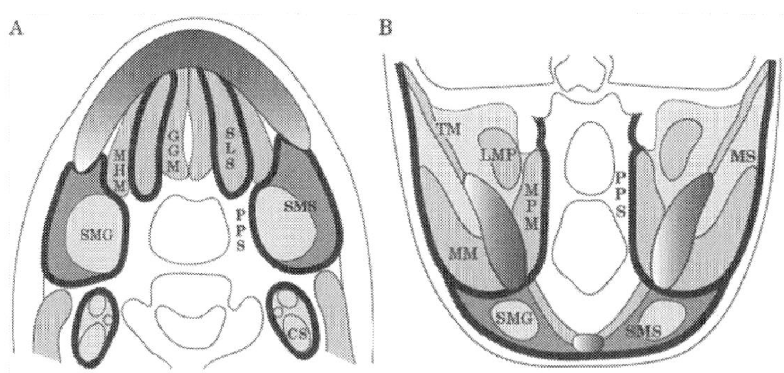

Figure 1. Anatomy of the fascial spaces in axial (A) and coronal (B) images. SMS: submandibular space; SLS: sublingual space; PPS: parapharyngeal space; CS: carotid space; MS: masticatory space. SMG: submandibular gland; GGM: genioglossus muscle; MHM: mylohyoid muscle; MM: masseter muscle; MPM: medial pterygoid muscle; LPM: lateral pterygoid muscle; TM: temporal muscle.

The superficial fascia a component of the fatty subcutaneous tissue and the deep cervical fascia is an important anatomic structure, determining the location and course of spread within the soft tissues of the neck.

2.1. Deep cervical fascia

The deep cervical fascia is divided into three layers: the superficial layer, the visceral or middle layer, and the pre-vertebral or deep layer.

The superficial layer of the deep cervical fascia encircles the neck, enveloping the sternocleidomastoid and trapezius muscles and the muscles of mastication, along with the submandibular and parotid salivary glands. It extends from the nuchal line of the skull, mastoid processes, and mandible inferiorly to the scapula, clavicle, and lower cervical vertebrae.

The middle layer of the deep cervical fascia encloses the anterior viscera of the neck (thyroid gland, larynx, trachea, and pharynx) and the strap muscles. It attaches to the skull base and extends into the mediastinum.

The deep layer of the deep cervical fascia is divided into the pre-vertebral and alar divisions. The pre-vertebral division tightly encloses the spine and paraspinous muscles. Ventrally, it lies immediately anterior to the vertebral bodies, forming the anterior wall of the pre-vertebral space. It extends from the base of the skull to the coccyx.

The alar division of the deep layer of the deep cervical fascia lies between the pre-vertebral division and the middle layer of the deep cervical fascia. It extends from the skull base to the mediastinum. The carotid sheath is made of contributions from all three layers of the deep cervical fascia and envelops the carotid artery, jugular vein, and vagus nerve.[21, 22]

2.2. Fascialspaces

The parapharyngeal space fascia is in an area of fatty areolar tissue with complex fascial margins that lies in a central location in the deep face. It extends from the skull base to the hyoid bone, containing only fat tissue, branches of the trigeminal nerve, and the pterygoid venous plexus. Posterior to the parapharyngeal space is the carotid space. All three layers of deep cervical fascia contribute to the carotid sheath that circumscribe this space.

The carotid space extends from the skull base to the aortic arch. Its suprahyoid contents include the internal carotid artery, jugular vein, cranial nerves IX–XII, and deep cervical lymph node chain.

The retropharyngeal space is a posterior midline space that has the middle layer of deep cervical fascia as its anterior margin and the deep layer of deep cervical fascia as its posterior and lateral margins. It extends from the skull base to the level of the T3 vertebral body.[21, 23]

The danger space lies posterior to the retropharyngeal space and is separated from the retropharyngeal space by the alar fascia. The posterior margin of the danger space is the pre-vertebral division of the deep layer of the deep cervical fascia. The importance of the danger space, and the reason for its name, is that it extends from the skull base to the level of the diaphragm, providing a pathway into the posterior mediastinum and pleural spaces. Infections of danger space most commonly occurs when an abscess in the retropharyngeal space ruptures through the alar fascia.[21, 23-31]

3. Teeth involved in fascial infections

Invasive dental manipulation is known to cause bacteremia and generally considered high-risk procedures for the spread of infection in susceptible patients.[31-48] Sato et al., has shown that the main origin of maxillofacial infections were odontogenic (79.31%), followed by trauma (10.7%), immunosuppression (1.6%), pathologies (1.6%), and other causes (8%).[49] Seppänen et al., also reiterated that the most common dental procedures that precede odontogenic infection complications are: tooth extraction (60%), endodontic treatment (20%), dental implant surgery (8%), restorative treatment (8%) and dental plaque and calculus removal (4%).[50-52]

Lower third molars are more frequently involved in odontogenic infections when compared with other teeth. Flynn et al., presented in their prospective study with 37 consecutive hospitalized patients, a 68% prevalence rate of this group of teeth in association with odontogenic infections, followed by other lower posterior teeth (premolars, first and second molars), without anterior teeth involvement.[13] Third molar removal is one of the most regular dentoalveolar surgical procedures.[10, 26, 52-65] With an 80% prevalence of retained third molars in the adult population,[23] appropriate treatment, and especially prophylactic third molar removal remains a key focus of interest in healthcare with both medical and economic dimensions. It is generally accepted that substantial risks may arise both from third molar removal,[6, 29, 37, 60, 66, 67] as well as from a "wait and see "policy.[4, 11, 14, 25, 33, 44, 65]

4. Microbiological involvement

The severe infections of odontogenic origin frequently involve a complex polymicrobial mix of aerobes, facultative aerobes and strict anaerobes working together. Some species like *Peptostreptococcus, Staphylococcus, Lactobacillus, Prevotella, Treponema, Fusobacterium, Veillonella, Actinomyces, Bacteroide* ssp. and oral *Streptococcus* sp. are frequently associated with infections of odontogenic origin.[13, 36, 43, 46, 48, 56] Sakamoto et al., reported 17 different species collected from a single surgical site.[48] Flynn et al., isolated 90 different strains of microorganisms in 37 patients, and of these, 17 were penicillin-resistant.[13] Other species can be easily found at the infection sites, but generally, they reflect the indigenous microflora of the oral cavity. Routine culture and sensitivity testing for minor oral infections does not appear to be justified, however, when an infection involves anatomic spaces of moderate or greater severity, or when there is significant medical/immune compromise, the tests become important to the outcome.

5. Pathway of facial and cervical infections of odontogenic origins

5.1. Fascial infections derived from mandibular odontogenic origins

Infections originating in the facial planes of the head and neck spread downward along the cervical fascia, facilitated by gravity, breathing, and negative intrathoracic pressure. Knowledge of the facial spaces and fascial planes is essential for understanding the propagation, pathways, symptoms, and complications of cervical infections.[4, 47] Although the pattern of spread varies among patients, a relatively constant trend in the distribution of infection into the spaces seem to be evident. Some studies clearly demonstrated that the masticatory space is the most prevalent site for odontogenic infection spread. Taken together with the finding that the masticatory space encompasses the posterior mandibular body, ramus, and a part of the alveolar bones of the maxilla, this suggests that the masticatory space may be the initial site of spread of odontogenic infection. This contention was further supported by the finding that mandibular infection more frequently involved the masseter and medial pterygoid muscles (located in the lower compartment of the masticatory space where the mandible is included) than the temporalis and lateral pterygoid muscles (located in the upper compartment of the space where part of the maxilla is included).[3]

The spaces adjacent to the masticatory space are the parotid space posteriorly, the parapharyngeal space medially, and the submandibular and sublingual spaces inferiorly (Figure 1).[48] The parapharyngeal space occupies the central position among the masticatory, parotid, and carotid vascular spaces. Therefore, infections in the parapharyngeal space may originate from any adjacent space. A fascia extends from the posterior superior margin of the medial pterygoid muscle to the base of the skull to separate the masticatory space from the parapharyngeal space.[49] In this way, it is possible to believe that infection spreading from the masticatory space into the parapharyngeal space may pass via the medial pterygoid muscle. Yonetsu et al., found that 100% of patients with parapharyngeal space involvement also had the medial pterygoid muscle affected, and 79% of patients with infection in the medial pterygoid muscle area had concomitant involvement of the parapharyngeal space. However, in none of their cases spread from the submandibular into the pharyngeal spaces.[3]

The parotid space abuts the posterior masticatory space and is enveloped by a layer of the deep cervical fascia.[50] Yonetsu et al., demonstrated that odontogenic infection may extend into the parotid space, via the masticatory space.[3] The retropharyngeal space connects the skull base to the upper mediastinum and contains loose fatty tissue in its infrahyoid portion. Thus, the retropharyngeal space is considered to be important due to its proximity to the airway and because infections in this space may cause mediastinitis, bronchial erosion, and septicemia.[3, 50] The vertebral and vascular spaces are thought to be rarely involved by head and neck infection.[51]

The infection spread occurs when accumulated pus perforates bone at the weakest and thinnest part. In the mandible, the lingual aspect of the molar region represents the easiest way.[4, 52] If odontogenic infection perforates this portion of bone, it will spread into the sublingual or submandibular space. As these spaces are partially separated by a thin sheet of mylohyoid muscle, infection in either space easily spreads into the other. It is generally believed that the midline enables free communication from either the sublingual or submandibular space.[3, 50]

Delineating the maxillary spread pattern is quite difficult, because limited data is available regarding its infections.[3] Nevertheless, it is plausible to consider that the observed difference in the spread profile between maxillary and mandibular infections may be due to differences in the distance between the original focal area in jaw bones and each of the spaces. For instance, maxillary infection was associated with temporalis muscle involvement more often than mandibular infection. Maxillary infection also spreads first to the masticatory space, but the temporalis and lateral pterygoid muscles are predominant targets for the infection. Involvement of the sublingual and submandibular spaces is rare. Otherwise, odontogenic infection arising in the mandible spreads first to the masticatory space. The masseter and medial pterygoid muscles in the masticatory space are most frequently involved. Thereafter, the infection spreads medially into the parapharyngeal space and posteriorly into the parotid space. Involvement of the sublingual and submandibular spaces seems to occur directly from the primary site of mandibular infection.[3]

There are complex pathways which allow infection to spread along the facial and neck structures. Thus, it is important for dental practitioners to know more about the possibility of a dental intervention to be a cause of severe infections.

The sequence of odontogenic infection spread that most commonly occurs is:

1. The masticatory space is the primary site of spread from mandibular infection.
2. The parotid and pharyngeal spaces are the secondary sites of spread from the masticatory space.
3. Mandibular infection spreads directly to the sublingual and submandibular spaces, and
4. Maxillary infection spreads to the deep facial and neck spaces in a different way from that of mandibular infection (Figure 2).

5.2. Fascial infections derived from maxillary odontogenic origins

The pattern of maxillary infection spread differs from that of the mandible. Generally, the main maxillary spaces involved were found to be the buccal maxillary (19.05%) and canine (15.24%).[49] According to Yonetsu et al., the temporalis muscle was involved in 100% of the patients with maxillary infection. The involvement of the temporalis muscle in mandibular infections occurred only in 26% of the patients. The downward spread into the sublingual and submandibular spaces from maxillary infections did not occur. The lateral pterygoid and masseter muscles were frequently involved (86%) as in the cases of mandibular infection. Other spaces were also involved, but less frequently. The buccal space was involved in 57% of the patients with maxillary infection[66] (Figure 2).

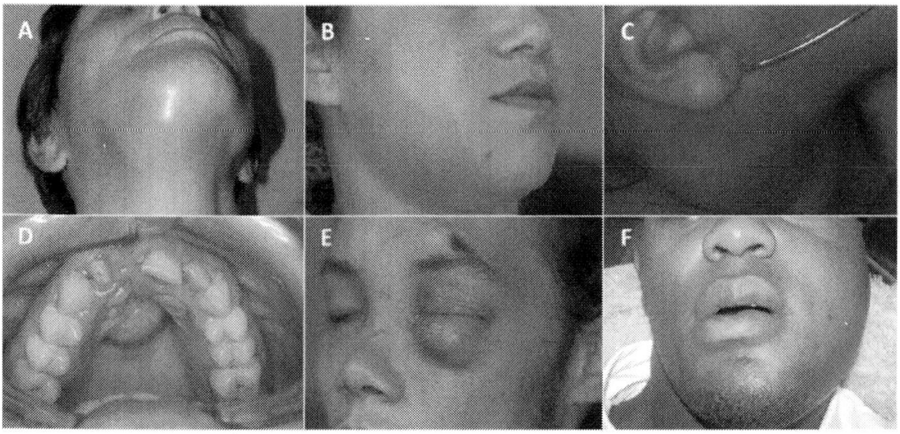

Figure 2. Different locations of odontogenic infections. (A) Submandibular and sublingual region. (B) Submandibular region. (C) Cervical region. (D) Palate. (E) Orbital region. (F) Submandibular and buccal region.

6. Causes of infections

6.1. Pericoronitis

Pericoronitis is an infection of the gingiva of a partially erupted tooth. The most frequent form of pericoronitis is caused by the partially erupted lower third molar, mainly due to the favorable niche that is created once the mucous cap covering the molar becomes retentive and deep enough to trap food particles and reduce the oxygen potential. These factors create the perfect microenvironment for the onset and subsequent development of a recurrent infectious, inflammatory condition caused by polymicrobial microorganisms, especially strict anaerobes. [19] Third molar pericoronitis may appear in either of its two acute variations, namely serous and suppurative, as well as in its chronic form; when either of the two acute forms previously mentioned stays untreated.

6.2. Periapical lesions/Intra-oral abscess

The most significant clinical condition of all bacterial infections of periapical origin is the so-called acute apical periodontitis.[16] It is usually the result of purulent pulpitis that spreads into the periapical space, therefore, it appears in the course of pulpal disease. In acute apical periodontitis there is an accumulation of pus inside the apical space of the tooth involved. This condition is commonly underestimated by dental practitioners in terms of its morbidity and mortality.[46] (Figure 3)

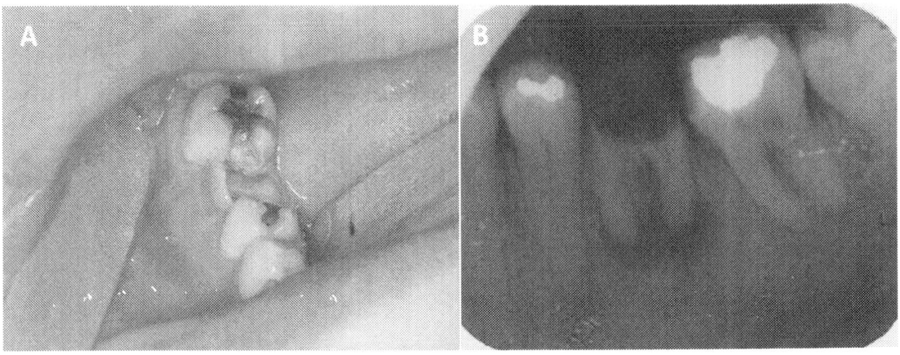

Figure 3. Clinical (A) and radiographic(B) aspects of a periapical lesion.

6.3. Infection of sublingual, submental and submandibular spaces (Ludwig's Angina)

Ludwig's angina is a rapidly spreading cellulitis that may produce upper airway obstruction, often leading to death. The most common source of Ludwig's angina is an odontogenic infection, from one or more grossly decayed, infected teeth, and is usually as a result of a native oral mixed aerobic-anaerobic flora. The patient with Ludwig's angina presents severe and obvious extra oral swellings including bilateral submandibular, submental, and sublingual spaces. Elevation and displacement of the tongue, trismus, drooling of saliva, airway obstruction, sore throat, dysphagia and/or dyspnea are commonly present. With extensive use of drainage and antibiotics, most facial infections have satisfactory outcome before they have a chance to progress to Ludwig's angina.[1] (Figure 4)

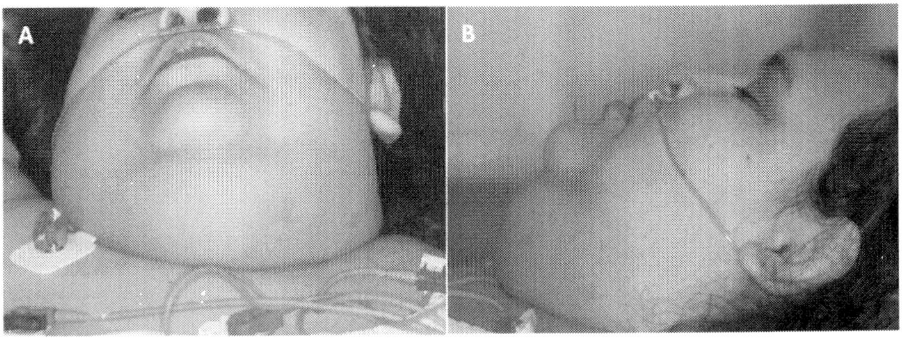

Figure 4. Clinical presentation of Ludwig's angina.

6.4. Cervical cellutis

Cervical cellulitis is most commonly from odontogenic origin and despite modern antibiotic therapy, cases with an initial delay in diagnosis and treatment may still result in this life-threatening situation.[17, 58-60] Odontogenic infections are usually locally confined, self-limiting processes. However, under certain circumstances, like anatomical variations or suppression of the immune system of some patients, these infections may pass through the bony, muscular, and mucosal barriers and spread into contiguous and distant spaces, resulting in severe fulminating infections in the body cavities.[60]

When cervical cellulitis involves the parapharyngeal, retropharyngeal, and viscerovascular spaces, the purulent process has easy access to the mediastinum, pericardium, and thorax, thereby increasing mortality rates.[13, 17, 58-60] Because of the fulminant nature of descending cervical cellulitis with mediastinal complications, prompt recognition followed by broad-spectrum antibiotic therapy, immediate surgical intervention, and intensive medical support are required.[13, 61]

The second and third mandibular molars are the teeth most frequently implicated in the cause of odontogenic deep neck infections.[17, 58, 60, 61] Because their roots lie below the mylohyoid muscle, medial perforation of a periapical abscess has immediate access to the submandibular space. Then, a collection of pus in the neck spreads along the cervical fascial planes, resulting in complications.[13]

6.5. Descending Necrotizing Mediastinitis (DNM)

Acute purulent mediastinitis occasionally develops as a complication of odontogenic infection, in which case it is denominated descending necrotizing mediastinitis.[17] This is a serious infection involving the connective tissue that fills the interpleural spaces and surrounds the median thoracic organs. It is one of the most dreaded and the most lethal form of mediastinitis, which occurs as a complication of oropharyngeal abscesses or as a complication of cervical trauma, with severe cervical infection spreading along the fascial planes into the mediastinum. As infection spreads along deep cervical fascial planes into the mediastinum, widespread cellulitis, necrosis, abscess formation, and sepsis may concomitantly occur. The delay of diagnosis and late or incomplete drainage of the mediastinum are the main causes for high mortality rates associated with this condition.[4]

Even with the use of computed tomography scanning or magnetic resonance examination, aggressive drainage, and modern antibiotic treatment, the mortality rate of descending necrotizing mediastinitis remains high. Surgical management, particularly the optimal form of mediastinal drainage, remains controversial with support ranging from cervical drainage alone to cervical drainage and routine thoracotomy.

6.6. Necrotizing fasciitis

Abscesses of the peritonsillar region are among the most common deep abscesses of the head and neck. Although rare, complications resulting from this disease may be life threatening.

One of the most dangerous complications is necrotizing fasciitis, which is a rare soft tissue infection characterized by progressive destruction of fascia and adipose tissue that may not involve the skin.[62, 63] Necrotizing fasciitis is characterized by its fulminating, devastating, and rapid-progressing course.[64] Diabetes mellitus, burns and malnutrition are common predisposing factors. Initially, cervical necrotizing fasciitis is predominantly characterized by a "simple" infection in the upper aerodigestive tract like pharyngitis or even tonsillitis. Typically, the general condition gets worse within a very short period of time with cardiovascular decompensation due to a toxic shock-like condition. Cervical necrotizing fasciitis initially involves the superficial muscular system and superficial fascial planes of the head and neck or it may result from a deep soft tissue infection, such as odontogenic infections or even pharyngitis, which spreads along the deep fascial planes.

If the disease is not recognized in time the infection can rapidly involve the great vessels or mediastinum, producing systemic toxicity and sepsis.[65, 66] The basis of successful treatment comprises aggressive surgical debridement and drainage of the involved necrotic fascia and tissue along with intensive broad-spectrum intravenous antibiotic coverage.[63]

7. Signs and symptoms

The current signs and symptoms presented by patients with severe infections from odontogenic origin are crucial factors for the patient's life maintenance. Sato et al., has shown in their eight-year retrospective study that cases of odontogenic infections call for immediate therapeutics, either clinical or surgical, with precise daily or long-term monitoring of patients until complete resolution of the clinical infection status is reached. The most frequent signs and symptoms found in these patients were trismus (43.33%), fever (28.10%), dysphagy (25.24%), pain (24.76%), and swelling (20%), all of which are classic signs of a dire clinical situation.26

8. Imaging

Imaging plays an essential role in the diagnosis and management of head and neck infections since, by clinical examination alone. It is often difficult to determine if a swollen neck is due to cellulitis or an abscess; the location, extent or source of the infection, and whether the process is self-limited or if it is potentially life-threatening is also clinically unclear.[21]

Radiographs of the cervical segment and the chest may be useful in the demonstration of subcutaneous emphysema in the form of vertical, linear, clear bands of gas extending from the cervical spaces into the mediastinum. The lateral radiograph of the neck can reveal a prevertebral soft tissue opacity pushing the trachea anteriorly. Chest radiograph can demonstrate a widened mediastinum and pleural effusion. However, the modest diagnostic sensibility of cervical and chest plain film should call immediately for computed tomography scanning or a magnetic resonance of the cervicothoracic areas.[2, 17, 67, 68]

Any patient with neck swelling and/or pain from dental infection should have a computed tomography exam of the neck and chest to evaluate the spread of infection. Computed tomography examination and neck evaluation include: diffuse thickening of the cutis and subcutis and reticular enhancement of the subcutaneous fat of the face and neck; thickening and/or enhancement of cervical fasciae; asymmetric thickening or enhancement of cervical muscles, reactive lymphadenopathy; septic vascular thrombosis and fluid collections with or without gas. Mediastinal computed tomography findings include: streaky enhancement of mediastinal fat, fluid collections with or without gas, pericardial effusion and pleural effusion.[21]

9. Treatment

Treatment of odontogenic infections includes diagnosis and management of the causative factor, drainage when necessary (Figures 5-6) and, usually, prescription of appropriate antibiotics. It is imperative that the source of infection be addressed immediately. In addition, the patient's medical status must be optimized. The patient's fluid and nutrition status should also be addressed, as many patients with odontogenic infections have decreased oral intake due to pain and difficulty in chewing or swallowing. The clinician must be aware of the most likely causative organisms and prescribe the narrowest spectrum of antibiotics that will cover all possible offending organisms.

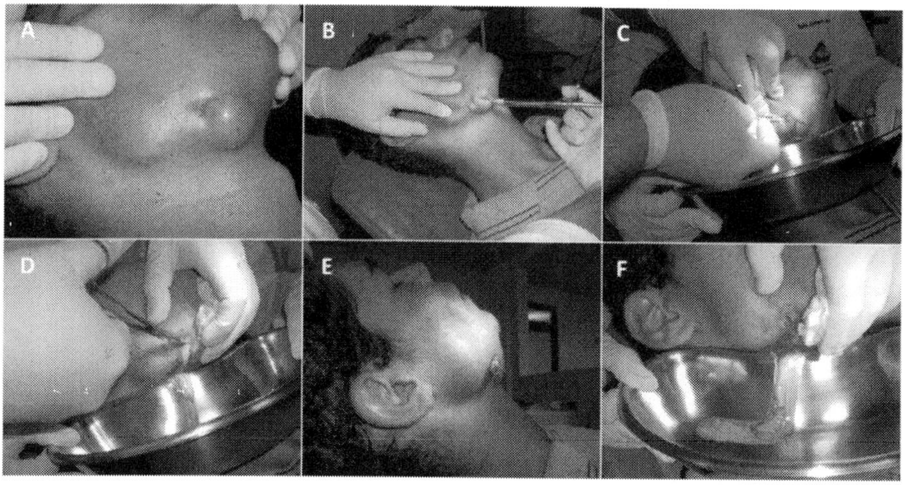

Figure 5. Sequence of drainage of odontogenic infection – case 1. Note that the most dependent part (under the swelling) must be incised not the thin most swollen part (to prevent scarring).

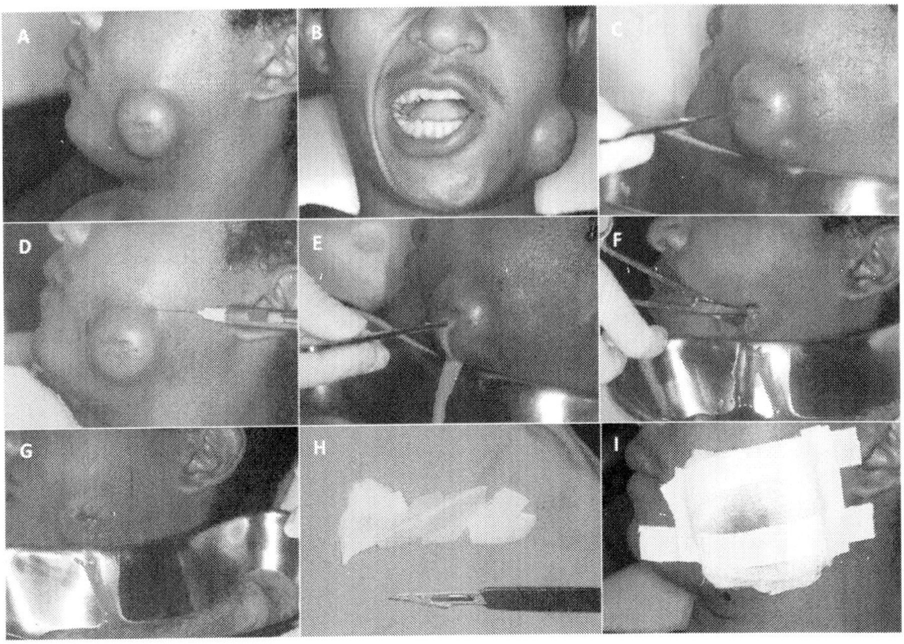

Figure 6. Figure 6: Sequence of drainage of odontogenic infection – case 2.

10. Conclusions

A simple tooth infection, especially in diabetics, immunocompromised, or debilitated patients should not be underestimated in its ability to cause severe infections. Furthermore, even non-invasive dental manipulations may also precipitate systemic spread. Facial and cervical infections are potentially lethal complications. However, with good knowledge of the anatomic pathways of the infection, early diagnosis, attention to airway maintenance, aggressive intravenous antibiotic therapy, surgical intervention and careful postoperative management, the infectious process should have a satisfactory outcome. The practitioner must be alert to the particularities of infections from odontogenic origin, as well as to the facial and cervical spaces anatomy, because these structures are crucial for the patient's life and play important roles during the execution of treatment procedures.

Acknowledgements

The authors would like to thank Analice Giovani Pereira for the support during the writing of the chapter and selection of clinical cases.

Author details

Flaviana Soares Rocha[1], Jonas Dantas Batista[1*], Cláudia Jordão Silva[1], Roberto Bernardino Júnior[2] and Luis Henrique Araújo Raposo[3]

*Address all correspondence to: jonasdantasbat@gmail.com

1 Department of Oral and Maxillofacial Surgery and Implantology – School of Dentistry - Federal University of Uberlândia – UFU, Brazil

2 Department of Human Anatomy - Biomedical Science Institute - Federal University of Uberlândia – UFU, Brazil

3 Department of Occlusion, Fixed Prostheses, and Dental Materials – School of Dentistry - Federal University of Uberlândia – UFU., Brazil

References

[1] Abramowicz S, Abramowicz JS, Dolwick MF. Severe life threatening maxillofacial infection in pregnancy presented as Ludwig's angina. Infect Dis ObstetGynecol 2006: 2006: 51931.

[2] Ariji Y, Gotoh M, Kimura Y, Naitoh M, Kurita K, Natsume N, *et al.* Odontogenic infection pathway to the submandibular space: imaging assessment. Int J Oral MaxillofacSurg 2002: 31: 165-169.

[3] Yonetsu K, Izumi M, Nakamura T. Deep facial infections of odontogenic origin: CT assessment of pathways of space involvement. AJNR Am J Neuroradiol 1998: 19: 123-128.

[4] Mihos P, Potaris K, Gakidis I, Papadakis D, Rallis G. Management of descending necrotizing mediastinitis. J Oral MaxillofacSurg 2004: 62: 966-972.

[5] Haug RH, Hoffman MJ, Indresano AT. An epidemiologic and anatomic survey of odontogenic infections. J Oral MaxillofacSurg 1991: 49: 976-980.

[6] Indresano AT, Haug RH, Hoffman MJ. The third molar as a cause of deep space infections. J Oral MaxillofacSurg 1992: 50: 33-35; discussion 35-36.

[7] Ohshima A, Ariji Y, Goto M, Izumi M, Naitoh M, Kurita K, *et al.* Anatomical considerations for the spread of odontogenic infection originating from the pericoronitis of impacted mandibular third molar: computed tomographic analyses. Oral Surg Oral Med Oral Pathol Oral RadiolEndod 2004: 98: 589-597.

[8] Gosney MA, Preston AJ, Corkhill J, Millns B, Martin MV. Pseudomonasaeruginosasepticaemiafroman oral source. Br Dent J 1999: 187: 639-640.

[9] Seppanen L, Lauhio A, Lindqvist C, Suuronen R, Rautemaa R. Analysis of systemic and local odontogenic infection complications requiring hospital care. J Infect 2008: 57: 116-122.

[10] Bergmann OJ. Oral infections and septicemia in immunocompromised patients with hematologic malignancies. J ClinMicrobiol 1988: 26: 2105-2109.

[11] Wilson W, Taubert KA, Gewitz M, Lockhart PB, Baddour LM, Levison M, *et al.* Prevention of infective endocarditis: guidelines from the American Heart Association: a guideline from the American Heart Association Rheumatic Fever, Endocarditis and Kawasaki Disease Committee, Council on Cardiovascular Disease in the Young, and the Council on Clinical Cardiology, Council on Cardiovascular Surgery and Anesthesia, and the Quality of Care and Outcomes Research Interdisciplinary Working Group. J Am Dent Assoc 2007: 138: 739-745, 747-760.

[12] Harrison GA, Schultz TA, Schaberg SJ. Deep neck infection complicated by diabetes mellitus: Report of a case. Oral Surg Oral Med Oral Pathol 1983: 55: 133-137.

[13] Sugata T, Fujita Y, Myoken Y, Fujioka Y. Cervical cellulitis with mediastinitis from an odontogenic infection complicated by diabetes mellitus: report of a case. J Oral MaxillofacSurg 1997: 55: 864-869.

[14] Ueta E, Osaki T, Yoneda K, Yamamoto T. Prevalence of diabetes mellitus in odontogenic infections and oral candidiasis: an analysis of neutrophil suppression. J Oral Pathol Med 1993: 22: 168-174.

[15] Carter L, Lowis E. Death from overwhelming odontogenic sepsis: a case report. Br Dent J 2007: 203: 241-242.

[16] Green AW, Flower EA, New NE. Mortality associated with odontogenic infection! Br Dent J 2001: 190: 529-530.

[17] Estrera AS, Landay MJ, Grisham JM, Sinn DP, Platt MR. Descending necrotizing mediastinitis. SurgGynecolObstet 1983: 157: 545-552.

[18] Mathieu D, Neviere R, Teillon C, Chagnon JL, Lebleu N, Wattel F. Cervical necrotizing fasciitis: clinical manifestations and management. Clin Infect Dis 1995: 21: 51-56.

[19] Sakamoto H, Aoki T, Kise Y, Watanabe D, Sasaki J. Descending necrotizing mediastinitis due to odontogenic infections. Oral Surg Oral Med Oral Pathol Oral RadiolEndod 2000: 89: 412-419.

[20] Wheatley MJ, Stirling MC, Kirsh MM, Gago O, Orringer MB. Descending necrotizing mediastinitis: transcervical drainage is not enough. Ann ThoracSurg 1990: 49: 780-784.

[21] Pinto A, Scaglione M, Scuderi MG, Tortora G, Daniele S, Romano L. Infections of the neck leading to descending necrotizing mediastinitis: Role of multi-detector row computed tomography. Eur J Radiol 2008: 65: 389-394.

[22] Smith JK, Armao DM, Specter BB, Castillo M. Danger space infection: infection of the neck leading to descending necrotizing mediastinitis. EmergRadiol 1999: 6: 129-132.

[23] Harnsberger HR, Osborn AG. Differential diagnosis of head and neck lesions based on their space of origin. 1. The suprahyoid part of the neck. AJR Am J Roentgenol 1991: 157: 147-154.

[24] Lockhart PB, Brennan MT, Kent ML, Norton HJ, Weinrib DA. Impact of amoxicillin prophylaxis on the incidence, nature, and duration of bacteremia in children after intubation and dental procedures. Circulation 2004: 109: 2878-2884.

[25] Rajasuo A, Nyfors S, Kanervo A, Jousimies-Somer H, Lindqvist C, Suuronen R. Bacteremia after plate removal and tooth extraction. Int J Oral MaxillofacSurg 2004: 33: 356-360.

[26] Sato FR, Hajala FA, Freire Filho FW, Moreira RW, de Moraes M. Eight-year retrospective study of odontogenic origin infections in a postgraduation program on oral and maxillofacial surgery. J Oral MaxillofacSurg 2009: 67: 1092-1097.

[27] Flynn TR, Shanti RM, Levi MH, Adamo AK, Kraut RA, Trieger N. Severe odontogenic infections, part 1: prospective report. J Oral MaxillofacSurg 2006: 64: 1093-1103.

[28] Eklund SA, Pittman JL. Third-molar removal patterns in an insured population. J Am Dent Assoc 2001: 132: 469-475.

[29] Kunkel M, Morbach T, Kleis W, Wagner W. Third molar complications requiring hospitalization. Oral Surg Oral Med Oral Pathol Oral RadiolEndod 2006: 102: 300-306.

[30] Worrall SF, Riden K, Haskell R, Corrigan AM. UK National Third Molar project: the initial report. Br J Oral MaxillofacSurg 1998: 36: 14-18.

[31] Hugoson A, Kugelberg CF. The prevalence of third molars in a Swedish population. An epidemiological study. Community Dent Health 1988: 5: 121-138.

[32] Bui CH, Seldin EB, Dodson TB. Types, frequencies, and risk factors for complications after third molar extraction. J Oral MaxillofacSurg 2003: 61: 1379-1389.

[33] Libersa P, Roze D, Cachart T, Libersa JC. Immediate and late mandibular fractures after third molar removal. J Oral MaxillofacSurg 2002: 60: 163-165; discussion 165-166.

[34] Moghadam HG, Caminiti MF. Life-threatening hemorrhage after extraction of third molars:case report and management protocol. J Can Dent Assoc 2002: 68: 670-674.

[35] Valmaseda-Castellon E, Berini-Aytes L, Gay-Escoda C. Inferior alveolar nerve damage after lower third molar surgical extraction: a prospective study of 1117 surgical extractions. Oral Surg Oral Med Oral Pathol Oral RadiolEndod 2001: 92: 377-383.

[36] Yoshii T, Hamamoto Y, Muraoka S, Kohjitani A, Teranobu O, Furudoi S, *et al.* Incidence of deep fascial space infection after surgical removal of the mandibular third molars. J Infect Chemother 2001: 7: 55-57.

[37] Blakey GH, Marciani RD, Haug RH, Phillips C, Offenbacher S, Pabla T, *et al.* Periodontal pathology associated with asymptomatic third molars. J Oral MaxillofacSurg 2002: 60: 1227- 1233.

[38] Eliasson S, Heimdahl A, Nordenram A. Pathological changes related to long-term impaction of third molars. A radiographic study.Int J Oral MaxillofacSurg 1989: 18: 210-212.

[39] Fuselier JC, Ellis EE, 3rd, Dodson TB. Do mandibular third molars alter the risk of angle fracture? J Oral MaxillofacSurg 2002: 60: 514-518.

[40] Knutsson K, Brehmer B, Lysell L, Rohlin M. Pathoses associated with mandibular third molars subjected to removal. Oral Surg Oral Med Oral Pathol Oral RadiolEndod 1996: 82: 10- 17.

[41] Manganaro AM, Cross SE, Startzell JM. Carcinoma arising in a dentigerous cyst with neckmetastasis. Head Neck 1997: 19: 436-439.

[42] Punwutikorn J, Waikakul A, Ochareon P. Symptoms of unerupted mandibular third molars. Oral Surg Oral Med Oral Pathol Oral RadiolEndod 1999: 87: 305-310.

[43] Yamaoka M, Furusawa K, Ikeda M, Hasegawa T. Root resorption of mandibular second molar teeth associated with the presence of the third molars. Aust Dent J 1999: 44: 112-116.

[44] Leone SA, Edenfield MJ, Cohen ME. Correlation of acute pericoronitis and the position of the mandibular third molar. Oral Surg Oral Med Oral Pathol 1986: 62: 245-250.

[45] Venta I, Turtola L, Murtomaa H, Ylipaavalniemi P. Third molars as an acute problem in Finnish university students. Oral Surg Oral Med Oral Pathol 1993: 76: 135-140.

[46] Robertson D, Smith AJ. The microbiology of the acute dental abscess. J Med Microbiol 2009: 58: 155-162.

[47] Zachariades N, Mezitis M, Stavrinidis P, Konsolaki-Agouridaki E. Mediastinitis, thoracic empyema, and pericarditis as complications of a dental abscess: report of a case. J Oral MaxillofacSurg 1988: 46: 493-495.

[48] Braun IF, Hoffman JC, Jr. Computed tomography of the buccomasseteric region: 1. Anatomy. AJNR Am J Neuroradiol 1984: 5: 605-610.

[49] Curtin HD. Separation of the masticator space from the parapharyngeal space. Radiology 1987: 163: 195-204.

[50] Paparella MM, Shumrick KA. Otolaryngology: Head and Neck. Philadelphia: WB Saunders, 1993: 2545-2563.

[51] Nyberg DA, Jeffrey RB, Brant-Zawadzki M, Federle M, Dillon W. Computed tomography of cervical infections. J Comput Assist Tomogr 1985: 9: 288-296.

[52] Lindner HH. The anatomy of the fasciae of the face and neck with particular reference to the spread and treatment of intraoral infections (Ludwig's) that have progressed into adjacent fascial spaces. Ann Surg 1986: 204: 705-714.

[53] Gutierrez-Perez JL. Third molar infections. Med Oral Patol Oral Cir Bucal 2004: 9 Suppl: 122-125; 120-122.

[54] Dogan N, Orhan K, Gunaydin Y, Koymen R, Okcu K, Ucok O. Unerupted mandibular third molars: symptoms, associated pathologies, and indications for removal in a Turkish population. Quintessence Int 2007: 38: e497-505.

[55] Peltroche-Llacsahuanga H, Reichhart E, Schmitt W, Lutticken R, Haase G. Investigation of infectious organisms causing pericoronitis of the mandibular third molar. J Oral MaxillofacSurg 2000: 58: 611-616.

[56] Gonzalez-Moles MA, Gonzalez NM. Bacterial infections of pulp and periodontal origin. Med Oral Patol Oral Cir Bucal 2004: 9 Suppl: 34-36; 32-34.

[57] Marple BF. Ludwig angina: a review of current airway management. Arch Otolaryngol Head Neck Surg 1999: 125: 596-599.

[58] Rubin MM, Cozzi GM. Fatal necrotizing mediastinitis as a complication of an odontogenic infection. J Oral MaxillofacSurg 1987: 45: 529-533.

[59] Garatea-Crelgo J, Gay-Escoda C. Mediastinitis from odontogenic infection. Report of three cases and review of the literature.Int J Oral MaxillofacSurg 1991: 20: 65-68.

[60] Zeitoun IM, Dhanarajani PJ. Cervical cellulitis and mediastinitis caused by odontogenic infections: report of two cases and review of literature. J Oral MaxillofacSurg 1995: 53: 203- 208.

[61] Maisel RH, Karlen R. Cervical necrotizing fasciitis. Laryngoscope 1994: 104: 795-798.

[62] Sellers BJ, Woods ML, Morris SE, Saffle JR. Necrotizing group A streptococcal infections associated with streptococcal toxic shock syndrome. Am J Surg 1996: 172: 523-527; discussion 527-528.

[63] Skitarelic N, Mladina R, Morovic M, Skitarelic N. Cervical necrotizing fasciitis: sources and outcomes. Infection 2003: 31: 39-44.

[64] Tung-Yiu W, Jehn-Shyun H, Ching-Hung C, Hung-An C. Cervical necrotizing fasciitis of odontogenic origin: a report of 11 cases. J Oral MaxillofacSurg 2000: 58: 1347-1352; discussion 1353.

[65] Lalwani AK, Kaplan MJ. Mediastinal and thoracic complications of necrotizing fasciitis of the head and neck. Head Neck 1991: 13: 531-539.

[66] Shindo ML, Nalbone VP, Dougherty WR. Necrotizing fasciitis of the face. Laryngoscope 1997: 107: 1071-1079.

[67] Novellas S, Kechabtia K, Chevallier P, Sedat J, Bruneton JN. Descending necrotizing mediastinitis: a rare pathology to keep in mind.Clin Imaging 2005: 29: 138-140.

[68] Schuknecht B, Stergiou G, Graetz K. Masticator space abscess derived from odontogenic infection: imaging manifestation and pathways of extension depicted by CT and MR in 30 patients. EurRadiol 2008: 18: 1972-1979.

[69] Tsunoda R, Suda S, Fukaya T, Saito K. Descending necrotizing mediastinitis caused by an odontogenic infection: a case report. J Oral MaxillofacSurg 2000: 58: 240-242.

Section 6

Diagnosis and Treatment of Sleep Apnea

Chapter 17

Orthodontic Considerations in Obstructive Sleep Apnea — State of the Art

Hakima Aghoutan, Sana Alami, Samir Diouny and
Farid Bourzgui

Additional information is available at the end of the chapter

http://dx.doi.org/10.5772/59086

1. Introduction

Obstructive Sleep Apnea (OSA) was described as early as 1837 in "The Posthumous Papers of the Pickwick Club". Dickens, a British author, described "Joe", the main character, as a fat boy who falls asleep easily and involuntarily (Figure 1). [1]

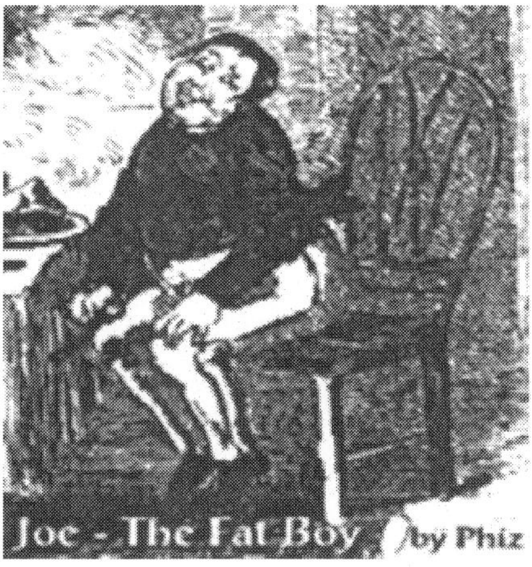

In The Pickwick Papers (c. 1836–1837)

Figure 1. Artist (Hablot Knight Browne- Phiz) rendering of Joe, Charles Dickens' character.

Later on, Osler (1914) used the term "Pickwickian syndrome" to describe obese and sleepy patients, in homage to Dickens' character "Joe". As early as 1956, Bickelmann et al [2] reported that the "Pickwickian syndrome" was associated with extreme obesity and alveolar hypoventilation.

Gastaut's research group described three different types of apnea, namely, obstructive apnea central apnea, and mixed apnea. In 1973, Guilleminault introduced the apnea-hypopnea index (AHI), which refers to the total number of apnea and hypopnea episodes per hour of sleep, and proved, along with Dement, that obesity is not a prerequisite for OSA. In 1977, Guilleminault and Dement used the term "sleep apnea syndrome", in association with hypertension and electrocardiographic pathologies. [3]

Recently, much research on OSA has been conducted with a view to help elucidate the characteristic features of OSA. Sleep is a process through which the body restores energy used during the day. Not much is known about its biological purpose, but its evaluation can be undertaken by muscle and brain electrical activity, and ocular movement. Good-quality sleep entails several functions; these include physical recovery, biochemical refreshment, memory consolidation and psychological well-being. [4]

In adults, sleep is regulated by a cycle of five periods. The first four periods belong to non-rapid eye movement sleep (light and deep stage) and the fifth period is named the rapid-eye-movement (REM) or paradoxical sleep (active stage). The progression from the first stage to the RAM constitutes one sleep cycle. Generally, there are four to six sleep cycles per night; during which activities of the brain, muscles, and the cardio-respiratory system fluctuate (Figure 2, 3). [4]

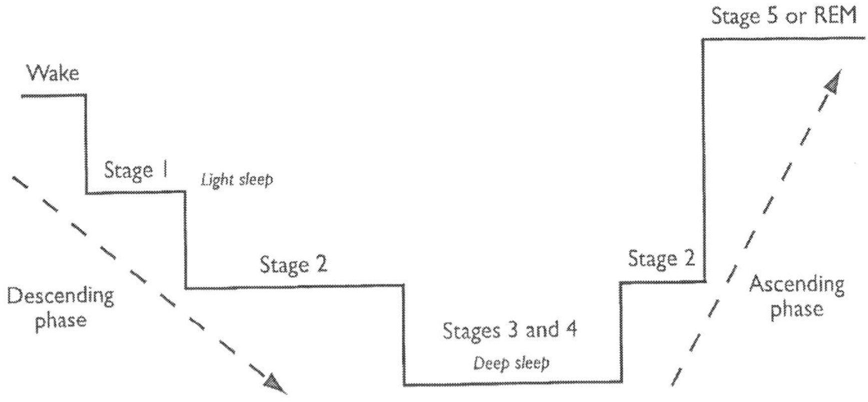

Figure 2. A sleep cycle (non-REM to REM stages). [4]

During these sleep stages, several sleeping disorders can occur. International classification of Sleep Disorders (ICSD-3), revisited in 2014, includes the following broad categories: [5]

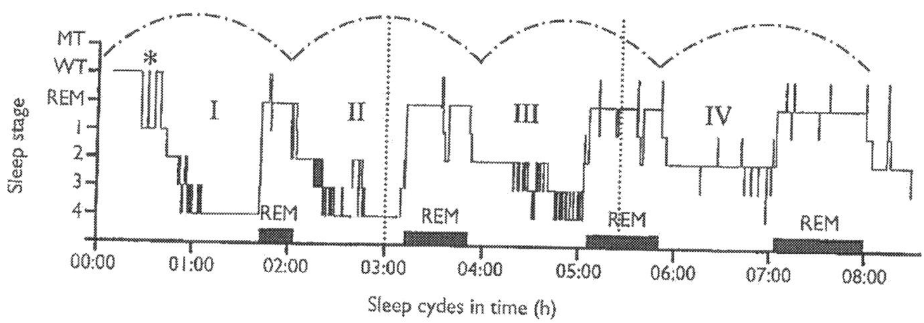

Figure 3. Consecutive wave of non REM to REM sleep cycles (I to IV). Throughout the night, REM becomes longer than slow wave sleep (stage 3and 4). MT: movement time, WT: wake time. [4]

- Insomnia
- Sleep related-breathing disorders
- hypersomnomlence Central disorders
- Circadian rhythm sleep-wake disorders
- Parasomnias
- Sleep related-movement disorders

Sleep apnea is the most common sleep disorder related to breathing. There are 3 types of sleep apnea: Obstructive, central, and mixed (a combination of both forms). Obstructive sleep apnea (OSA) is caused by partial or complete obstruction at multiple levels of the upper airway, producing reduction (hypopnea), or cessation (apnea) of airflow. Due to the lack of adequate alveolar ventilation, oxygen saturation may drop and partial pressure of CO2 may occasionally increase. Snoring and sleep fragmentation are common with OSA that can be graded as mild, moderate and severe.[6] Adults and children are equally affected. However, the prevalence, etiology and pathophysiology of the disorder differ from one group to another. It is important to note that the physiopathology and etiology of OSA are poorly understood.

Furthermore, OSA is associated with neuropsychological impairment, sexual dysfunction, metabolic and cardiovascular co-morbidities; and causes an increase in mortality. Quality of life and economic potential are also affected: snoring affects the sleeping pattern of the partner, and frequent arousals at night result in relative sleep deprivation and can cause excessive daytime sleepiness, loss of concentration and motor vehicle accidents.[4]-[7] Therefore, OSA is regarded as a public health condition and increases the consumption of health care resources.

Continuous positive airway pressure (CPAP) is considered a golden standard treatment; oral appliances and surgical procedures for upper airway soft tissues and maxilla-mandibular advancement are other alternatives. Hence OSA treatment requires a multidisciplinary management. [8] Orthodontists, sleep specialists and surgeons should all be involved in managing and treating OSA. This chapter gives a comprehensive account of the literature on OSA and underlines the role of orthodontists in managing OSA with a view to improve the physical, mental and social status of patients diagnosed with OSA.

2. OSA epidemiology

2.1. Prevalence

Due to various definitions of respiratory events and differences in study design, contradictory variable prevalence rates of OSA are reported. The American Academy of Sleep Medicine published the first guidelines to standardize the definition of OSA; however, the standardization of OSA definition only expanded the diagnostic criteria.[1] According to the Wisconsin sleep cohort study, the estimated prevalence of moderate to severe sleep breathing disorder in the United States for the period of 1988–2011 ranged from 3% to 17% in adults depending on sex and age; OSA seemed to affect especially middle-aged and elderly men and has increased substantially over the last two decades in the US. [9] In Morocco, however, OSA prevalence ranges from 5, 4% to 7, and 9% in the general population. [10] De Backer (2013) reported that epidemiological studies investigating the prevalence of OSA are all biased because there is a lack of a uniform definition. He also indicated that the prevalence of an AHI of >5 events per hour in the general population (without taking into account symptoms of sleepiness) has been estimated to be 24% in the male population. When symptoms of sleepiness are also taken into account, this prevalence goes down to 4% in males and 2% in females. [11]

2.2. Risk factors

In the literature on OSA, most researches agree that risk factors for OSA include obesity, upper airway and craniofacial abnormalities, gender, age, alcohol consumption and cigarette smoking. [12] Obesity, particularly central or upper body fat distribution, with increased neck circumference (collar size) is a main risk factor for OSA. But this association may be less important with the elderly. In non-obese patients, craniofacial abnormality like micrognathia and retrognathia may also be considered as a risk factor leading to OSA. [13]

Aging is also associated with higher OSA prevalence. Still, it is not clear if OSA in the elderly compared to middle-aged adults manifests itself the same way; middle age and over-weight adult men seem to have the highest prevalence of OSA. However, after menopause, prevalence seems to be the same for both women and men. [1]Some studies have examined craniofacial features among different ethnic groups; their objective was to investigate whether ethnicity differences had an effect on the prevalence of OSA. These studies reported an increased risk of OSA among African-Americans, Latinos and Asians. [14]-[17] Wong et al. (2005) claimed that the hyoid bone was located more caudally in Chinese subjects and may be a severity indicator in this population. [18] In addition, OSA prevalence seems to be much higher in patients with cardiac or metabolic disorders than in the general population. Other factors such as heredity, hormonal change, sedative hypnotics and supine sleep position have also been described as risk conditions for developing OSA. [11, 12]

2.3. Mortality and morbidity

Epidemiologic data have shown a strong association between untreated obstructive sleep apnea and incident cardio and cerebrovascular morbidity and mortality. [19, 20] These co-morbid conditions may be due, in part, to common risk factors (i.e. obesity and hypertension), and also to hypoxemia-hypercapnia, which can lead to vascular dysfunctions. [21] In an18-year mortality follow-up conducted on the population-based Wisconsin Sleep Cohort sample (n = 1522), Young et al. found a significant mortality risk with untreated sleep breathing disorder (SBD). They underscored the need for early diagnosis and treatment of SBD, indicated by frequent episodes of apnea and hypopnea, regardless of sleepiness symptoms.[20]A recent review of OSA in adults reported an increased risk of morbidity and mortality associated with OSA, which reached its peak at 55 years of age. [12], This association seems to disappear after 70 yrs. [22]Sampaio et al., 2012 suggested that women revealed more psychological morbidity associated with OSAS. Therefore, it seems extremely important to look at women as potential patients for sleep apnea. [23] However, Gozal and Kheirandish-Gozal highlighted the potential interaction between gene polymorphisms, organ vulnerability, and the phenotypic expression of OSA and suggested that it should be identified and incorporated into future prediction schemes of morbidity risks associated with OSA. [24]

3. OSA pathophysiology

In recent years, the understanding of the pathophysiology of sleep-breathing disorder has improved. Central nervous system regulation of breathing is now recognized as a significant contributor to the pathogenesis of OSA. To understand the pathophysiologic mechanisms that contribute to OSA, an overview of anatomical and physiological aspects of upper airway is in order.

3.1. Upper airway anatomy and physiology

The upper airway is a complex, multifunctional, and dynamic neuro-mechanical system. It is defined as the passageway for gas and food, beginning at the mouth and nose and ending at the epiglottis and vocal cords. It is composed of bony structures (maxilla, mandible and hyoid bone) and soft tissues (tonsils, soft palate, tongue, uvula, pharyngeal muscle, para-pharyngeal fat pads and lateral wall of the pharynx). The mandible and hyoid bone are the principal craniofacial bone structures that determine the dimensions of the upper airways. Soft tissues form the walls of the upper airways and they are supported by bone structures.[1, 25] The upper airways are typically divided into three segments: The nasopharynx (end of the nasal septum to the margin of the soft palate), the oropharynx (free margin of the soft palate to the tip of the epiglottis), divided into the retropalatal and retroglossal regions, and the hypopharynx (tip of the epiglottis to the vocal cords) (Figure 4).

The pharynx has several functions that enter into competition with each other; it requires patency and closure.[1, 4] It serves the neurological (speech, taste, smell), but also gastro-intestinal and respiratory system (chewing, swallowing, breathing).Speech and swallowing

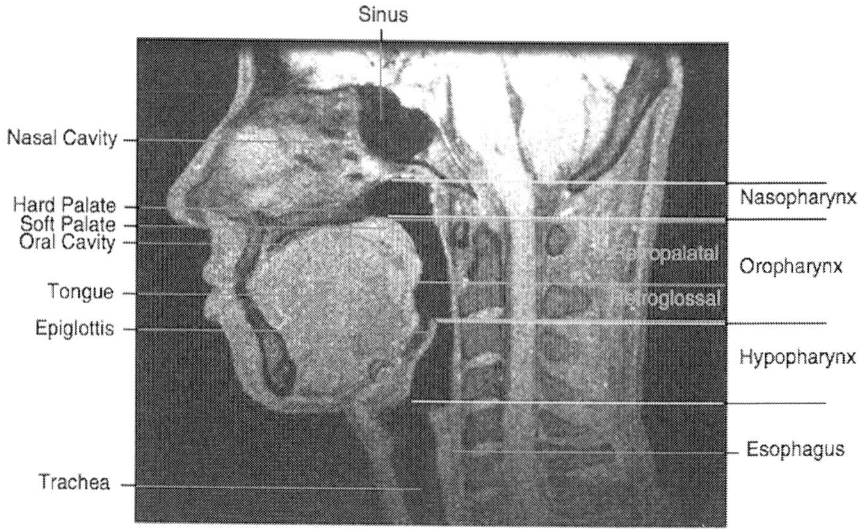

Figure 4. Sagittal magnetic resonance imaging of airway and division of oropharynx. (Clete A. Kushida)

require that the upper airway be collapsible. However, during breathing, the pharynx must remain patent.

Oropharynx and hypopharynx compose the collapsible portion of the pharynx. Due to the absence of bone and cartilage in these segments, their lumen patency, during awakening and sleep, depends heavily on muscle activity and intrinsic airway collapsibility, which is dictated by a combination of passive mechanical properties and active neural mechanisms.

During inspiration, negative intra-thoracic pressure is transmitted to the upper airways, resulting in a reduction in the transverse area of the pharynx. [25] The permeability of the upper airways is maintained through the balance between opposing forces from factors that collapse the airway and those that promote its patency. This is called "the balance of pressure concept" and involves the following determinants (Figure 5): [1,4, 26]

- The baseline pharyngeal area, determined by both craniofacial and soft tissue structures;
- The compliance or collapsibility of the airway;
- The negative intraluminal pressure within the airway (intraluminal pressure), transmitted from inspiratory muscles (the diaphragm, the external intercostal muscles....), that tends to narrow the airway;
- The pressure acting on the outside surface of the pharyngeal wall (tissue pressure), which also tends to collapse the airway such as compression by the lateral pharyngeal and submandibular fat pad and a large tongue confined to a small oral cavity;

- The positive extra-luminal pressure from the abduction force of the pharyngeal dilator muscles, which is directed outwards, and functions to increase cross-sectional area.

Pharyngeal dilating muscles can be divided into four groups: [1, 4]

- Muscles influencing hyoid bone position such as geniohyoid and sternohyoid
- Muscles of tongue: Genioglossus is the largest and the most important muscle
- Muscles of the palate such as tensor palatini and levator palatini
- Muscles protruding the mandible, principally the pterygoid muscles

In normal individuals in awake state, the upper airway dimensions remain practically constant throughout inspiration by neuromotor mechanisms, like reflex muscle activation in response to stimuli such as sub-atmospheric pressure and hypercapnia. However, during sleep, neuromotor tone decreases and upper airway resistance increases considerably especially in sleep onset and REM stages. These physiologic variations are counteracted by a reduction of diaphragm and intercostal muscles activity and thus a decrease in inspiratory pressure. This tendency for the human upper airway to collapse predisposes it to abnormal deformation during sleep, mainly in susceptible individuals. [1,4, 27]

OSA results from a combination of structural upper airway narrowing and abnormal upper airway neuromotor tone. It is believed that the upper airways collapse more easily in OSA patients and occurs at slightly negative intra-thoracic pressures or even positive pressures. [27] Narrowing can occur in more than one site. The retropalatal or velopharyngeal region is the most common site; but the collapse usually extends to other locations. Since REM sleep is associated with greater muscle hypotonia compared to non-REM sleep, sleep-breathing disorder is more likely to occur during REM sleep. [13] In addition, the sleep-awake state in the pathogenesis of OSA is important to highlight. OSA patients, even with the most severe apnea, have generally no respiratory dysfunction during wakefulness through compensatory systems. [28]

According to recent studies on OSA pathophysiology, anatomical factors are not the whole story. The coordination between collapsing and dilating forces is an important concept and there is increasing evidence that the quantity and pattern of ventilation plays a substantial role in airway collapse [29] as well as the presence of upper airway neuropathology. [28] In addition, not all individuals with OSA have the same anatomical features. Thus, OSA pathophysiological factors are usually divided into three categories, whose complex interplay may explain the variable response to treatment:

1. Anatomic factors that effectively reduce airway caliber;
2. Non-anatomic factors that promote increased upper airway collapsibility and include: mechanical factors that are passive and related to tissues properties; and
3. neurological factors that change with the state of awakening or sleep

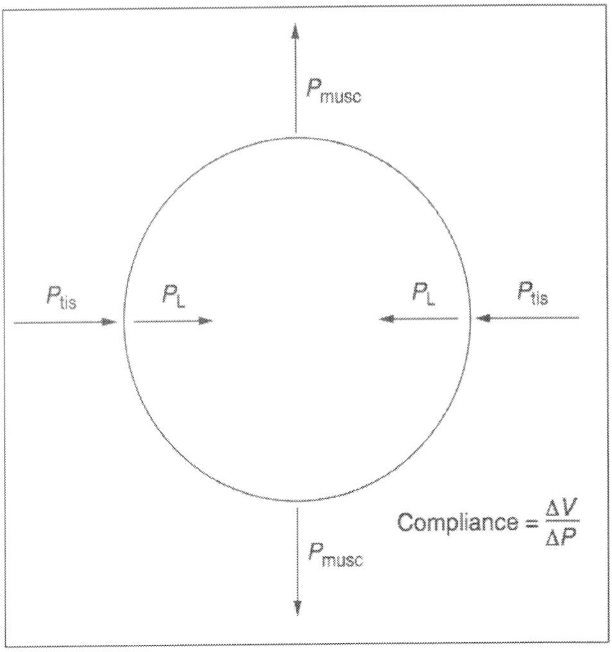

Figure 5. Determinants of upper airway caliber. PL = intraluminal pressure; Ptis = pressure in the tissues surrounding the pharyngeal wall; Pmusc = pressure exerted by the pharyngeal dilating muscles; V = change in volume; P = change in pressure. [1, 26]

3.2. Anatomic factors in OSA

There have been a number of studies comparing anatomic features of OSA patients and normal individuals. Upper airway imaging techniques such as cephalometry, acoustic reflection, nasopharyngoscopy, computed tomography and magnetic resonance imaging, have greatly improved the understanding of OSA biomechanical aspect, and guided treatment modalities.

Over the past several decades, many studies have demonstrated that patients with OSA have significant craniofacial and upper airway abnormalities when compared with age matched and sex matched controls. [17, 30]

Typical abnormalities include retroposition of the mandible and maxilla, shorter mandibular body length, longer anterior facial height, steeper and shorter anterior cranial base.... [1, 4, 13, 17]

However recent studies have shown no strong evidence for a direct causal relationship between sagittal and vertical craniofacial features and sleep-breathing disorder. In contrast, transverse width in the maxilla has a real impact with strong support for a narrow maxilla in OSA patients. [31]-[32] In addition, there is theoretical evidence that the size and the shape of the upper airway are also important and influence upper airway collapsibility.[4, 13] Imaging studies have shown reduced nasopharyngeal and oropharyngeal sagittal dimensions in OSA cases, associated with longer soft palate and longer airway. Indeed, the upper airway long axis of OSA patients is likely to be oriented transversely compared to the wide, elliptically shaped airway of normal controls.[33]-[35]

Lung volume is also reported to influence upper airway caliber and compliance.[13, 29] Decreased lung volume results in a caudal traction effect, which decreases the pharynx area and increases its resistance and its collapsibility due to a loss of tracheal tug.

Nasal airway pressure required to maintain airway patency is defined as the critical closing pressure (P_{crit}). [4] It has been demonstrated that P_{crit} is related to anatomical features and lung volumes, and shown to correlate with soft palate length in obese patients and airway length and hyoid-mandibular distance in non-obese patients [13]

On the other hand, the magnitude of extra luminal tissue pressure depends on the interaction of the upper airway soft tissues and the bony compartment size (Figure 6).[36] According to this model, soft tissues excess like in obesity, or restriction in bony compartment size such as retrognathia or both can lead to tissue pressure increase, thereby reducing airway caliber and predisposing to OSA. Soft tissues excess can be seen in case of tongue, soft palate and pharyngeal wall volume augmentation; but also in adenoids and tonsils lymphoid tissue hypertrophy.

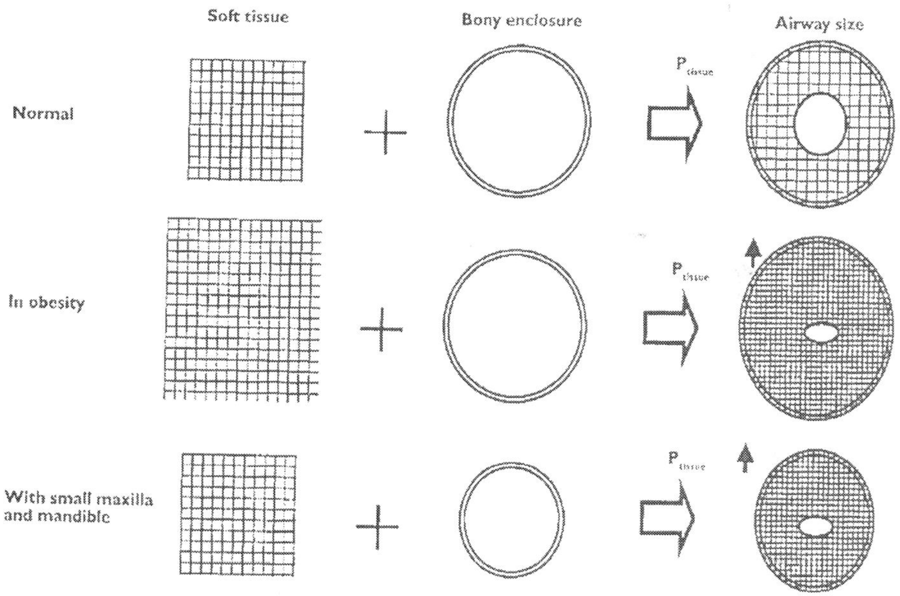

Figure 6. Figure 6: OSA pathophysiology: schematic explanation for anatomic factors interaction to regulate extraluminal tissues pressure (P_{tissue}) [36]

Despite the relationship between structural features and function, some patients with OSA do not have clear anatomic abnormalities. Evidence for a direct causal relationship between craniofacial structure and OSAs has yet to be elucidated because several methodological deficiencies in the literature and lack of research standardization methods and treatment success definitions have been highlighted.

3.3. Non-anatomic factors

This category includes all factors underlying collapsibility. They are divided into pure mechanic and neurologic factors. In OSA patients, airway dilation appears less coordinated than normal subjects and intrinsic mechanical properties of airway tissues are altered (Figure 7). [30, 37]

The respiratory control pattern generator responsible for automatic control ventilation is located into the brainstem. Respiratory rhythm is regulated by chemoreceptors and neural input from the upper airway and lungs to the brainstem neuronal network.[4] Instability of ventilatory control contributes to OSA pathophysiology by leading to periodic breathing and compromising airway patency during the ventilatory cycle. [28] It has also been suggested that upper airway inflammation and trauma caused by snoring and the hypoxia caused by intermittent upper airway collapse may impair the sensory pathways (upper airway mucosa) and the activation of neuromuscular reflexes (pharyngeal dilator muscles) rendering the upper airway prone to collapse. [38]

Other factors that may contribute to OSA pathophysiology include head posture, vascular supply to the mucosa and tissues surrounding the airway and arousal threshold.

Strohl et al. (2012) [39] reported that changes in blood pressure and/or pharyngeal muscles vascularity could affect airway stability and patency. Mucosal blood flow may either help resist distortion or contribute to narrowing if engorged.

On the other hand, flexion and extension of the neck affect the mechanics of the upper airway because the axis of rotation for extension and flexion is behind the airway. Thus, altered sleep position, mainly supine, may increase upper airway collapsibility and predispose to OSA particularly in adults because of tongue base prolapse. [40] In contrast, OSA children breathe better in the supine than in the prone position; this may be true because obstruction in children occurs usually at the level of the adenoids or soft palate rather than at the level of the tongue [1]

Although arousal is known to reinstate ventilation and thus to be protective in OSA, it is not essential to terminate an obstructive event. Low arousal threshold can exacerbate instability and worsen OSA.[1, 41] However, some authors who believe, that poor sleep is a secondary cause of OSA have rejected this claim. [29]

OSA has been shown to aggregate significantly within families. Genetic factors are likely to determine upper airway anatomy, neuromuscular activity and ventilatory control stability; these factors produce the phenotype of the OSA syndrome.[1, 4, 25, 42].

In sum, it is probably reliable to conclude that, in OSA individuals, there is a multiplicity of coexisting factors interacting to varying degrees at night; and everyone has biological sus-

http://dx.doi.org/10.5772/59086

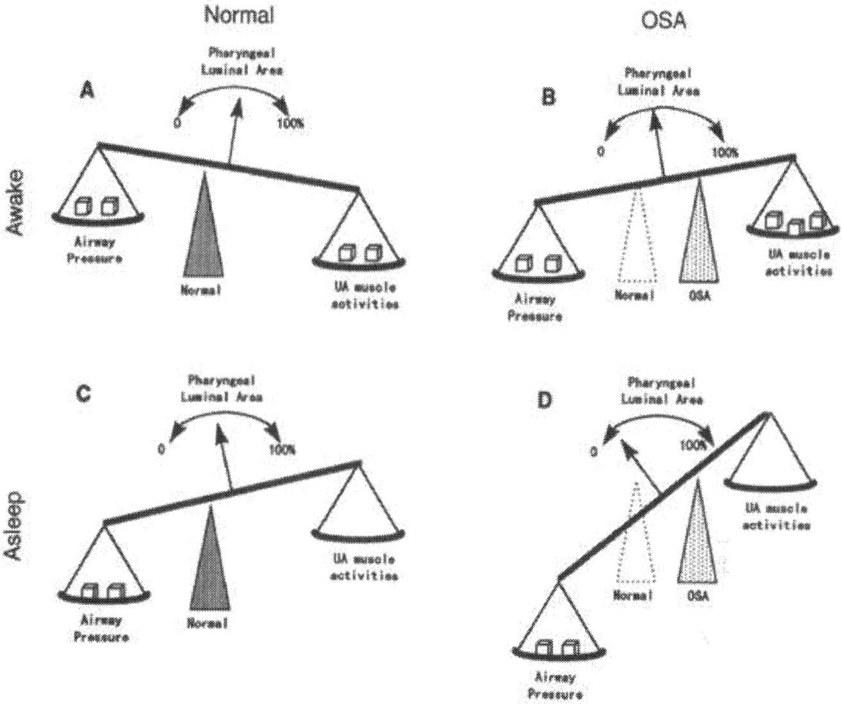

Figure 7. Schematic model proposed by Isono et al., 1997 [30] and explaining pharyngeal airway patency: When a wake, upper airway (UA) muscle activity compensates the depression forces exerted by the air, both in normal subjects (A) and the OSA (B) for which activity is most important. During sleep, activity decrease generates too much imbalance in the apneic and causes collapse (D). In panels B and D (subject with OSAS) the fulcrum that represents intrinsic properties of the pharynx, is to the right of the normal subject (A and C)

ceptibility and responds differently to environmental predisposing factors. Because OSA is a public health problem, its treatment should target the specific pathophysiologic processes that contribute to the collapse of the upper airway, in an attempt to alleviate symptoms and modify the long-term health consequences.

4. OSA diagnosis

4.1. Definitions

Aimed at maximal standardization and better care of patients, a task force of the American Academy of Sleep Medicine (AASM) has recommended terminology and standards of practice for recording sleep and breathing, and assigned evidence-based definitions for abnormal events, parameters and disorders. [43] These definitions are still valid today.

4.1.1. Respiratory events

Apnea is defined as cessation of airflow at the nose and mouth for 10 seconds or more with an arterial oxygen desaturation of 2% to 4%. Apnea is central, obstructive or mixed. The distinction between central and obstructive apnea is essential in determining the most appropriate treatment. During obstructive apnea, patients display respiratory effort without being able to ventilate because of upper airway obstruction, whereas central apnea occurs in the absence of ventilatory effort. Mixed apnea is initially started without ventilatory effort (as a 'central' pattern), and ends as obstructive with resumption of ventilatory efforts.

Hypopnea is defined as a decrease in airflow for 10 seconds or more with a concomitant drop in arterial oxygen saturation. AASM distinguish two situations of hypopnea events:

- A clear decrease (> 50%) from baseline in the amplitude of a valid measure of breathing during sleep;
- Or an amplitude reduction (< 50%) associated with either an oxyhemoglobin desaturation (> 3%) or an arousal. [4]

The exact magnitude of desaturation for a hypopnea varies in the literature. In routine clinical practice, it may not be necessary to differentiate apneas from hypopneas when both have similar pathophysiological consequences.[13] It is recommended to associate these two events in the form of an index of apnea / hypopneas (AHI).

4.1.1.1. Apnea and Hypopnea Indices (AHI)

This index, also termed respiratory disturbance index (RDI), refers to the total number of apnea and hypopnea episodes per hour of sleep. It is calculated by dividing the total number of apneas/hypopneas during a recording period by the total sleep time. AHI is usually employed to quantify OSA severity, but also to compare individual patient data with normative as well as pre-treatment and post-treatment values.

4.1.2. Obstructive sleep apnea syndrome

As noted previously, OSA is characterized by repeated partial or complete collapses of the upper airway during sleep, which precludes or reduces airway flow. It is associated with excessive daytime somnolence, sleep fragmentation and adverse sequelae attributable to frequent obstructive apneas or hypopneas during sleep. According to the AASM, OSA refers to an AHI ≥ 5 associated to one or both of these two criteria:

- Excessive daytime sleepiness (EDS) not explained by other factors
- Manifestation of at least two of following symptoms that should co-exist:
- Daily severe snoring
- Choking or suffocation during sleep
- Fragmented and non-restorative sleep

- Diurnal tiredness
- Concentration difficulties
- Nocturia

However, the presence of 15 or more obstructive respiratory events per hour of sleep in the absence of sleep related symptoms is enough proof for the diagnosis of OSA due to the greater association of this severity of obstruction with important consequences such as increased cardiovascular disease risk.[44] Two indicators must be taken into account for severity estimation of OSA: AHI and the importance of diurnal hyper-somnolence after exclusion of another cause of sleepiness. Patients in normal sleep have an AHI of 5 or less. Patients with mild sleep apnea have an AHI of 5 to 15, with moderate sleep apnea typically 15 to 30 events and severe apnea 30 or more events per hour.

4.2. OSA clinical approach

Despite its high estimated prevalence, awareness of OSA remains insufficient in the community.[4] Health professionals, including orthodontists, should not disregard the risk factors of OSA and should detect and diagnose this disorder. OSA screening should be based on sleep-oriented history and physical examination in conjunction with objective tests. When diagnosed, OSA severity level must be determined for an effective treatment decision.[44]

4.2.1. Physical examination

According to the AASM, sleep history is sought to evaluate OSA symptoms and to determine patients who present high-risk levels. A sleep examination is directed at modifying the OSA probability based on the history, looking for associated or complicating disease, and excluding other potential causes for symptoms.

Clinical assessment must encompass all sleep and physical features of the patient that may provide helpful guidance for screening this condition such as:

4.2.1.1. Excessive Daytime Sleepiness (EDS)

EDS is caused by sleep fragmentation due to frequent arousals at night. It is still a very subjective symptom that overlaps significantly with other factors such as tiredness and lethargy. [4] Epidemiological studies estimate EDS prevalence at 8% to 30% in the general population. [45]Sleepiness may occur during "passive" conditions, such as watching television or, in severe forms, during "active" conditions, such as conversation or driving. Several instruments have been developed to measure EDS. Currently, the most useful instrument is the Epworth Sleepiness Scale.[46] This questionnaire provides sleep propensity measure and has good test–retest reliability. It should be described with regards to onset, situation, and chronicity of sleep problems (Figure 8). [45]Objective laboratory sleep tests, like multiple sleep latency test (MSLT) or maintenance of wakefulness test (MWT) are also used for EDS assessment, but their limits are principally related to their costs and duration.

Epworth Sleepiness Scale

Name: ______________________ Today's date: __________

Your age (Yrs): __________ Your sex (Male = M, Female = F): ______

How likely are you to doze off or fall asleep in the following situations, in contrast to feeling just tired?

This refers to your usual way of life in recent times.

Even if you haven't done some of these things recently try to work out how they would have affected you.

Use the following scale to choose the **most appropriate number** for each situation:

0 = would **never** doze
1 = **slight chance** of dozing
2 = **moderate chance** of dozing
3 = **high chance** of dozing

It is important that you answer each question as best you can.

Situation	**Chance of Dozing (0-3)**
Sitting and reading	___
Watching TV	___
Sitting, inactive in a public place (e.g. a theatre or a meeting)	___
As a passenger in a car for an hour without a break	___
Lying down to rest in the afternoon when circumstances permit	___
Sitting and talking to someone	___
Sitting quietly after a lunch without alcohol	___
In a car, while stopped for a few minutes in the traffic	___

THANK YOU FOR YOUR COOPERATION

Figure 8. Figure 8. 1997 version of Epworth sleepiness scale. [47]. A score > 10 is consistent with EDS, and a score >16 indicates a high level of EDS.

4.2.1.2. *Snoring and witnessed apneas with choking or gasping*

The presence of snoring alone is a poor predictor of OSA. Thus, it must be correlated with other accompanying clinical features. Similarly, snoring absence does not exclude OSA. If severe, snoring can affect social relationship and become one of the main complaints of patients. Talking to the partner and family members can be very helpful; they can often report signs, such as apnea or falling asleep unintentionally (that the patient may be unaware of or deny). Therefore, patients can report awakening during choking episodes. But this is less common among females. OSA can also be associated with array of nocturnal and daytime symptoms that are not necessarily specific to this affection, but can complete its clinical pattern and give an idea about its impact on patients' functionalities. One can cite poor sleep quality, morning headaches, impaired memory, failed concentration, nocturia, and depression....[4]

4.2.1.3. *Obesity*

Obesity is the main predisposing factor for OSA. It is usually quantified by BMI (Body Mass Index). Increased BMI is closely correlated to OSA likelihood and severity. [4, 13] Additionally, central obesity (i.e. fat around the neck and waist), evaluated by neck circumference and hip-to-waist ratio, is simple clinical measurements that seem most predictive for SDB. There is no evidenced threshold value for these measurements, but a BMI ≥ 30 kg/m^2 and a neck circumference >17 inches in men and >16 inches in women are habitually used as critical values.[4] Moreover, a study found that waist-hip ratio is the most reliable correlate of OSA in both sexes; while neck circumference is an independent risk factor for males. [48]To establish OSA diagnosis, obesity indicators alone are not sufficient and further diagnostic testing is needed. [26]

4.2.1.4. *Craniofacial examination*

Clinical examination should include anatomical features of craniofacial and oropharyngeal structures as they can compromise airway patency. Particular attention should be paid to upper airway narrowing signs such as tonsillar hypertrophy especially in children, nasal obstruction, macroglossia with dental impressions at the edge of the tongue, elongated uvula or soft palate inflammation. [44, 45] Oropharyngeal crowding can be assessed using the modified Mallampati classification designed originally by anesthetists to grade intubation difficulty (Figure 9). [49]

Other conditions that should be searched for when examining potential OSA patients are skeletal abnormalities because they are high risk factors among either obese or non-obese individuals. Actually, retrognathia, micrognathia, maxilla deficiency with high arched/narrow hard palate, longer anterior facial height, cranial base abnormalities or inferior hyoid bone position should be evaluated as they may suggest the presence of OSA. Cephalometric radiographs enable health professionals to obtain quantitative measures of these features. [50]

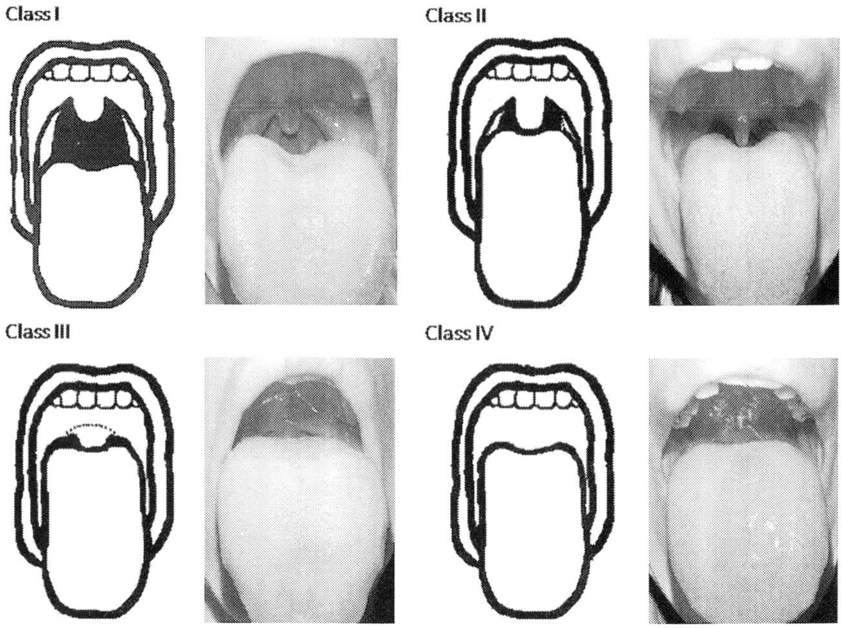

Figure 9. Modified Mallampati classification of oropharyngeal visualization. Class I: Soft palate, tonsils, pillars, and uvula, are clearly visible. Class II: Soft palate, pillars, and uvula are visible. Class III: only part of soft palate and base of uvula are visible. Class IV: Soft palate is not visible at all. 49

4.2.1.5. Associated comorbidities

A clinical examination should not ignore respiratory, cardiovascular, and neurologic systems. In this area, medication history must be taken into account especially with regard to drugs that are associated with OSA (Barbiturates, Benzodiazepines...), those that sedate and/or decrease respiratory drive (Antihistamines, Antispasmodics, Anxiolytics, Muscle relaxants...) and those that impair sleep onset or maintenance (Anticholesterol agents, Appetite suppressants, Benzodiazepines, Caffeine, Nicotine, Diuretics...). Furthermore, since hypertension is described as independently associated with OSA, blood pressure has been integrated into several clinical prediction rules for sleep apnea. [22, 44]

4.2.2. Objective testing

To establish OSA severity, objective testing is required. There are two accepted methods: laboratory polysomnography (PSG) and home testing with portable monitors (PM)

Polysomnography is the golden standard method for diagnosing OSA. It records sleep-breathing pattern and oxygen saturation overnight via a minimum of 12 channels of physiological signal such as electroencephalogram, electrocardiogram, electromyogram, oronasal airflow, electroocculogram, respiratory effort, body position and oxygen saturation. This examination provides AHI by monitoring apnea and hypopnea occurrence. Clinical interpretation of OSA severity is based, in addition to AHI, on factors like oxygen desaturation and sleep fragmentation degrees. In general, a single night PSG is sufficient to make an appropriate OSA diagnosis. However, some variability can be identified in recordings between the first and the second night of a PSG, a phenomenon known as the "first night effect". This may be due to factors such as sleep position and alcohol [44, 51]

Unlike PSG that is expensive and labor intensive, PM is performed at home and thus offers greater convenience for patients. Nonetheless, this procedure has some limits related to the lack of supervision, which can affect its reliability, but also to the impossibility to detect other sleep disorders such central apnea or nocturnal epilepsy. The choice between PSG and PM should take into consideration resource limitations and pre-test clinical evaluation. Thus, PSG could be performed if PM is technically inadequate or fails to establish OSA patients with a high pre-test probability.[44]

Furthermore, numerous imaging modalities are available for 2D or 3D craniofacial and airway study. They have potential usefulness in understanding the pathogenesis of sleep- breathing disorder, and planning of treatment (adenoidectomy, orthognathic surgery), but their routine use in the evaluation and diagnosis of OSA is limited. All diagnosis components previously studied (clinical examination and diagnostic testing) should be discussed with patients to establish a program including risk factors, consequences, but also treatment options/outcomes of OSA in the context of disease severity and patients' expectations.[44]

5. Treatment of OSA syndrome

Therapeutic approach of OSA requires interdisciplinary communication among healthcare professionals and long-term management with a regular follow-up. Patient adherence to therapy, potential side effects and further stability of results must be continually monitored. On the other hand, outcomes assessment should be performed after all therapy has been undertaken. The criteria used to determine successful treatment of OSA varies widely. A task force of AASM have reported some indicators for assessment of treatment results; these include resolution of sleepiness, OSA specific quality of life measures, patient and spousal satisfaction, adherence to therapy, avoidance of factors worsening disease, obtaining an adequate amount of sleep, practicing proper sleep hygiene and weight loss for overweight/obese patients. Objectively, clinicians strive to achieve at least 50% reduction in the baseline AHI in addition to reduction in AHI to <5 events per hour or <10 events per hour. However, less stringent definitions can be adopted. Treatment modalities of OSA can be divided into surgical and non-surgical treatment to which adjunctive therapies can be associated. Less invasive treatment should be selected whenever possible. Also, patients must be advised about surgical success rates and complications, the availability of alternative options and their levels of effectiveness. [52, 53]

5.1. Non-surgical treatments of OSA

This category includes continuous positive airway pressure (CPAP), behavior modifications, and oral appliances.

5.1.1. Continuous positive airway pressure (Figure 10)

First described by Sullivan in 1981, CPAP was to become the golden standard of moderate to severe OSA treatment. [54].It consists of delivering, during sleep, compressed air into the airway to keep it open, by positive pressure across the airway walls and pneumatic splinting effect. CPAP can be applied through oral, nasal or oro-nasal interface; and the optimal level of positive airway pressure is determined by full-night, attended in-laboratory PSG. Successful therapy with CPAP depends greatly on individual patient acceptance and compliance that can fall for numerous reasons including functioning noise, discomfort, feelings of claustrophobia, and skin irritation. Thus, CPAP prescription requires explanation of benefits and medical reasons for its use. Patients should also be informed about the function and maintenance of equipment. According to the American college of Physician (ACP), moderate quality evidence has showed that CPAP improves sleep measurement in patients with at least moderate OSA (AHI > 15events/h), and there are no data to determine which patients benefit most from specific treatment strategies. [55] However, OSA remains at present the preferred treatment for OSA, as it could effectively reduce AHI and arousal index scores, and increase the minimum oxygen saturation. Finally, if CPAP use fails, based on objective monitoring and symptom evaluation, more efforts should be implemented to improve PAP use or consider alternative therapies.

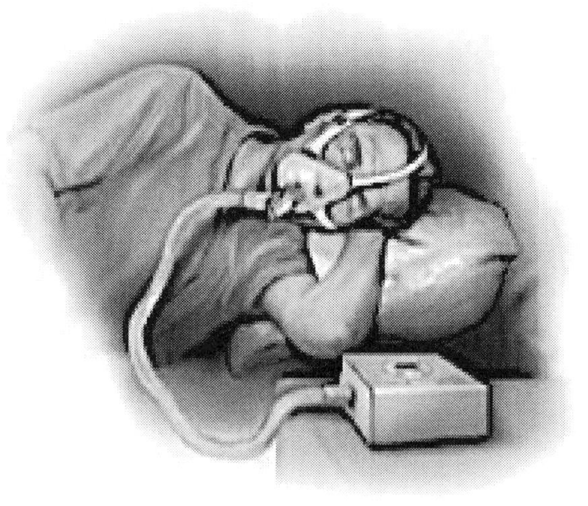

Figure 10. CPAP device requiring the use of mask interface, sealed tubing and flow generator providing airflow. [56]

5.1.2. Behavior modifications or conservative treatments

Behavior strategy includes all practices that enhance life routines and hygiene. It involves weight loss (ideally to a BMI of 25 kg/m2 or less), positional therapy, and avoidance of smoking, alcohol and sedatives 3h before sleep. Weight loss has been shown to improve AHI in obese patients with OSA. It is recommended for all overweight OSA patients and should be combined with a primary treatment for OSA. Sleeping in the supine position can affect airway size and patency with a decrease in the area of the lateral dimension of upper airway. Positional therapy keeps the patient in a non-supine position by positioning device like alarm, pillow, back-pack or tennis ball is an effective secondary therapy or can be a supplement to primary therapies for OSA in patients who have a low AHI in the non-supine position. To ascertain treatment outcomes, indicators, such as self-reported compliance, objective position monitoring, are used. However, studies argue that CPAP is still superior to positional therapy in reducing the severity of sleep apnea and increasing the oxygen saturation level during sleep in patients with positional OSA. [50]-[57]

5.1.3. Oral appliances (figure 11-13)

Pierre Robin was the first orthodontist to have used oral appliances (OAs) in the 1900s for glossoptosis. Since the 80s, these oral devices were used as a non-invasive treatment for OSA. This therapy has proven to be effective in reducing the apnea and hypopnea index, improving oxygen saturation during sleep, and reducing snoring. OAs are recommended as an alternative therapy to CPAP for mild to moderate OSA patients with CPAP adverse effects or for those who do not tolerate or adhere to CPAP or those who refuse surgery. They are also appropriate for patients with primary snoring, who do not respond to treatment with behavioral measures such as weight loss or sleep position change. [44, 50]-[58]

Both Mandibular advancement devices (MADs) and tongue-retaining devices were described (TRD). But MADs are the most commonly used and evaluated in the literature. Orthodontists must indicate the most appropriate design of MADs for each patient, depending on dental history and complete examination of the stomatognathic system (soft tissues, dental occlusion, masticatory muscles and the temporomandibular joint). MADs cover the upper and lower teeth and hold the mandible in an advanced position with respect to the resting position. The appliance is constructed, adjusted, and gradually titrated (advanced forward) over several weeks until the snoring and daytime sleepiness are reduced to an acceptable level, or the patient cannot tolerate further advancement. They are worn during sleep and they act by enlarging obstructed upper airway by moving the mandible and tongue anteriorly and then the activation of airway dilator muscles. Craniofacial changes induced by OA were evaluated using cephalometric analysis. Significant modifications were reported: Retroclination of the maxillary incisors, proclination of the mandibular incisors, increased lower facial height, and changes in molar relationship. Loss of edema, caused by snoring and repetitive apneas, associating OAs seems to result in palatal length decrease and pharyngeal area increase. OAs have some side effects: Dry mouth, excessive salivation, jaw discomfort, myofacial pain and tooth grinding. However, they are frequently reported as mild, acceptable, and transient.

Another inconvenience of OAs is the time needed for titration, which makes it a second choice for severe or high symptomatic OSA treatment. [58]

The Academy of Dental Sleep Medicine suggested the use of cephalograms as a diagnostic aid at the initial dental examination of every patient receiving OA treatment. In addition, some cephalometric predictors like longer maxilla, shorter soft palate and decreased distance between mandibular plane and hyoid bone have been related to successful MAD treatment of OSA. [4]

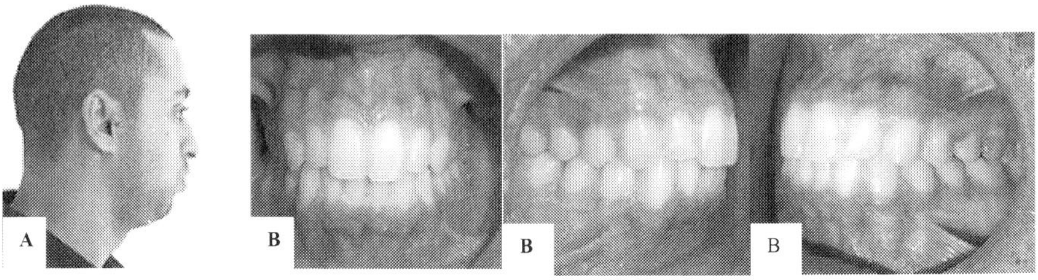

Figure 11. A 27-year-old man with mild OSA: initial profile view (A), and initial occlusal views (B). We can note a severe retrognathia compensated with a class I dental occlusion.

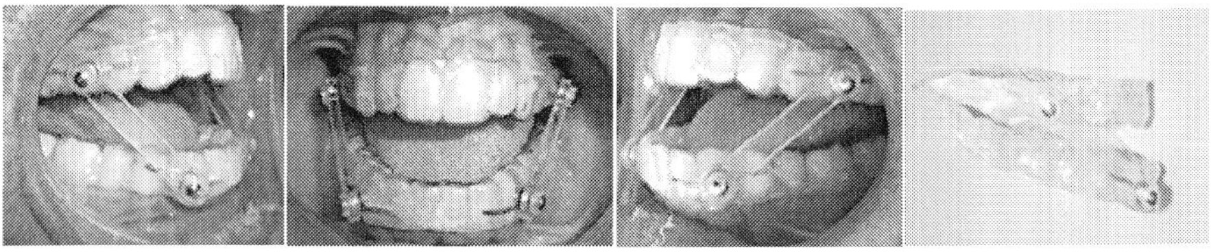

Figure 12. A MAD device was indicated for night.

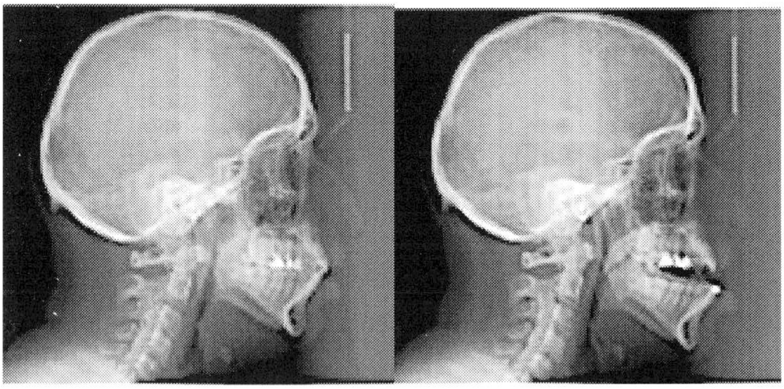

Figure 13. Lateral Cephalograms before (left) and after (right) oral appliance positioning showing change in hyoid bone position and slight enlargement of retroglossal area of pharynx

5.2. Surgical treatments of OSA

Surgical management was the first therapeutic modality employed to treat SDB by placement of a tracheotomy tube to bypass upper airway obstruction in Pickwickian patients. Currently, there are numerous surgical approaches to upper airway treatment in OSA, which consist of upper airway tissue reduction or reconstruction at different levels. OSA surgical management often involves several procedures that can be at times multi-phased or a combination of multi-level simultaneous surgeries. The selection of the most adequate surgery entails a meticulous preoperative multidisciplinary assessment and rests on the surgeon's experience. [59]

OSA surgery should be determined after clinical diagnosis and severity assessment by objective testing. It is recommended for patients who are medically and psychologically able to tolerate the operation ; primary surgery is advocated in mild OSA and severe obstructing anatomy feasible to treat surgically such as tonsillar hypertrophy and nasal obstruction; surgery is recommended secondarily in cases of ineffective treatment or intolerance to the other non-invasive therapies in mild, moderate and severe OSA. Surgical treatment involves evaluation of three anatomic sections of the airway for detection of collapse-related abnormalities namely:

1. the nose (alar cartilage deformities, septal deviations, enlarged turbinates, nasal floor constriction),
2. the retropalatal area (lymphoid hyperplasia, retrusive maxilla, long palate) and
3. the retroglossal area and the tongue (mandibular retrognathia).

Thus, surgical procedures can be classified as intra-pharyngeal or skeletal. Intra-pharyngeal surgery includes all procedures directed towards soft tissues of upper airway, the most common being uvulopalatopharyngoplasty (UPPP). Hard tissues surgery includes maxillo-mandibular advancement (MMA) (Figures 14-16) and genioglossus advancement (GGA) (Figure 17)

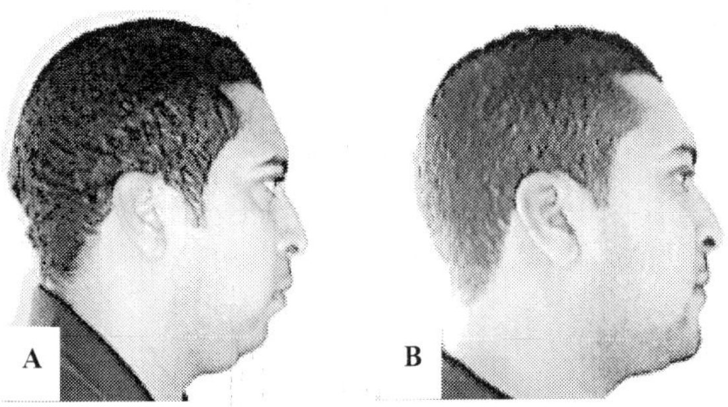

Figure 14. Profile views of a 34-year-old man with severe OSA. A: before treatment, B: after OSA management including orthognathic surgery (mandibular advancement osteotomy)

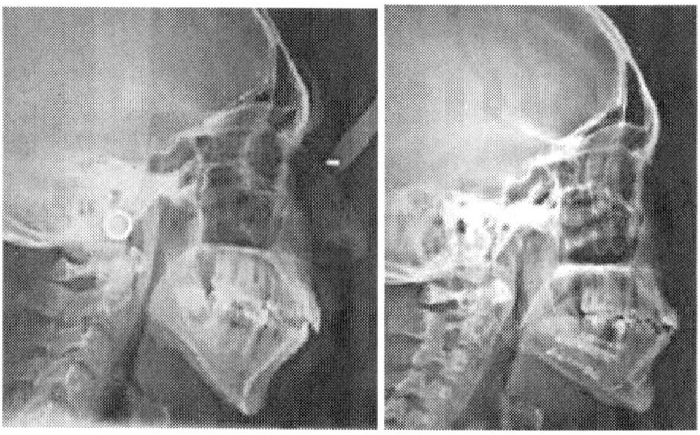

Figure 15. lateral cephalograms showing posterior airway space enlargement Before treatment (left) and after surgical mandibular advancement (right)

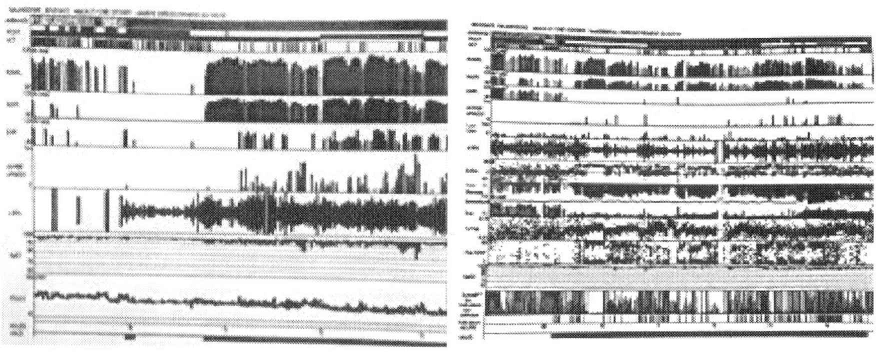

Figure 16. PSG registration: before treatment (left) and after mandibular advancement and adenoidectomy (right).

5.2.1. Sleep parameters evaluation for this clinical case

Before treatment: total number of obstructive apnea events: 51, number of total hypopnea events: 30, AHI: 30/h, desaturation index: 27/h. BMI: 24 Kg/m^2 (Severe OSA).

After treatment: total number of obstructive apnea events: 22, total number of hypopnea events: 108, AHI: 22, desaturation index: 2/h, BMI: 25 Kg/m^2. Moderate OSA.

Powell et al. have created a two-phase directed protocol (Powell-Riley surgical protocol) for surgical treatment of upper airway obstruction at several levels in order to avoid unnecessary surgery. Phase I surgery is designed essentially to treat the upper airway soft tissue (nose, palate, and tongue base) without dental occlusion or facial skeleton modifications. Clinical response is assessed, after adequate healing, four to six months following surgery by PSG. Persistent OSA requires phase II surgery indications. Phase II surgery refers to maxilla-

http://dx.doi.org/10.5772/59086

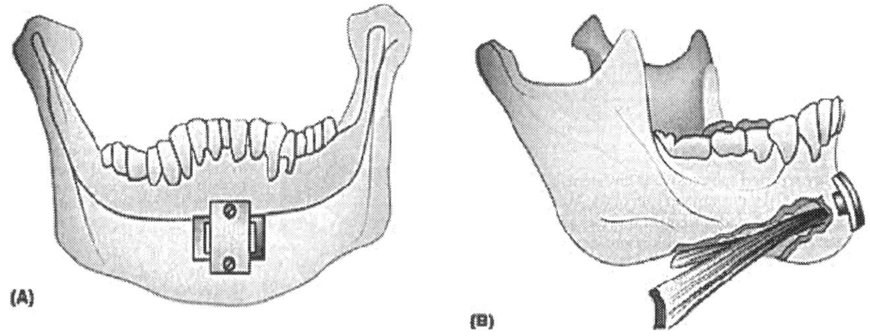

Figure 17. Genioglossus advancement technique. (A): rectangular osteotomy is created in the anterior mandible. (B) : The genial tubercle and the attached genioglossus muscle are advanced anteriorly. The bony fragment is rotated 90° to overlap the inferior border of the mandible and secured to the mandible with a titanium screw. [59]

mandibular advancement osteotomy, which physically creates more space for the tongue, thus enlarging the posterior airway space. [59]

UPPP has been developed to alleviate isolated obstructing tissues of the soft palate, lateral pharyngeal walls, and tonsils. However, according to ACP, it does not reliably normalize AHI when treating moderate to severe OSA, as a sole procedure. Furthermore, with regards to MMA, there is a need for more understanding of the relative risks and benefits of MMA compared to other treatment modalities. CPAP or OAs should generally be suggested ahead of MMA if the patient is consenting. These recommendations do not corroborate with other findings having reported a success rate of 89% obtained by physically expanding the facial skeletal framework and increasing tissue tension, which decreases velopharyngeal and suprahyoid musculature collapsibility. [53, 61]

Complications of maxilla-mandibular advancement surgery have been reported, including side effects such as neurosensory deficit, infection, bleeding, or temporomandibular joint problems; but patients' satisfaction is reported to be as high as 95%. Finally, long-term stability depends on the body mass index, the amount of skeletal advancement, and the skill and experience of the surgeon.[60, 61]

The palatal implant is a new treatment option for snoring that emerged in 2003. It is composed of polyethylene terephthalate, a biocompatible material, and inserted into the soft palate to reduce vibration and collapsibility by stiffening the soft palate, thus reducing palatal flutter and snoring. Additional stiffening of the palate is achieved by fibrosis and formation of capsule in response to the inflammatory reaction. Studies have showed that they may be effective in some patients with mild obstructive sleep apnea, who cannot tolerate or do not adhere to positive airway pressure therapy, or in whom oral appliances have been considered and found to be ineffective or undesirable. However, at the present time, it is difficult to predict if it will be a reliably effective intervention or not. [55, 59, 62]

5.3. Adjunctive treatment

5.3.1. Pharmacological therapy

A wide range of medication targeting OSA treatment has been explored in the literature. Except for hypothyroidism or acromegaly in which medication can improve AHI, there are no really effective pharmacotherapies for OSA. Topical nasal corticosteroids can be used in patients with OSA and concomitant rhinitis especially in children, and thus may be a useful adjunct to primary therapies for OSA. In addition, Modafinil, a psychostimulant, is recommended for the treatment of residual excessive daytime sleepiness despite effective PAP treatment and absence of other evident causes for their sleepiness. [44, 63]

A Cochrane review issued in 2013 showed insufficient evidence to recommend any systemic pharmacological treatment for OSA; drug therapy needs to be targeted depending on the presence or absence of obesity and the predominance of OSA in a particular sleep stage. The review also reported that among all drugs evaluated, Donepezil is the most promising for further research. [64]

5.3.2. Bariatric surgery

Bariatric surgery consists of a variety of operative techniques performed to promote weight reduction such reducing gastric banding, gastric and jujenoileal bypass or gastroplasty. It is often recommended for treatment of morbid obesity, particularly when associated with other medical complications (BMI ≥ 35 kg/m2) or those with a BMI ≥ 35 kg/m2 when dietary efforts fail at weight control. Therefore women seem likely to be candidates for this method of weight loss. [44, 65]

6. Obstructive sleep apnea syndrome in orthodontic practice

As cited above, OSA is associated with numerous craniofacial abnormalities. Orthodontics improvement of dento-facial morphology may have a positive impact on OSA components. Orthodontic professionals should provide treatment for OSA patients as well as diagnose potential OSA patients. Medical history and clinical examination allows orthodontists to identify the risk factors of OSA or signs related to OSA (obesity, allergy, nasal dysfunction, maxillary constriction, retrognathia, long uvula, mouth breathing...) or record some symptoms reported by patients. Moreover, several imaging modalities (lateral and frontal cephalogram, cone beam computed tomography, MRI.) can assist Orthodontic professionals in assessment of this condition.

Orthodontic management of OSA syndrome could be provided to children as a preventive and interceptive modal or to adults by an interdisciplinary management. A significant number of children suffering from respiratory problems and obstructive sleep apnea have nasal obstruction associated with a narrow maxilla that may increase nasal resistance and alter the tongue posture, leading to a narrowing of the retroglossal airway and OSA. Maxillary expansion with orthopedic appliances is very effective in these cases allowing for an increase of nasal cavity dimension. It can be combined with adenotonsillectomy for best results in children with OSA associated with adenotonsillar hypertrophy. [4, 66, 67] Among adults, this expansion can be attained by RME or surgically assisted RME and has been reported to reduce snoring and hyper-somnolence.

Maxillomandibular advancement can also be provided either by surgery or orthopedic systems as therapeutic or preventive measure in OSA cases. A good finishing of dental occlusion is desirable. On the other hand, It has been suggested [68] that the improvement observed in the respiratory symptoms with surgical MMA, namely apnea/hypopnea episodes, should be correlated with SNA increase after surgery which may help maxillofacial surgeons establish selective criteria for the surgical approach to sleep apnea syndrome patients. Mandibular advancement in case of retrognathia can be accomplished by oral appliances in adulthood, functional appliance therapy in younger patients, mandibular distraction osteogenesis or osteotomies, and is among the most frequently used approaches in OSA management.

Orthodontists can also have a role in the treatment of OSA consequences especially those with nocturnal bruxism, which differs from stress-related bruxism. Sleep bruxism has been shown to be prevalent in children, and correlated with sleep disturbances (microarousals). It is characterized by rhythmic masticatory muscle activity and may be related to the patients' attempt to improve airway patency during episodes of oxygen desaturation via co-activation of jaw opening and closing muscles. Its management requires use of night splints and restorative dentistry.

In brief, although the bi-directional cause and effect relationship between OSA and craniofacial abnormalities remains to be proven, early identification and treatment of dentofacial disorders may enhance OSA management with respect to preventive and curative approaches. Interdisciplinary professional communication is crucial for the success of global OSA management.

7. Conclusion

OSA is a common breathing disorder, which affects all age groups. It is a serious public health problem. Because of its potential pathophysiological consequences, it associates alteration of quality of life, decreased economic potential and increased morbidity and mortality in affected patients. Assessment of OSA requires a thorough clinical examination as well as overnight testing to determine PSA presence and severity before initiating treatment. Polysomnography remains the most common and reliable test for OSA diagnosis. Additionally, several imaging modalities can be used for upper airway structure and function during wakefulness and sleep. Treatment modalities of OSA are aimed at increasing life expectancy, decreasing disease problems and improving the quality of life. CPAP is still the mainstay for treatment of moderate to severe OSA. However, medical or surgical alternatives can be used in case of failure or non-compliance of the patients.

OSA is also a condition that orthodontists may encounter in their daily practice; thus, they are in a better position to diagnose and treat it using a multidisciplinary approach and management.

Author details

Hakima Aghoutan[1*], Sana Alami[1], Samir Diouny[2] and Farid Bourzgui[1]

*Address all correspondence to: hakimadental@yahoo.fr

1 Department of Dento-facial Orthopedics, Faculty of Dental Medicine. Hassan II Ain Chok University. Casablanca, Morocco

2 Chouaib Doukkali University, Faculty of Letters and Human Sciences, El Jadida, Morocco

References

[1] Kushida CA. Obstructive sleep apnea: Pathophysiology, comorbidities, and consequences. Informa Healthcare USA, Inc. 2007

[2] Bickelmann AG, Burwell CS, Robin ED, Whaley RD. Extreme obesity associated with alveolar hypoventilation- a Pickwickian syndrome. Am J Med 1956; 21(5): 811-18.

[3] Guilleminault C, Dement WC. 235 cases of excessive daytime sleepiness. Diagnosis and tentative classification. J Neurol Sci 1977; 31(1): 13-27.

[4] Lavigne GJ, Cistulli PA, Smitn MT. Sleep medicine for dentists. A practical overview. Quitessence Publishing Co, Inc 2009

[5] International classification of sleep disorders. 3rd ed, American academy of sleep medicine, Darien IL 2014

[6] American Academy of Sleep Medicine Task Force. Sleep-related breathing disorders in adults: recommendations for syndrome definition and measurement techniques in clinical research. Sleep 1999; 22:667-89.

[7] Giannasi LC, Magini M, Costa MS and al. Oral appliance treatment for obstructive sleep apnea in a partly edentulous patient. Am J Orthod Dentofacial Orthop 2010; 137: 548-51

[8] Mason M, Welsh EJ, Smith I. Drug therapy for obstructive sleep apnoea in adults. Cochrane Database of Systematic Reviews 2013, Issue 5. Art. No.: CD003002. DOI: 10.1002/14651858.CD003002.pub3.

[9] Peppard PE, Young T, Barnet JH et al. Increased Prevalence of Sleep-Disordered Breathing in Adults. Am J Epidemiol. 2013; 177(9): 1006-14

[10] Laraqui O, Laraqui S, Manar N, et al. Screening and prevalence of obstructive sleep apnea syndrome among health professionals in Morocco. Archives des maladies professionnelles et de l'environnement. 2013; 74(2): 178-85

[11] De BackerW. Obstructive sleep apnea/hypopnea syndrome. Panminerva Med. 2013; 55(2): 191-5.

[12] Lurie A. Obstructive sleep apnea in adults: epidemiology, clinical presentation, and treatment options. Adv Cardiol. 2011; 46:1-42.

[13] Johnson JT, Gluckman JL, Sanders MM. Management of Obstructive Sleep Apnea. Martin Dunitz Ltd, 2002

[14] Ip MS, Lam B, Lauder IJ, et al. A community study of sleep-disordered breathing in middle-aged Chinese men in Hong Kong. Chest 2001; 119(1): 62–69.

[15] Scharf SM, Seiden L, DeMore J, et al. Racial differences in clinical presentation of patients with sleep-disordered breathing. Sleep & breathing = Schlaf & Atmung 2004; 8(4): 173–183.

[16] Lam B, Ip MS, Tench E, et al. Craniofacial profile in Asian and white subjects with obstructive sleep apnoea. Thorax 2005; 60(6): 504–510.

[17] Liu Y, Lowe AA, Zeng X et al. Cephalometric comparisons between Chinese and Caucasian patients with obstructive sleep apnea. Am J Orthod Dentofacial Orthop 2000; 117: 479-85

[18] Wong ML, Sandham A, Ang PK, et al. Craniofacial morphology, head posture, and nasal respiratory resistance in obstructive sleep apnoea: an inter-ethnic comparison. Eur J Orthod 2005; 27(1): 91–97.

[19] Basner RC. Cardiovascular Morbidity and Obstructive Sleep Apnea. N Engl J Med 2014; 370(24): 2339-41.

[20] Young T, Finn L, Peppard PE, Szklo-Coxe M, et al. Sleep Disordered Breathing and Mortality: Eighteen-Year Follow-up of the Wisconsin Sleep Cohort. Sleep 2008; 31(8): 1071-78.

[21] Gagnon K, Baril AA, Gagnon JF, et al. Cognitive impairment in obstructive sleep apnea. Pathol Biol (Paris) (2014), http:// dx.doi.org/10.1016/j.patbio.2014.05.015

[22] Dauvilliers Y, Arnulf I, d'Ortho MP et al. Which pretherapeutic evaluation of a newly diagnosed patient with obstructive sleep apnea syndrome? Rev Mal Respir 2010; 27 (Suppl 3): S124-36

[23] Sampaio R, Pereira MG, Winck JC. Psychological morbidity, illness representations, and quality of life in female and male patients with obstructive sleep apnea syndrome. Psychol Health Med. 2012; 17(2): 136-49

[24] Gozal D, Kheirandish-Gozal L. Cardiovascular Morbidity in Obstructive Sleep Apnea: Oxidative Stress, Inflammation, and Much More. Am J Respir Crit Care Med 2008; 177:369-375.

[25] Martins AB, Tufik S, Moura SM. Physiopathology of obstructive sleep apnea-hypopnea syndrome. J Bras Pneumol. 2007; 33(1): 93-100.

[26] Koenig SM, Suratt P. Obstructive sleep apnea: the syndrome. In Johnson JT. (ed.) Management of Obstructive Sleep Apnea. Martin Dunitz Ltd, 2002. p 3-20.

[27] Ayappa I, Rapoport DM. The upper airway in sleep: physiology of the pharynx. Sleep Med Ver. 2003; 7(1): 9-33.

[28] Fogel RB, Malhotra A, White DP. Sleep - 2: Pathophysiology of obstructive sleep apnoea/hypopnoea syndrome. Thorax 2004; 59: 159-63.

[29] Susarla SM, Thomas RJ, Abramson ZR et al.: Biomechanics of the upper airway: Changing concepts in the pathogenesis of obstructive sleep apnea. Int. J. Oral Maxillofac. Surg. 2010; 39: 1149–1159.

[30] Isono S, Remmers JE, Tanaka A, et al. Anatomy of pharynx in patients with obstructive sleep apnea and in normal subjects. J Appl Physiol 1997; 82(4): 1319-26.

[31] Katyal V, Pamula Y, Martin AJ, et al. Craniofacial and upper airway morphology in pediatric sleep-disordered breathing: systematic review and meta-analysis. Am J Orthod Dentofacial Orthop 2013; 143: 20-30.

[32] Katyal V, Pamula Y, Daynes CN et al. Craniofacial and upper airway morphology in pediatric sleep-disordered breathing and changes in quality of life with rapid maxillary expansion. Am J Orthod Dentofacial Orthop 2013; 144: 860-71

[33] Patel NP, Schwab RJ. Upper Airway Imaging. In Kushida CA. (ed.) Obstructive sleep apnea: diagnosis and treatment. Informa Healthcare USA, Inc. 2007. P61-88

[34] Leiter JC. Upper airway shape: is it important in the pathogenesis of obstructive sleep apnea? Am J Respir Crit Care Med 1996; 153: 894–8.

[35] Abramson Z, Susarla S, August M, et al. Three-dimensional computed tomographic analysis of airway anatomy in patients with obstructive sleep apnea. J Oral Maxillofac Surg 2010; 68: 354–362.

[36] Watanabe T, Isono S, Tanaka A et al. Contribution of body habitus and craniofacial characteristics to segmental closing pressures of the passive pharynx in patients with Sleep-disordered breathing. Am J Respir Crit Care Med 2002; 165 (2): 260–5.

[37] Bilston LE, Gandevia SC. Biomechanical properties of the human upper airway and their effect on its behavior during breathing and in obstructive sleep apnea. J Appl Phyiol 2014; 116: 314-24

[38] Tsai YJ, Ramar K, Liang YJ. Peripheral neuropathology of the upper airway in obstructive sleep apnea syndrome. Sleep Med Rev 2013; 17: 161-8

[39] Strohl KP, Butler JP, Malhotra A. Mechanical properties of the upper airway. Compr Physiol 2012 Jul; 2(3):1853-72

[40] Joostenab SA, O'Driscolla DM, Bergerb PJ. Supine position related obstructive sleep apnea in adults: Pathogenesis and treatment. Sleep Medicine Reviews 2014; 18: 7-17

[41] Younes M. Role of arousals in the pathogenesis of obstructive sleep apnea. Am J Respir Crit Care Med. 2004; 169(5): 623–33.

[42] Redline S, Tishler PV. The genetics of sleep apnea. Sleep Med Rev. 2000; 4(6): 583-602.

[43] Sleep-related breathing disorders in adults: recommendations for syndrome definition and measurement techniques in clinical research. The Report of an American Academy of Sleep Medicine Task Force. Sleep 1999; 22 (5): 667-89.

[44] Epstein LJ, Kristo D, Strollo PJ et al. Clinical Guideline for the Evaluation, Management and Long-term Care of Obstructive Sleep Apnea in Adults. Adult Obstructive Sleep Apnea Task Force of the American Academy of Sleep Medicine. J Clin Sleep Med 2009; 5(3): 263-76

[45] Ramsey R, Khanna A, Strohl K P. History and Physical Examination. In Kushida CA. (ed.) Obstructive sleep apnea: diagnosis and treatment. Informa Healthcare USA, Inc. 2007 p1-20

[46] Johns WW.A new method for measuring daytime sleepiness: the Epworth sleepiness scale. Sleep1999; 14(6):540-5

[47] The Epworth Sleepiness Scale The Official website of the Epworth Sleepiness Scale by Dr Murray Johns. http://epworthsleepinessscale.com/1997-version-ess/ (Accessed 16 August 2014)

[48] Lim YH, Choi J, Kim KR, et al. Sex-Specific Characteristics of Anthropometry in Patients With Obstructive Sleep Apnea: Neck Circumference and Waist-Hip Ratio. Ann Otol Rhinol Laryngol. 2014; 123(7): 517-23.

[49] Huang HH, Lee MS, ShihYL et al. Modified mallampati classification as a clinical predictor of peroral esophagogastroduodenoscopy tolerance. BMC Gastroenterol. 2011; 11: 12. doi: 10.1186/1471-230X-11-12.

[50] Prabhat KC, Goyal L, Bey A e al. Recent advances in the management of obstructive sleep apnea; the dental perspective. J Nat Sci Biol Med. 2012; 3(2): 113-18

[51] Yaggi HK, Strohl KP. Adult obstructive sleep apnea/hypopnea syndrome: definitions, risk factors, and pathogenesis. Clin Chest Med 2010; 31: 179-86.

[52] Fukuda T, Tsuiki S, Kobayashi M. Selection of response criteria affects the success rate of oral appliance treatment for obstructive sleep apnea. Sleep Med 2014; 15 (3): 367-70

[53] Aurora RN, Casey KR, Kristo D, et al. Practice Parameters for the Surgical Modifications of the Upper Airway for Obstructive Sleep Apnea in Adults. Sleep 2010; 33 (10): 1408-13

[54] Sullivan CE, Issa FG, Berthon-Jones M, et al. Reversal of obstructive sleep apnoea by continuous positive airway pressure applied through the nares. Lancet 1981; 1: 862-5.

[55] Qaseem A, Holty JEC, Owens DK, et al. Management of obstructive sleep apnea in adults: A clinical practice guideline from the American College of physicians. Ann Intern Med. 2013; 159 (7): 471-83

[56] Nucleus Medical Media. Sleep Apnea. Nucleus Catalog. April 3 2009 10:20 EDT. Available at: http://www.nucleuscatalog.com/sleep-apnea/view-item?ItemID=11086. Accessed 19 Aug 2014.

[57] Ha SN, Hirai HW, Tsoi KF. Comparison of positional therapy versus continuous positive airway pressure in patients with positional obstructive sleep apnea: A meta-analysis of randomized trials. Sleep Med Rev 2014; 18:19-24

[58] De Almeida FR, Lowe AA, Sung JO, et al. Long-term sequellae of oral appliance therapy in obstructive sleep apnea patients: Part 1. Cephalometric analysis. Am J Orthod Dentofacial Orthop 2006; 129: 195-204

[59] Sesso DM, Powell NB, Riley RW et al. Upper Airway Surgery in the Adult. In Kushida CA. (ed.) Obstructive sleep apnea: diagnosis and treatment. Informa Healthcare USA, Inc. 2007 p191-215

[60] Jacobson RL, Schendel SA. Treating obstructive sleep apnea: The case for surgery. Am J Orthod Dentofacial Orthop 2012; 142: 434-42

[61] Li KK. Maxillomandibular advancement for obstructive sleep apnea. J Oral Maxillofac Surg 2011; 69 (3): 687-94.

[62] Lee LA, Yu JF, Lo YL, Chen NH, et al. Comparative Effects of Snoring Sound between Two Minimally Invasive Surgeries in the Treatment of Snoring: A Randomized Controlled Trial. PLoS One. 2014; 9(5): e97186. doi: 10.1371/journal.pone.0097186.

[63] Tan HL, Gozal D, Kheirandish-Gozal L. Obstructive sleep apnea in children: a critical update. Nat Sci sleep 2013; 5: 109-23.

[64] Mason M, Welsh EJ, Smith I. Drug therapy for obstructive sleep apnoea in adults. Cochrane Database of Systematic Reviews 2013, Issue 5. Art. No.: CD003002. DOI: 10.1002/14651858.CD003002.pub3.

[65] Krishnan V, Collop NA. Gender Differences in Obstructive Sleep Apnea. In Kushida CA. (ed.) Obstructive sleep apnea: diagnosis and treatment. Informa Healthcare USA, Inc. 2007 p: 247-60

[66] Pirelli P, Saponara M, De Rosa C et al. Orthodontics and Obstructive Sleep Apnea in Children. Medical Clinics of North America 2010; 94 (3): 517-29et al

[67] Villa M, Rizzoli A, Miano S, Malagola C. Efficacy of rapid maxillary expansion in children with obstructive sleep apnea syndrome: 36 months of follow-up. Sleep Breath 2011; 15: 179-84.

[68] Ronchi P, Cinquini V, Ambrosoli A, et al. Maxillomandibular Advancement in Obstructive Sleep Apnea Syndrome Patients: a Restrospective Study on the Sagittal Cephalometric Variables. Oral Maxillofac Res 2013; (4): 2. doi: 10.5037/jomr.2013.4205

Chapter 18

Telegnathic Surgery for Obstructive Sleep Apnea

Dina Ameen

Additional information is available at the end of the chapter

http://dx.doi.org/10.5772/59276

1. Introduction

Obstructive sleep apnea (OSA) is a repetitive partial or complete upper airway collapse during sleep. It is defined as reparative episodes of hypopnea or apnea for at least 10 seconds in association with more than 2 % decrease in oxygen hemoglobin saturation. OSA along with snoring and upper airway resistant syndrome fall into a broad category of sleep related breathing disorder (SBD). The incidence of OSA is up to 9% of women and 24% of men aged 30–60y. Adverse consequences of OSA include: excessive daytime sleepiness (EDS), hypertension, ischemic heart disease, metabolic syndrome, stroke and death. There are many modalities for OSA treatment; conservative approach includes weight reduction, positioning devices, continuous airway pressure (CPAP), and oral appliances. Due to a large percentage of noncompliance with the conservative approach, surgical treatment is a valid option of OSA treatment.

Surgical options are tracheostomy, uvulopalatopharyngoplasty, palatal pillars, radiofrequency ablation of soft palate or tongue, anterior mandibular osteotomy, hypoid suspension, tongue reduction, tongue suspension and telegnathic surgery (maxillomandibular advancement). This chapter provides an overview in OSA surgical treatment.

2. Sleep stages

During normal sleep, the stages are:

1st stage is non-rapid eye movement (non-REM), lasting 70-90 minutes. The non-REM is the quiet sleep, which is consists of 4 stages.45-50% of total sleep is stage 2. Delta sleep is stages 3 and 4, which are a deeper sleep marked by the increasing appearance of high-amplitude slow waves. There is generalized slowness in all activities in non-REM sleep stage.

2nd **stage** rapid eye movement (REM) stage will follow for 20 minutes. REM stage represents the deep sleep stage; it follows the non-REM stage with 20-25% of total sleep. During average night REM to non-REM ratio is 4:6 with intervals 60-90 minutes. Physiologic changes during REM are generalized muscle atonia except for ocular muscles, increase temperature, blood flow and oxygen use in the brain as well as increase in heart rate, blood pressure and respiration with dramatic fluctuations. Respiration is controlled by 2-control systems; metabolic and behavioral. Non-REM is predominantly controlled by the metabolic control system, which is influenced by hypoxia and hypercapnia. On the other hand during the REM sleep, behavioral control system is predominant. OSA usually occurs during stage 3, 4 and REM, which are the deep sleep stages, and that is because of blunt responses to hypoxia and hypercapnia along with the generalized muscle atonia; pharyngeal wall muscles may collapse [1] [2].

3. Anatomy

Upper airway obstructions can occur anywhere in the nasopharynx, oropharynx and hypopharynx. Nasopharyngeal obstruction examples are nasal septum deviation, nasal polyps and rhinosinusitis; they can cause mild OSA [3]. Most common sites of airway collapse occur in the hypopharynx [4]. It extends from the soft palate to the epiglottis; anteriorly it is formed by the base of the tongue and soft palate, while pharyngeal constrictor muscles form the posterior borders. Studies show that tongue volume and lateral walls of the pharynx are independent risks to OSA. There are many craniofacial abnormalities that cause OSA. Even a minimal change in maxillary or mandibular position can lead to upper airway collapse. OSA patients could have one or more of the following anatomical variations:

A retro-position of the mandible or the maxilla, micrognathia, long soft palate, increased thickness of the soft palate, macroglossia (large tongue) and differences in hyoid bone position [5].

The success of surgical treatment is depending on the recognition of the level of obstruction. There is a special surgical procedure for each site of obstruction.

4. Diagnosis

Many diagnostic tools can be used, yet physical examination is very important. A through physical examination of the nose, oral cavity, pharynx and neck should be done. Endoscopy gives clinicians visual assessment to the upper airway and may show possible sites of collapse. Endoscopic Mullar maneuver is a useful procedure for OSA[6].The best results obtained by instructing the patient to lie down in supine position then inspire maximally then with closed nose and mouth, while placing the endoscope at the level of supraglottis, the examiner will be able to visualize the degree of pharyngeal collapse. Increase in negative pressure in the pharynx will demonstrate the point of collapse. Standardized performance and documentation is advocated to prevent any inter-investigator variability [7]. There are many classifications

http://dx.doi.org/10.5772/59276

for upper airway obstruction; Fujita's classification system described patterns of upper airway obstruction in OSA patients in 1985. Fujita classified airway obstruction into 3 types namely:

Type 1. Isolated palatal obstruction,

Type 2. Isolated retrolingual obstruction, and

Type 3. Palatal and retrolingual obstruction

Recently other modifications to Fujita classification were advocated by adding more details for the base of the tongue [8].

Polysomnography (PSG) is still the golden standard to establish OSA diagnosis. It can be used as a diagnostic tool as well as to assess therapeutic efficacy of a given treatment modality including weight loss, CPAP, oral appliances and MMA. It is usually done in a sleep clinic, as the patient should sleep at least for 4 hours, and the electroencephalogram (EEG), electrooculogram (EOG), electromyogram (EMG), and electrocardiogram (ECG) will be monitored [9].

There are many imaging studies proposed to evaluate the upper airway such as CT, MRI, dynamic scanning protocols e.g. ultrafast CT or MRI [7]. In oral and maxillofacial clinics cephalometric x-ray is still one of the most common x-rays used to diagnose and to evaluate treatment along with orthopantomogram (OPG). Both are a simple 2D image commonly used by oral and maxillofacial surgeon. It helps to detect posterior airway obstruction caused by skeletal disharmony. Examples of some important cephalometric measurements are:

- Sella nasion A point (SAN) 82 °
- Sella nasion B point (SAB) 80°
- Posterior airway space (PAS) 11mm
- Posterior nasal spine-palate (PNS-P) 35mm
- Mandibular plane-hyoid (MP-H) 15mm

OPG is used before any skeletal surgery to estimate the location of vital structures such as inferior alveolar nerve, mental foramen and apices of anterior teeth [10].

5. Risk factors and systemic complications

The incidence of OSA is different between men and women; most epidemiological studies reports male predominance with 5-8:1 ratio [11]. Male predominance is due to the sex related differences in upper airway anatomy and function, plus the differences in ventilator response to arousals from sleep [12]. But menopause women show a similar incidence to men because hormonal influences which play an important role in pathogenesis of OSA [13]. The other important risk factor is body mass index (BMI); the Wisconsin Sleep Cohort Study shows that one standard deviation difference in body mass index (BMI) was associated with a four-fold increase in disease prevalence [14] [15]. Partial or complete airway obstruction for more than

10 seconds will lead to decrease oxygen supply to vital organs such as the heart and brain which result in many sign and symptoms. Excessive daytime sleepiness, memory loss, impaired concentration, morning headache, decreased manual dexterity, libido and decrease sexual performance [16].

Systemic complications of OSA includes cardiovascular and neurocognitive disorders and death. Periods of apnea, prevent effective gaseous exchange at the alveoli which lead to hypoxia and hypercapnia. Apnea dependent hypoxia and hypercapnia increase sympathetic neural tone, which in turn cause vasoconstriction and increase in sympathetic nerve activity. Sympathetic nerve function rises progressively during apnea and is enhanced further by arousal. Increase in the sympathetic tone is the major cause of cardiovascular complications. OSA is associated with hypertension [16-18], arrhythmia, myocardial infarction [16, 19, 20], and congestive heart failure [16]. During the obstruction episodes there are marked changes in blood flow in cerebral arteries. Netzer et al reported 80% changes in cerebral blood flow in cerebral arteries [21]. During periods of apnea there is rapid increase in cerebral blood flow followed by rapid fall to below baseline levels after apnea periods. Fluctuation in cerebral blood flow along with many physiologic changes may lead to stroke [16]. Mortality rate of OSA can reach up to 30% in 15 years if left untreated [22]. Excessive daytime sleepiness could contribute to high rates of road traffic accidents. Studies show RTA among OSA patients is 1.3 to 7 times higher than the general population [23, 24].

6. Orthognathic surgery vs. telegnathic surgery

Maxillomandibular advancement is considered a telegnathic surgery, which involves maxillary and mandibular osteotomies to enlarge posterior airway space. Telegnathic surgery is derived from the Greek words *tele,* which means "over a distance," and *gnathis,* which relates to the jaws, whereas orthognathic surgery is derived from the Greek words, ortho, which means, "to straighten," and *gnathis meaning "jaw"*. OSA patients are usually middle age, obese, mostly males with significant comorbid medical conditions; on the other hand patients with dentofacial abnormalities are young with no sex prevalence (male or female) and usually in a good health.

There are no major differences in the surgical techniques although the goals of therapy are different. In orthognathic surgery the goal is to correct the occlusion and improve esthetics while in telegnathic surgery the optimal goal is to relieve upper airway obstruction. Orthodontic treatment is a must for all patients with dentofacial deformities who are going for orthognathic surgery. In OSA patients accepting the existing bite can be used if the patient does not want to go through the lengthy orthodontic treatment. Surgical movement in the orthognathic surgery patient are dependent upon the esthetic requirement as well as occlusion correction, whereas in OSA patients a larger surgical movement of the maxilla and mandible should be done (up to 10mm) with the main concern being opening the posterior airway space [25, 26].

7. Classification

Respiratory disturbance index (RDI) represents the number of obstructive respiratory events per hour of sleep. An RDI of 5 is the upper limit of normal.

RDI= (apnea+hypopnea ÷ total sleep time) × 60 [27].

OSA is classified into mild, moderate and severe depending on the respiratory disturbance index (RDI) and oxyhemoglobin desaturation (SaO_2).

Mild OSA is when RDI 10-30 and SaO_2 >90%,

Moderate OSA is when RDI 30-50 and SaO_2 >85%, and

Severe OSA is when RDI >50 and SaO_2 <60% [28].

8. Treatment options

8.1. Conservative treatment

After diagnosis of OSA, conservative treatment is indicated. It includes weight reduction, positional treatment, CPAP and oral appliances. Increase in BMI is a risk factor for OSA. Although high BMI is a risk factor for OSA, 30% of OSA patients are not obese. BMI is defined as the weight in kilograms divided by the height in meters squared (kg/m^2). Overweight is considered when BMI of more than 25 kg/m^2 while obese is a BMI of more than 30 kg/m^2. Constriction of the hypopharynx and oropharynx are due to increase in neck circumference and increased fatty deposits in the peripharyngeal area [29]. In the Wisconsin Sleep Cohort Study, a 10% weight gain predicted a 32% increase in AHI, whereas a 10% weight loss predicted a 26% decrease in AHI [14].

Continuous positive airway pressure (CPAP) or nasal Continuous Positive Airway Pressures (nCPAP) are effective treatments for OSA. They are the 1st line treatment strategies when the patient is diagnosed with OSA. CPAP/ nCPAP work as a pneumatic splint to open the airway via tight fitting facemask or nasal mask and oxygen pump. There are many studies reporting the success of CPAP treatment. CPAP can stop and reverse all OSA complications. Treatments with CPAP result in decreased sympathetic tone, which will lead to decrease in blood pressure, AHI, oxygen desaturation and improve sleep efficiency, [30-32]. CPAP compliance however is only 65-80%, with 8% to 15% of patients stopping the treatment after the first night. This low compliance rate is due to many associated complications such as nasal dryness and congestion, sinus discomfort, massive epistaxis, skin rash and conjunctivitis from air leak. These complications plus the physical discomfort, noise and difficult transporting the unit lowers the CPAP tolerance [33,34].

OSA patients should be advised not to sleep in supine position; gravity is a factor that can cause upper airway collapse. Positional behavioral therapy is to educate the patient to alter their sleep position by using a pillow or body belt; patients can alter their sleeping to a more lateral position that could open the airway and reduce collapsibility [35].

Mild to moderate OSA patients who are unable to tolerate CPAP can be treated with oral appliances. It simply prevents the mandible and associated muscles from going backward during sleep; some appliances actually advance the mandible from centric occlusion. Oral appliances should be adjusted on a periodic basis to prevent occlusal disturbances and temporomandibular joint dysfunction [36].

8.2. Surgical options

1969 Kuhlo et al was the first to recommend tracheostomy for OSA treatment [37]. Although tracheostomy is the most effective surgical procedure to treat OSA, it has morbidity and many adverse effects on the quality of life namely wound infection, stenosis and bleeding. Because of this many surgical techniques have developed to treat OSA. Based on the level of obstruction there are many surgical options; for example nasal surgeries such as septoplasty, turbinoplasty, polypectomy, adenectomy and tonsillectomy will address nasal obstruction. There are several palatal surgeries to address retropalatal obstruction for example: uvulopalatopharyngoplasty (UPPP), uvulopalatopharyngoplasty laser assisted (UPPP-LA), palatal pillar implants, radiofrequency ablation of the soft palate, and many others. Tongue operations like tongue suspension, radiofrequency ablation of the tongue, genial tubercle advancement with or without hyoid suspension are used for retrolingual obstruction. On the other hand maxillo-mandibular advancement with or without combined procedures address retropalatal and retrolingual levels of obstruction [26] [38].

The following section of this chapter will address some surgical techniques.

8.3. OSA treatment protocols

Successful OSA treatments depend on the recognition of the level of obstruction. Stanford University Sleep Disorders and Research Center proposed a protocol for OSA based on the site of obstruction.

Phase I protocol includes: UPPP, genioglossus advancement, and/or hyoid suspension then

Phase II protocol maxillomandibular advancement if the patient fails phase I treatment. MMA can be used to treat OSA as a primary or secondary procedure. MMA is considered primary when it is the 1st surgical procedure done to address multi-level of obstruction, when MMA done after phase one treatment it is called secondary MMA. Recently some surgeons prefer MMA advancement as the 1st surgical procedure especially if the patient has maxillary or mandibular deficiencies [26,39]. MMA is indicated if the diagnosis is confirmed severe OSA with RDI >50 and $SaO_2 < 60\%$, non-compliance or tolerance to CPAP, retroglossal obstruction, failure to respond to other surgical treatment such as UPPP and maxillomandibular hypoplasia [1].

8.4. Uvulopalatopharyngoplasty

Historically UPPP was an available option instead of tracheostomy until the recent expansion in surgical treatment of OSA. In 1981 Fujita et al introduced the concept of uvulopalatopharyngoplasty (UPPP) to enlarge retropalatal airway. UPPP involves partial excision of the uvula and redundant pharyngeal and palatal tissues, with primary closure of the anterior and posterior pillars under general anesthesia [40]. In 1991 O'Leary and Millman modify Fujita UPPP by excising the palatopharyngeus muscle [41]. Uvulopalatal flap is another modification published in 1996 by Powell et al [42]. UPPP complications range from velopharyngeal insufficiency, dysphagia (difficulty swallowing), voice changes, and death from general anesthesia [43]. With the advances in laser surgery uvulopalatopharyngoplasty–laser assisted (UPPP-LA) was developed using the same principle of scalpel UPPP [44]. Variable success rates reported in the literature is up to 70% and 78% respectively [45, 46]. Other studies show only 40 % success in eliminating snoring [47].

Today UPPP or UPPP-LA is rarely used as a single treatment modality; this is primarily due to the understanding of multilevel obstruction in most OSA patients. It is usually part of a staged protocol for OSA treatment [48]. UPPP can be performed with genioglossus advancement or with MMA. Hendler and Barry in 2001 published their data about 41 OSA patients; 33 of them treated with combined UPPP and modified mortised genioglossus advancement while the others had MMA combined procedures. All patients had pre-operative and post-operative polysomnography to evaluate treatment success. They reported comparable success rate of 86% in both groups concluding that UPPP/mortised genioglossus advancement is effective for the treatment of obstructive sleep apnea. Maxillomandibular advancement is effective for treating severe sleep apnea, and MMA can be done combined with UPPP/mortised genioglossus advancement in some cases as long as it is indicated in order to avoid multiple procedures [49].

8.5. Genioglossus advancement

Genioglossus muscle is a major pharyngeal dilator that plays an important role in OSA pathophysiology. In 1984 Riley et al. first reported advancing the genial tubercle with its genioglossus muscle attachment. The procedure was called inferior sagittal osteotomy [50]. If hyoid suspension to the inferior mandible is done at the same time it is called genioglossus advancement-hyoid myotomy [51]; the later was modified by suspending the hyoid to the thyroid cartilage. By advancing the genioglossus muscle the tension will increase at the tongue base thereby stabilize the hypopharyngeal airway [52]. In 1991 Riley et al modified the technique by limiting the osteotomy to a rectangular window and called it anterior mandibular osteotomy; this modification decreased anterior mandibular fracture [53]. In 2000, Lee and Woodson introduced a circular osteotomy of the genial tubercle [54]. All these modifications were done to address postoperative complications such as bone necrosis and anterior teeth pulp necrosis. Inferior sagittal osteotomy is indicated for patients with a deficient mandible in anteroposterior dimension, it involves genial tubercle advancement with the inferior border of the mandible while the occlusal relations ship is unchanged. On the other hand anterior mandibular osteotomy is indicated for patients with normal mandibular anteroposterior dimension [52]; it requires careful assessment of the genial tubercle, based on a study done by Mintz et al [55] on 14 human skulls, the superior border of the genial tubercle is 6.45 mm inferior to the apices of central incisors with 35.4% of the genial tubercle were located less than 5mm inferiorly. After estimating genial tubercle location a rectangular window osteotomy is performed leaving the inferior border of the mandible intact then advancing the segment to stabilize the hypopharyngeal airway. It will require a 90 degree rotation of the osteotomized segment and placing the lingual cortical plate anterior to the buccal/labial cortical plate [52]. Trephine osteotomy approach is another technique using the same concept but with trephine burr in an attempt to decrease post-operative complications (anterior teeth roots amputation) [54]. Foltán and René [56] published a follow-up of 31 patients who had genioglossus advancement by the modified genioplasty with hyoid myotomy. They reported 74% success rate showed by significant dropping in RDI and oxygen desaturation index. Genioglossus advancement with or without hyoid suspension is a valid technique to treat OSA; it could be performed alone or as an adjunct to UPPP [57]. Another technique to address retrolingual obstruction is tongue base surgeries. Tongue suspension is a revisable minimally invasive surgery performed via submental incision. By introducing a large suture into the base of the tongue and suspending the tongue to the mandibular lingual surface. Omur et al reported high success (81.81%)of tongue base surgery with UPPP. They conclude that tongue base suspension combined with UPPP has been shown to reduce RDI better than UPPP alone [58].

8.6. Maxillomandibular advancement

It is well recognized that patients with maxillomandibular deficiencies will ultimately develop OSA; from this observation MMA is advocated for OSA treatment even in patients with normal skeletal proportion [59]. MMA will increase the posterior airway dimension by physically expanding the skeletal structure. The forward movement of the maxillomandibular complex improves the tension and collapsibility of the velopharyngeal and suprahyoid muscles [60] [61]. Since the majority of OSA patients are middle age with a saggy and droopy soft tissue; forwarded movement of the mandibulomaxillary complex will not only bypass the obstruction; it will also provide facial rejuvenation by augmenting soft tissue support [62]. MMA has many advantages such as decrease number of surgeries needed by utilizing one surgery to bypass several sites of obstructions (by performing Le Fort I advancement; it will open the nasal valve and consequently improve air flow, tighten the soft palate and pharyngeal muscles at the same time while mandibular advancement will tighten genioglossus and suprahyoid muscles), avoid the need for tracheostomy in the postoperative period and ultimately decrease medical costs by decreasing hospital stay. If the patient will undergo simultaneous MMA and soft tissue procedure such as UPPP or tongue reduction surgeries; temporary tracheostomy may be indicated to ensure patent airway. Other indications for temporary tracheostomy are difficult airway, RDI >60 and Sao2 <60, morbid obesity and significant craniofacial abnormality [1] [59]. MMA is considered one of the most successful treatment modalities for OSA after tracheostomy and CPAP [63] [64]. MMA success rate is very high comparing to other surgical treatment. Riley et al [65] reported the largest MMA series with success rate of 98%. In 2004 Dattilo and Drooger [66] reported 93% success rate in 14 of 15 cases, whereas Hochban et al in 1997 reported 97% success rate in 37 of 38 cases [67].

MMA as a surgical techniques per se is the same as classical orthognathic surgery it involve maxillary Le Fort I advancement and mandibular advancement simultaneously. The amount of advancement is usually 10mm - the maximum amount of possible advancement. There are some differences that should be considered with MMA e.g. vascular supply, bone healing and the need of adjunctive surgical procedures. Most of MMA candidate patients had unsuccessful UPPP; palatal scar may cause difficulty in advancing the maxilla or compromise its blood supply. Patients treated with UPPP may have or be at risk for velopharyngeal insufficiency (VPI). Advancing the maxilla may theoretically cause VPI or worsen existing VPI. During MMA surgery, based on cephalometrics and model surgery, the mandible is advanced first; this is because the amount of advancement is arbitrary and without any considerations of the maxillary incisors esthetic position or functional occlusion. [1,59,68]

Holty and Guilleminault published a meta-analysis of 53 reports describing 627 OSA patients with maxillomandibular advancement for the treatment of obstructive sleep apnea; they concluded that major and minor complication rates for MMA were 1.0% and 3.1%, respectively with cardiac complications as the most major complications. Facial paresthesia is the most common complication after MMA with 86% of cases resolved by 12 months after surgery. No postoperative deaths were reported. Most subjects reported satisfaction after MMA with improvements in quality of life measures [69]. Patients with poor response to MMA often have had UPPP. The possible cause is failure of the airway to stretch laterally in the retropalatal area caused by soft palate scarring from the previous surgery, making the tissues of the lateral pharyngeal walls stiffer and thus less responsive to advancement [1,59].

9. Distraction osteogenesis and OSA

Recently, many surgeons suggest distraction osteogenesis for treating OSA. Distraction osteogenesis has many advantages over the traditional MMA surgical technique; better soft tissue adaptation, elimination of the need of a bone graft, less soft tissue dissection and better stability. On the other hand, lengthy treatment and the need of postoperative orthodontic treatment are the disadvantages of this kind of treatment [70] [71].

10. Summary

OSA surgical treatment success is primarily dependent on careful diagnosis and recognition of levels of obstruction. Many surgical protocols are there in the literature. MMA along with tracheostomy are the most successful surgical procedures to treat OSA.

	Orthognathic surgery	Telegnathic surgery
Sex	Male or female	Male
Age	Young	Middle age or older
Health	Usually healthy	Many medical comorbidities
Surgical goal	Correct the occlusion and improve esthetics	Relive upper airway obstruction.
Type of movement	Depend on the dentofacial deformity	Maxillomandibular advancement
Amount of movement	Depend of the esthetic position of maxillary central incisors and facial esthetic	Up to 10mm advancement
Orthodontic treatment	Must	Might accept the existing bite

Table 1. Differences between Orthognathic and Telegnathic surgery

	RDI=(apnea+hypopnea ÷ total sleep time) × 60	SaO_2
Mild	10-30	>90%
Moderate	30-50	>85%
Severe	>50	<60%

Table 2. OSA classification

Conservative / medical treatment	Surgical treatment
Weight reduction	Tracheostomy
CPAP, nCPAP	Nasal surgeries
Positional device	Palatal surgeries
Oral appliances	Tongue surgeries
	Skeletal surgeries

Table 3. OSA Treatment

Author details

Dina Ameen*

Address all correspondence to: dr.dinaameen@gmail.com

Clinical Fellow at the University of Alabama at Birmingham, USA

References

[1] Waite P D. Obstructive sleep apnea A review of the pathophysiology and surgical management. Oral Surgery Oral Medicine Oral Pathology ; 85(4).

[2] Boudewyns AN, Van de Heyning. Site of upper airway obstruction in obstructive apnoea and influence of sleep stage. Eur Respir J. 1997; 10(11): p. 2566–72.

[3] Georgalas C. The role of the nose in snoring and obstructive sleep apnoea: an update. Eur Arch Otorhinolaryngol. 2011; 268(9): p. 1365-73.

[4] Schwab RJ, Gefter WB, Hoffman EA, et al. Dynamic upper airway imaging during awake respiration in normal subjects and patients with sleep disordered breathing. Am Rev Respir Dis. 1993; 148(5): p. 1385–400.

[5] Chebbo A, Tfaili A, Ghamande S. Anatomy and Physiology of Obstructive Sleep Apnea. Sleep Med Clin. 2013; 8: p. 425–431.

[6] Hsu PP, Tan AK, Tan BY, et al. Uvulopalatopharyngoplasty outcome assessment with quantitative computer-assisted videoendoscopic airway analysis. Acta Otolaryngol. 2007;(127): p. 65-70.

[7] Boris A Stuck, Joachim T Maurer. Airway evaluation in obstructive sleep apnea. Sleep Medicine Reviews. 2008;(12): p. 411-436.

[8] Kent E. Moore, and Ceib Phillips. A Practical Method for Describing Patterns of Tongue-Base Narrowing (Modification of Fujita) in Awake Adult Patients With Obstructive Sleep Apnea. J Oral Maxillofac Surg. 2002;(60): p. 252-260.

[9] Mansoor Madani, Marcella Frank, Ryan Lloyd, Dessislava I. Dimitrova, Farideh Madani. Polysomnography Versus Home Sleep Study: Overview and Clinical Application. Atlas Oral Maxillofacial Surg Clin N Am. 2007; 15: p. 101-109.

[10] Nuntigar Sonsuwan, Sirithorn Suchachaisri, Ladda Chaloeykitti. The relationships between cephalometric parameters and severity of obstructive sleep apnea. Auris Nasus Larynx. 2011; 38: p. 83-87.

[11] Tishler, Larkin, Schluchter,Redline. Incidence of sleep disordered breathing in an urban adult population: the relative importance of risk factors in the development of sleep-disordered breathing. AJMA. 2003;(289): p. 2230-2237.

[12] Strohl KP, Redline S. Recognition of obstructive sleep apnea. Am J Respir Crit Care Med. 1996;(154): p. 279-289.

[13] Bixler EO, Vgontzas AN, Lin HM, et al. Prevalence of sleep-disordered breathing in women: effects of gender. Am J Respir Crit Care Med. 2001;(163): p. 608-613.

[14] Young T, Palta M, Dempsey J, et al. The occurrence of sleep-disordered breathing among middle-aged adults. N Engl J Med. 1993;(328): p. 1230-1235.

[15] Peppard PE, Young T, Palta M, et al. Longitudinal study of moderate weight change and sleep-disordered breathing. JAMA. 2000;(284): p. 3015-3021.

[16] Jacek Wolf, Joanna Lewicka, Krzysztof Narkiewicz. Obstructive sleep apnea: An update on mechanisms and cardiovascular consequences. Nutrition, Metabolism & Cardiovascular Diseases. 2007; 17: p. 233-240.

[17] Bixler EO, Vgontzas AN, Lin HM, Ten Have T, Leiby BE, Vela-Bueno A, et al. Association of hypertension and sleep-disordered breathing. Arch of Intern Med. 2000; (160): p. 2289-95.

[18] Nieto FJ, Young TB, Bonnie KL, Shahar E, Samet JM, Redline S, et al. Association of sleep-disordered breathing, sleep apnea, and hypertension in a large community-based study. JAMA. 2000;(283): p. 1829-36.

[19] Peled N, Abinader EG, Pillar G, Sharif D, Lavie P. Nocturnal ischemic events in patients with obstructive sleep apnea syndrome and ischemic heart disease effects of continuous positive air pressure treatment. J Am Coll Cardiol. 1999;(34): p. 1744-9.

[20] Sahar E, Whitney CW, Redline S, Lee ET, Newman AB,Nieto FJ, et al. Sleep disordered breathing and cardiovascular disease. Cross-sectional results of the sleep heart study. AM J Respir Crit Care Med. 2001;(163): p. 19-25.

[21] Netzer N, Werner P, Jochums I, Lehmann M, Strohl KP. Blood flow of the middle cerebral artery with sleep-disordered breathing:correlation with obstructive hypopneas. Stroke 1998;29:7-93.

[22] Young T, Finn L, Peppard PE, et al. Sleep disordered breathing and mortality: eighteen-year follow-up of the Wisconsin sleep cohort. Sleep. 2008;: p. 1071-8.

[23] Findley LJ, Unverzagt ME, Suratt PM. Automobile accidents involving patients with obstructive sleep apnea. Am Rev Respir Dis. 1998;: p. 138-337.

[24] Vidya Krishnan, Susheel P. Patil. Obstructive Sleep Apnea and Transportation: Medicolegal Issues. Sleep Med Clin. 2013; 8: p. 591–605.

[25] Lars Andersson Karl-Erik Kahnberg, M. Anthony (Tony) Pogrel.Oral and Maxillofacial Surgery : Blackwell Publishing Ltd ; 2010.

[26] Bagheri SC. Current therapy of Oral & Maxillofacial Surgery: Saunders ; 2012.

[27] John G. Park,Kannan Ramar, and Eric J. Olson. Updates on Definition, Consequences, and Management of Obstructive Sleep Apnea. Mayo Clin Proc. 2011 jun: p. 549-555.

[28] Institute for Clinical Systems Improvement web site. Healthcare guideline: Diagnosis and treatment of obstructive sleep apnea in adults. [Online].; 2008.

[29] Hoffstein V, Mateika S. Differences in abdominal and neck circumferences in patients with and without obstructive sleep apnea. Eur Respir J. 1992;(5): p. 377-381.

[30] Giles TL. Continuous positive airways pressure for obstructive sleep apnea in adults. 2006 oct: p. CD005308.

[31] Pepperell JC, Ramdassingh-Dow S, Crosthwaite N, Mullins R, Jenkinson C, Stradling JR, et al. Ambulatory blood pressure after therapeutic and subtherapeutic nasal continuous positive airway pressure for obstructive sleep apnoea: a randomised parallel trial. Lancet. 2002;(359): p. 204-10.

[32] Bonsignore MR, Parati G, Insalaco G, Marrone O, Castiglioni P, Romano S, et al. Continuous positive airway pressure treatment improves baroreflex control of heart rate during sleep in severe obstructive sleep apnea syndrome. Am J Respir Crit Care Med. 2002;(166): p. 279-86.

[33] Waldhorn RE, TW Herrick, MC Nguyen, AE O'Donnell, J Sordero, Potolicchio SJ. Long term compliance with nasal continuous positive airway pressure therapy of obstructive sleep apnea. Chest. 1990;(97): p. 33-38.

[34] Wells RD, Freedland KE, Carney RM, Duntley SP, Stepanski EJ. Adherence, reports of benefits, and depression among patients treated with continuous positive airway pressure. Psychosomatic Medicine. 2007; 65(5): p. 449-454.

[35] Raphael C. Heinzer, Cyril Pellaton, Vincianne Rey, Andrea. Rossetti, Gianpaolo Lecciso,José Haba-Rubio, Mehdi Tafti, Gilles Lavigne. Positional therapy for obstructive sleep apnea: An objective measurement of patients' usage and efficacy at home. Sleep Medicine. 2012;(13): p. 425-428.

[36] Tatsuya Fukuda, Satoru Tsuiki, Mina Kobayashi, Hideaki Nakayama, Yuichi Inoue. Selection of response criteria affects the success rate of oral appliance treatment for obstructive sleep apnea. Sleep Medicine. 2014;(15): p. 367–370.

[37] Kuhlo W, Doll E, Frank MD. Erfolgreiche Behandlungeines Pickwick-Syndroms durch eine Dauertrachealkanüle. Dtsch Med Wochenschr. 1969;(94): p. 1286-90.

[38] Macario Camacho et al. Surgical Treatment of Obstructive Sleep Apnea. Sleep Med Clin. 2013;(8): p. 495-503.

[39] Hillel D. Ephros, Mansoor Madani, Brett M. Geller, Robert J. DeFalco. Developing a Protocol for the Surgical Management of Snoring and Obstructive Sleep Apnea. Atlas Oral Maxillofacial Surg Clin N Am. 2007;(15): p. 89–100.

[40] Fujita S, Conway W, Zorick F, et al. Surgical correction of anatomic abnormalities of obstructive sleep apnea syndrome: uvulopalatopharyngoplasty. Otolaryngol Head Neck Surg. 1981;(89): p. 923 – 34.

[41] O'Leary MJ, Millman RP. Technical modification of uvulopalatopharyngoplasty: the role of the palatopharyngeus. Laryngoscope. 1991;(101): p. 1332 – 5.

[42] Powell N, Riley R, Guilleminault C, Troell R. A reversible uvulopalatal flap for snoring and sleep apnea syndrome. Sleep. 1996;(19): p. 593 – 9.

[43] Kezirian EJ. Incidence of serious complicaions after uvulopalatopharyngoplasty. Laryngoscope. 2004; 114(3): p. 450-453.

[44] Madani M. Laser assisted uvulopalatopharyngoplasty (LA-UPPP) for the treatment of snoring and mild to moderate obstructive sleep apnea. Atlas Oral Maxillofac Surg Clin North Am. 2007; 15(2): p. 129-137.

[45] Madani M. Complications of laser-assisted uvulopalatopharyngoplasty (LA-UPPP) and radiofrequency treatments of snoring and chronic nasal congestion: a 10-year review of 5,600 patients. J Oral Maxillofac Surg. 2004; 62(11): p. 1351-1362.

[46] Li HY, Wang PC, Lee LA, Chen NH, Fang TJ. Prediction of uvulopalatopharyngoplasty outcome: anatomy-based staging system versus severity-based staging system. Sleep. 2006; 29(12): p. 1537-1541.

[47] Lyngkaran T, Kanaglaingam J, Rajeswaran R, Georgalas C, Kotecha B. Long-term out- comes of laser-assisted uvulopalatoplasty in 168 patients with snoring. J Laryngol Otol. 2006; 120(11): p. 932-938.

[48] Walenczak I, Siekiewicz A, Rogowski M, Swietek M. The evaluation of the effectiveness of uvulopalatopharyngoplasy in the treatment of selected patients with mild to moderate obstructive sleep apnea—one year of postoperative follow up. Pol Merkur Lekarski. 2007; 22(132): p. 529-531.

[49] Hendler, Barry H. A protocol for uvulopalatopharyngoplasty, mortised genioplasty, and maxillomandibular advancement in patients with obstructive sleep apnea: An analysis of 40 cases. Journal of oral and maxillofacial surgery. 2001; 59(8): p. 892.

[50] Powell NB, Riley RW, Guilleminault C. Maxillofacial surgical techniques for hypopharyngeal obstruction in obstructive sleep apnea. Operative techniques. Otolaryngol Head Neck Surg. 1991;(2): p. 112 – 9.

[51] Riley RN. Powell NB, Guilleminault C. Inferior sagittal osteotomy of the mandible with hyoid suspension: a new procedure for obstructive sleep apnea. Otolaryngol Head Neck Surg. 1986;(94): p. 589.

[52] N. Ray Lee, Mansoor Madani. Genioglossus Muscle Advancement Techniques for Obstructive Sleep Apnea. Atlas Oral Maxillofacial Surg Clin N Am. 2007; 15: p. 179-192.

[53] Riley RW, Powell NB, Guillaminault C. Obstructive sleep apnea and the hyoid: a revised surgical procedure. Otolaryngol Head Neck Surg. 1994;(111): p. 717-21.

[54] Lee NR, Woodson T. Genioglossus muscle advancement via a trephine osteotomy approach. Operative techniques. Otolaryngol Head Neck Surg. 2000;(11): p. 50-4.

[55] Mintz SM, Ettinger AC, Geist JR, et al. Anatomic relationship of the genial tubercles to the dentition as determined by cross-sectional tomography. J Oral Maxillofac Surg. 1995;(53): p. 1324.

[56] Foltán, René. Genioglossus advancement and hyoid myotomy in treating obstructive sleep apnoea syndrome–A follow-up study. Journal of craniomaxillofacial surgery. 2007;(35): p. 246.

[57] YIN, S. Genioglossus advancement and hyoid suspension plus uvulopalatopharyngoplasty for severe OSAHS. Otolaryngology head and neck surgery. 2007; 136(4): p. 626.

[58] Mehmet Omur, Dilaver Ozturan, Feyzi Elez, Celal Unver, Sabri Derman. Tongue Base Suspension Combined With UPPP in Severe OSA Patients. Otolaryngology–Head and Neck Surgery. 2005;(133): p. -218223.

[59] Louis T. George, H. Dexter Barber, Brian M. Smith. Maxillomandibular Advancement Surgery: An Alternative Treatment Option for Obstructive Sleep Apnea. Atlas Oral Maxillofacial Surg Clin N Am. 2007;(15): p. 163–177.

[60] Fairburn SC, Waite PD, Vilos G, et al. Three-dimensional changes in upper airways of patients with obstructive sleep apnea following maxillomandibular advancement. J Oral Maxillofac Surg. 2007;(65): p. 6-12.

[61] Li KK, Guilleminault C, Riley RW, Powell NB. Obstructive sleep apnea and maxillomandibular advancement: an assessment of airway changes using radiographic and nasopharyngoscopic examinations. J Oral Maxillofac Surg. 2002;(60): p. 526–30.

[62] Li KK, Riley RW, Powell NB, et al. Patient's perception of the facial appearance after maxillomandibular advancement for obstructive sleep apnea syndrome. J Oral Maxillofac Surg. 2001;(59): p. 377–80.

[63] Waite PD, Shettar SM. Maxillomandibular advancement surgery: a cure for obstructive sleep apnea syndrome. Oral Maxillofac Surg Clin North Am. 1995;(7): p. 327–36.

[64] Li KK. Surgical management of obstructive sleep apnea. Clin Chest Med. 2003;(24): p. 365–70.

[65] Riley RW, Powell NB, Guilleminalt C. Obstructive sleep apnea syndrome: A review of 306 consecutively treated surgical patients. Otolaryngol Head Neck Surg. 1993; (108): p. 117.

[66] Dattilo DJ, Drooger SA. Outcome assessment of patients under- going maxillofacial procedures for the treatment of sleep apnea: Comparison of subjective and objective results. J Oral Maxillofac Surg. 200;(62): p. 164.

[67] Hochban W, Conradt R, Bradenburg U, et al. Plast Reconstr Surg. Surgical maxillofacial treatment of obstructive sleep apnea. 1997;(99): p. 619.

[68] Scott B. Boyd. Management of Obstructive Sleep Apnea by Maxillomandibular Advancement. Oral Maxillofacial Surg Clin N Am. 2009;(21): p. 447–457.

[69] Jon-Erik C. Holty, Christian Guilleminault. Holty CG. Maxillomandibular advancement for the treatment of obstructive sleep apnea: A systematic review and meta-analysis. Sleep Medicine Reviews. 2010;(14): p. 287–297.

[70] Kasey K. Li, Nelson B. Powell, Robert W. Riley, Christian Guilleminault. Distraction Osteogenesis in Adult Obstructive Sleep Apnea Surgery: A Preliminary Report. J Oral Maxillofac Surg. 2002;(60): p. 6-10.

[71] Stevan H. Thompson, Michael Quinn, Joseph I. Helman, Dale A. Baur. Maxillomandibular Distraction Osteogenesis Advancement for the Treatment of Obstructive Sleep Apnea. J Oral Maxillofac Surg. 2007;(65): p. 1427-1429.

Section 7

Diagnosis and Management of Ankylosis of the Temporomandibular Joint

Chapter 19

Comprehensive Management of Temporomandibular Joint Ankylosis — State of the Art

Hossein Behnia, Azita Tehranchi and
Farnaz Younessian

Additional information is available at the end of the chapter

http://dx.doi.org/10.5772/59165

1. Introduction

Temporomandibular joint (TMJ) ankylosis is one of the most challenging TMJ disorders that can negatively affect oral related daily functions like mastication, speech and hygiene [1,2]. The accepted definition of ankylosis is the bony or fibrous tissue fusion between articular surfaces including the meniscus, glenoid fossa and condylar heads [3]. Consequently, jaw functions like the maximal incisal opening (MIO) and lateral excursive movements progressively decrease. This chapter describes the most important issues of early and late management of TMJ ankylosis in both children and adults.

2. Etiology and pathogenesis of TMJ ankylosis

Trauma to the TMJ has been cited as the most common underlying reason responsible for ankylosis; however, local infections (e.g. otitis media) and systemic disorders (e.g. rheumatoid arthritis) also can also cause unilateral or bilateral TMJ ankylosis in some cases [4-7]. By improving the immediate management protocol of condylar fracture and proper application of antibiotics to fully address ear infections, the prevalence of ankylosis has decreased significantly in recent years. In addition to the common etiologic factors of TMJ condylar ankylosis, some affected infants with unknown etiological factors have been reported in the literature (Figure 1 a-c) [8].

The pathogenesis of the TMJ ankylosis is described by a sequence of events. The increased intra-articular vascular supply at the traumatized joint develops fibrosis and ultimately

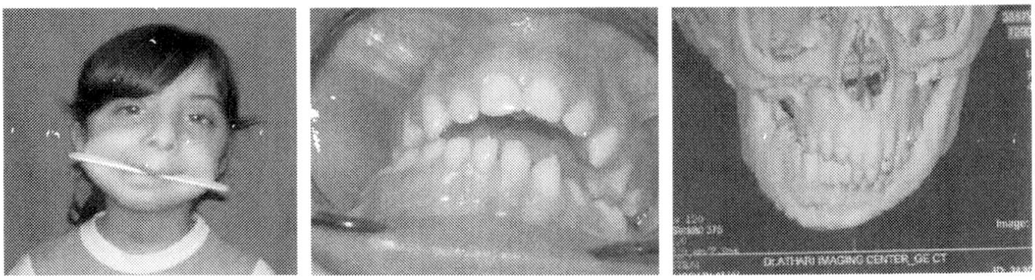

a b c

Figure 1. A 5-year-old girl with bilateral condylar ankylosis of unknown etiology (no history of trauma or infection). a) Extraoral facial photograph of the patient demonstrate the upper occlusal canting with the help of a tongue depressor, b) Intraoral photograph shows midline deviation, mandibular shift and increased overjet of the patient, c) three dimensional cone beam computer reconstruction of the patient demonstrates the facial asymmetry.

excessive localized bone formation [4]. Most of the animal studies consider intra-capsular hematoma as the main underlying reason for development of the ankylotic mass following trauma. Observed hemorrhage contains different cellular pathways activated by bone morphogenic proteins (BMPs) and tumoral growth factors (TGFs) [9]. However, a study on human subjects, revealed that hematoma in the joint space does not always result in bony ankylosis [2]. This excessive bone mass does not have a neoplastic nature, but has the potential of continual growth [10]. The presence of abnormal bony mass may restrict mandibular movement, which subsequently may lead in loss of the functional matrix of bone and muscle interaction, and consequently result in growth failure [11]. Inadequately treated or excessive treatment of condylar fractures may lead to growth retardation or growth excess, respectively [3]. Therefore, the best treatment steps for post-traumatic ankylosis and resulting growth abnormality is prevention.

3. Diagnosis and clinical features of TMJ ankylosis

Maximum mouth opening in the presence of pain or without it is a clinical indicator of traumatized condyles [12]. In addition to routine extra and intraoral photographs, supplemental diagnostic records may be needed for complete diagnosis of each case. Towne's projection, posteroanterior and cone beam CT (3D) radiographs are commonly used for this purpose (Figure 2 a, b).

Due to the flexibility of bone, it is possible to open the mandible to some extent, particularly in unilateral ankylotic cases [13]. Long-standing TMJ ankylosis can result in functional loss and facial deformity of affected individuals. In growing patients (mostly under 15 years) lack of adequate growth at the condyles, which are the main growth centers of the mandible, forward and downward movement of the mandible does not occur [13]. This growth retardation can result in a distorted mandibular structure in all three dimensions, highlighted mostly on sagittal views. Furthermore, deepening of the antegonial notch following continuous subperiosteal bone formation at the angles may be seen in most of the affected. However,

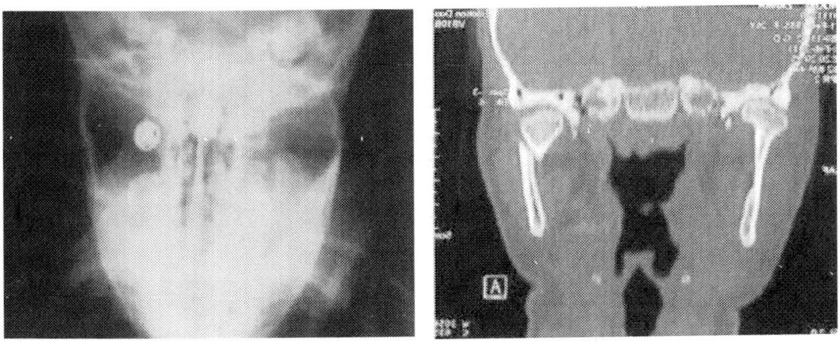

a b

Figure 2. a) Posteroanterior view of a condylar neck fracture, b) Coronal section of computer tomography scan of another adult patient with unilateral condylar fracture on the right side.

ankylosis in patients older than 15 years of age experience mild facial deformities concomitant with significant functional loss. Depending on the type of ankylosis (unilateral or bilateral) clinical features can vary.

In the case of unilateral ankylosis, the patient also develops a mandibular asymmetry and subdivision malocclusion [14]. Furthermore, in unilateral cases canting of the upper occlusal surface thought to be caused by compensatory vertical eruption of the posterior maxillary teeth ipsilateral to the restricted condyle is seen (Figure 3 a-c). On the other hand, in bilateral ankylosis, more limited range of interincisal opening and absence of maxillary occlusal canting is observed. Patients with bilateral ankylosis develop retrognathia, short posterior facial height and openbite with possible upper airway obstruction and severely convex facial profile (Figure 4 a, b) [15].

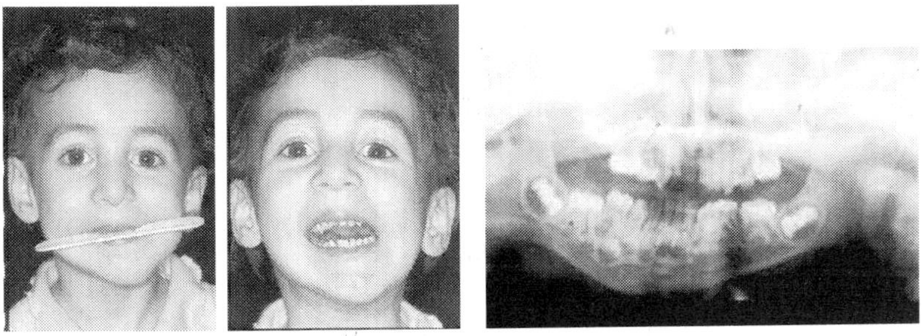

a b c

Figure 3. A 3-year-old girl with unilateral condylar ankylosis following trauma at birth, a) on facial examination, the patient presented with facial asymmetry, shortened ramus height, jaw deviation and the chin was noticeably deviated to the left and the maxilla was canted downward on the right side. b) The mandibular border became flat and elongated on the unaffected side and round on the affected side. The asymmetry is usually the least at the cranial base area and becomes worse at the lower parts including the chin.

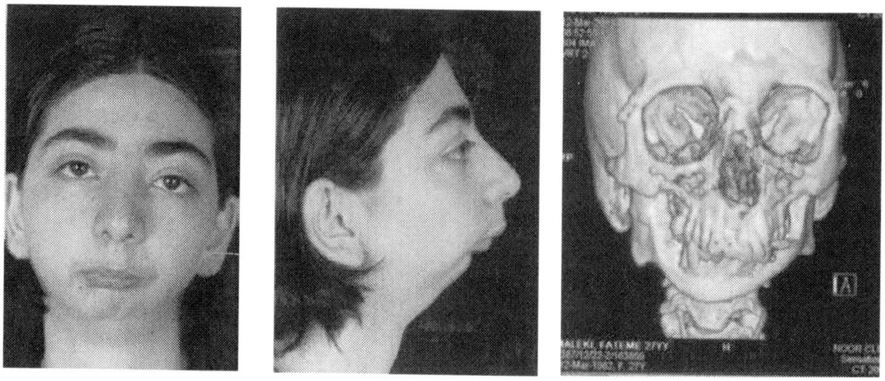

a b c

Figure 4. An 18-year-old girl with bilateral condylar ankylosis. a) Long term effect of bilateral condylar ankylosis in a growing adolescent, which result in limited mouth opening, micrognathia and absent neck chin angle. b) The profile view is helpful to assess anteroposterior and vertical facial imbalance as well as aid in the determination of etiology of the asymmetry. C) 3D CT scan.

Prevention of TMJ ankylosis following trauma:

Regaining normal range of mandibular movement should begin as soon as possible after trauma. Many clinicians recommended a few days [5-7] of no-intervention immediately after the injury. This phase allows resolution of pain and swelling of the TMJ before reestablishment of normal range of movement [16]. However, care must be taken not to overextend this phase regarding ankylosis development. Excellent compliance of the affected individuals with physiotherapy and functional appliances immediately after trauma is an essential part of future growth and development. Failure to achieve a high level of compliance to physiotherapy and application of intraoral appliances, increase the risk of future ankylosis, which would be more problematic for patients as time passes.

3.1. Early management in childhood

Prevention of the ankylosis of the traumatized condyles requires maintenance of the normal range of movement. In most cases, if the normal range of movement can be achieved, the TMJ will heal without any functional complication. When the patient is able to reach maximal opening, even in the presence of pain, the simplest prevention regimen would be insertion of a removable appliance, which guides the mandible into its correct position during closure. The design and fabrication of different types of removable appliances depends on the clinical situation of each patient, but commonly all are fabricated from a construction bite in which advances the mandible on the affected side more than the contralateral side in addition to concise maxillary and mandibular midlines. The major difficulty with construction bite is that the clinician must be able to guide the mandible to the proper position, rapidly and accurately. Different types of appliances and various combinations of components can be incorporated in these appliances to meet individual requirements. Depending on compliance and age of the affected child, we use four different techniques:

1. Two simple removable Hawley appliances attached together while the patient is in centric occlusion (CO) guiding the lower jaw to symmetric position (Figure 5).

2. Fixed functional appliance with the aid of cement luting agent on the primary molars bands for more secure retention (Figure 6-a).

3. Usage of bi-zygomatic suspension wires in more severe cases in the absence of patient compliance and inadequate intraoral retention of the appliance.

4. Interdental Kobayashi wires with guiding interarch elastics, in cases of excessive restricted mandibular movement, which do not permit the clinician to take an impression (Figure 6-b).

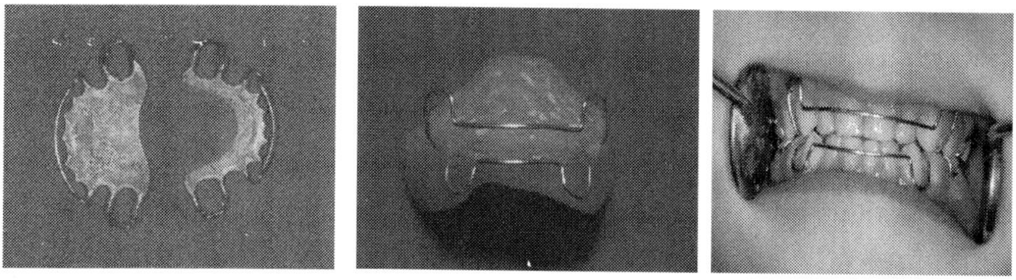

a b c

Figure 5. Two simple removable Hawley appliances attached together is the most common appliance used to guide the patient into symmetric position.

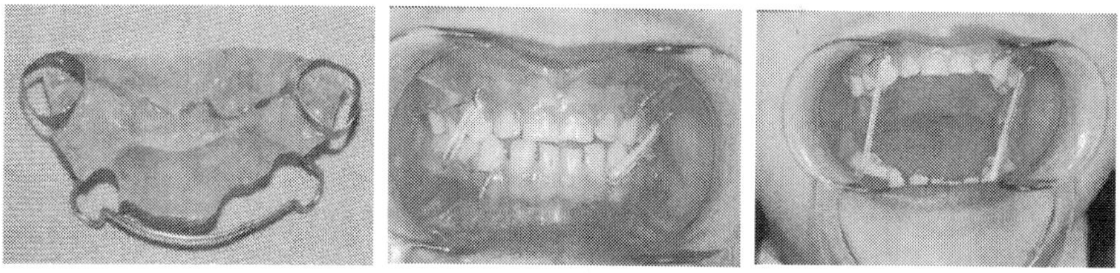

a b c

Figure 6. a) Fixed functional appliance with molar bands that can hold the mandible in its correct position full-time, b and c) Interdental Kobayashi wires and guiding interarch orthodontic elastics.

Despite the improvements, removable appliances are not a practical way to manage more severe situations that require extra manipulation of the TMJ fracture. A closed reduction often is useful to re-establish normal jaw function as a next step [17]. In fact, if the fractured condyle is still within the articular fossa, there is an opportunity to heal in a quite adequate functional position, only by maintaining the occlusion. This technique is preferred over open reduction due to high success rate, less complications and technical problems and also less remnant facial scars [18]. However, clinical decision on the most appropriate type of treatment must be made considering different individualized factors like patient age, medical history, risk of infection, and risk of chronic pain, risk of scarring or nerve injury, and also presence of other concomitant facial, mandibular or cranial fractures [19]. Conservative management of condylar fractures is still the preferred option, however, in rare cases of condylar displacement into the middle cranial fossa, or lateral extracapsular displacement of the fractured segment, open reduction is selected [17]. The advantages of open treatment for condylar fractures would be the possibility of restoring the anatomical position of the fragments and disc, and subsequently immediate functional movement of the jaw, which greatly avoids the development of ankylosis of the traumatized joint [20].

3.1.1. *Treatment*

3.1.1.1. *Unilateral condylar fracture*

A 4-year-old boy was brought in approximately five hours after being hit on the left side of the face. He complained of pain on the left side (Figure 7 a). The impressions of upper and lower arch with limited jaw opening were performed and an attached upper and lower Hawley appliance was fabricated to guide the patient into correct closure (Figure 7 b). The condyle of the affected side healed and positive outcomes were maintained during a 1-year follow-up (Figure 7 c and Figure 8 a, b).

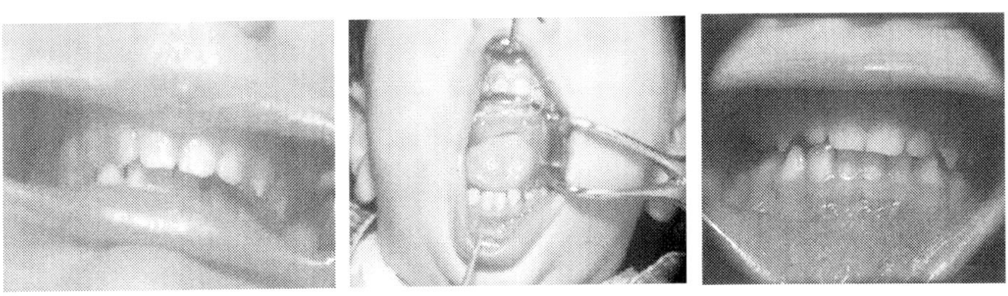

a b c

Figure 7. a) Pretreatment intraoral photograph shows inability of the patient to open the mouth. b) Removable appliance inserted for further guidance of the lower arch. c) Frontal facial view at the end of active treatment.

3.2. Early management in adulthood

Sometimes adult patients suffer severe trauma to the condyles, particularly as a part of a catastrophic event [21]. Although, because of absence of required growth in later stages of life, this restricted condylar growth might not result in severe facial deformities, but it may result in limited mandibular function. Recent improvements in treatment techniques including advent

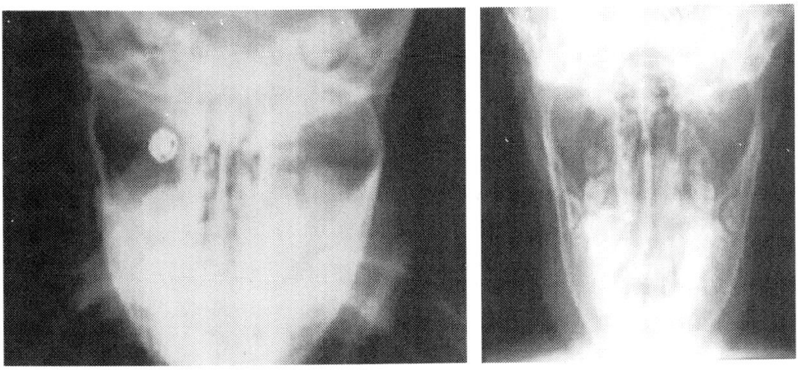

a b

Figure 8. Same patient shown in Figure 7. a) Note the presence of condylar neck fracture at posteroanterior projection radiograph immediately before treatment with removable appliance. b) Follow-up radiograph of the patient which reveals adequate alignment of the fractured bony segment after 1-year.

of temporary anchorage devices (TAD) can help clinicians manage the other jaw fractures presenting with the traumatized condyles. In contrast to the traditional techniques like intermaxillary wire fixations, application of TADs does not restrict the range of normal functional movements. In addition, comparing their application in growing patients, TADs could be inserted in mature bony structures of the jaws without any additional risk regarding possible damage to un-erupted dental crypts. This approach removes the necessity of presence of enough remaining dentition to be used as guidance of jaw movements (Figure 9 a-c). With the help of these TADs and temporary light interarch elastics one can guide directional remodeling of traumatized condylar segments, in a manner similar to removable appliances [21].

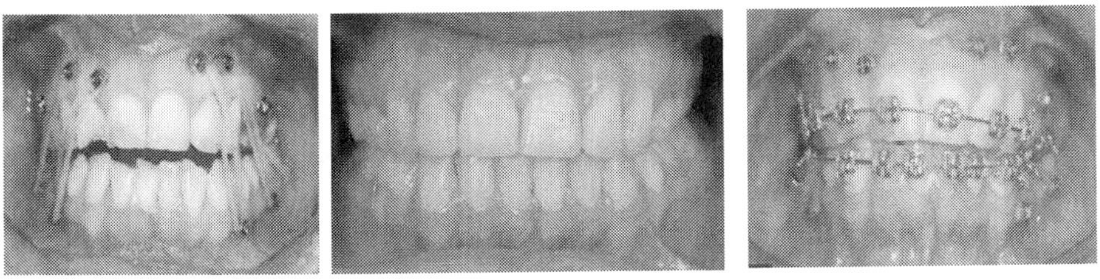

a b c

Figure 9. a) Settling of the occlusion and guidance of proper healing procedure by means of TADs and light intermaxillary elastics in an adult patient, b) orthodontic brackets were bonded on teeth to correct the remaining dental malposition, c) final treatment result (From Tehranchi A: Rapid, conservative, multidisciplinary miniscrew-assisted approach for treatment of mandibular fractures following plane crash Dent Res J. 2013 Sep-Oct; 10: 678–684).

4. Management of TMJ ankylosis

Treatment of TMJ ankylosis is an excellent example of an important principle in the timing of the treatment: because of devastating effects on future growth, presence of condylar ankylosis in growing patients is an indication for early treatment; in contrast, condylar ankylosis in adult patients must be treated considering the extent of functional limitation of mandibular movement. In many clinical situations pain is uncommon and limited range of opening is the first sign of condylar ankylosis, usually noticed by dental practitioners [22].

4.1. Management of TMJ ankylosis without severe dentofacial deformity

To date, various treatment approaches have been described to achieve successful management of ankylosis [23-24]; however no single treatment with uniformly successful results has been assigned for all cases [4, 25-26]. The optimum selection of an adequate technique depends directly on the details of clinical situation of the patients and is highlighted particularly in patients' growing phase, since their consequent facial deformity could be significantly worsened during growth [27]. In the aforementioned patients, orthopedic treatment with functional appliances following surgical release of ankylosis is highly recommended.

Possible treatment modalities for cases without severe facial deformities include surgical excision of an ankylotic mass, gap arthroplasty and interpositional arthroplasty [16, 24]. These techniques may be supplemented by application of different autogenous or alloplastic materials to reconstruct the ramus and affected condylar segments [28-29].

The first treatment option is gap arthroplasty, which increases the gap between the articular cavity and ramus by means of a simple bone division (Figure 10). The modifications of this technique including increasing the gap alone to reduce the re-ankylosis may not be clinically effective [30].

The second category, interpositional arthroplasty addresses the main drawbacks of the first method, which is high recurrence rate [31]. In this technique, surgeons try to fill the gap with autogenous graft materials including skin, dermis, flap of temporal muscle, cartilage or even alloplastic materials like silastic (Figure 11 a-c). The placement of these materials prevents the recurrence possibility. TMJ reconstruction is the third treatment option commonly done by means of a costochondral graft. However, other autogenous graft sources like clavicular osteochondral graft, coronoid process graft or alloplastic condylar implants can be used to reconstruct the lost segments. Autogenous sources present donor site morbidity; however alloplastic grafts are procedures with significant disadvantages of implant fracture of foreign body reaction. Between autogenous sources, costochondral grafts represent the most variable growth behavior, particularly in growing children, as compared to coronoid process graft, which demonstrate more predictable growth behavior.

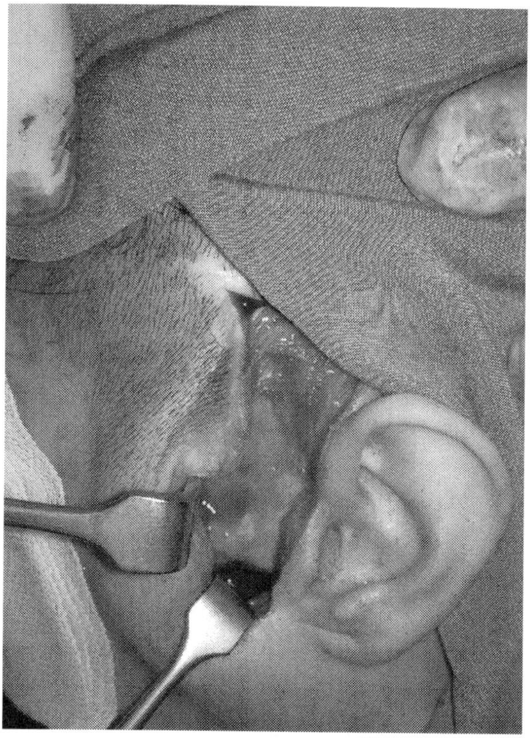

Figure 10. Intra-operative view demonstrating gap arthroplasty technique.

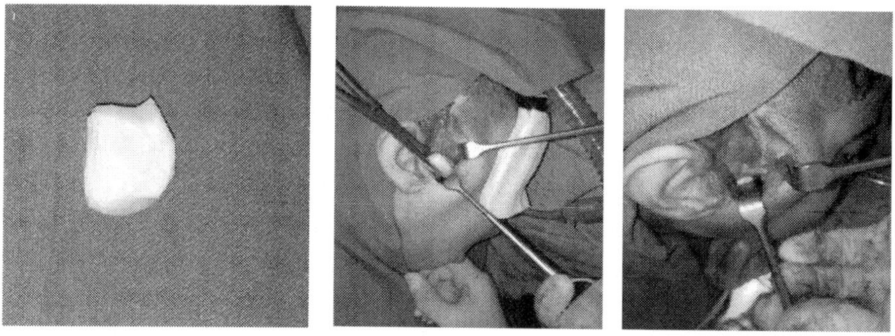

a b c

Figure 11. Interpositional arthroplasty of an ankylotic condyle by means of square-shaped silastic graft material, a) Selected alloplastic silastic-based graft material, b) Insertion of the alloplastic silastic material, c) final position of the alloplastic material filling up the entire space created by the gap arthroplasty.

An approved international surgical protocol consists of 9-steps to take before and after surgery.

1. Aggressive total resection of the ankylotic segment in the condylar TMJ region. Recently, complete excision of the bony mass has been questioned regarding the increasing probability of the recurrence rate [10]. The underlying postulation was that leaving the opposing bony cut surface of the condyles after complete excision increase the amount of clot formation on dead space, which ultimately results in the formation of dense fibrous bridges that impede future mandibular movement [32]. Partial osteotomy of the region with minimal clot formation has been cited as a more potent surgical approach [32].

2. Coronoidectomy on the affected side (ipsilateral) which usually elongates in long-standing ankylosis and prevents intra-operative maximal opening because of the restriction. The autogenous bone achieved by this step can be used as a source of graft material to re-establish the ramus height of the affected side.

3. If the above-mentioned procedures do not result in normal maximum opening (more than 35 mm) without excessive force, the opposite coronoid (contralateral) must also be removed.

4. Lining of the joint with temporalis fascia or the remaining disk [16]

Remnants of the meniscus can serve as a barrier to prevent direct bony contacts and further fusion between condylar heads and glenoid fossa. However, there is controversy in the literature regarding the main role of the disc on the development of ankylosis [7]. In many traumatized cases, it has been shown that the ankylosis can occur even in the presence of an intact meniscus in the joint space [33-34].

5. Reconstruction of the ramus segment with costochondral grafts in growing patients if possible using rigid fixation (Figure 12 a-c),

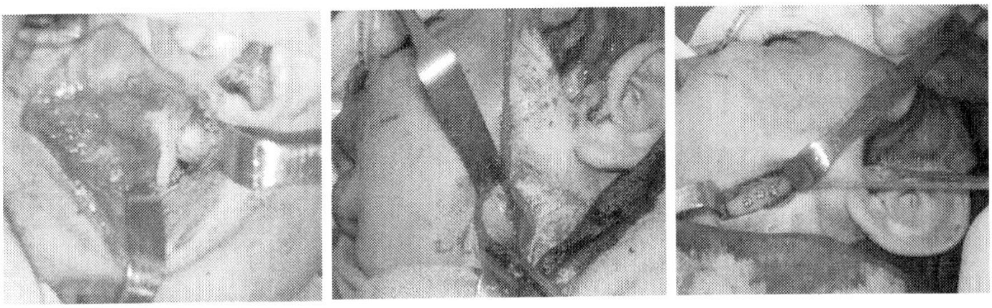

a b c

Figure 12. Intraoperative photographs of a patient with TMJ reconstruction treatment plan, a) extraoral access to the TMJ ankylotic mass through a preauricular excision, b) submandibular incision for placement of fixation plates over the costochondral graft, c) after aggressive excision of the ankylotic mass and fixation of the costochondral graft by means of fixation screws.

6. Intra-operative open bite creation on the affected side to permit settling of the bone graft, which should be maintained by a hybrid orthodontic appliance for 3-6 months (Figure 13 a) [35]. Simple removable functional appliance (Hybrid) with lingual and buccal shields on the affected side to encourage dental eruption and a bite block on the contralateral side to impede the eruption (Figure 13 b). In adult cases, however, considering the absence of passive dental eruption, the open bite should be managed by means of orthodontic brackets and light intermaxillary elastics (Figure 14 a, b).

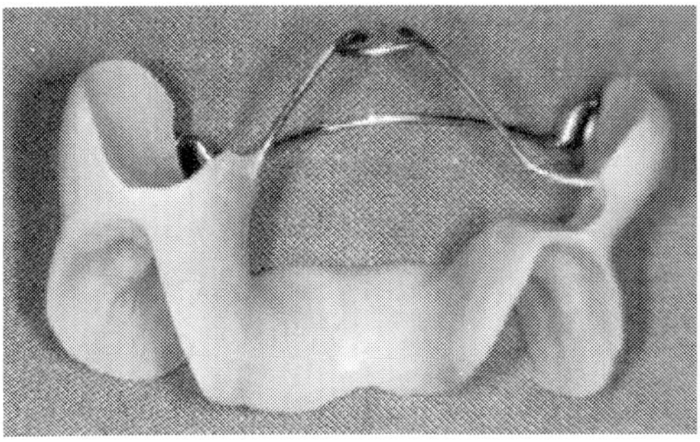

a

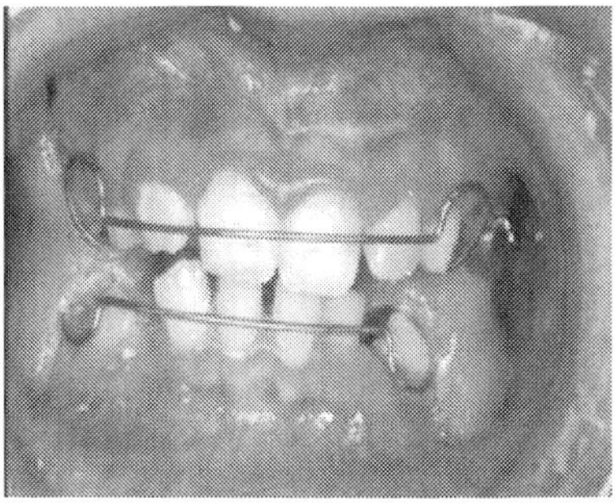

b

Figure 13. a) A hybrid functional appliance consist of two set of shields (lingual and buccal) to faciiitate dental eruption on the affected side and acrylic bite block to impede dental eruption on the opposite site, b) A hybrid functional appliance in place

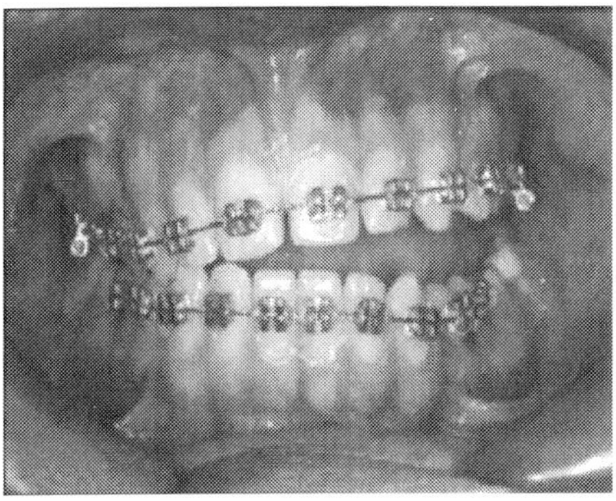

a

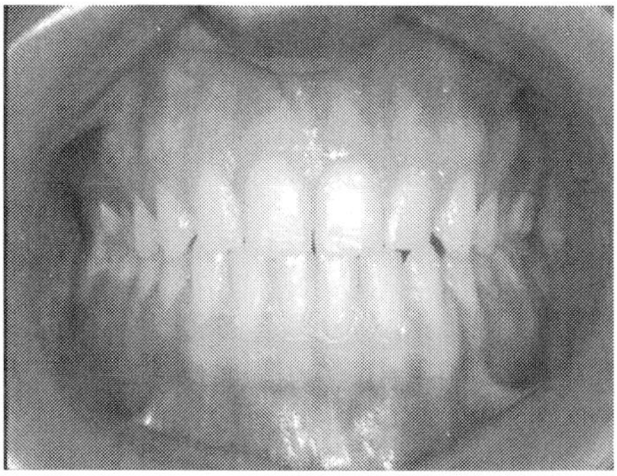

b

Figure 14. a) Bonding of orthodontic brackets on the upper and lower arch to correct the openbite on the affected side; note the degree of anterior open bite, b) Intraoral photograph of the final occlusion (From Behnia H: A Textbook of Advanced Oral and Maxillofacial Surgery ISBN 978-953-51-1146-7. chapter 16, Distraction Osteogenesis; 2013).

7. Early mobilization with a short period of intermaxillary fixation (not more than 3 weeks),

8. Supportive adjunctive therapy including physiotherapy with strict follow up to prevent the re-ankylosis phenomena. This therapy disrupts and prevents adhesions and soft tissue contraction in the healing stage (Figure 15 a-c).

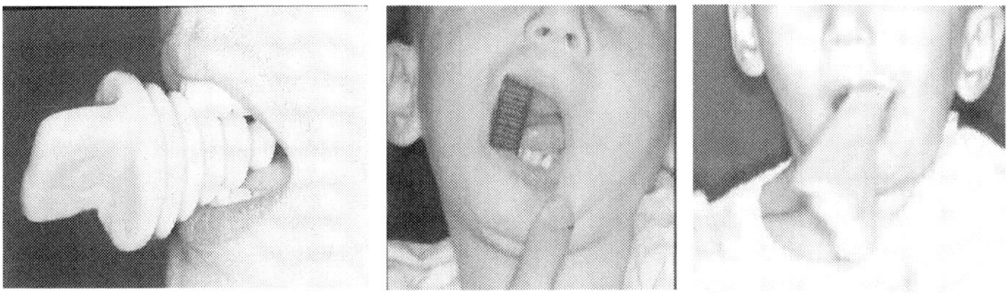

a b c

Figure 15. a-c) Adjunctive physiotherapy appliances that are used as aiding appliances during the physiotherapy phase.

9. Additional corrective surgery at the later stages when growth is completed

Recurrence of ankylosis and restricted mandibular movement are the most common complications after surgical management of the ankylotic mass. Following surgical protocol and also adequate compliance with postoperative adjunctive therapy might prevent these complications [31]. The final postoperative result is dependent directly on the selected surgical procedure, surgical technique, and attention to postsurgical physiotherapy.

4.1.1. Treatment

4.1.1.1. Unilateral condylar ankylosis

A 5-year-old girl with a history of left condylar trauma at age 2, with progressive facial asymmetry and deviation of the dental midlines due to left condylar ankylosis (Figure 16 a). There was no history of any other congenital malformation or childhood illness. On clinical examination her jaw deviated slightly to the left on closure and showed limited right lateral excursion. The ankylotic mass of the left condyle was demonstrated clearly on the MRI (Figure 16 b). An autogenous costochondral graft to reconstruct the left condyle had been done at age 5, which left an intraoperative open bite on the left side (Figure 16 c, d). A removable functional hybrid appliance was provided for the patient immediately after surgery to maintain the graft in a suitable position and let the posterior teeth on contralateral side erupt. This appliance opened the bite on the left side and brought the chin to the midline (Figure 16 e). The patient cooperated very well in the postsurgical phase with removable appliance and functional exercises of the jaws. One year after the orthodontic phase, the patient demonstrated an acceptable occlusion and facial symmetry (Figure 16 f).

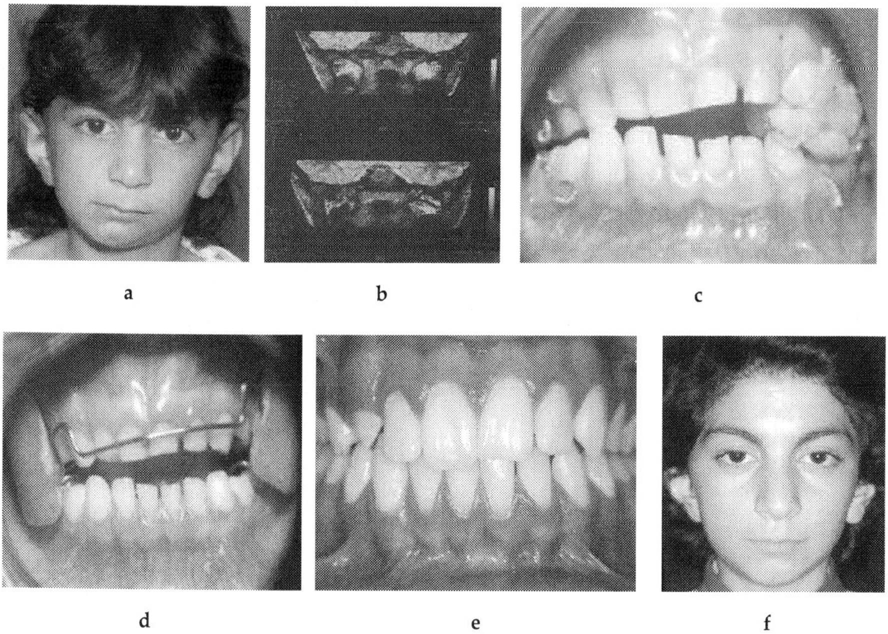

Figure 16. a) Facial view of a 5 year-old boy, b) MRI before any orthodontic intervention, c) postoperative openbite immediately after surgery to free the ankylotic condyle, d) Insertion of a hybrid functional appliance for differential dental eruption, e) occlusion of the patient. The remarkable improvement from unilateral condylar ankylosis and subsequent normal symmetric growth of facial structure was achieved. The functional appliance was also worn at night during the growth period. f) Final facial view

4.2. Management of temporomandibular joint ankylosis combined with severe dentofacial deformity

Patients with a history of persistent ankylosis usually demonstrate significant facial asymmetry. In addition to previously described surgery to release the ankylotic mass, these patients usually should undergo a second procedure to compensate developed facial asymmetries. This second procedure can range from a conservative genioplasty to orthognathic surgery of both jaws. Recently, distraction osteogenesis has become popular as another possible treatment option for the second phase [36]. However, precise monitoring of the distraction direction is an important consideration during this procedure. The final result of the distraction osteogenesis must be maintained via help of other functional appliances in growing patients [37]. Other adjunctive cosmetic surgical techniques like fat injection also can be applied to compensate the remaining asymmetry of the face [30].

Surgical treatment with costochondral graft (CCG) and distraction osteogenesis (DO) in cases with temporomandibular joint ankylosis associated with severe dentofacial deformities is usually effective and quite reliable (Figure 17 a,b). Most of the assigned patients had significant mandibular retrognathia and asymmetry. Distraction usually started on day 7 after surgery.

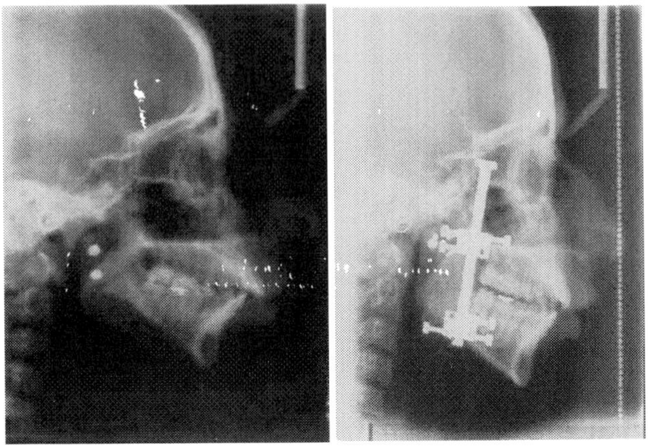

Figure 17. A case with unilateral distraction osteogenesis after receiving costochondral graft. Lateral cephalometry of the patient before (left) and after (right) distractor insertion.

4.2.1. Treatment

4.2.1.1. Bilateral condylar ankylosis

A 21-year-old male with a history of trauma at age 9, presented severe mandibular deficiency, micrognathia with restricted excursive and protrusive mandibular movement secondary to bilateral condylar ankylosis (Figure 18 a). The dental history of the patient revealed that, he had previously undergone an autogenous costochondral graft after bilateral condylectomy one year later, but re-ankylosis occurred. This whole procedure was repeated again one year after failure; however it did not fully address the patient's problem.

The treatment plan was to lengthen the mandible with bilateral distraction osteogenesis, which could advance the soft tissue volume simultaneously. Orthodontic treatment including extraction of first premolars on both sides due to preparation of adequate overjet was conducted on both sides. The extraction space was subsequently closed with moderate anchorage on both sides. Circumferential osteotomies were done on both side of the ramus and unilateral extraoral distractors (multiguided Leibinger) and were fixed in place (Figure 18 b). Considering the asymmetric representation of mandibular retrusion, the amount of mandibular advancement in the distraction phase was not equal on the right and left sides. During distraction phase, posterior open bite developed on the right side which was corrected by continuous application of cross elastic traction via fixed orthodontics (Figure 18 c). Upper and lower Hawley retainers with embedded wire on the occlusal surface of the upper posterior teeth were provided for the patient after finishing orthodontic treatment.

http://dx.doi.org/10.5772/59165

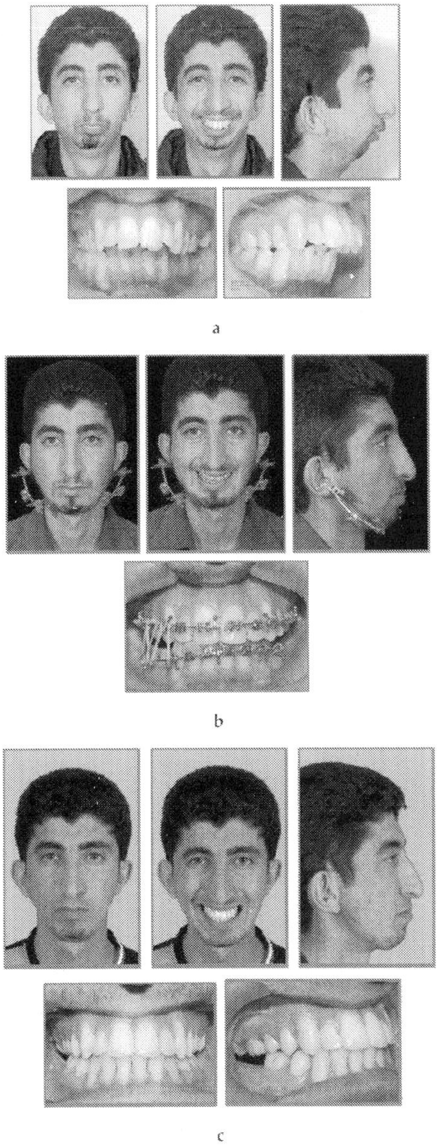

Figure 18. a) Pre-distraction facial and intraoral appearance. Significant mandibular deficiency is apparent. b) Circumferential osteotomies were made at the body of the right and left ramus and then custom-made unidirectional extraoral distractors were fixed in place. The mandible was advanced by 7 mm. The posterior open bite was created at the right side as a result of mandibular lengthening. Orthodontic triangle elastics were used concomitant with fixed orthodontic appliance to manage the posterior right open bite. c) Frontal facial view after debonding.

5. Complications after surgery

Although significant complications in the postoperative phase subsequent to surgery are not dramatic, it varies from mild pain to more serious persisting pain with restricted jaw movement and re-ankylosis. These unexpected adverse events and complications after surgery are mostly divided into two broad categories; those related to re-ankylosis and those related to the overgrowth of the cartilaginous autograft [38].

In the literature, there are two main reasons for re-ankylosis after surgical release including inadequate resection of the ankylotic mass intraoperatively and also, absence of patient compliance regarding post-operative jaw exercises [39-40]. The higher rate of reported re-ankylosis in children comparing to adults may be due to poor compliance to aggressive post-operative physiotherapy [4]. Complete diagnostic assessment of the ankylotic area, based on preoperative imaging examinations, is necessary to determine the extent of bony fusion and the length of the coronoid process on both sides [38]. The extent of bony fusion in both sagittal and coronal planes should be studied carefully to prevent any serious complication of facial nerve and maxillary artery injuries. Adequate mouth opening must be checked intraoperatively as a clinical indicator of successful surgery. Further ipsilateral or contralateral coronoidectomy with or without soft tissue release may need to be performed to achieve required mouth opening [38]. Growth behavior of inserted grafts including under and overgrowth may also present some complications in later stages of treatment. The role of jaw mobility exercises at home and at physiotherapy in prevention of re-ankylosis cannot be over-emphasized in children or adults. The preventive approach should be strict adhesion to surgical protocol and post-operative physiotherapy requirements, monitored by both the orthodontist and surgeon (Figure 19).

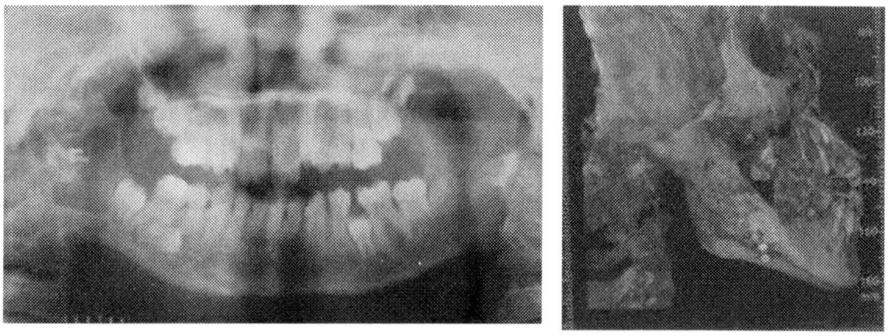

a b

Figure 19. a) Panoramic radiograph of re-ankylosis after previous costochondral grafting b) 3D CT showing complete bony ankylosis of the right condyle.

However, if the re-ankylosis occurs, the best option for its management depends directly on the type of ankylosis. Bony re-ankylosis needs additional surgical procedures. Fibrosis re-ankylosis may be managed by means of progressive jaw mobility exercises that can be delivered through different approaches. Some removable appliances may help clinicians overcome this problem (Figure 20 a-d). If the patient cannot comply with these techniques, the surgeon should help them by initiating physiotherapy under local anesthesia.

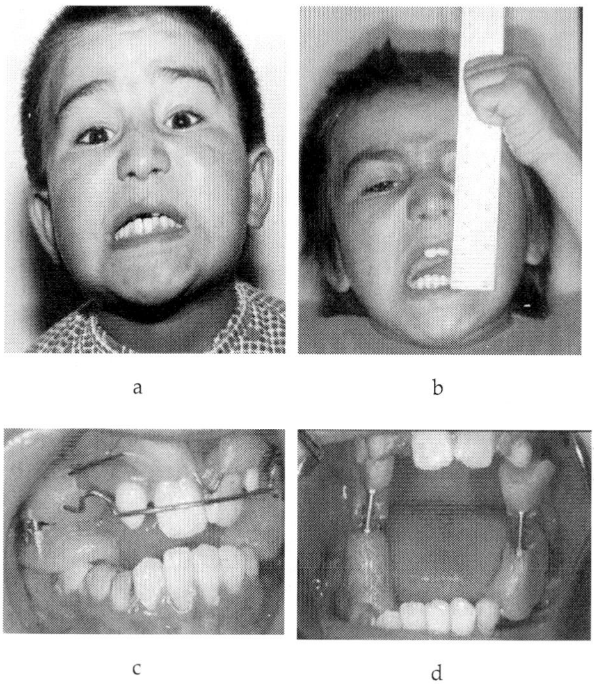

Figure 20. A 5-year-old with bilateral condylar ankylosis following a traumatic event. He underwent a surgical procedure to release the ankylotic condyles, which involved bilateral coronoidectomy also, a) Restricted opening secondary to re-ankylosis, b) Intraoral appliance consisting of labial pads, and acrylic posterior bite plates that incorporate two vertical-direction screws, c) The patient was asked to open the screw once a day, d) Because of the fibrosis type of ankylosis, the patient was able to open his mouth significantly more after treatment.

5.1. Treatment

5.1.1. Unilateral condylar overgrowth

A 29-year-old man was seen for treatment of severe facial asymmetry secondary to right condylar overgrowth (Figure 21 a-e). There was a history of TMJ ankylosis of the right condyle at age 3. Three years later, the patient underwent an autogenous costochondral graft to reconstruct the right mandibular condyle. The condylar structure was composed of the cartilage part of rib graft. As reported by the patient, the condylar overgrowth initiated approximately four years after graft surgery, when he was 10 years old, which lead to a marked facial asymmetry. On clinical examination there was chin deviation and midline divergence (mandibular dental midline shift). On functional evaluation of the patient, there was a significant restriction on full range of anterior and transverse jaw motion, with deviation upon opening. The treatment plan was to remove the condylar overgrowth through a preauricular incision (Figure 21 f, g). Postoperative facial photography and panoramic view showed significant improvement in facial symmetry at 18 month follow up (Figure 21 h-k).

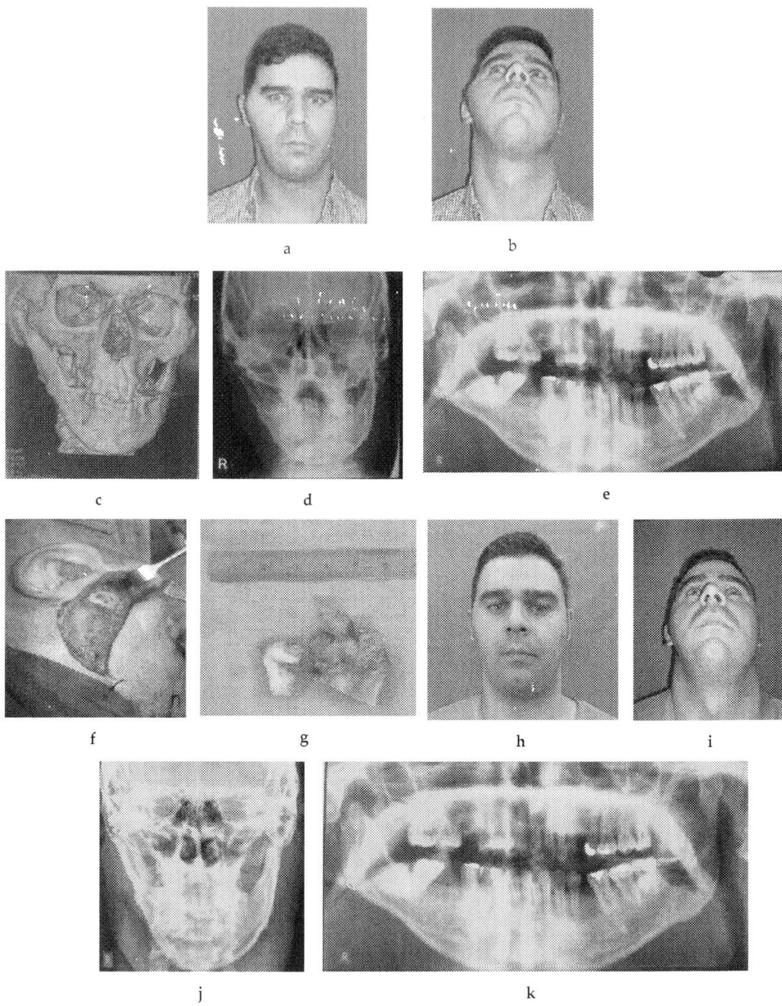

Figure 21. Male aged 29 years, a,b) severe facial asymmetry secondary to right condylar overgrowth is apparent, c-e) 3D computed tomography, posteroanterior and panoramic radiographs of the patient before surgical procedure, f) intra-operative view of the right condylar overgrowth mass, g) excess part of overgrowth of the condyle. h,i) postoperative clinical appearance of the patient after surgical removal of condylar overgrowth mass, j,k) Final posteroanterior and panoramic radiographs of the patient following 18 months follow up.

http://dx.doi.org/10.5772/59165

Acknowledgements

The authors thank staff of Orthodontic, Pediatric and Oral and Maxillofacial Surgery departments for general support and treatment procedures of the presented cases.

Author details

Hossein Behnia[1*], Azita Tehranchi[2] and Farnaz Younessian[3]

*Address all correspondence to: behnia_h@hotmail.com

1 Dentofacial Deformity Research Center, Research Institute of Dental Sciences, Department of Oral and Maxillofacial Surgery, School of Dentistry, Shahid Beheshti University of Medical Sciences, Tehran, Iran

2 Dental Research Center, Research Institute of Dental Sciences, Department of Orthodontics, School of Dentistry, Shahid Beheshti University of Medical Sciences, Tehran, Iran

3 Dentofacial Deformity Research Center, Research Institute of Dental Sciences, School of Dentistry, Shahid Beheshti University of Medical Sciences, Tehran, Iran

References

[1] Ingawalé S, Goswami T. Temporomandibular joint: disorders, treatments, and biomechanics. Annals of biomedical engineering. 2009;37(5):976-96.

[2] Oztan HY, Ulusal BG, Aytemiz C. The role of trauma on temporomandibular joint ankylosis and mandibular growth retardation: an experimental study. Journal of Craniofacial Surgery. 2004;15(2):274-82.

[3] Long X, Li X, Cheng Y, Yang X, Qin L, Qiao Y, et al. Preservation of disc for treatment of traumatic temporomandibular joint ankylosis. Journal of oral and maxillofacial surgery. 2005;63(7):897-902.

[4] Kaban LB, Perrott DH, Fisher K. A protocol for management of temporomandibular joint ankylosis. Journal of Oral and Maxillofacial Surgery. 1990;48(11):1145-51.

[5] Guralnick W, Kaban L. Surgical treatment of mandibular hypomobility. Journal of oral surgery (American Dental Association: 1965). 1976;34(4):343-8.

[6] Topazian R. Etiology of ankylosis of temporomandibular joint: analysis of 44 cases. Journal of oral surgery, anesthesia, and hospital dental service. 1964;22:227-33.

[7] Sawhney CP. Bony ankylosis of the temporomandibular joint: follow-up of 70 patients treated with arthroplasty and acrylic spacer interposition. Plastic and reconstructive surgery. 1986;77(1):29.

[8] Behnia H, Shamse MG. Congenital unilateral fusion of the mandibular and maxillary alveolar ridges, temporomandibular joint, and coronoid process: A case report. Journal of oral and maxillofacial surgery. 1996;54(6):773-6.

[9] Deckers MM, van Bezooijen RL, van der Horst G, Hoogendam J, van der Bent C, Papapoulos SE, et al. Bone morphogenetic proteins stimulate angiogenesis through osteoblast-derived vascular endothelial growth factor A. Endocrinology. 2002;143(4): 1545-53.

[10] Salins PC. New perspectives in the management of cranio-mandibular ankylosis. International Journal of Oral & Maxillofacial Surgery. 2000;29(5):337-40.

[11] Zhang Y, He D. Clinical investigation of early post-traumatic temporomandibular joint ankylosis and the role of repositioning discs in treatment. International journal of oral and maxillofacial surgery. 2006;35(12):1096-101.

[12] Chossegros C, Guyot L, Cheynet F, Blanc J, Cannoni P. Full-thickness skin graft interposition after tempormomandibular joint ankylosis surgery. International Journal of Oral & Maxillofacial Surgery. 1999;28(5):330-4.

[13] Engel MB. Condylar growth and mandibular deformities. The Angle Orthodontist. 1948;18(3):132-4.

[14] Manganello-Souza L, Mariani P. Temporomandibular joint ankylosis: report of 14 cases. International journal of oral and maxillofacial surgery. 2003;32(1):24-9.

[15] El-Sheikh M, Medra A, Warda M. Bird face deformity secondary to bilateral temporomandibular joint ankylosis. Journal of Cranio-Maxillofacial Surgery. 1996;24(2): 96-103.

[16] Su-Gwan K. Treatment of temporomandibular joint ankylosis with temporalis muscle and fascia flap. International journal of oral and maxillofacial surgery. 2001;30(3): 189-93.

[17] Zide MF, Kent JN. Indications for open reduction of mandibular condyle fractures. Journal of Oral and Maxillofacial Surgery. 1983;41(2):89-98.

[18] Nacht JL, Ecker ML, Chung SM, Lotke PA, Das M. Supracondylar fractures of the humerus in children treated by closed reduction and percutaneous pinning. Clinical orthopaedics and related research. 1983;177:203-9.

[19] Brandt MT, Haug RH. Open versus closed reduction of adult mandibular condyle fractures: a review of the literature regarding the evolution of current thoughts on management. Journal of Oral and Maxillofacial Surgery. 2003;61(11):1324-32.

[20] Boffano P, Benech R, Gallesio C, Arcuri F, Benech A. Current Opinions on Surgical Treatment of Fractures of the Condylar Head. Craniomaxillofacial Trauma and Reconstruction. (EFirst).

[21] Tehranchi A, Behnia H, Younessian F, Ghochani MS. Rapid, conservative, multidisciplinary miniscrew-assisted approach for treatment of mandibular fractures following plane crash. Dental research journal. 2013;10(5):678.

[22] Rishiraj B, McFadden LR. Treatment of temporomandibular joint ankylosis: a case report. Journal-Canadian Dental Association. 2001;67(11):659-63.

[23] Norman JE. Ankylosis of the temporomandibular joint. Australian dental journal. 1978;23(1):56-66.

[24] Moorthy AP, Finch L. Interpositional arthroplasty for ankylosis of the temporomandibular joint. Oral Surgery, Oral Medicine, Oral Pathology. 1983;55(6):545-52.

[25] Roychoudhury A, Parkash H, Trikha A. Functional restoration by gap arthroplasty in temporomandibular joint ankylosis: a report of 50 cases. Oral Surgery, Oral Medicine, Oral Pathology, Oral Radiology, and Endodontology. 1999;87(2):166-9.

[26] Erdem E, Alkan A. The use of acrylic marbles for interposition arthroplasty in the treatment of temporomandibular joint ankylosis: follow-up of 47 cases. International journal of oral and maxillofacial surgery. 2001;30(1):32-6.

[27] Tehranchi A, Behnia H. Treatment of mandibular asymmetry by distraction osteogenesis and orthodontics: a report of four cases. The Angle Orthodontist. 2000;70(2): 165-74.

[28] Lindqvist C, Pihakari A, Tasanen A, Hampf G. Autogenous costochondral grafts in temporomandibular joint arthroplasty: A survey of 66 arthroplasties in 60 patients. Journal of maxillofacial surgery. 1986;14:143-9.

[29] Saeed N, Kent J. A retrospective study of the costochondral graft in TMJ reconstruction. International journal of oral and maxillofacial surgery. 2003;32(6):606-9.

[30] Dimitroulis G. The interpositional dermis-fat graft in the management of temporomandibular joint ankylosis. International journal of oral and maxillofacial surgery. 2004;33(8):755-60.

[31] Topazian RG. Comparison of gap and interposition arthroplasty in the treatment of temporomandibular joint ankylosis. Journal of oral surgery (American Dental Association: 1965). 1966;24(5):405-9.

[32] Ko E, Chen M, Hsu M, Huang E, Lai S. Intraoral approach for arthroplasty for correction of TMJ ankylosis. International journal of oral and maxillofacial surgery. 2009;38(12):1256-62.

[33] Ferretti C, Bryant R, Becker P, Lawrence C. Temporomandibular joint morphology following post-traumatic ankylosis in 26 patients. International journal of oral and maxillofacial surgery. 2005;34(4):376-81.

[34] Goss AN, Bosanquet AG. The arthroscopic appearance of acute temporomandibular joint trauma. Journal of Oral and Maxillofacial Surgery. 1990;48(8):780-3.

[35] Behnia H, Motamedi MHK, Tehranchi A. Use of activator appliances in pediatric patients treated with costochondral grafts for temporomandibular joint ankylosis: analysis of 13 cases. Journal of oral and maxillofacial surgery. 1997;55(12):1408-14.

[36] Behnia H, Tehranchi A, Morad G. Distraction Osteogenesis. 2013.

[37] Tehranchi A, Behnia H. Facial symmetry after distraction osteogenesis and orthodontic therapy. American Journal of Orthodontics and Dentofacial Orthopedics. 2001;120(2):149-53.

[38] Jagannathan M, Munoli AV. Unfavourable results in temporomandibular joint ankylosis surgery. Indian journal of plastic surgery: official publication of the Association of Plastic Surgeons of India. 2013;46(2):235.

[39] Arakeri G, Kusanale A, Zaki GA, Brennan PA. Pathogenesis of post-traumatic ankylosis of the temporomandibular joint: a critical review. British Journal of Oral and Maxillofacial Surgery. 2012;50(1):8-12.

[40] Kaban LB, Bouchard C, Troulis MJ. A protocol for management of temporomandibular joint ankylosis in children. Journal of Oral and Maxillofacial Surgery. 2009;67(9):1966-78.

Section 8

Diagnosis and Management of Frontal Sinus Fractures

Chapter 20

Contemporary Management of Frontal Sinus Injuries and Frontal Bone Fractures

Petr Schütz, Hussein Hassan Hamed Ibrahim and Bashar Rajab

Additional information is available at the end of the chapter

http://dx.doi.org/10.5772/59096

1. Introduction

Frontal bone (FB) fractures are found in about 12% of craniomaxillofacial trauma patients. [1, 2] They are more strongly associated with concomitant brain injuries than other facial fractures, which is the reflection of the amount of energy required to produce a fracture in this region. Recently, increase in the incidence of FB fractures was reported, while the incidence of fractures of other facial sites decreased. [3] This increase in frontal bone fractures (FBFs) incidence may be related to the emergence of causes other than road traffic accidents (RTAs), especially all terrain vehicle (ATV) accidents. The aims of FBF treatment are restoration of facial appearance, restoration of skull integrity and protection of brain, and prevention of late complications. The most important factor in management of FBF is involvement of frontal sinus (FS). Despite the relative frequency of FS injuries, there is no general consensus about their optimal management and numerous treatment algorithms were published during the recent years. The purpose of this chapter is to provide an overview of advances in surgical management of traumatized FS and to share our experience with this type of injury.

2. Development and growth of the frontal bone

Ossification of the intra-membranous calvarial bones depends on the presence of the brain; in its absence (anencephaly), no bony calvarium forms. A pair of FBs appears from single primary ossification centers, forming in the region of each superciliary arch at the 8th week post-conception. Three pairs of secondary centers appear later in the zygomatic processes, nasal spine and trochlear fossae. Fusion between these centers is complete at 6 to 7 months post-conception. At birth, the frontal bones are separated by the metopic suture. Synostotic fusion of this suture usually starts about the 2nd year and unites the frontal bones into a single bone by 7 years of age. The metopic suture persists into adulthood in 10 to 15% of skulls. In such cases, the frontal sinuses are absent or hypoplastic. [4]

The cranial and facial bones are first made of fibrous connective tissue. In the third month of fetal development, fibroblasts become more specialized and differentiate into osteoblasts, which produce bone matrix. From each center of ossification, bone growth radiates outward as calcium salts are deposited in the collagen model of the bone. This process is not complete at birth; a baby has areas of fibrous connective tissue remaining between the bones of the skull. These are called fontanels, which permit compression of the baby's head during birth without breaking the still thin cranial bones. The fontanels also permit the growth of the brain after birth. By the age of 2 years, all the fontanels have become ossified. [5]

Growth of the calvarial bones is a combination of suture growth, surface apposition and resorption (remodeling), and centrifugal displacement by the expanding brain. The proportions attributable to the various growth mechanisms vary by age. Accretion to the calvarial bones is predominantly sutural until about the 4th year of life, after which surface apposition and remodeling become increasingly important.

The bones of the newborn calvarium are unilaminar and lack diploë. From about 4 years of age, lamellar compaction of cancellous trabeculae forms the inner and outer tables of the cranial bones. The tables become continuously more distinct into adulthood. This differential bone structure creates a high stiffness - to - weight ratio, with no relative increase in the mineral content of cranial bone from birth to adulthood. Whereas the behavior of the inner table is related primarily to the brain and intracranial pressures, the outer table is more responsive to extracranial muscular and buttressing forces. The internal plate becomes stable at 6 to 7 years of age, reflecting the near cessation of cerebral growth. The thickening of the frontal bone in the midline at the glabella results from separation of the inner and outer tables with invasion of the FS between the cortical plates. Growth of the external plate during childhood produces the superciliary arches and other bony landmarks that are all absent in the neonatal skull. [4]

FS is a small out-pouching at birth and undergoes almost all of its development thereafter. The FS may develop from one or several different sites (primary pneumatization): as a rudiment of the ethmoid air cells, as a mucosal pocket in or near the frontal recess, as an invagination of the frontal recess, or from the superior middle meatus. The process starts 3 to 4 months post conception, but they do not yet invade the frontal bone. Secondary pneumatization takes place between the ages of 6 months to 2 years postnatally and it develops laterally and vertically. FS itself cannot be identified radiographically until approximately the age of 6 to 8 years, and most pneumatization is completed by the time the child is 12 to 16 years- old, but it continues until the age of 40. [4,6] In 10% of persons, FS develops unilaterally, in 5% it is a rudimentary structure, and in 4% it is absent altogether, so that almost one-fifth of individuals have aberrant sinus development (Figure 1).[7]

http://dx.doi.org/10.5772/59096

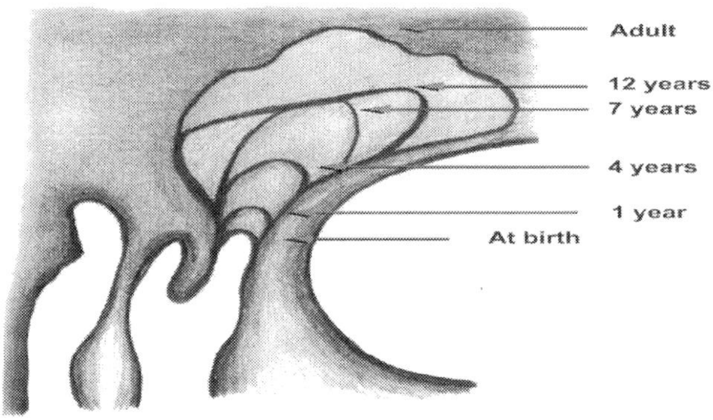

Figure 1. Postnatal development of the frontal sinus.

3. Frontal bone anatomy

The frontal bone forms the forehead and the anterior part of the top of the skull, the anterior cranial fossa and the roofs of the orbits. It consists of two parts, vertical called the squamous part and horizontal called the orbital part. From the nasion FB extends approximately 12.5 cm superiorly, 8.0 cm laterally, and 5.5 cm posteriorly. [8]

The squamous part has a convex outer surface which forms the main substance of the forehead and the anterior part of the vault of the skull. The squamous part of FB has the nasal notch which articulates with the nasal bone on either side of the middle line and more laterally with the frontal process of maxilla and with the lacrimal bone. The squamous part of the frontal bone consists of two layers of compact bone separated by a layer of cancellous bone (the diploë) which contains red bone marrow and a number of diploic veins.

Its outer surface shows the following features:

Frontal eminences are the most prominent parts of FB.

Superciliary arches, thick curved ridges lie little above the medial portions of the supraorbital margins. They are well developed in males and less marked or even totally absent in females.

Supraorbital margins, which form the upper boundaries of the orbits, end laterally at each side in the zygomatic processes of the FB. They have the supraorbital notches at the junctions of the middle and intermediate thirds. In some cases there may be foramina instead of notches. Supratrochlear foramina are located medially to the supraorbital foramina or notches and laterally to the nasal bones. The smooth area of the frontal bone just above the root of the nose is called the glabella. Temporal line, a well-marked ridge, runs from the zygomatic process of FB upward and backward (Figure 2).

The inner surface of the squamous part is concave and forms the anterior cranial fossa.

The sagittal groove lies in the upper part of the middle line. The two edges of this groove unite below to form a ridge - the frontal crest. The sagittal groove accommodates the anterior part of the venous superior sagittal sinus.

The frontal crest gives attachment to the falx cerebri, a fold of dura matter. The frontal crest ends below in a small hole called the foramen caecum between the frontal and the ethmoid bone. The foramen caecum does not usually transmit any structure but may transmit a vein from the nose to the superior sagittal sinus. [5, 8, 9]

The orbital parts of the FB extend laterally from the nasal notch, become concave and form the orbital roofs. A spine or concavity exists along the medial anterior orbital roof, where the trochlea of the superior oblique muscle is attached. The arched roofs of the orbits are separated from one another by a median gap called the ethmoid notch. In the intact skull the ethmoid notch is filled by the cribriform plate of ethmoid bone. The margins of the ethmoid notch of the frontal bone contain many half cells which unite with corresponding half cells on the upper surface of the ethmoid bone to form together the ethmoid air cells (Figure 2).

The frontal bone articulates with 12 other cranial bones: two parietals, two nasals, two maxillae, two lacrimal, two zygomatic, the sphenoid and the ethmoid. The bones are separated by sutures which hold the bones firmly together in the mature skull. Occasionally the squamous part of FB may be separated into two halves by a midline metopic suture persistent from early childhood. Normally, two halves of the frontal bone unite completely by the 8th year.

The arterial blood supply to the frontal bone is by the supraorbital, anterior superficial temporal, anterior cerebral and middle meningeal arteries. The venous drainage is transosseous through the anastomosis of vessels of the subcutaneous, orbital, and intracranial structures. The primary venous drainage is through the supratrochlear, supraorbital, superficial temporal, frontal diploic (veins of Breschet), superior ophthalmic, and superior sagittal sinuses. [4, 10, 11]

The frontal sinus may consist of one or more compartments, depending on the source of pneumatization. The inter-sinus septum, which separates the left and right cavities of the sinus, is continuous with the crista galli and cribriform plate inferiorly. The septum is usually deviating from the midline sagittal plane. FSs vary in size in different people. The average height of the sinuses is 32 mm, and their average width is 26 mm. The surface area is approximately 720 mm^2. [6-8, 12] The FS is in critical approximation to anatomical structures, which underscores the importance of its management in injury. Posteriorly, the cribriform plate, dura mater, and frontal lobes of brain are in close apposition to one another and to the posterior wall of the sinus. The dura is densely adherent to the deep surface of the posterior table and becomes more adherent and thinner along the caudal edge, where it turns to cover the fovea ethmoidalis. [13] The lateral floor of the FS is the roof of the orbit, whereas the medial floor of the frontal sinus contains the opening of the nasofrontal duct. Each sinus opens into the anterior part of the corresponding nasal middle meatus by the ethmoidal infundibulum or nasofrontal duct (NFD), traversing the anterior part of the ethmoid labyrinth. Anatomically significant variations exist in the width, length, and shape of the NFD. The duct opening usually lies in the posteromedial floor of the sinus. It is a funnel shaped constriction that passes between the

http://dx.doi.org/10.5772/59096

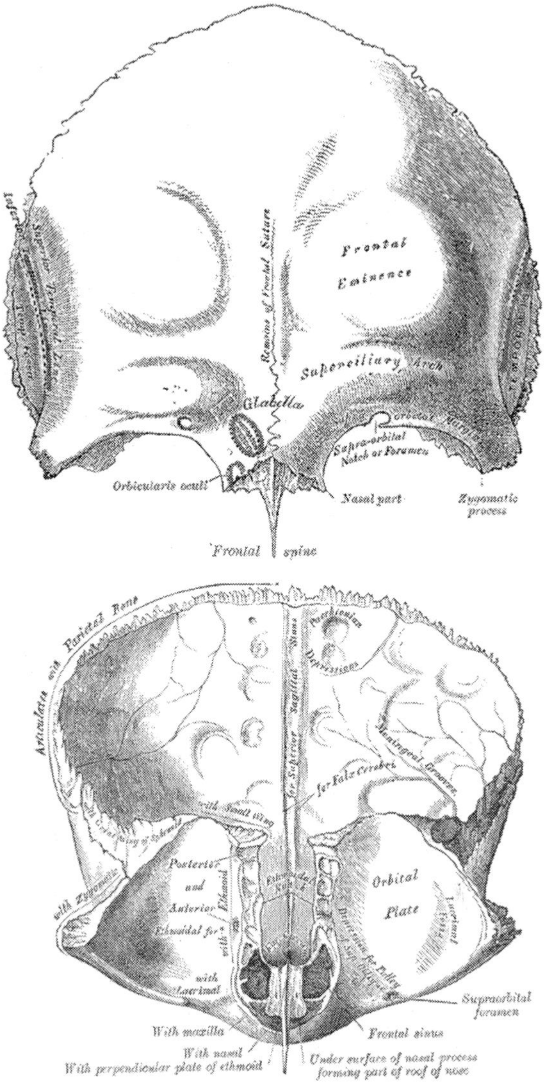

Figure 2. Frontal bone (Gray's Anatomy)

cancellous part of the anterior wall underlying the glabella and the anterior ethmoidal cells. Its course is highly variable, running caudally from a few millimeters to up to 2 cm. The NFD terminates at the uncinate process in the nasal cavity, which is a thin bone plate that is covered on either side by mucosa. When the uncinate process is attached to the lamina papyracea, the drainage is medial to the uncinate process through the middle meatus. This type of drainage pattern is seen in 66-88 % of cases. When the uncinate process attaches superiorly to more medial structures (middle turbinate, cribriform, or skull base), the drainage of the sinus is lateral to the uncinate process. This type of drainage pattern is seen in 12-34% of cases. A true identifiable duct may be absent in up to 85% of FSs. In this situation, the FS drains indirectly through ethmoid air cells to the middle meatus. Therefore, some investigators chose the term *nasofrontal outflow tract* (NFOT) or *frontal sinus outflow tract* (FSOT) for the drainage path of the FS (Figure 3). [7, 12-18]

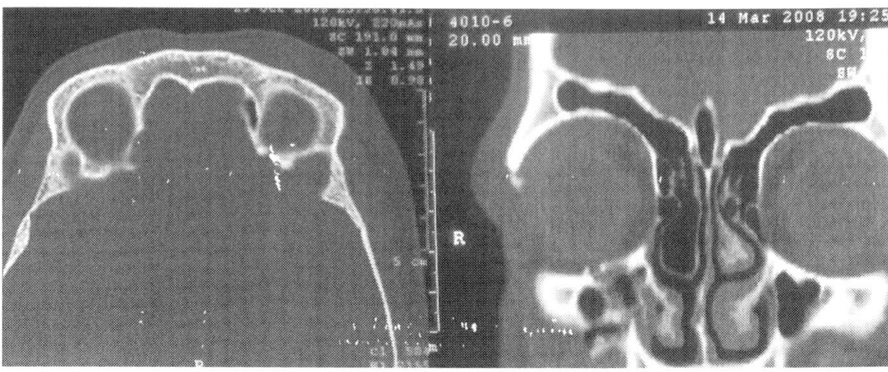

Figure 3. Opposite extremes of frontal sinus development; aplasia (left) versus hypertrophy (right).

4. Frontal sinus physiology

The mucosa of the frontal sinus consists of pseudostratified ciliated epithelium, mucus producing goblet cells, a thin basement membrane, and a thin lamina propria that contains seromucous glands. It covers the entire surface of the sinus and ranges in thickness from 0.07 to 2.0 mm. When the mucosa is healthy, a blanket of mucin overlies the epithelium. The cilia beat at 250 cycles/min. The mucin blanket flows in a spiral fashion in a medial-to-lateral direction; the flow is slowest at the roof and fastest at the NFD. The mucin empties at the NFD at a daily rate of 5.0 g/cm2. [14, 19, 20,]

The frontal sinus is unique in that it is the only sinus that has a recirculation phenomenon. The mucus travels along the lateral side of the sinus and turns medially over the sinus floor and down the lateral frontal recess wall. Of the secretion, 60% is directed back into the sinus cavity as it reaches the frontal recess. [13] Clinically significant anatomical structures of the mucosa of the frontal sinus are the foramina of Breschet, first described over 60 years ago. These foramina are sites of venous drainage of the mucosa and can serve as the route of intracranial spread of infection. The mucosa is found deeply penetrating these foramina. If mucosa is not completely removed microscopically from these foramina in obliteration or cranialization procedures, there is a high risk of mucocele formation. [13]

5. Frontal sinus pathology and concept of "safe sinus"

Pathology of FS is rare but most commonly is associated with trauma, which causes fracture of the frontal sinus walls.

Fractures of FS have many forms and a variety of classifications. Basically, they can be classified as anterior or posterior wall fractures. These fractures can be simple with no displacement, or complex displaced and comminuted with or without brain injury. Displaced anterior wall fracture usually leads to a simple aesthetic deformity. Posterior wall fracture usually results from high impact injury and bears a risk of placing the intracranial content in direct communication with the nasal cavity. A complicating factor is involvement of the NFOT. Its obstruction can lead to mucus retention and late infectious complications. [21]

A more detailed classification of the frontal sinus fractures which is suggested by many authors [22-25] and can be as follows:

Anterior wall fractures:

Anterior wall fractures with no displacement

Anterior wall fractures with displacement and intact FSOT.

Anterior wall fracture with displacement and FSOT injury.

Posterior wall fractures:

Posterior wall fracture without displacement and no cerebro-spinal fluid (CSF) leak.

Posterior wall fractures without displacement and positive CSF leak.

Posterior wall fracture with displacement and no CSF leak.

Posterior wall fracture with displacement and positive CSF leak.

Infection of the sinus, which causes sinusitis, may give rise to serious complications due to the proximity of FS to the cranial cavity, orbit, and nasal cavity. Complications can develop into orbital cellulitis, epidural abscess, subdural abscess, meningitis, and in long-term into mucopyocele.

Mucocele formation is a complication, which can develop years after trauma and the symptoms may go unnoticed for a long period of time. [26] Therefore it is desirable to treat injured FS in such way as to make it "safe". This means either to obliterate it completely including all mucosa lining, or to restore it to the functional state with unobstructed NFOT.

6. Diagnosis of frontal bone fracture

6.1. Physical examination

Findings suggestive of FBF include tenderness, paresthesia, forehead abrasions, lacerations, contour irregularities and hematoma. Forehead lacerations should be examined under sterile conditions to assess the integrity of the underlying bone. Through-and-through injuries of the frontal sinus have high morbidity, and prompt surgical treatment is indicated. Conscious patients should be questioned regarding the presence of watery rhinorrhea or salty-tasting postnasal dripping suspicious for CSF leak. Suspicious fluid can be grossly evaluated bedside with a "halo test". The bloody fluid is allowed to drip onto filter paper. If CSF is present, it will diffuse faster than blood and result in a clear halo around the blood. Glucose or β2-transferrin are the laboratory tests to confirm a CSF leak. [27]

6.2. Radiological examination

Plain radiographs do not adequately characterize FS fractures. Computed tomography (CT) is the gold standard for the assessment of FS injuries. Advances in the equipment used for CT imaging can now produce reformatted images of a very high quality. Patients are scanned in one axial plane, in a supine position with thin cut spiral CT, creating data set allowing generation of reformatted and reconstructed diagnostic images. Sagittal reconstructions can be made to evaluate the posterior wall defect. Special importance belongs to evaluation of the involvement and severity FSOT. [28]

Gross outflow tract obstruction (fracture fragments lying in the tract) can be observed in some cases. FSOT injury is strongly suggested when the CT scan demonstrates the involvement of the base of FS, the anterior ethmoid complex, or both. Fracture in the floor of the sinus can be seen best with sagittal and coronal views, anterior ethmoid cell injury with coronal more than axial views, and obstruction best with the coronal view (occasionally axial).Thus, the naso-frontal tract complex should be evaluated in the axial, coronal and sagittal planes. Unfortunately, the involvement of the FSOT is not always easily discernible with CT imaging. [16] Three-dimensional (3D) reconstructions may help to visualize the external contour deformity as well as associated facial skeleton injuries.

7. Historic development of operative methods

The evolvement of surgical methods dealing with diseased or injured FS is described in several publications. The following summary is based on synopsis of two of them [1, 13]. In the preantibiotic era frontal sinusitis and its complications were fearsome, with high morbidity and mortality secondary to intracranial spread. The first reported procedure on FS for a mucopyocele was performed by *Wells* in 1870. Operations of limited extent involved puncturing the anterior table, some with limited removal of the mucosa, packing of the sinus or creation of an external draining sinus tract.

In 1898 *Reidel* first described ablation of the anterior sinus wall. This radical, disfiguring operation involved removal of the frontal bone and supraorbital bar to the posterior table of the frontal sinus. *Killian* modified this approach in 1904 by preserving the supraorbital rims to improve the patient's appearance but still removing the anterior table and contents of FS and then collapsing the skin to the posterior table of FS. The Killian procedure produced less disfigurement but had significant rates of failure because of persistent disease at the nasofrontal ducts and incomplete removal of all FS mucosa. The next significant advance was the *Lynch* operation, described in 1921. The floor of FS and ethmoids were removed and the mucosa extirpated through a medial periorbital incision in an effort to re-establish drainage. Complete removal of the mucosa via this approach proved difficult. Disappointing results were also due to re-stenosis of NFD, either by scarring or by herniation of the orbital tissues into the created communication with the nasal cavity. Several modifications using stents and mucoperiosteal flaps were devised later in an attempt to maintain patency of this artificial conduit.

In 1955, *Bergara and Itoiz* described the osteoplastic approach, which consisted of first defining the extent of FS and then elevating the anterior sinus wall on an inferior pedicle of periosteum. This provided adequate surgical access to allow for visualization and complete removal of the sinus mucosa and obliteration of the remaining sinus with autologous free fat grafts. It also improved forehead cosmesis. The osteoplastic flap operation has been subsequently modified for use in trauma of the frontal sinus by elevating the pericranium with the scalp flap and exploring the frontal sinus by removal of the free bone fragments.

Later studies published by *Goodale* (1958) and *Montgomery* (1964) recognized the importance of NFD injury and popularized obliteration of FS with autologous fat. A variety of materials such as bone, muscle, fascia, and hydroxyapatite have been successfully used to obliterate the sinus cavity by later authors. In 1974, *Nadell and Kline* described a procedure to primarily reconstruct depressed frontal skull fractures involving the sinus and cribriform plates.

Donald and Bernstein (1982) described a cranialization, procedure in which the intracranial contents were isolated from the nose and the sinus was completely ablated. They validated this approach in a cat model by demonstrating respiratory mucosa regrowth and an infection rate of 44% with untreated posterior table defects.

8. Surgical approaches to frontal bone

8.1. Traumatic wounds

Only in exceptional cases an existing traumatic wound can be used to address an isolated fracture of the anterior FS wall. It can be considered in limited injuries without involvement of the FSOT and/or the medial orbital rim, in the absence of other associated regional craniofacial injuries (Figure 4). [13]

8.2. Coronal incision

The main purpose of coronal approach is to avoid visible facial scars. Coronal incision more or less follows the course of the coronal suture of the neurocranium, which joins FB to the parietal bones. Therefore in the literature frequently encountered term *bicoronal incision* is a misnomer, because there is just one coronal suture on the skull. Acceptable alternative term is *bitemporal incision*. The extent and design of the incision depends on the targeted anatomic area and intended surgical procedure. A fully developed coronal flap with preauricular or postauricular extensions provides access to FB, zygomatic arches, bodies of the zygomatic bones,

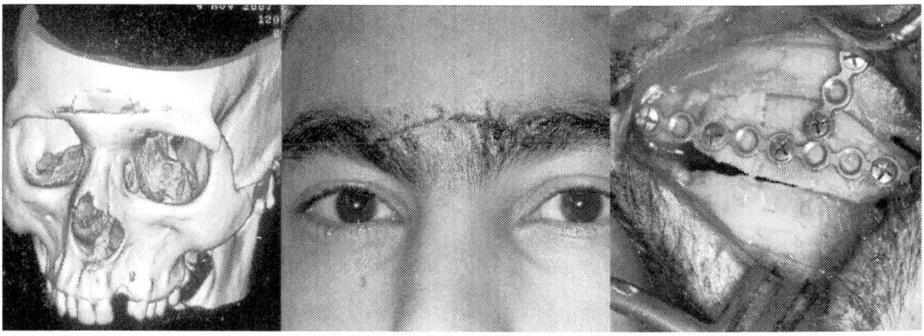

Figure 4. Industrial accident; re-opening of traumatic wound for fracture exposure

medial, superior and lateral orbital margins and much of the corresponding orbital walls, as well as nasal bones. Via preauricular extension it is possible to address the temporomandibular joint and the upper neck of the condylar process of the mandible. Coronal incision also allows harvesting of calvarial bone grafts. There is general agreement that it is not necessary to shave the hair, however shaving facilitates wound closure. In female patients with long hair, who are understandably more distressed by prospect of hair shaving, the hair can be divided by a comb and braided. Alternatively, 2 cm wide strip of shaven skin is sufficient. In consenting male patients there is no harm in a complete hair shave, which makes suturing of the flap much more comfortable and subsequent wound care easier and more hygienic (Figure 5).

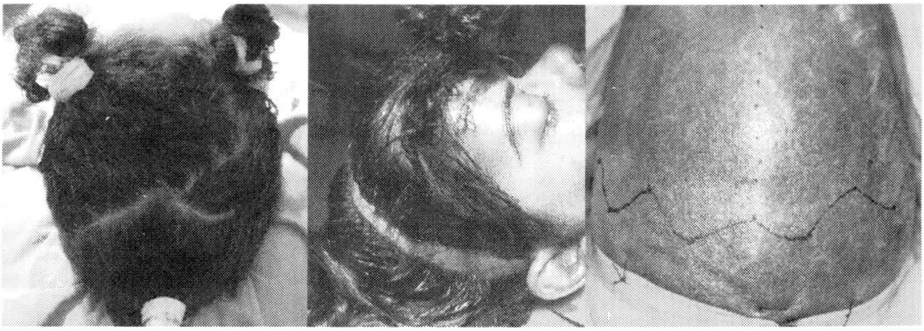

Figure 5. Scalp preparation for coronal incision: hair braiding, strip shaving and full head shave.

After proper skin disinfection and draping the planned line of incision is marked with a surgical pen. The incision line runs from ear to ear across the top of the head in either straight, anteriorly curved, sinusoid or zigzag fashion. There is always some hair loss in the incision line and the scar is much less prominent if it is not straight, especially in a patient with a short hair-cut and when the hair is wet (Figure 6).

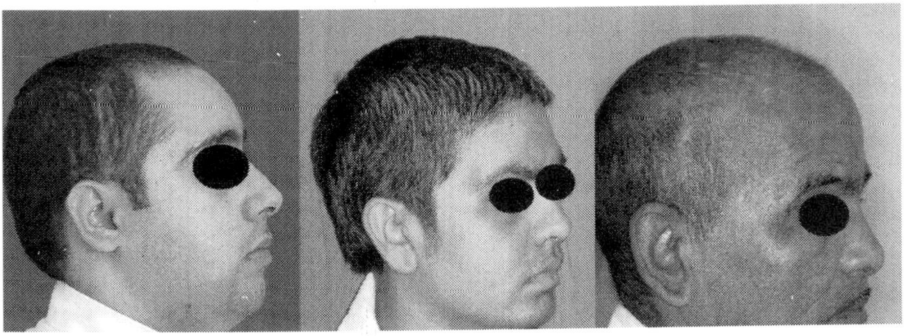

Figure 6. Straight incision is more prominent in closely cropped hair, while zigzag incision gives good results even in bald scalps.

The inferior extent of the incision depends on the target region. When desired exposure is limited FB, it is sufficient to confine the incision to the level of upper ear attachment. The placement of the incision line should take into consideration future balding patterns in men, and anterior migration of the scar due to growth of the cranium in young children. There is no advantage in placing the incision more ventrally, because the extent of exposure is given by the caudal extent of the incision: the lowest points define the axis around which the flap will rotate. Sufficient dorsal extension will also preserve the deep branch of the supraorbital nerve and avoid sensory loss behind a too-anteriorly placed incision. It is desirable to make the incision of the scalp parallel to the hair follicles. Avoiding the transection of hair follicles avoids alopecia at the edges of the wound. [13]

Vascularization of the scalp is very rich and due to the presence of subcutaneous fibrous septa the vessels gape and bleed profusely when cut. To reduce the initial bleeding and make establishment of the proper dissection level easier, the sub-galeal layer is infiltrated with saline or diluted local anesthetic with vasoconstrictor (e.g. adrenalin 1:200 000). The incision starts on the top of the head and progresses step by step latero-caudally to both sides, while arresting bleeding after each step. Hemostasis is mainly achieved by compression of wound margins by Raney clips, Tessier scalp clamps, or running interlocking silk sutures. Use of electrocautery should be minimized and only bipolar coagulation should be employed to protect hair follicles.

The three superficial layers of the scalp (skin, subcutaneous layer and galeal aponeurotica) make up one functional unit. [29] The incision penetrates through these layers and stops just above the pericranium inside the fourth layer of loose areolar tissue (subgalea fascia). Dissection inside this level is initially facilitated by undermining the incision line with a spreading hemostat. Below the superior temporal line the galea continues as temporoparietal fascia. The dissection should be kept below this fascia, just on the top of temporalis fascia, which can be identified as a tough white glistening layer. Branches of superficial temporal artery and vein are usually transected here and need to be ligated or cauterized. After the whole length of the incision has been developed to the proper depth, the scalp is pulled forward with a pair of cat paw retractors and the flap is dissected further by reverse cutting with a large blade until it can be turned inside out (Figure 7).

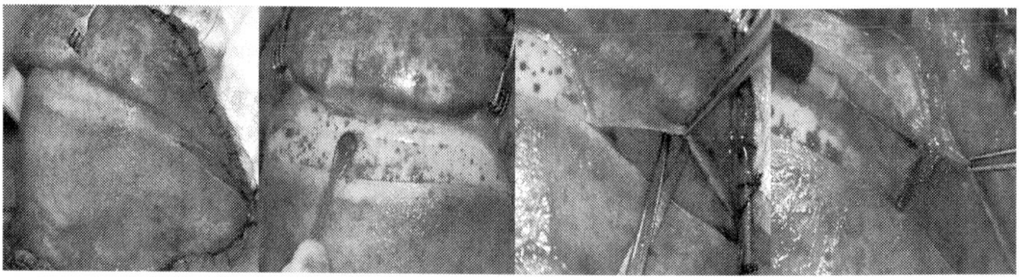

Figure 7. Dissection of coronal flap: subperiosteal dissection over top of skull, dissection under temporalis fascia below the level of the temporal line. In this case pericranial flap is not developed.

Anterior dissection progresses to the point where the base of the flap dissected so far reaches a 45º angle with the zygomatic arches. The temporal and zygomatic branches of the facial nerve leave the parotid gland and cross close to the periosteum of the zygomatic arch into the temporoparietal fascia, 15–28 mm ventral to the external acoustic meatus. [30] To protect them, further dissection in the temporal areas must continue under the temporalis fascia. The temporalis fascia is incised over the root of the zygoma and the incision progresses firstly through the external leaflet of fascia, just over the temporal fat pad. Above the line of fusion of external and deep layer of temporalis fascia the dissection progressed just above the temporalis muscle fibers, alongside the base of the developing flap, to the superior temporal line. At this point it is necessary to consider if a pericranial flap will be needed for anterior cranial fossa repair or sinus obliteration. If this is the case, its design must be incorporated into the periosteal dissection instead of cutting the periosteum straight across the frontal bone. If pericranial flap is not needed, right and left incisions in the temporalis fascia are connected by incising the pericranium between them. The forward dissection of the coronal flap continues in the subpericranial level, then subfascial level over the temporalis muscles and temporalis fat pads. The connection between the periosteum and temporalis fascia at the superior temporal line is firmly adherent to the underlying bone and requires sharp dissection, which is best done by diathermy in cutting mode (Figure 8).

When the dissection reaches the orbital margins, careful attention is paid to identification and freeing of the supraorbital neurovascular bundles. This is easy if only supraorbital notches are present. If the bundles pass through supraorbital foramina, these must be converted into notches by resecting the foramina's inferior margins with a fine chisel. The periosteum must be subsequently elevated beyond the orbital margin and inside the orbital cavity to allow free retraction of the flap. [31] The contentious point of the above described technique is the dissection in the temporal area. If the dissection proceeds as described, it jeopardizes innervation and vascularization of the temporal fat pad. It can lead to postoperative temporal hollowing as a consequence of a fat atrophy. [13] For this reason some authors prefer to keep the dissection completely above temporalis fascia, but "maintaining the integrity of tempor-

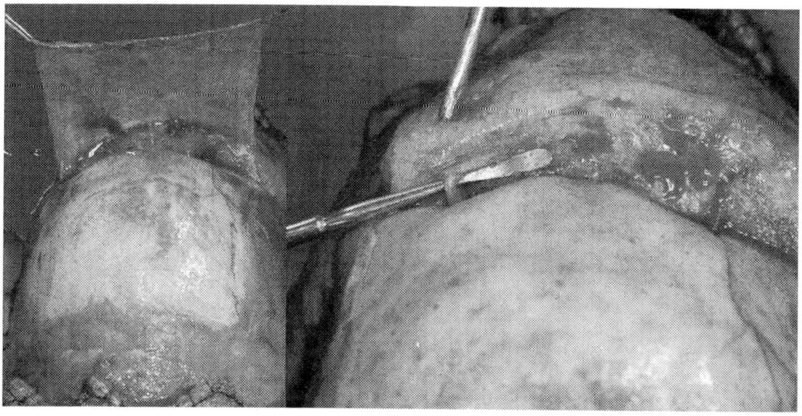

Figure 8. Elevation of pericranial flap and release of supraorbital nerve.

oparietal fascia" to protect the facial nerve branches. [32] To overcome this dilemma between jeopardizing either the facial nerve or temporal fat pad, *Luo et al.* recently described an alternative dissection technique: the supratemporalis approach. The temporal fascia was incised 5-6 cm up the zygomatic arch. The flap was composed of skin, subcutaneous fat, temporoparietal fascia, temporal fascia, and temporal fat pad on the surface of the temporalis muscle. The authors operated 40 cases with no temporal fossa depression observed in any of them. [33]

8.3. Alternative skin incisions

The coronal scalp approach provides excellent operative field exposure and results in a hidden scar. However, it is also associated with certain disadvantages and complications. These include longer operating times, increased blood loss, scalp hematoma, postoperative infection, a large scar with related alopecia, potential injury to the branches of the facial nerve with frontalis muscle paresis and brow ptosis, injury to auriculotemporal, supraorbital and supratrochlear nerves with numbness and paresthesia, parietal scalp pain, temporal fossa depression, scar irregularities and ptosis of facial soft tissues. [13, 34, 35] In attempts to avoid these problems different simplified methods of surgical access were reported for management of uncomplicated anterior table FS fractures. If the posterior table is involved then the technique is contraindicated. Also FSOT must be intact. Careful selection of patients is vital. A small skin incision can be made parallel to the margin of the eyebrow to approach the fracture. It is often possible to introduce a small periosteal elevator through the inferior edge of the fracture. If this is not possible, a 5 mm burr hole is created near or on the fracture site. A narrow periosteal elevator is introduced into FS and fracture is reduced with careful pressure. The bony opening may be used to confirm adequate reduction endoscopically. [34] A similar technique with wider exposure of fracture utilizes an upper blepharoplasty incision. [44] Another alternative approach is incision through the frontalis rhytid crease. [36]

9. Current operative methods of frontal sinus management

According to the clinical presentation of the fractures, treatment can range from reconstruction of the sinus walls to obliteration or cranialization. The degree of the displacement of the facture and the involvement of FSOT and/or the brain will determine the type of management of the fracture.

9.1. Reconstruction of frontal sinus

Common treatment for simple FS fracture without FSOT involvement requires adequate surgical exposure, an anatomic reduction and plating. Frontal sinus function and anatomy can be preserved this way in the majority of cases. [1]

9.1.1. Open methods

The surgical approach is usually through coronal incision or alternatively through existing lacerations if access is adequate. [37] After complete exposure of the fracture it is necessary to remove fragments of the anterior sinus wall to gain unobstructed access and to be able to evaluate integrity of posterior sinus wall, FSOT and sinus mucosa. In case of comminuted fracture with multiple fragments these can be lifted using periosteal elevator or small bone hook. Reduction of noncomminuted, compressed fractures can be challenging. When the convex surface of the frontal bone is fractured, it goes through a compression phase before it becomes concave. Fracture reduction requires enough force to pull the bone fragments back through the compression phase. [38] It may be necessary to remove bone from fracture line using cutting burr and widen it to gain enough space and relieve pressure for lifting of impacted fragment. It can be helpful to place a screw in the depressed segment, grasp it with a heavy hemostat, and pull upward - technique similar to use of Carrol-Girard screw for zygoma reduction. It is important to record orientation of removed fragments to prevent confusion during reassembly. Placing the fragments atop a drawing of the fracture will help to maintain the anatomic orientation of each fragment. Damaged or diseased mucosa of sinus should be removed as well as mucosa covering mobilized fragments, but intact mucosa should be left undisturbed.

FSOT can be visually evaluated and if there is doubt about its patency, it can be tested by application of flurescein or diluted methylene blue followed by inspection of nasal contents. Any suspicion of blockage of FSOT as evidenced by preoperative imaging studies or by intraoperative inspection and testing warrants treatment by sinus obliteration. Sinus preservation with duct reconstruction with the help of drainage tube or stent has been attempted in the past [39-41]. Unfortunately, a rate of stenosis of the duct following stent removal can be as high as 30%. [28] Recently there has been tendency to preserve and reconstruct sinuses despite injuries of FSOT with the help of endoscopic sinus surgery (ESS). [42]The final step is reassembly of fragments and reconstruction of anterior sinus wall using microplates or miniplates. Small gaps (4 to 10 mm) can be reconstructed with titanium mesh (Figure 9). [38]

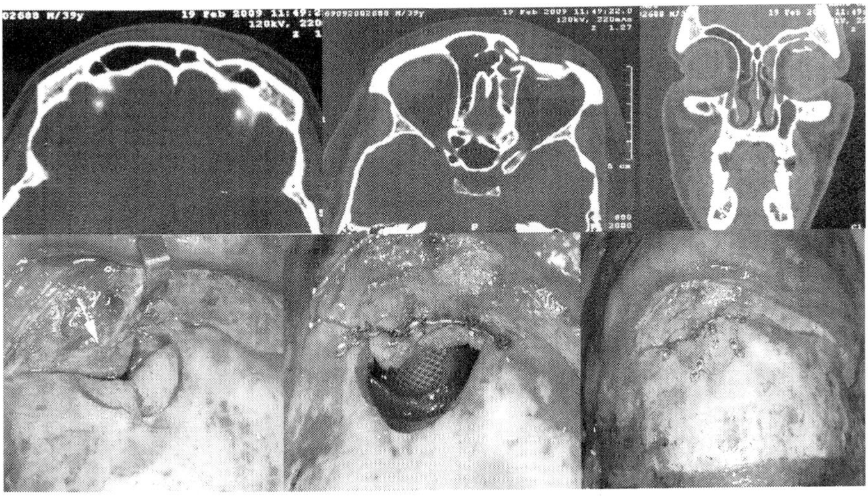

Figure 9. Fracture of FS with displacement of fragment into left orbit. Fragment is impinging on levator palpebrae superioris and displacing the globe. Reconstruction of orbital roof with titanium mesh after removal of the fragment.

9.1.2. Endoscopic methods

Throughout all surgical fields, less invasive approaches have been employed to decrease the potential morbidity of traditional open procedures. Endoscopic procedures and their applications for management of FS fractures allow for more conservative management and sinus preservation in selected patients. [43] Trephination and endoscopic visualization of FS can be useful to assess the frontal recess as well as the extent of any posterior table injury. Skin incision is placed midway between the medial canthus and the glabella and a small cutting burr is used to open a 4- to 5-mm frontal sinusotomy. The posterior table and nasofrontal recess can be examined with a 0-degree and/or 30-degree endoscope. A Valsalva maneuver can assist with the diagnosis of a CSF leak. [44, 45]

Shumrick reported on endoscopic reduction of FS fractures on 19 patients. The author's technique is similar endoscopic forehead lifting, with one central and two lateral hairline incisions. The forehead soft tissues are elevated subperiosteally, and the fractures are visualized by means of a 30-degree endoscope. An attempt is made to elevate the fragments with endoscopic elevators. However, it is usually necessary to approach the fragments directly through small forehead incisions (preferably hidden in the brow). The fractures are elevated using percutaneous nerve hooks, or by drilling into the fragments and grabbing them with threaded Steinmann pins. With gentle retraction, the fragments often elevate into a reduced position and are stable without the need for rigid fixation. Residual surface irregularities can be camouflaged with patches of Vicryl mesh. In four patients endoscopic fracture repair was unsuccessful, the fracture segments were unstable. These cases were converted to an open approach with coronal incisions and rigid fixation. The described technique is appropriate only for anterior wall FS fractures that have several large segments without extensive comminution. [44]

Alternative technique of endoscopic transnasal reduction in combination with balloon support has also been reported. [45]

Endoscopic technique can also be used for camouflage of cosmetic deformity resulting from untreated depressed anterior table FS fractures above the orbital rim. The repair is performed 2 to 4 months after the injury when all forehead swelling has resolved. A 3-5 cm parasagittal working incision should be placed above the fracture, 3 cm behind the hairline and carried through the periosteum onto bone. A 1-2 cm subperiosteal endoscope incision is then placed at the same height, 6 cm medial to the working incision. Using an endoscopic brow lift elevator and external palpation, subperiosteal dissection is performed down to the level of the fracture and the periosteum is carefully elevated over the defect. Once the limits of the fracture have been visualized, alloplastic implant is fitted to the defect and fixed with self-drilling screws transcutaneously. [38]

Another usage of endoscopic surgery is reestablishing of patency of compromised FSOT. The endoscopic surgery can be either part of primary FS management or can be kept in reserve for delayed FSOT recanalization, should the obstruction develop or not resolve postoperatively. [42, 45]

9.2. Obliteration of the frontal sinus

The principle of FS obliteration is turning it into self-contained cavity devoid completely of mucosa, including microscopic remnants and extensions into pits of Breschet, and filling it by choice of material, or leaving it empty for spontaneous ossification. After gaining satisfactory access through some of the above mentioned surgical approaches, the anterior wall of sinus is removed and preserved for later reconstruction. This can be achieved by careful removal of fractured fragments. It is important to record orientation of removed fragments to prevent confusion during reassembly. Placing the fragments atop a drawing of the fracture will help to maintain the anatomic orientation of each fragment. With incomplete fractures, it is often necessary to remove the intact remainder of the anterior table or to perform formal frontal sinusotomy. To keep the bone cut within the confine of FS and prevent violation of intracranial space, it is necessary to mark the extent of the sinus. This can be done using pre-prepared sterilized film cut out or tin template based on posteroanterior skull x-ray in Caldwell projection with the patient placed 1.8 meters (6 feet) from the x-ray tube. [46] Alternatively, one tine of a two-pronged instrument, like tweezers, artery forceps or bipolar cautery can be placed through defect or trephination on each side of the anterior table. The internal tine is then used to probe the periphery of the sinus, while the outer tine is used to mark its outline. Another technique involves trans-illumination with a light source inserted into a fracture line. [38] Intraoperative navigation is the most accurate but requires specialized equipment. Sometimes it is possible to preserve contralateral FS if the contralateral sinus is not injured and the interlining septum remains intact. After the limits of the sinus have been defined, miniplates can be pre-applied, spanning the osteotomy site. This allows accurate re-approximation of the bone fragments at the end of the procedure. During osteotomy, a burr or a saw should be angled toward the sinus cavity to avoid intracranial penetration. Care should be taken to avoid obliteration of the predrilled miniplate holes while performing the osteotomy. After complete exposure of the sinus, integrity of the posterior table is evaluated. If it is stable and free of large defects, sinus obliteration is acceptable. All sinus mucosa must be meticulously removed from all walls of the sinus. This applies also to temporarily removed fractured or osteotomized segments of anterior sinus wall. Inner walls of FS are reduced with a large cutting burr and smaller diamond burrs, as the surgeon proceeds deeper into the sinus. Access to the peripheral extensions of the sinus, especially above the orbital roofs, can be extremely difficult in patients with pronounced pneumatization. Special attention must be paid to the scalloped areas deep in the sinus. If the orbital roof has significant convexity, it may be necessary to remove a portion of the roof to gain access the posterior sinus mucosa. After complete removal of the sinus mucosa, the mucosa of the FS infundibulum is elevated and inverted into the frontal recess. A small temporalis muscle or pericranium plug is then placed over the FSOT to obliterate it. It can be held in place by packed oxycellulose (Surgicel®) or fibrin glue. Finally two bone chips obtained from the calvarium can be inserted to complete isolation of FS from the nasal cavity. [, 38] The FSOT can be further secured using the pedicled pericranial flap, which is rotated into the sinus. The rest of the sinus is packed with autologous or alloplastic material and anterior wall of FS is reassembled and stabilized with titanium miniplates. A number of autogenous and alloplastic materials have been used as fillers in FS obliteration.

Autogenous fat is probably the most widely used and has the longest tradition [47]. The advantages of fat grafts include ease of harvest, minimal donor site morbidity, ample available volume, and favorable handling characteristics. However, complication rate was reported as high as 18% [48]. Magnetic resonance study 24 months post-operatively found vital fatty tissue in only 6 out of 11 cases of obliteration of FS via an osteoplastic approach. Fatty necrosis occurred five times; whereas in four cases a transformation into granulation tissue and in one case into connective tissue could be seen [49].The harvest of the fat is performed using sterile technique: the surgeon will rescrub and a separate set of instruments that have not come in contact with the infected field is used. A transverse incision is made in the left lower abdominal quadrant, and subcutaneous fat is removed. Alternatively, a periumbilical incision can also be made. Bleeding is controlled using monopolar cautery, but excessive cauterization should be avoided because it may harm the fat cells and result in graft failure. Drainage of the abdomen is usually not necessary. [46]

Autogenous muscle graft harvested from temporalis muscle has advantage of being located within the operative field and being available in adequate volume. Like autogenous fat graft, this nonvascularized graft undergoes necrosis and eventual replacement by fibrous tissue. Donor site morbidity, including temporal hollowing and trismus, is unacceptable. [37]

Autogenous bone graft for FS obliteration was first described in 1969 [50]. Since then, cancellous bone grafts, most often harvested from the ilium, have been widely used as a filler material. Cancellous bone promotes re-ossification from both the periphery of the defect and centrally. The main contributions of the grafts are their osteoconductive properties and osteoinductive factors that are released from them during the process of resorption. [51] Another advantage of cancellous bone over adipose or muscle tissue for obliteration is that it is easier to distinguish radiographically in postoperative period between resorption, infection, and mucocele formation.[13,37] The greatest disadvantage to the use of cancellous bone grafts lies with the potential donor site morbidity. [52] Much more comfortable and safer is to harvest bone chips from adjacent calvarium. It can be done using bone scraper. In case the harvested amount of bone is not sufficient for filling of a large sinus, it can be augmented by admixture of bone substitute such as demineralized bone matrix (Figure 10) [53].

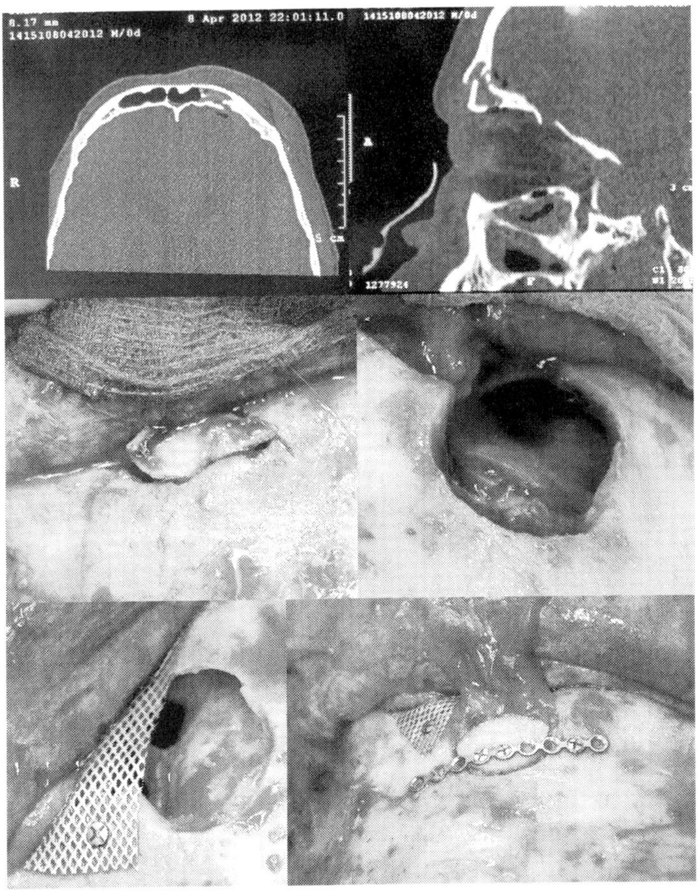

Figure 10. Fracture of left FS with minimal defect in posterior sinus wall and displacement of supraorbital rim. Reconstruction with titanium mesh and obliteration of the left FS with small pericranial flap.

Pericranial flap has been widely used in anterior cranial fossa repair, reconstruction of the middle third of face defects, full-thickness scalp defects, and orbital defects. It is composed of the skull periosteum and the subgaleal fascia. The anteriorly based flap receives its blood supply from the supraorbital and supratrochlear arteries. Branches of the superficial temporal artery supply the laterally based flap. In contrast to all other avascular grafts used for sinus obliteration, the anteriorly based pericranial flap is composed of a well-vascularized tissue. The high vascularity makes this flap less prone to infections and turns it into an ideal method for obliteration of an infected cavity in a contaminated surgical field. [54]

Allografts like lyophilized cartilage [55] have the advantage of unlimited availability and lack of donor site morbidity. They are easy to handle, well adaptable to the defect, and thus reduce the operative time. Nevertheless, a failure in revascularization or subsequent osseointegration may occur, with associated risk of infection and extrusion [56]. Allogenic transplantation may be associated with increased risk of transmitting such diseases as hepatitis, AIDS or bovine spongiform encephalopathy.

Alloplastic materials._Methyl methacrylate_ has been widely used alloplastic material since its introduction in 1940. It is well tolerated by soft tissues and has a density similar to bone, low thermal conductivity, and acceptable strength. However, the material produces a significant exothermic reaction during polymerization and foreign body reaction has been noted when it is polymerized in contact with tissue. [57]

Hydroxyapatite is a nonceramic calcium phosphate substance (_BoneSource, Stryker Leibinger_). It has osteoconductive properties, may be contoured to a defect, adheres to adjacent bone, has the ability to resist mucosal ingrowth, is resistant to infection, and is gradually replaced by native bone without a loss of volume. It has been investigated in experimental and clinical frontal sinus obliteration, but no long term observation results were reported [58]. Currently the use of hydroxyapatite cement in FS is not recommended. Significant problems related to material failure have been reported. [37]

Glass-ionomer cement is a hybrid glass polymer composite consisting of inorganic glass particles in an insoluble hydrogel matrix and bonded by ionic cross-links, hydrogen bridges, and chain entanglements. It is widely used in dentistry and also has been used in frontal sinus reconstruction [59]. However, because of severe complications after using glass ionomer cement next to dura mater this material has been taken off the market. [51]

Proplast, a polytetrafluoroethylene (_Teflon_) polymer with vitreous carbon fibers with pore sizes of 200 to 500 μm, is extremely porous to body fluids. Fibrous tissue ingrowth occurs rapidly and acts to mechanically stabilize the material. The material can cause a mild foreign body reaction. [51, 60]

Glass ceramic_(bioactive glass)_ has proved biocompatible, non-toxic and bone conducting material for occlusion of bone cavities. Total accurate obliteration of the sinus is achieved with different sizes of granules and blocks. Uneventful recovery and clinical outcome were seen in 92% of patients. Histopathological samples revealed a healing process progressing from the fibrous tissue phase to bone formation with scattered fibrous tissue and granule remnants. Bone produced by replacement of material was similar to natural frontal bone. Microbiologic cultures obtained with histological samples revealed no growth of bacteria. [61, 62]

Spontaneous obliteration was reported long ago by Samoilenko (1913), who found obliteration by osteofibrous ingrowth in an experimental study on cats and dogs. His results were confirmed by later experimental studies that found subsequent replacement of obliterated FSs by cancellous bone to a variable degree. [51] Because FS after removal of all of its mucosa and occluding the nasofrontal duct is nothing more than an isolated bone cavity, it is not irrational to expect its gradual ossification. [63]

9.3. Cranialization of the frontal sinus

Cranialization is the most radical method of FS management. It can be considered an extension of obliteration procedure with complete removal of the posterior table. In effect, it increases the volume of anterior cranial fossa at the expense of cranialized FS, and the brain is allowed to expand into this additional extradural dead space. Because intracranial space is entered, and there is a possibility of encountering dura and brain injury, cranialization should always be performed in cooperation with a neurosurgeon. The approach to FS cranialization should be as a rule performed via a coronal incision. This approach provides wide access to the entire upper facial skeleton, allowing repair of associated naso-orbito-ethmoid fractures. Furthermore, it allows dissection of a pericranial flap and harvesting of split calvarial bone grafts when necessary. [32] Maintaining integrity of the pericranial flap is critical for isolation of expanded intracranial space from FSOT and ethmoid cells.

Cranialization can be achieved either through sinusotomy as described in previous segment dealing with FS obliteration [13], or through frontal craniotomy. The choice is usually dependent on the degree of brain damage and preference of the neurosurgeon. [39]

In the former case, once access to the posterior table has been achieved, this is removed carefully in pieces with a rongeur. Larger pieces are saved in moist gauze for possible use replacing defects in the anterior table, instead of separately harvested bone grafts. When the dura is exposed, any adherent posterior table bone fragments should be carefully dissected off. The brain should be gently retracted and the remaining posterior table bone is then removed using straight and angled (Kerrison) rongeurs. Small overhangs at the periphery of the sinus should be smoothed completely, using a cutting burrs and the posterior table edge should be made flush with the anterior sinus walls, floor, and anterior cranial fossa. [32]

In most cases cranialization is performed through frontal craniotomy. This will allow thorough evaluation and repair of dural lacerations, immediate reconstruction of the orbital roof, medial orbital wall, or naso-orbito-ethmoidal fractures. [37] If a craniotomy has been performed, the portions of the posterior table associated with the craniotomy bone flap can be removed easily and safely, working on a sterile side table. [32] Also split calvarial bone grafts can be harvested from inner compacta of the craniotomy bone flap. Care should be taken during craniotomy to maintain the integrity of the cribriform plate and to avoid injury to the sagittal sinus. Once all the sinus mucosa and the posterior bony table have been removed the nonviable bone, soft tissue or damaged brain, are debrided and dural lacerations repaired. The next step is a reconstruction of the orbital roof, naso-orbital-ethmoid complex, or cribriform plate/fovea ethmoidalis, as necessary. Establishing a secure barrier between the cranial fossa and the nose is mandatory to prevent CSF leak and meningitis, but also to prevent ascending regrowth of the sinonasal mucosa with late mucocele. The frontal recess and FSOT are occluded as previously described in FS obliteration. Pericranial flap is sutured as far back as possible to the cranial base dura over the anterior cranial fossa to provide additional isolating layer of vascularized tissue. Because the wide pedicle of this flap will prevent the access to supraorbital rims, glabella and nasal skeleton, osteosynthesis of these parts must be completed first. A small bony defect (slit) must be left between supraorbital rims and inferior margin of repositioned craniotomy flap to prevent compression and ischemia of the pericranial flap. After repositioning of craniotomy flap the anterior table of FS is reconstructed as described in FS reconstruction section previously (Figure 11).

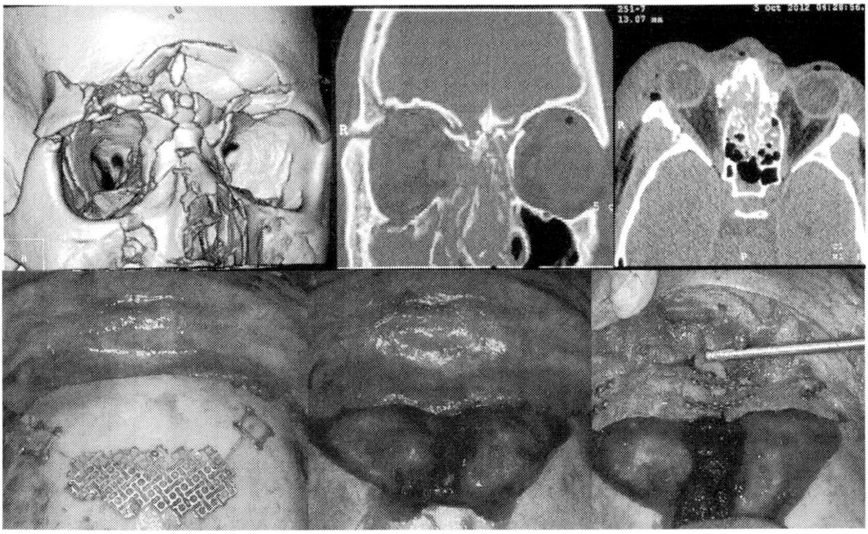

Figure 11. Severe comminuted fracture involving anterior cranial fossa, supraorbital rims and naso-orbito-ethmoidal complex. Nasal dorsum, supraorbital rims and glabella are reconstructed with bone grafts harvested from inner corticalis of craniotomy flap. Pericranial flap covers anterior cranial fossa.

10. Indications and treatment algorithms

Injured FS can be managed in four basic ways: 1-observation, 2-exploration and fracture reduction without or with internal fixation, 3- obliteration and 4-cranialization. [13] The choice of method is dependent on following factors:

a. Involvement of anterior, posterior or both walls of the sinus.

b. b) Degree of displacement and comminution.

c. Involvement and patency of fronto-nasal communication - FSOT.

d. Involvement and degree of displacement of sinus floor – orbital roof.

e. Presence or absence of CSF leak.

f. Associated neurological injuries

Other circumstances important for treatment planning are associated facial injuries, patient's general health condition, expected compliance and availability for follow-up, as well as availability of specialized services that could help in solving complications, namely endoscopic sinus surgery.

Degree and combination of anterior and posterior table, with or without FSOT involvement, would best help to determine the management protocol for FSFs, from observation to surgery [28, 38].

Improvement in diagnostic imaging, especially introduction of CT, and surgical technology has led to a wide variety of philosophies, protocols, and procedures. There is no universal agreement as to how the best achieve treatment goals, and no consensus on when surgical intervention is indicated. The choice of surgical method largely depends on the extent of the injury, the status of the FSOT and presence or absence of CSF leak. [63, 64] Most surgeons agree that nondisplaced fractures should be treated non-operatively. Management of patients with more complex injuries remains controversial. Many of the previously published reports are of poor quality (level 4 evidence) and represent retrospective case series consisting of highly censored samples with little reference given to exclusion or inclusion criteria. Additionally, most previous reports fail to include patients who were treated non-operatively, so little is known about the outcome of these patients or the relative frequency of procedures in the context of a population of trauma patients. [1]

10.1. Anterior table fractures without FSOT involvement

Nondisplaced or minimally displaced (less 2 mm) anterior table fractures can be observed. The risk of an aesthetic deformity increases with the degree of displacement (>2 mm). An endoscopic repair or repair through alternative skin incision may be indicated in this patient population. However, many authors found it to be technically challenging.

Another option is to assess the degree of deformity after all facial edema has resolved. At this point, the patient can make an informed decision as to whether he/she desires surgical intervention, which can be endoscopic camouflage. A significant number of patients will opt for no surgical intervention. [27]

More complex anterior table fractures and those extending below the orbital rim may require open reduction using a coronal incision. The presence of improperly reduced bone segments, comminuted sequestrae, foreign bodies, devitalized and torn sinus mucosa expose the patient to a greater risk of infectious complications. [39] Reconstruction of the anterior wall using miniplates is a procedure virtually free of significant complications when the FSOT is patent.

10.2. Anterior table fractures with FSOT involvement

This is the point, where controversy about appropriate treatment of FS injuries begins. The traditional treatment for FS fractures with FSOT involvement is obliteration followed by anterior table reconstruction. [23,64] Some authors are not only strong proponents of obliteration, but employ this method also for some cases on nondisplaced anterior table fractures with FSOT involvement and even cranialize patients with nondisplaced and displaced fractures with FSOT involvement. [65]

On the other hand, the advancement in endoscopic surgery of frontal recess and modern imaging has enabled sinus preservation as a viable alternative to FS obliteration in cases with suspected FSOT involvement in the fracture. High-resolution, thin-section CT with sagittal reformatting may evaluate the involvement and severity of injury of the FSOT preoperatively and help in planning of its management. Sinus preservation may apply for displaced anterior wall FS fractures, even with concomitant minimally displaced posterior wall fractures, and without significant intracranial injury or persistent CSF leak. [28]

Thong and Lee [42] reported on primary endoscopic management. Patients with depressed anterior table FS fractures that involved FSOT were managed by ORIF via a coronal incision plus endoscopic fronto-ethmoidectomy with removal of any obstructing bony fragments, and insertion of a stent into the fronto-ethmoidal recess. Middle meatal nasal packs were left in situ for 1 week and patients were discharged home with prophylactic antibiotics. Frontal stents were removed after 1 month. Patients were followed up by regular endoscopic surveillance and CT scans were performed annually. There were no complications.

Smith at al. [45] treated 14 patients with FS and concurrent facial fractures. Seven patients were included in the modified treatment algorithm. Postoperatively, 5 patients had spontaneous FS ventilation. Two patients, both of whom had naso-orbito-ethmoid fractures, had persistent FSOT obstruction. These patients were successfully managed with an endoscopic FS procedure. The decision to repair, obliterate, or cranialize the sinus is often made intraoperatively, based on the extent of FSOT obstruction found during the procedure. [37]

10.3. Posterior table fractures

The primary decision criteria for surgical intervention are the degree of fracture displacement and the presence of a CSF leak. Traditionally as a rule of thumb, a width of the posterior table displacement is considered significant. [14, 32]

10.3.1. Fractures without significant displacement

Patients with posterior table displacement less than one table width and no CSF leak may be observed. Long-term follow-up with repeat CT scans at 2 months and 1 year is appropriate to rule out mucocele formation. If a CSF leak is present at time of injury, 1 week of observation is indicated; 50% will resolve spontaneously. The methods of conservative treatment include complete bed rest with oral acetazolamide 250 mg every 8 hours, prescription of laxatives and prophylactic antibiotics, and avoidance of breath holding and straining. Acetazolamide is a carbonic anhydrase inhibitor and is intended to reduce CSF secretion. Laxatives are given to prevent increases in intracranial pressure caused by constipation, and antibiotics to prevent infection. CSF drainage can be performed if the patient has intracranial infection or rapid leakage. Persistent leak openings in the posterior wall of the frontal sinus warrant repair via craniotomy. CT cisternography facilitate highly accurate preoperative localization of the fistula. [66]

10.3.2. Fractures with significant displacement

Patients with posterior table displacement greater than one table width, no CSF leak, and only mild comminution should be considered for sinus obliteration. More severe injuries, with a frank CSF leak and/or moderate to severe comminution, will likely require removal of posterior table bone to repair the dural tear. If the injury or surgical repair results in disruption of more than 25 to 30% of the posterior table, sinus cranialization should be considered. [32]

10.4. Treatment algorithms

In an effort to optimize functional and cosmetic outcomes in complex clinical situations, while minimizing serious short- and long-term sequelae, algorithms were developed to determine which patients should receive operative intervention and which frontal sinus procedure is most appropriate in a given case. Following are examples of such algorithms placing emphasis on different aspects of FSF characteristics:

It seems to be obvious that all these algorithms are to some extent simplified. To develop algorithm taking into account all possible characteristics and circumstances would probably result in a too -complicated diagram.

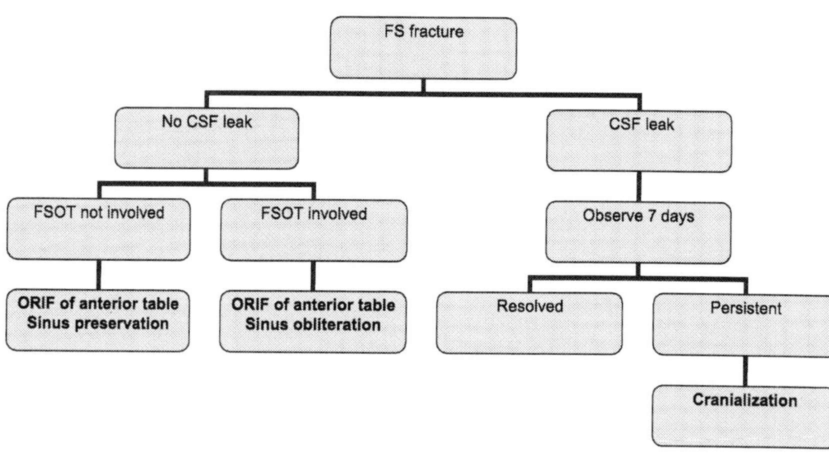

According to Chen et al., 2006 [64]

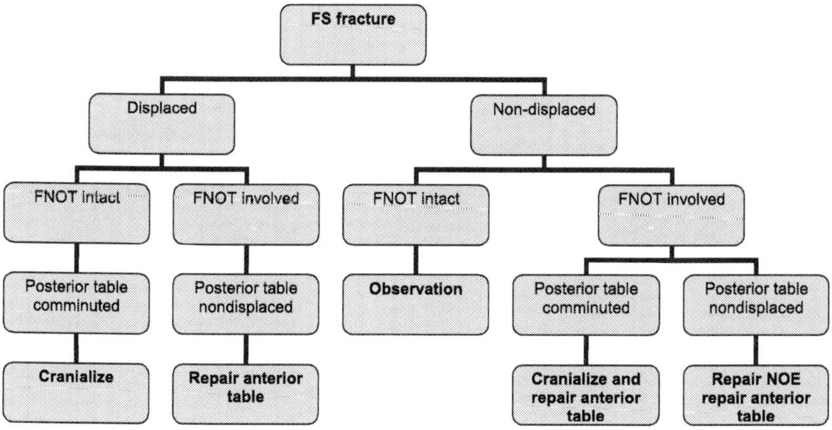

According to Bell et al., 2007 [37]

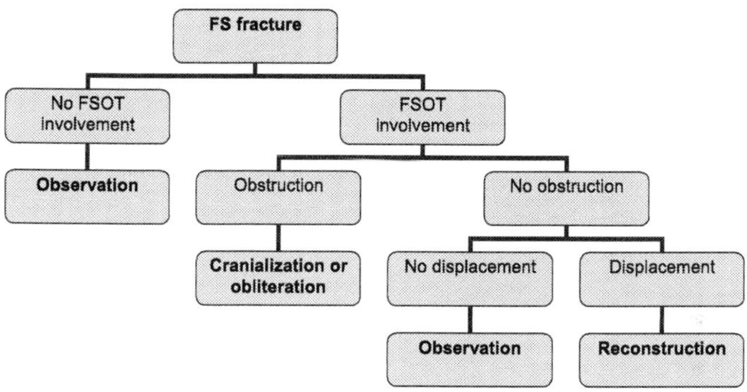

According to Rodriguez at al., 2008 [65]

11. Complications of frontal sinus fractures

Frontal sinus fractures carry a risk of complications, which can be characterized as early or late. Complication rates for patients with FS fractures range from 10% to 17%. [67] The most serious are early infectious complications that can endanger patient's life. There is a greater urgency of operative treatment in cases where intracranial infection can develop through potential communication of the neurocranium with the non-sterile sinuses. Bellamy et al. [68] found that delay in repair beyond 48 hours was associated with a greater than fourfold increased risk of serious infection, even when controlling for clinical and statistical confounders. However, FS fracture patients often present with other, more severe intracranial and bodily injuries. Thus, definitive management is often delayed until the patient's neurologic and medical condition has stabilized. Several additional factors are associated with serious infection, among them use of an external cerebrospinal fluid drainage catheter and soft-tissue infection that predisposes to deeper infection in these patients.

The recommendation of 7-days waiting period for management of persistent CSF leaks was borne out of historical studies that predate the modern research. According to recent opinion, there is no evidence to support 7 days as a particularly important threshold for cerebrospinal fluid leak management to prevent intracranial infection. [68]

The efficacy of antibiotic prophylaxis, especially beyond the perioperative period, in frontal sinus and skull base injury remains unclear. The risks of antibiotic use, evolving drug resistances and associated patient and epidemiologic costs require careful evaluation. To date, there is no standard of care for postoperative antibiotic administration, though many surgeons continue to administer antibiotics beyond the immediate perioperative period.[68] A variety of adverse events can occur after fixation of a frontal sinus fracture, such as frontal sinusitis, mucocele, mucopyocele, cerebrospinal fluid leakage, deformity, hardware infection, headache, and chronic pain in the area of the injury.[67] Potentially life threatening late complications include thrombosis of the cavernous sinus, encephalitis, mucopyocele, or brain abscess. [21] In the literature there is no consensus regarding the follow-up. Because of the possible long period after trauma until complications, namely mucocele, develops, some advise to continue to follow these patients for a lifetime. Others suggest a follow-up period of 5 or 7 years. [26]

12. Our experience in treatment of frontal bone fractures

12.1. Patients' demographics

During a period of 10 years beginning from 2004 we treated 188 males (90%) and 22 females (10%) admitted with diagnosis of FBF. The most frequent etiology overall was road traffic accidents (43%), followed by falls from heights (26%) and impact of fast moving objects (11%). Fifty injuries (24%) were work-related, most of them falls from heights at construction sites. However, in females 70% of accidents were caused by falls from heights. These female patients were mostly domestic helpers, who either tried to commit suicide or avoid abuse (Graphs 1and 2).

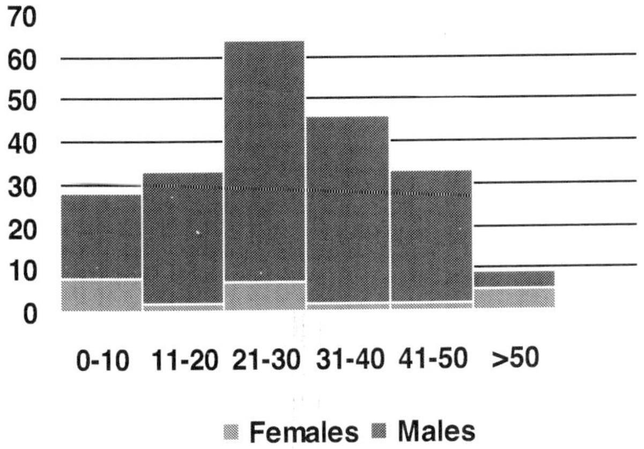

Graph 1. Age and sex distribution

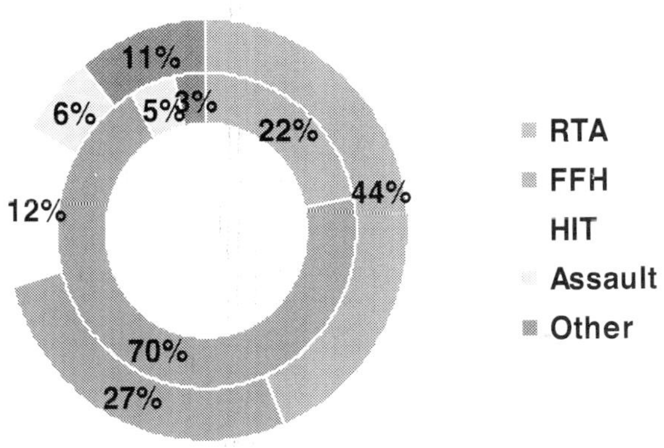

Graph 2. Etiology distribution by sex: males; outer circle, females; inner circle

12.2. Associated injuries

Solitary FBF was found in 116 patients, 82 patients suffered concomitant midfacial fracture(s), 3 patients associated mandibular fracture and 9 patients had panfacial fractures. Central nervous injury was found in 80 patients, of whom 11 died. Seven of these fatalities were polytraumatized with multiple non-head fractures and internal organ injuries. Non-head injuries were found altogether in 74 patients. Serious ocular injuries (bulbus rupture and/or traumatic optic neuropathy) were present in 14 patients (below).

Brain injury, contusion, edema, bleeding (died)	80 (11)
Non-facial fractures (spine)	68 (17)
Eye injuries	14
Internal organ injuries	9

12.3. Our classification scheme

We founded our classification solely on CT examination. We did not attempt to include involvement of FSOT, because its CT evaluation is often not reliable. Decisions based on status of FSOT were done intraoperatively. We had five types namely:

Type 1	Outside frontal sinus (Figure 12)
Type 2	Non-displaced, involving one or both frontal sinus walls (Figure 13)
Type 3	Displaced anterior sinus wall, posterior wall intact or nondisplaced (Figure 14)
Type 4	Displaced anterior + posterior sinus wall (Figure 15)
Type 5	Displaced posterior sinus wall, anterior wall intact or non-displaced (Figure 16)

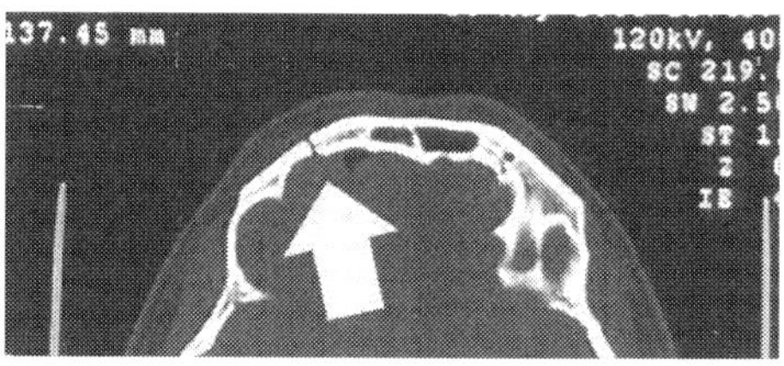

Figure 12. Type 1: fracture outside sinus.

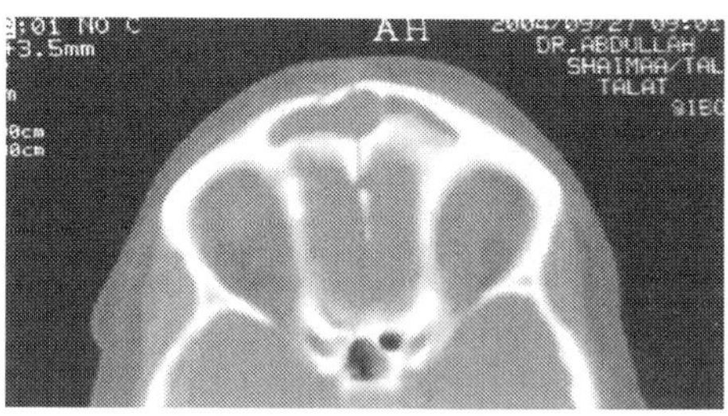

Figure 13. Type 2: nondisplaced fracture involving anterior and/or posterior sinus wall.

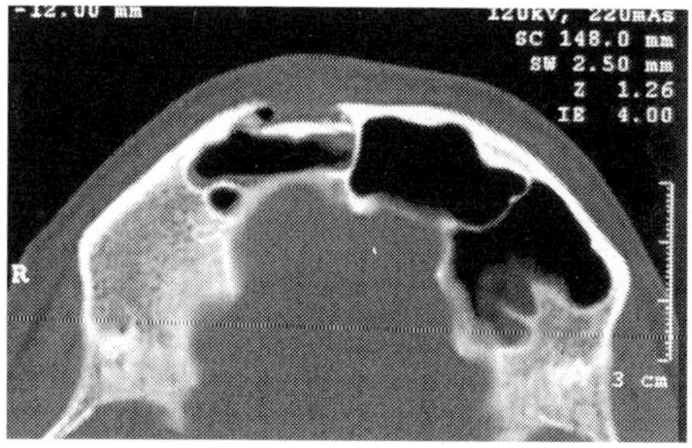

Figure 14. Type 3: displaced fracture of anterior sinus wall with posterior sinus wall intact or undisplaced.

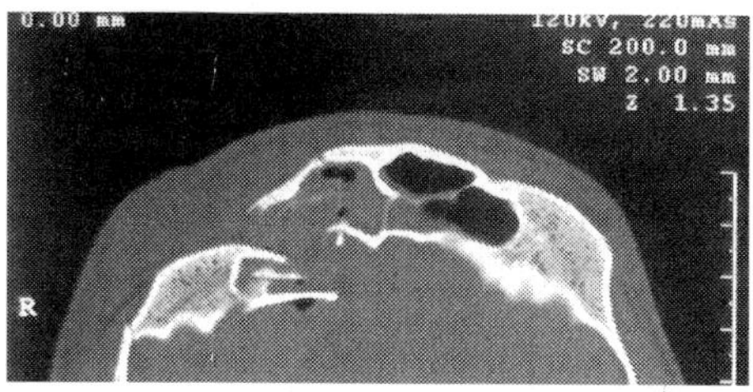

Figure 15. Type 4: displaced fracture of both anterior and posterior sinus walls.

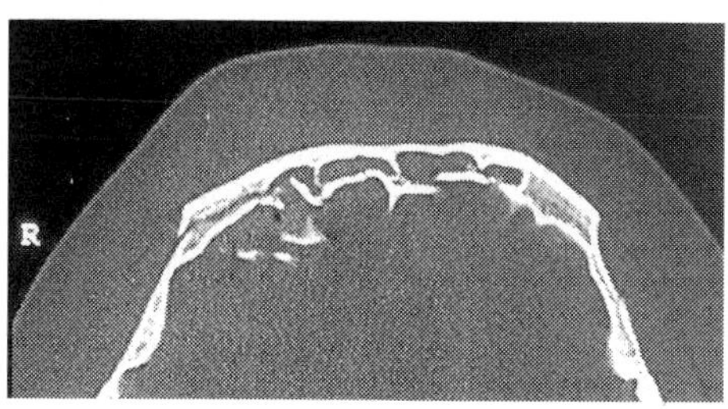

Figure 16. Type 5: displaced and comminuted posterior sinus wall with anterior wall intact or nondisplaced.

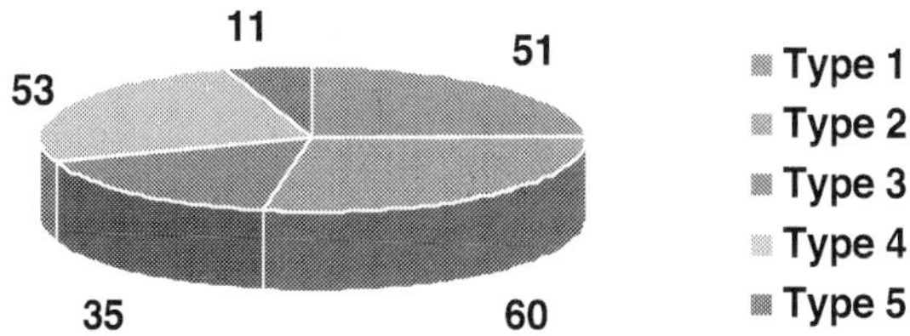

Graph 3. Distribution by types of fracture.

12.4. Surgical procedures

From patients with **Type 1** injuries 4 patients died due to concomitant CNS trauma. Two patients were operated: both of them were children with severe disruption of FB and the purpose of surgeries was to repair calvarial defects. Only one patient from **Type 2** group was operated to remove a foreign body from the FS. In patients with **Type 3** fractures, there was the highest relative incidence of operative treatment: 24 patients were operated with 1 sinus obliteration and 23 anterior wall reconstructions.

Type 4 group had 33 operated patients, 31 of them received cranialization and 2 obliteration of FS. Dural tears were found in 21 patients in this group despite only 5 cases of CSF leak noticed preoperatively.

Type 5 group had the lowest relative incidence of operated cases and only 4 patients were operated. In five cases we were not able to reach an agreement with neurosurgery service about the indication to operate. The overview of operative treatment and reasons for not operating cases are given in the following table.

Type	No.	CSF leak	CNS injury	Other injuries	Operated	Died	Refused	Unfit	Transfer	Neurosurgeon Disagree
1	51	2	18	20	2	4	-	-	-	-
2	60	0	18	23	1	0	-	-	-	-
3	35	0	6	6	24	0	7	4	-	-
4	53	5	33	19	33	7	6	3	3	1
5	11	1	5	0	4	0	1	1	-	5
Σ	**210**	**8**	**80**	**68**	**64**	**11**	**14**	**8**	**3**	**6**

12.5. Discussion

Surprisingly, only one of our operated patients developed an early infectious complication-soft tissue abscess in the vicinity of the orbital rim, which responded to local incision and antibiotic treatment. The other 2 patients had persistent postoperative CSF leakage and were successfully treated by lumbar drain and bed rest. Similar to other studies we were not able to maintain long term follow-up in the majority of operated cases, not mentioning conservatively managed cases. Supposedly, had serious complication developed and the patient was still living in Kuwait, he/she would have looked for help in our unit, like other maxillofacial trauma patients, who are usually refused even simple tooth extraction in other facilities other than ours once the patient's trauma history is known to a care provider.

We recognize the importance of close cooperation with the neurosurgery service in instances of cranio-facial injuries. However, we sometimes run into difficulties when deciding on indications for operative treatment in patients who are in good general condition and without signs of external deformity or CSF leakage. These are mainly patients with type 5 injuries. More often than not a neurosurgeon takes only short term perspective on a case without consideration of possible development of late complications many years later.

Author details

Petr Schütz*, Hussein Hassan Hamed Ibrahim and Bashar Rajab

*Address all correspondence to: petrschutz@yahoo.com

Al-Farwaniya Dental Center, Al-Farwaniya Hospital, Ministry of Health, State of Kuwait

References

[1] Bell RB, Dierks EJ, Brar P, Potter JK, Potter BE. A protocol for the management of frontal sinus fractures emphasizing sinus preservation. Journal of Oral and Maxillofacial Surgery 2007;65(5):825-839.

[2] Mithani SK, St-Hilaire H, Brooke BS, Smith IM, Bluebond-Langner R, Rodriguez ED. Predictable patterns of intracranial and cervical spine injury in craniomaxillofacial trauma: analysis of 4786 patients. Plastic and Reconstructive Surgery 2009;123(4): 1293-1301. doi: 10.1097/PRS.0b013e31819e26f2.

[3] Roden KS1, Tong W, Surrusco M, Shockley WW, Van Aalst JA, Hultman CS. Changing characteristics of facial fractures treated at a regional, level 1 trauma center, from 2005 to 2010: an assessment of patient demographics, referral patterns, etiology of injury, anatomic location, and clinical outcomes. Annals of Plastic Surgery 2012;68(5): 461-466. doi: 10.1097/SAP.0b013e31823b69dd.

[4] Sperber GH, Guttmann GD, Sperber SM. Craniofacial Development. BC Decker Inc, 2001

[5] Scanlon VC; Sanders T: Essentials of anatomy and physiology. F.A. Davis, 5th ed., 2007.

[6] Brown WA, Molleson TI, Chinn S. Enlargement of the frontal sinus. Annals of Human Biology 1984;11:221–226.

[7] McLaughlin RB, Rehl RM, Jr., Lanza DC. Clinically relevant frontal sinus anatomy and physiology. Otolaryngologic Clinics of North America. 2001;34(1):1-22.

[8] Williams P, Warwick R. The paranasal sinuses. In: Warwick R, ed. Gray's anatomy. WB Saunders 1980.

[9] Saladin: Anatomy & Physiology: The Unity of Form and Function, Third Edition, The McGraw–Hill Companies, 2003.

[10] El-Rakhawy MT. Illustrative anatomy head and neck. Al Al-Bayt University 2002

[11] Salentijn L. Anatomy and embryology. In: Freidman W, ed. Surgery of the paranasal sinuses. W. B. Saunders 1985; p. 15–19.

[12] Urken ML, Som PM, Lawson W, et al. The abnormally large frontal sinus. I. A practical method for its determination based upon an analysis of 100 normal patients. Laryngoscope 1987;97(5):602–605.

[13] Manolidis S, Hollier LH Jr. Management of frontal sinus fractures. Plastic and Reconstructive Surgery. 2007;120(Suppl 2):32S-48S.

[14] Rohrich RJ, Hollier LH. Management of frontal sinus fractures. Changing concepts. Clinics in Plastic Surgery 1992;19(1):219–232.

[15] Harris, L, Marano GD, and McCorkle D. Nasofrontal duct: CT in frontal sinus trauma. Radiology 1987;165(1)195-198.

[16] Stanwix MG, Nam AJ, Manson PN, Mirvis S, Rodriguez ED. Critical computed tomographic diagnostic criteria for frontal sinus fractures. Journal of Oral and Maxillofacial Surgery 2010;68(11):2714-2722. doi: 10.1016/j.joms.2010.05.019.

[17] Kennedy DW, Senior BA. Endoscopic sinus surgery: A review. Otolaryngologic Clinics of North America 1997;30(3)313-330.

[18] Landsberg R, Friedman M. A computer-assisted anatomical study of the nasofrontal region. Laryngoscope 2001;111(12)2135-2130.

[19] Rohrich RJ, Hollier L. The role of the nasofrontal duct in frontal sinus fracture management. Journal of Cranio-maxillofacial Trauma 1996;2(1):31–40.

[20] Tos M, Mogensen C, Novotny Z. Quantitative histologic features of the normal frontal sinus. Archives of Otolaryngology 1980;106(3):143–148.

[21] Tiwari P, Higuera S, Thornton J, Hollier LH. The management of frontal sinus fractures. Journal of Oral and Maxillofacial Surgery 2005;63(9):1354-1360.

[22] Laskin D, Abubaker A. Decision Making in Oral and Maxillofacial Surgery. Quintenssence; 2007. p74-76.

[23] Stevens M, Kline SN: Management of frontal sinus fractures. Journal of Cranio-maxillofacial Trauma. 1995;1(1):29-37.

[24] Stanley RB Jr, Becker TS. Injuries of the nasofrontal orifices in frontal sinus fractures. Laryngoscope. 1987;97(6):728-731.

[25] Stanley RB Jr. Management of severe frontobasilar skull fractures. Otolaryngologic Clinics of North America. 1991;24(1):139-150.

[26] Koudstaal MJ, van der Wal KG, Bijvoet HW, Vincent AJ, Poublon RM. Post-trauma mucocele formation in the frontal sinus; a rationale of follow-up. International Journal of Oral and Maxillofacial Surgery 2004;33(8):751-754.

[27] Strong EB. Frontal sinus fractures: current concepts. CraniomaxillofacialTrauma&Reconstruction 2009;2(3):161-175. doi: 10.1055/s-0029-1234020.

[28] Koento T. Current advances in sinus preservation for the management of frontal sinus fractures. Current Opinion in Otolaryngology & Head and Neck Surgery 2012;20(4):274-279. doi: 10.1097/MOO.0b013e328355a54a.

[29] Tremolada C, Candiani P, Signorini M, Vigano M, Donati L. The surgical anatomy of the subcutaneous fascial system of the scalp. Annals of Plastic Surgery 1994;32(1):8–14.

[30] Miloro M, Redlinger S, Pennington DM, Kolodge T. In situ location of the temporal branch of the facial nerve. Journal of Oral and Maxillofacial Surgery 2007;65(12): 2466–2469.

[31] Schütz P, Andersson L: Midfacial fractures. In: Andersson L, Kahnberg KE, Pogrel MA (Eds.): Oral and Maxillofacial Surgery. Wiley-Blackwell, 2010.

[32] Ruggiero FP, Zender CA. Frontal sinus cranialization. Operative Techniques in Otolaryngology – Head and Neck Surgery 2010;21(1):143-146.

[33] Luo W, Wang L, Jing W, Zheng X, Long J, Tian W, Liu L. A new coronal scalp technique to treat craniofacial fracture: the supratemporalis approach. Oral Surgery, Oral Medicine, Oral Pathology and Oral Radiology 2012;113(2):177-1782. doi: 10.1016/j.tripleo.2011.01.037.

[34] Meiklejohn BD, Lynham A, Borgna SC. A simplified approach for the reduction of specific closed anterior table frontal sinus fractures. British Journal of Oral and Maxillofacial Surgery 2014 52(1):81-84. doi: 10.1016/j.bjoms.2013.09.012.

[35] Rontal ML. State of the art in craniomaxillofacial trauma: frontal sinus. Current Opinion in Otolaryngology & Head and Neck Surgery. 2008;16(4):381-386. doi: 10.1097/MOO.0b013e328308672c.

[36] Noury M, Dunn RM, Lalikos JF, Fudem GM, Rothkopf DM. Frontal sinus repair through a frontalis rhytid approach. Annals of Plastic Surgery. 2011;66(5):457-459. doi: 10.1097/SAP.0b013e3182185f14.

[37] Bell RB. Management of frontal sinus fractures. Oral and Maxillofacial Surgery Clinics of North America, 2009;21(2):227-242. doi: 10.1016/j.coms.2008.12.003.

[38] Strong EB. Frontal sinus fractures. Operative Techniques in Otolaryngology – Head and Neck Surgery 2008;19(2):151-160.

[39] Gerbino G, Roccia F, Benech A, Caldarelli C. Analysis of 158 frontal sinus fractures: current surgical management and complications. Journal of Cranio-maxillo-facial Surgery 2000;28(3):133-139.

[40] Luce EA. Frontal sinus fractures: guidelines to management. Plastic and Reconstructive Surgery. 1987;80(4):500-510.

[41] Gabrielli MF, Gabrielli MA, Hochuli-Vieira E, Pereira-Fillho VA. Immediate reconstruction of frontal sinus fractures: review of 26 cases. Journal of Oral and Maxillofacial Surgery 2004;62(5):582-586.

[42] Thong JF, Lee J. Single-stage strategy for management of anterior table frontal sinus fractures involving the frontal sinus outflow tract. European Journal of Plastic Surgery 201;34(4):299–303.

[43] Carter KB Jr, Poetker DM, Rhee JS. Sinus preservation management for frontal sinus fractures in the endoscopic sinus surgery era: a systematic review. Craniomaxillofac ial Trauma & Reconstruction 2010;3(3):141-149. doi: 10.1055/s-0030-1262957.

[44] Shumrick KA. Endoscopic management of frontal sinus fractures. Otolaryngologic Clinics of North America 2007;40(2):329–336.

[45] Smith TL, Han JK, Loehrl TA, Rhee JS. Endoscopic management of the frontal recess in frontal sinus fractures: a shift in the paradigm? Laryngoscope. 2002 May;112(5): 784-90.

[46] Kim E, Duncavage J. Osteoplastic flap with and without fat obliteration. Operative Techniques in Otolaryngology – Head and Neck Surgery 2010;21(2):134-137.

[47] Goodale RL, Montgomery WW. Anterior osteoplastic frontal sinus operation. Five years' experience. Annals of Otology, Rhinology & Laryngology 1961;70(3):860-880.

[48] Hardy JM, Montgomery WW: Osteoplastic frontal sinusotomy: An analysis of 250 operations. Annals of Otology, Rhinology & Laryngology 1976;85(4):523-532.

[49] Keerl R, Weber R, Kahle G, Draf W, Constantinidis J, Saha A. Magnetic resonance imaging after frontal sinus surgery with fat obliteration. Journal of Laryngology & Otology 1995;109(11):1115-1119.

[50] Dickinson JT, Cipcic JA, Kamerer DB. Principles of frontal reconstruction. Laryngoscope1969;79(6):1019-1074.

[51] Weber R, Draf W, Kahle G, Kind M. Obliteration of the frontal sinus – state of the art and reflections on new materials Rhinology. 1999;37(1):1-15.

[52] Barone A, Ricci M, Mangano F, Covani U. Morbidity associated with iliac crest harvesting in the treatment of maxillary and mandibular atrophies: a 10-year analysis. Journal of Oral and Maxillofacial Surgery 2011;69(9):2298-2304. doi: 10.1016/j.joms.2011.01.014.

[53] Zubillaga Rodríguez I, Lora Pablos D, Falguera Uceda MI, Díez Lobato R, Sánchez Aniceto G. Frontal sinus obliteration after trauma: analysis of bone regeneration for two selected methods. International Journal of Oral and Maxillofacial Surgery 2014l; 43(7):827-833. doi: 10.1016/j.ijom.2014.02.012.

[54] Mlynarek AM, Seikaly H. Vascularized anteriorly based pericranial flap for frontal sinus obliteration. Operative Techniques in Otolaryngology – Head and Neck Surgery 2009;20(1),88-91.

[55] Sailer HF, Grätz KW, Kalavrezos ND: Frontal sinus fractures: Principles of treatment and long-term results after sinus obliteration with the use of lyophilized cartilage. Journal of Cranio-maxillo-facial Surgery 1998;26(4):235-242.

[56] Peltola MJ, Aitasalo KM, Aho AJ, Tirri T, Suonpää JT. Long-term microscopic and tissue analytical findings for 2 frontal sinus obliteration materials. Journal of Oral and Maxillofacial Surgery 2008;66(8):1699-1707. doi: 10.1016/j.joms.2007.11.020.

[57] Olson NR, Newman MH. Acrylic frontal cranioplasty. Archives of Otolaryngology 1969;89(5):774-777.

[58] Moeller CW, Petruzzelli GJ, Stankiewicz JA: Hydroxyapatite-based frontal sinus obliteration. Operative Techniques in Otolaryngology – Head and Neck Surgery 2010;21(2),147-149.

[59] Cole I, Dan N, Anker A. Bone replacement in head and neck surgery: a biocompatible alternative. The Australian and New Zealand Journal of Surgery 1996;66(7): 469-472.

[60] Schenck NL, Tomlinson MJ. Frontal sinus trauma: experimental reconstruction with proplast. Laryngoscope. 1977;87(3):398-407.

[61] Peltola M, Suonpää J, Aitasalo K, Varpula M, Yli-Urpo A, Happonen RP. Obliteration of the frontal sinus cavity with bioactive glass. Head & Neck 1998;20(4):315-319.

[62] Peltola M, Aitasalo K, Suonpää J, Varpula M, Yli-Urpo A. Bioactive glass S53P4 in frontal sinus obliteration: a long-term clinical experience. Head & Neck. 2006;28(9): 834-841.

[63] Kalavrezos N. Current trends in the management of frontal sinus fractures. Injury 2004;35(4):340—346.

[64] Chen KT, Chen CT, Mardini S, Tsay PK, Chen YR. Frontal sinus fractures: a treatment algorithm and assessment of outcomes based on 78 clinical cases. Plastic and Reconstructive Surgery. 2006;118(2):457-468.

[65] Rodriguez ED, Stanwix MG, Nam AJ, St Hilaire H, Simmons OP, Christy MR, Grant MP, Manson PN. Twenty-six-year experience treating frontal sinus fractures: a novel algorithm based on anatomical fracture pattern and failure of conventional techniques. Plastic and Reconstructive Surgery. 2008;122(6):1850-1866. doi: 10.1097/PRS. 0b013e31818d58ba.

[66] Liu P, Wu S, Li Z, Wang B. Surgical strategy for cerebrospinal fluid rhinorrhea repair. Neurosurgery. 2010;66(6 Suppl Operative):281-285; discussion 285-6. doi: 10.1227/01.NEU.0000369660.30126.02.

[67] Sivori LA 2nd, de Leeuw R, Morgan I, Cunningham LL Jr. Complications of frontal sinus fractures with emphasis on chronic craniofacial pain and its treatment: a review of 43 cases. Journal of Oral and Maxillofacial Surgery 2010;68(9):2041-2046. doi: 10.1016/j.joms.2010.05.041.

[68] Bellamy JL, Molendijk J, Reddy SK, Flores JM, Mundinger GS, Manson PN, Rodriguez ED, Dorafshar AH. Severe infectious complications following frontal sinus fracture: the impact of operative delay and perioperative antibiotic use. Plastic and Reconstructive Surgery 2013;132(1):154-162. doi: 10.1097/PRS.0b013e3182910b9b.

Chapter 21

Current Management of Frontal Sinus Injuries

Roozbeh Kahali and Alireza Tootoonchian

Additional information is available at the end of the chapter

http://dx.doi.org/10.5772/59968

1. Introduction

Frontal sinus fractures are relatively uncommon and are usually seen as a part of severe head injuries caused by high-velocity injuries. The management of frontal sinus fractures involves many difficulties since the frontal sinus is situated at the junction between the cranium and the face, and has anatomical features of both. Intracranial involvement should always be anticipated when upper facial trauma is suspected. Often the planning of how to treat frontal sinus fractures must actually be decided during the operation itself, because the fractures may extend more widely than predicted by pre-operative examination. Posterior wall fractures have more complications and a worse clinical outcome than fractures that only involve the anterior wall. Acute and chronic sinusitis, mucocele, mucopyocele, osteomyelitis, meningitis, and brain abscess are associated with frontal sinus injury. The purpose of this chapter is to present an overview of the frontal sinus fractures, associated injuries and a rationale for selecting surgical approach to frontal sinus injury.

2. Frontal sinus anatomy

The frontal sinus has a thick strong anterior wall, a thin fragile floor and a posterior wall. Its floor is the roof of the orbit. Its posterior wall forms the anteroinferior portion of the anterior wall of the anterior cranial fossa. Because the superior sagittal sinus lies against the posterior wall of the frontal sinus, it is vulnerable to injury in fracture dislocations of the posterior wall. Fortunately because of the toughness and resiliency of the dura, rupture of the superior sagittal sinus is uncommon, but when it occurs, the patient often dies of uncontrollable hemorrhage [1]. A vertical septum has commonly placed approximately in the center of the frontal sinus. In the case of highly developed orbital ethmoidal cells, the roofs of these cells make up the medial aspect of the frontal sinus floor. The nasofrontal ducts are located on either side of the frontal sinus. The opening of these structures is variable. They usually drain directly into the frontal recess, but they also may drain above the ethmoid infundibulum, into it or above the ethmoid bulla.

The frontal sinus is lined with pseudostratified ciliated columnar epithelium. The main source of blood supply to the frontal sinus is a diploic branch of the supraorbital artery [2].The frontal sinus also receives some blood supply from branches of the anterior ethmoidal artery [1].External venous drainage is through the angular and anterior facial veins. The deep drainage is through the foramen of Breschet which is located on the posterior wall of the sinus. This structure is responsible for communication with the subdural venous system in the subarachnoid space [1].

3. Frontal sinus fracture

A frontal sinus fracture is a common injury in patients who suffer high-energy trauma from motor vehicle accidents or altercations [3].The frontal sinus fracture accounts for 5–15% of all fractures of the maxillofacial area [4] and is often associated with neurological deficit and other facial fractures [3].The involvement of the brain is not uncommon. It has been suggested that more than 80% of the patients with a fracture of both the anterior and the posterior wall have intracranial injuries, such as hemorrhages and cerebral contusions [5].Pain is a common symptom in conscious patients with a frontal sinus fracture. Lacerations are seen in 50% of patients. About 25% of patients have a visible depression of the forehead [6]. Other possible symptoms are epistaxis, problems with vision, edema and paresthesia of the supraorbital region. Leakage of cerebrospinal fluid, due to damage of the dura, is a common finding [4].Computed tomography (CT) is the gold standard in diagnosing the degree of involvement of the frontal sinus [3].

4. Diagnosis of frontal sinus fracture

The physical examination of patients with frontal sinus fractures is difficult because of soft tissue swelling. The detection of cerebrospinal fluid rhinorrhea which indicates a posterior table injury with a dural tear is an important preoperative finding. CSF rhinorrhea is rarely detected because the fluid drains from the oropharynx. The surgeon should attempt to obtain a sample of this by having the patient lean forward to allow drainage from the nose and test the fluid for glucose or β-2 transferrin to confirm the diagnosis. Other signs of frontal sinus fracture include supraorbital nerve anesthesia and a depressed frontal region [7]. The most common associated finding is a laceration of the supraorbital ridge (Figure 1), glabella, or lower forehead [8]. These lacerations are often extensive and may be contaminated by foreign material [9].

Plain skull radiographs including the Caldwell and lateral views are occasionally used. Sinus pathology is strongly suspected when the radiograph demonstrates air-fluid levels, a diffusely cloudy sinus, or pneumocephalus. Accurate serial 1.5 mm cuts computed tomography (CT)

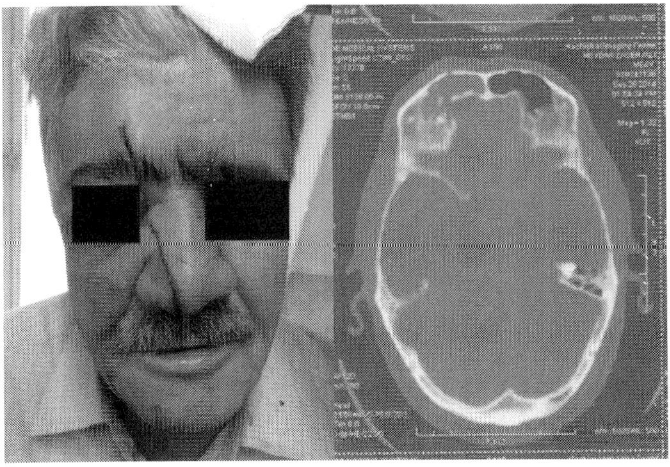

Figure 1. Left: A 52-year-old patient who has facial laceration due to an industrial accident. Right: CT scan of the same patient reveals both anterior and posterior table fractures of the frontal sinus.

imaging in both the axial (Figure 2) and coronal planes should be obtained in all cases to determine the degree of injury to the anterior and posterior tables and nasofrontal ducts [10]. The CT scan allows for visualization of the brain, face, and orbits as well, which is often necessary because of the high rate of associated injuries [9].

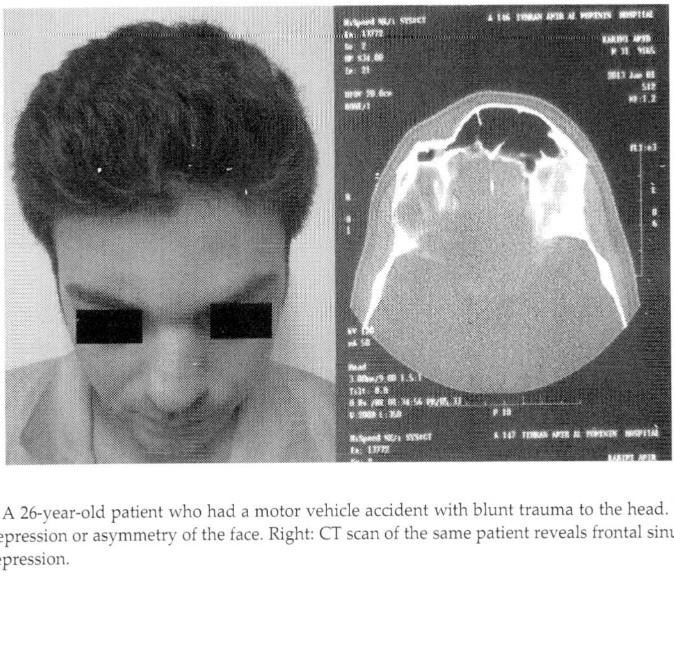

Figure 2. Left: A 26-year-old patient who had a motor vehicle accident with blunt trauma to the head. Note that there is no sign of depression or asymmetry of the face. Right: CT scan of the same patient reveals frontal sinus fracture with severe bone depression.

5. Treatment modalities

Isolation of the neurocranium, cessation of any CSF leak, prevention of early and delayed postoperative complications and restoration of the preoperative facial aesthetics are the aims of treatment of frontal sinus fractures. The integrity of the posterior wall and/or involvement of the nasofrontal duct are the factors influencing treatment. The integrity of the posterior wall is the main factor for the separation of the intracranial contents from the outer environment. The nasofrontal duct involvement is the decisive factor for the potential dysfunction of the sinus mucosa. Closed fractures of the anterior wall of the frontal sinus without displacement do not require surgical treatment and only observation is required. The treatment of depressed fracture of the anterior wall without involvement of the nasofrontal duct is simple elevation of the fracture and plate fixation. However, if the duct is involved, the treatment should include the obliteration of the sinus cavity after the sealing of the injured duct. In this way the frontal sinus is treated as an isolated cavity precluding any potential mucosal regrowth from the nasal epithelium. If the posterior wall is involved the determinant of successful management of the frontal sinus fracture is removal of the displaced bony fragments of the posterior sinus wall, restoration of the dural integrity and complete isolation of the brain from potential communication with the nose through the injured frontal sinus and cranialization of the frontal sinus [11].

6. Surgical approach

The most common approach is the bicoronal flap. It has several advantages including providing the best exposure of the frontal bone and the best cosmetic result in patients without alopecia. Its disadvantages are increased intraoperative blood loss and risk of injury to the frontal branch of the facial nerve. When using this approach, the hair is parted at the anticipated incision site and the tufts of parted hair are brought together and secured with small rubber bands on each side of the incision. Shaving of hair is not necessary. The incision site is infused with local anesthetic with 1:100,000 epinephrine in a subgaleal plane. The scalp is then incised from one temporal line to the other through the skin and subcutaneous tissues. A scalpel is used to incise the galea. Once the galea is violated, there will be an obvious separation between the galea and the pericranium. Bleeding from larger vessels should be tied off individually. The application of Raney clips minimizes the risk of bleeding. Finger dissection can then be used to elevate 2 to 3 cm on either sides of the incision, taking care to maintain the integrity of the pericranium. Overlying the temporalis muscle superiorly, the plane of dissection should remain in the loose areolar layer, which is deep to the temporoparietal fascia containing the frontal branch and superficial to the deep temporal fascia. In other areas overlying bone, the flap is raised in a plane immediately superficial to the pericranium. Carrying out the dissection in the correct anatomic plane minimizes the risk of injury to the frontal branch of the facial nerve. At the region of the zygomatic arch, the frontal branch of the facial nerve is most vulnerable to injury. If the dissection is carried within 1 to 2 cm of the arch, the plane of dissection should be one layer deeper in this area and dissection should be just deep to the superficial layer of the deep temporal fascia [12]. After the soft tissue has been retracted, the pericranium is incised several centimeters superior to the most superior aspect of the frontal sinus and raised inferiorly to a level approximately 1 cm below the inferior extent of the frontal sinus. Other options for incision include the midforehead and the gull wing incisions. These approaches offer decreased operative time, decreased blood loss, and decreased risk of injury to the frontal branch of the facial nerve. However, they also limit exposure, increase the incidence of damage of the ophthalmic branch of the trigeminal nerve, and leave more visible scars [13, 14].

7. Frontal recess fracture

Frontal recess fractures only result in disruption of the frontal sinus outflow tract. Regardless of anterior or posterior table injuries, frontal recess fractures that result in sinus outflow obstruction will require frontal sinus obliteration. Endoscopic frontal sinusotomy has also been described for the management of persistent obstruction. However, endoscopic frontal sinusotomy following frontal recess trauma is technically challenging and should only be considered in reliable patients.

8. Anterior table fracture

A displaced fracture of the anterior table is the most common type of frontal sinus injury [15] which leaves a contour deformity of the forehead. Anterior table fractures involving the nasal-orbital-ethmoidal area or supraorbital rim have a 25% to 50% incidence of nasofrontal duct involvement [16-19]. In general, operative exposure of an anterior table fracture should also include an intraoperative examination of the nasofrontal duct to evaluate for injury. Exposure is best achieved by using a bicoronal incision (Figure 3).

Once the coronal incision has been made and the anterior table exposed, sinusotomy must be planned. One prong of a bayonet forceps is placed inside the sinus to the maximum peripheral extent. The corresponding prong then reflects its position on the external surface of the outer table. A number 701 burr in a high-speed drill marks the perimeter adjacent to the bayonet forceps. After sinus marking is complete, the osteotomy is accomplished using either a drill or oscillating saw [20]. Once the frontal sinus has been entered, cultures are taken of any fluids encountered. At this point, nasofrontal duct patency can be evaluated with the placement of either fluorescein or methylene blue proximally at the ostium located medially at the sinus floor. If there is no evidence of nasofrontal duct obstruction, the fracture fragments should be reduced and fixated (Figure 4).

The severely comminuted anterior table is best repaired with a precontoured plate (Figure 5). If there is significant comminution of the anterior table with bone loss, split calvarial graft is the material of choice to address defects of the anterior table (Figure 6).The use of synthetic

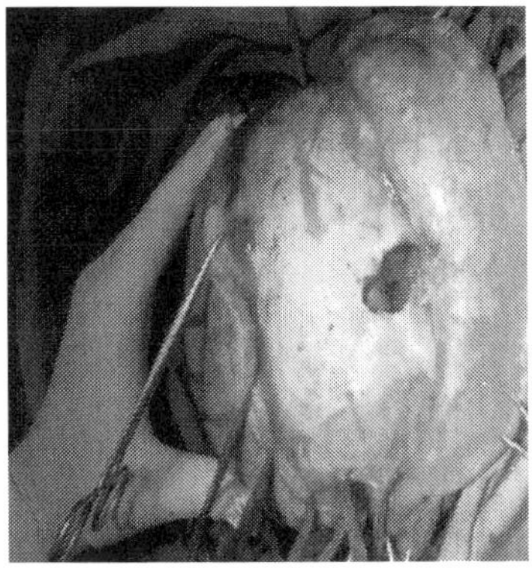

Figure 3. The frontal sinus fracture is approached via bicoronal incision

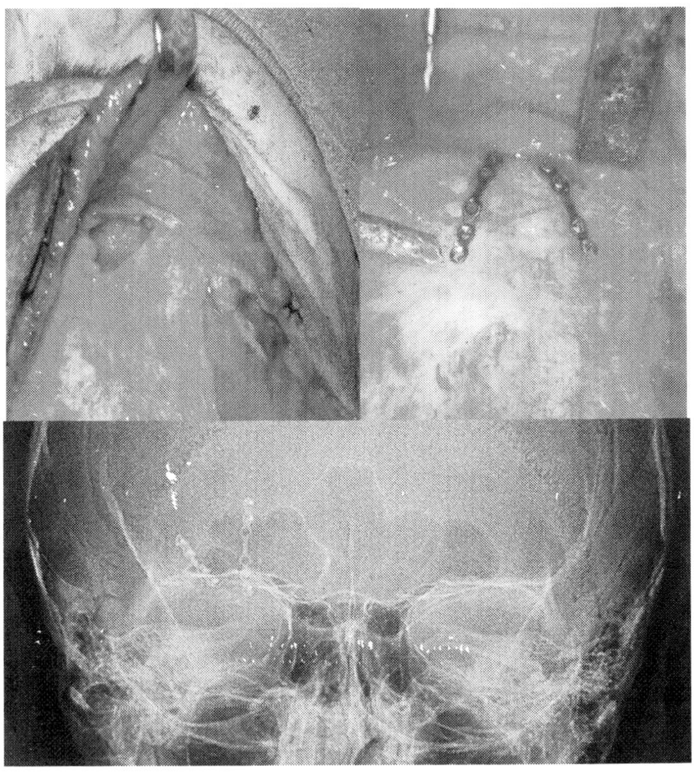

Figure 4. Left: Depressed fracture of the anterior table of the frontal sinus. Right: The fracture fragments are reduced and fixated by plates. Below: The postoperative radiograph of the patient.

materials, such as methyl methacrylate or even hydroxyapatite cements, is to be discouraged because of the risk of infection secondary to communication with the sinus floor [21].

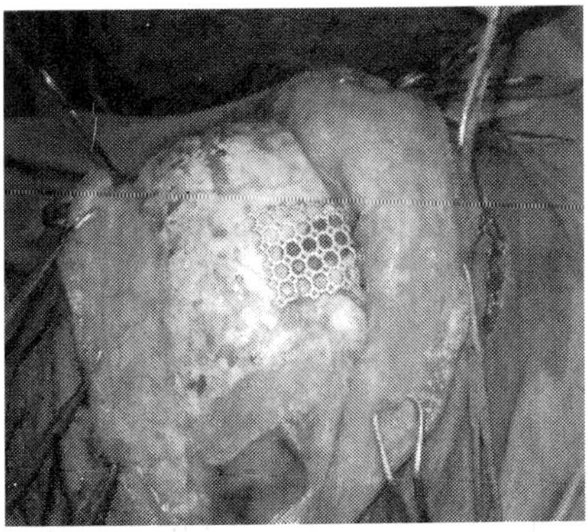

Figure 5. The severely comminuted anterior table is repaired with a titanium mesh

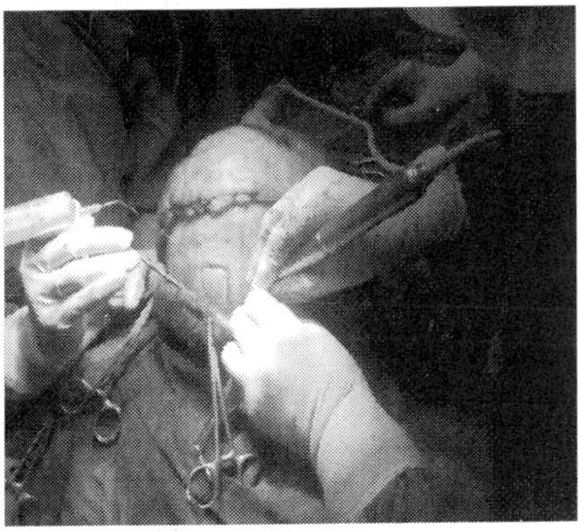

Figure 6. Split calvarial graft can be used for the repair of the severely comminuted anterior table

9. Fractures involving the nasofrontal duct

The anterior table fractures do not damage the nasofrontal duct unless there are concomitant nasal-orbital-ethmoidal complex or supraorbital fractures which extend into the sinus floor. A patent nasofrontal communication is necessary for the normal function of the frontal sinus. Therefore, treatment must either reestablish the communication or eliminate the sinus as a functional unit. If only one duct is injured, removal of the intersinus septum will allow mucus from the injured sinus to make its way to the uninjured side. Reconstruction of the duct requires long-term tenting (Figure 7) and mucosal flaps. However, in unilateral and bilateral nasofrontal duct injuries, obliteration of the frontal sinus is preferred. The procedure involves the removal of all mucous membrane and the inner cortical lining of the sinus and obliteration of the nasofrontal duct and the sinus. Mucocele formation is possible if the mucosa is inadequately removed during obliteration.

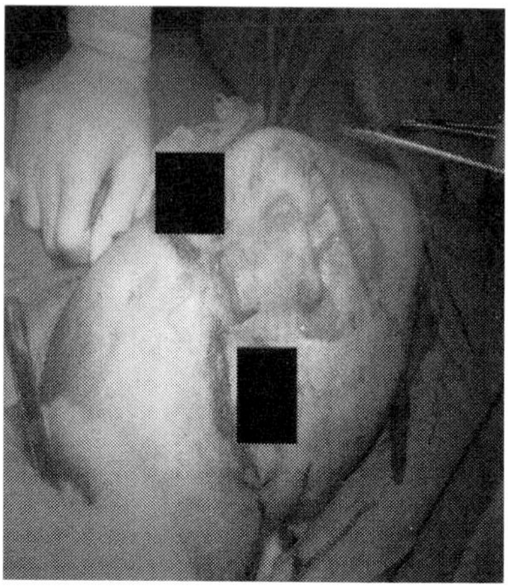

Figure 7. The frontal sinus approached with an open sky incision for reconstruction of the naso-frontal duct via stenting technique

10. Posterior table fracture

Extremely high-velocity injury may result in comminution of the posterior table with dural tearing. If this happens, the intracranial contents become in direct communication with nasal mucosa. In this setting, management principles are careful mucosal removal, nasofrontal duct occlusion and cranialization of the frontal sinus. The neurosurgeon repairs any associated intracranial injuries. The frontal lobes are then allowed to expand into the space where the frontal sinus once existed.

11. Frontal sinus obliteration

Obliteration of the sinus is performed by the use of various materials, such as fat, muscle, bone or hydroxyapatite. Meticulous removal of the entire mucosal lining is the most important element in successful frontal sinus obliteration. Permanent occlusion of frontal recess and complete obliteration of the sinus are essential in avoiding recurrence of infections and preventing possible complications [22].

Indications for frontal sinus obliteration include failure of endoscopic approaches to adequately communicate frontal sinus with the nasal cavity, loss of anterior bony table of the frontal sinus, severe fractures of floor of the frontal sinus and benign tumors [23]. The standard bicoronal incision is performed through the galea. The pericranium is incised as far posteriorly as possible, and a subperiosteal dissection is carried up to the supraorbital rim, preserving the supratrochlear and supraorbital neurovascular bundles. The frontal sinus is outlined. The anterior bony table is then removed. Sinus mucosa is meticulously exenterated with a periosteal elevator, and the interior of the sinus is carefully drilled with a medium-sized diamond burr. Nasofrontal ducts are then plugged with temporoparietal fascia and muscle. Obliteration of the frontal sinus is then performed with the previously mentioned materials (Figure 8).The anterior table plate is then replaced and plated.

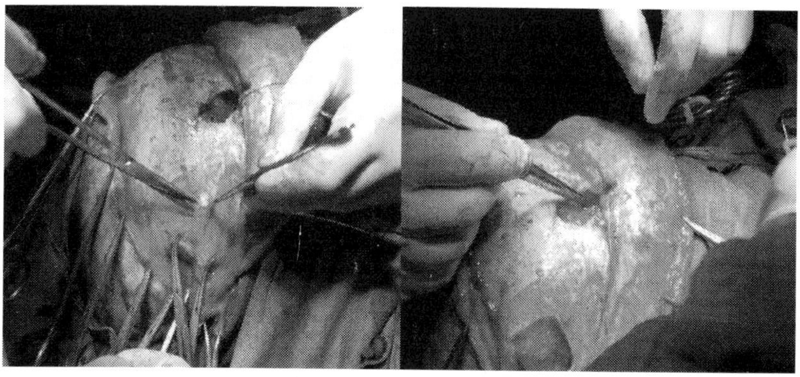

Figure 8. Left: Part of the temporalis muscle is excised for frontal sinus obliteration. Right: The frontal sinus is obliterated with muscle.

12. Frontal sinus cranialization

The primary indication for cranializing the frontal sinus is severe traumatic injury of the frontal sinus, with involvement of both the anterior and the posterior tables. Obliteration of the frontal sinus is an option in some cases but the loss of a substantial portion of the posterior table bone places the survival of a fat graft necessary for obliteration in doubt and makes cranialization more appropriate [24]. The presence of cerebrospinal fluid (CSF) rhinorrhea, the need for neurosurgical intervention, or simply an expectation of inadequate follow-up are all factors that may guide one towards cranialization. The approach to frontal sinus is performed via a bicoronal incision. Once access to the posterior table has been achieved, it is removed carefully in pieces with a rongeur. Larger pieces are saved for possible use replacing defects in the anterior table. Small overhangs at the periphery of the sinus should be smoothed completely, using a cutting burr. The end result of the removal of the posterior table bone is the elimination of the frontal sinus as a distinct space. This space is now encompassed within a new, larger anterior cranial fossa, with the anterior table as its anterior limit.

Once the entire posterior table has been removed, all sinus mucosa is taken out. This is done first bluntly, with a hemostat or forceps. Remnant mucosa is then eliminated using a diamond burr. Establishing a secure barrier between the cranial fossa and the nose is necessary to prevent CSF leak, meningitis, and ascending regrowth of the sinonasal mucosa. After the neurosurgery team has accomplished a watertight dural repair (Figure 9), and the bone and mucosa removal are complete, the most superior aspects of the frontal duct mucosa are elevated from the underlying bone and inverted downwards, toward the nose. The superior portions of the ducts are then packed off using bone, fascia, and muscle.

Abdominal fat harvested through a small paraumbilical incision is filled in around the dural closure, occupying intracranial dead space. Repair of the anterior table is essential for both structural and cosmetic concerns. Anatomic reductions are carried out with fixation.

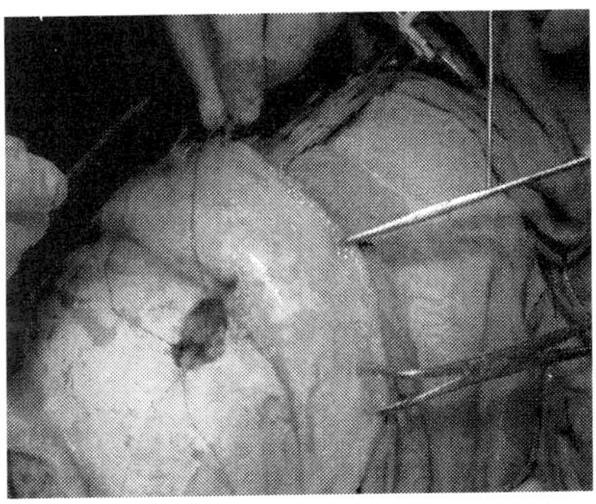

Figure 9. Water tight closure of the dura for prevention of CSF leakage

13. Flap closure

Closure of the coronal incision is performed in layers with interrupted 3-0 Vicryl stitches for the galea and deep dermis, and staples for the skin within the hairline. The skin outside the hairline is closed with interrupted 4-0 nylon stitches. Suction drains are generally avoided if immature dural closure is present. A neurosurgical head wrap is then applied.

14. Complications

Some complications of frontal sinus management relate to the surgical technique. The frontal branch of the facial nerve is vulnerable to injury during elevation of the coronal skin flap. The

http://dx.doi.org/10.5772/59968

result is paralysis of the ipsilateral forehead. This complication can be avoided by elevating the lateral aspects of the coronal flap in the proper plane. Too much disruption of the temporal fat pad during the lateral dissection can cause noticeable late temporal hollowing. A noticeable or widened scar from the coronal incision may develop. Other complications relate to the nature of the injury itself.CSF leak/rhinorrhea, with or without infectious consequences, may develop despite the fact that a watertight closure of the dura is performed. Management typically involves revision surgery, although nasal packing, bed rest, and CSF decompression via lumbar drain may be helpful adjuncts.

Appropriate management of meningitis relies on early recognition of signs, such as mental status changes, fever, and nuchal rigidity. When meningitis is detected, broad-spectrum antibiotics with CSF penetration should be employed empirically, with adjustments based on the subsequent cultures. A noticeable contour defect is always a possibility in the management of frontal sinus trauma. Meticulous reduction and fixation of all bone fragments and the appropriate use of bone grafts, titanium mesh, and bone cements are critically important for avoiding this complication.

The formation of a frontal mucocele, which may progress to mucopyocele, frontal bone osteomyelitis or endbrain abscess, are well-known complications of frontal sinus fractures.

15. Conclusion

The appropriate treatment of frontal sinus fractures is a controversial issue. Frontal sinus fractures represent only a small percentage of patients that require the evaluation by a comprehensive trauma service. The majority of patients will also present with concomitant facial fractures. A functional sinus can be preserved in the majority of patients, regardless of the degree of displacement, depending on the status of the nasofrontal duct, the amount of posterior table comminution, and the presence of significant neurologic injury or dural injuries. Frontal sinus obliteration is not a major component in the treatment of patients. The most important factor when treating a patient is to establish a secure barrier between the cranial fossa and the nose to prevent CSF leak, meningitis, and ascending regrowth of the sinonasal mucosa.

Author details

Roozbeh Kahali* and Alireza Tootoonchian

*Address all correspondence to: roozbehkahali@gmail.com

Department of Oral and Maxillofacial Surgery, Bouali Hospital, Islamic Azad University of Medical Sciences, Tehran, Iran

References

[1] Donald PJ. Frontal sinus fractures in otolaryngology, head and neck surgery. Cummings, ed. St. Louis: CV Mosby Co,1986:901

[2] Hollinshead WH. Anatomy for surgeons. Vol. 1. 3rd ed. New York: Harper & Row, 1982:249

[3] Manolidis S, HollierJr LH. Management of frontal sinus fractures. PlastReconstrSurg2007; 120(December (7 Suppl. 2)):32S–48S

[4] Gerbino G, Roccia F, Benech A, Caldarelli C.Analysis of 158 frontal sinus fractures: current surgical management and complications. J CraniomaxillofacSurg 2000;28(June (3)):133–9

[5] Dewall J. The ABCs of TBI.Evidence based guidelines for adult traumatic brain injury care. JEMS 2010;35(April (4)):54–61. quiz 63

[6] Manolidis S. Frontal sinus injuries: associated injuries and surgical management of 93patients. J Oral MaxillofacSurg 2004;62(July(7)):882–91

[7] Cantrell R: Fractures of the frontal sinus. Trans Pac Coast Otoophthalmol Soc Annu Meet 55:101, 1974

[8] Harris L, Marano G, McCorkle D: Nasofrontal duct: CT in frontal sinus trauma. Radiology 65:195, 1987

[9] Godin D, Miller R: Frontal sinus fractures. J La State Med Soc150:50, 1998

[10] Wallis A, Donald P: Frontal sinus fractures: A review of 72cases. Laryngoscope 98:593, 1988

[11] Donald PJ, Bernstein L. Compound frontal sinus injuries with intracranial penetration. Laryngoscope 1978;88:225-32

[12] Stuzin JM, Waystrom L, Kawamoto HK, et al: Anatomy of the frontal branch of the facial nerve: The significance of the temporal fat pad.PlastReconstrSurg 83:265-271, 1989

[13] Montgomery WW: State-of-the-art for osteoplastic frontal sinus operation.OtolaryngolClin North Am 34:167-177, 2001

[14] Hardy JM, Montgomery WW: Osteoplastic frontal sinusotomy—ananalysis of 250 operations. Ann Otolaryngol 85:523-532, 1976

[15] Sataloff R: Surgical management of the frontal sinus. Neurosurgery15:593, 1984

[16] Stevens M, Kline S: Management of frontal sinus fractures. J Craniomaxillofac Trauma 1:29, 1995

[17] Stanley R, Becker T: Injuries of the nasofrontal orifices in frontal sinus fractures. Laryngoscope 97:728, 1987

[18] Stanley R: Fractures of the frontal sinus. ClinPlastSurg 16:115,1989

[19] Stanley R: Management of severe frontobasilar skull fractures.OtolaryngolClin North Am 24:139, 1991

[20] Schmitz J, Lemke R, Smith B: The perimeter marking technique for rigid fixation of frontal sinus fractures: Procedure and report of cases. J Oral MaxillofacSurg 52:1120, 1994

[21] McGraw-Wall B: Frontal sinus fractures. Facial PlastSurg 14:59,1998

[22] Kennedy DW, Bolger WE, Zinreich SJ: Diseases of the Sinuses:Diagnosis, and Management. Hamilton and London, BC Decker, 2001

[23] Mendians AE, Marks SC: Outcome of frontal sinus obliteration.Laryngoscope 109:1495-1498, 1999

[24] Donald PJ, Ettin M: The safety of frontal sinus obliteration when sinus walls are missing. Laryngoscope 96:190-193, 1986

Section 9

Basics of Endoscopic Oral and Maxillofacial Surgery

Chapter 22

Endoscopic Oral and Maxillofacial Surgery

Gholamreza Shirani,
Shiva Solahaye Kahnamouii and
Mohammad Hosein Kalantar Motamedi

Additional information is available at the end of the chapter

http://dx.doi.org/10.5772/59160

1. Introduction

Endoscopy is the examination and inspection of the interior of body organs, joints or cavities through an endoscope. Endoscopic surgery uses scopes that go through small incisions or natural body openings to diagnose and treat disease. Another popular term is minimally invasive surgery (MIS), which emphasizes that diagnosis and treatment can be done with reduced body invasion. Endoscopes are revolutionary surgical tools that provide detailed video images, allowing visualization of internal structures through a skin incision the width of a thumb and an entry into the organ smaller than a pushpin. Small instruments that can cut, sample, or destroy abnormal tissue or tumors can also be passed through these tubes, allowing intricate surgery to be performed with little or no trauma. Endoscopy allows physicians to peer through the body's passageways.

Construction An endoscope uses two fiber optic lines. A "light fiber" carries light into the body cavity and an "image fiber" carries the image of the body cavity back to the physician's viewing lens. The portion of the endoscope inserted into the body may be rigid or flexible, depending upon the medical procedure. There is also a separate port to allow for administration of drugs, suction, and irrigation. This port may also be used to introduce small folding instruments such as scalpels, scissors, forceps, brushes, snares and baskets for tissue excision (removal), sampling, or other diagnostic and therapeutic work. They are inserted through different incisions and are used to perform the operation. Endoscopes may be used in conjunction with a camera or video recorder to document internal mages. New endoscopes have digital capabilities for manipulating and enhancing video images (Figures 1 and 2).

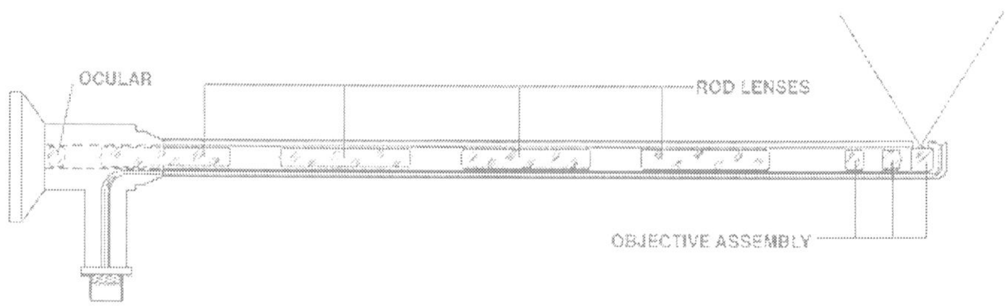

Figure 1. This figure shows an endoscope. The "image fiber" leads from the ocular (eye piece) to the inserted end of the scope. The "light fiber" is below and leads from the light source to the working end of the endoscope.

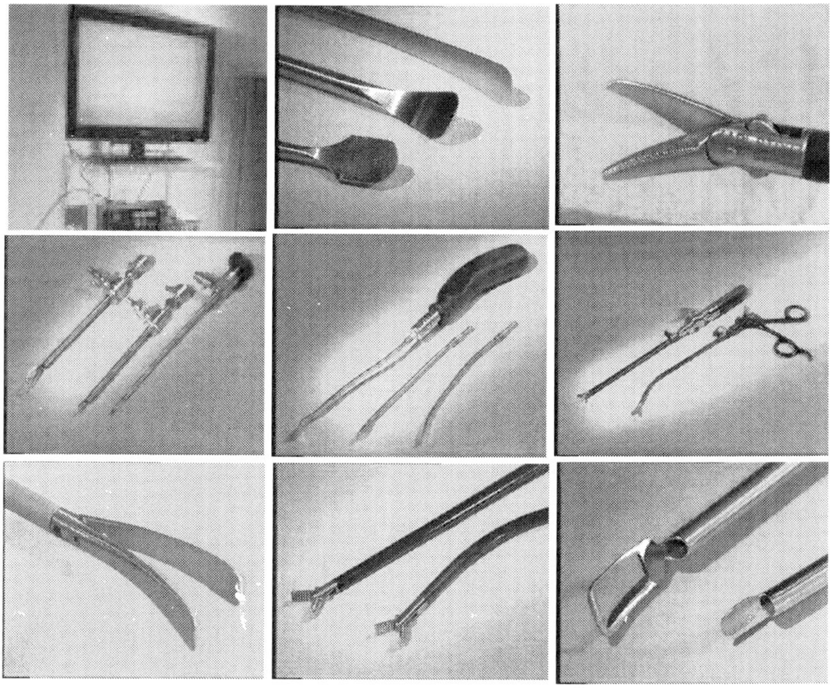

Figure 2. Endoscopic surgery equipment and instruments

1.1. Endoscopic plastic surgery

Endoscopic plastic surgery is one of the newest plastic surgery techniques. It allows surgeons to operate with fewer conspicuous incisions, reducing obvious scars. Improvements in technology have enabled surgeons to use endoscopy for many cosmetic procedures, including facelifts, forehead lifts, etc. Endoscopy can also be used in some reconstructive procedures. In many cases, the use of endoscopy results in shorter recovery.

Candidates must be in good health, have no active diseases or serious pre-existing medical conditions, and must have realistic expectations of the outcome of the surgery. Smoking, having recently quit smoking and being exposed to second-hand smoke are all contraindications. Primary and secondary smoking decreases blood flow to the body's tissues. This can result in prolonged wound healing, skin loss, infection, increased scarring, and a number of other complications depending on the kind of procedure performed.

The endoscope is merely a new tool to better achieve just that objective. Outcome enhancements initially predominated in aesthetic applications, but widespread use also in reconstructive endeavors has proved that today there is indeed a broad scope for minimally invasive surgery.

The goal of what today would be considered minimally invasive surgery may be to even surpass the outcomes possible with traditional open techniques, with diminished patient morbidity including accelerated recovery time and, at the same time, reducing overall healthcare costs. Initially conceived as a means to allow the direct examination of internal organs while avoiding large incisions, the origins of the clinical application of this concept can be traced back to Hippocrates in ~400 BC who used a rectal speculum to examine hemorrhoids.[1] The centuries to follow fostered slow, incremental improvements in instrumentation and light sources that would eventually allow the requisite access as well as proper illumination of the operative field. However, not until the 1950s did the advent of fiber-optic technology permit the transmission of light from an external light source along long, flexible glass or plastic threads so that a clear image could be obtained, yet now without risk of thermal injury.[1]

In 1990, ongoing research efforts at the University of Alabama at Birmingham culminated in reports of a broad clinical experience in endoscopy including endoscopic brow lift.[2] Nowhere were the early demands for minimally invasive surgery so prevalent than in cosmetic surgery.[3]

The interest in aesthetic endoscopic plastic surgery still predominates today, [4]-[11] and there is a concomitant explosion of novel applications in reconstructive surgery. An early thrust of the latter included relatively simple maneuvers such as the removal of benign lesions, decompressive fasciotomy for extremity compartment syndrome,[14] or retrieval of spare body parts such as tendon,[15] vein,[16] or nerve[17],[18] grafts. Congenital deformities such as torticollis[19] especially in the pediatric age group, [13] have been well suited to endoscopic correction, as the cosmetic result often is a major consideration. Acquired defects like facial fractures[20] may be directly or indirectly repaired. More complex indications for various tissue manipulations have included the safe placement of tissue expanders [21], [22] or harvest of local[23] or free adipofascial, muscle, and visceral flaps using endoscopic assistance. The realm in the future may be endoscopic robotic surgery for even greater precision, including not just the difficult and safe dissection of the vascular pedicles of all flaps but also the performance even of the microanastomoses themselves.[23], [24] The capability for all these tissue manipulations could someday then be routinely performed in any distant land or even on another planet, where the immediate availability and skills of a surgeon will no longer be a concern!

2. Endoscopic sinus surgery

The sinuses are air-filled holes in the skull. They are connected to the nose and can get infected leading to discharge, pain, etc. This may be caused by allergies, polyps, abnormal shape or swelling inside the nose. Medical therapies, such as antibiotics, steroids, nasal sprays and decongestants will often cure bouts of sinusitis. Sinus surgery is advocated in those patients who fail to improve after medication. There are circumstances when immediate sinus surgery is warranted. Tumors of the sinuses, whether benign or malignant, often require surgical removal. Surgery may be the only option for some patients whose sinus condition aggravates other medical problems such as asthma. Cancer or immunocompromised patients may require drainage for culture or for treatment of a fungal infection. In the past, surgeries requiring an incision under the lip (Caldwell-Luc) or face (external ethmoidectomy) were used to drain sinus cavities. Most procedures are now performed using endoscopic technology (via small cameras through the nose), eliminating the need for external incisions. Endoscopic sinus surgery uses small rods of light with a camera (endoscope) to operate through the nostrils into the sinuses (Figure 3).

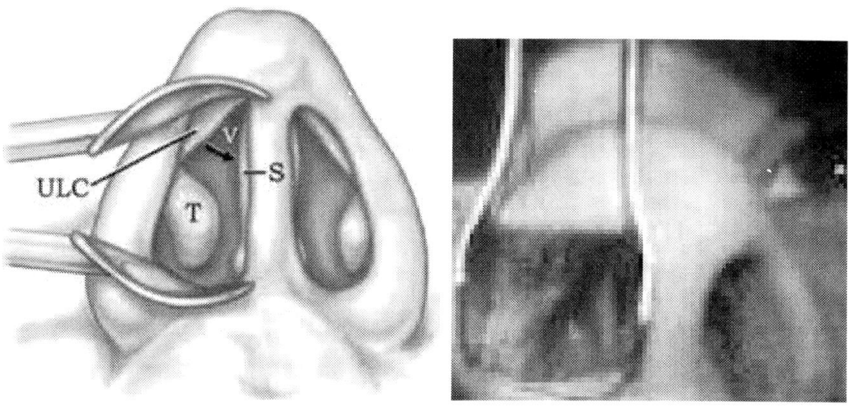

Figure 3. Entry to the sinus from the nostrils

This does not involve any incisions on the face, but may be combined with other external approaches, which may involve cuts. This surgery is usually done under general anesthesia for patient comfort. A CT scan will serve as a road map for the surgeon. ESS has presented a new philosophy allowing the surgeon to target the ostiumeatal complex (OMC). Obstruction of the OMC can lead to subsequent infection of the maxillary, frontal and sphenoid sinuses.

Accordingly, ESS removes thickened and diseased tissue blocking the OMC. Most of the healthy tissue in the sinuses is undisturbed allowing for faster and better overall recovery. Endoscopic surgery can also be utilized for removal of polyps, nasal masses and sometimes straightening the septum to improve nasal airflow.

2.1. Functional endoscopic sinus surgery

Functional endoscopic sinus surgery (FESS) is the mainstay in the surgical treatment of **sinusitis** and **nasal polyps**, including bacterial, fungal, recurrent, acute and chronic sinus problems. FESS is a relatively recent surgical procedure that uses nasal **endoscopes** (using **Hopkins rod lens technology**) through the nostrils to avoid cutting the skin. FESS came into existence through the pioneering work of Drs. Messerklinger (in 1960 to 1970's) and his assistant Stamberger who became chief of the ENT department in Graz, Austria. Other surgeons have made additional contributions (first published in the USA by Kennedy in 1985).[25]

By the early 1990's endoscopic sinus surgery become one of the most popular procedures. In their 1990 publication, Stamberger [26] mentioned operating 4500 patients, roughly 450 patients annually. Most procedures were very limited surgical procedures; diseased ethmoid compartments were operated on (usually the ethmoidal bulla), stenotic clefts were widened (uncinate process) and prechambers (agar nasi cells) to the frontal and maxillary sinuses were freed from disease.

2.2. Indications

The most common indication for endoscopic sinus surgery is "chronic rhinosinusitis". Chronic rhinosinusitis is a term applied to various nasal processes which involve inflammation of the nose and sinuses that do not adequately improve with medical management. Less common indications include (but are not limited to): recurrent infections (rather than chronic inflammation), complications of sinus infections, nasal polyps, mucoceles, chronic sinus headaches, impaired sense of smell, tumors of the nasal and sinus cavities, cerebrospinal fluid leaks, nasolacrimal duct obstruction, choanal atresia, and the need to decompress the orbit. Additionally, recent advances in endoscopic techniques allow the operator to provide access to areas of the brain and pituitary gland for neurosurgeons or to the orbits (eye sockets) for certain ophthalmology procedures.

2.3. Technique

The frontal, maxillary, and anterior ethmoid sinuses drain into the middle meatus. Posterior ethmoids drain into the superior meatus. Sphenoid sinuses drain into the sphenoethmoid recess. Telescopes with diameters of 4mm (adults) and 2.7mm (pediatrics) and with a variety of viewing angles (0 to 30, 45, 70, 90, and 120 degrees) provide good illumination of the inside of the nasal cavity and sinuses. High-definition cameras, monitors and a host of tiny articulating instruments aid in identifying and restoring the proper drainage and ventilation relationships between the nose and sinus cavities. Cultures and biopsies can be easily obtained to yield valuable diagnostic information to guide postoperative therapy for optimal long term results.

All the sinuses can be accessed at least to some degree by means of this device: The frontal sinuses located in the forehead, the maxillary sinuses in the cheek bones, the ethmoid sinuses between the orbits, and the sphenoid sinuses are located in the back of the nasal cavity at the base of the skull.

2.4. Extended approaches

Endoscopic access to pituitary tumors has been successfully accomplished for many years. More recently, further advanced techniques have allowed the paranasal sinuses to be a relatively low-morbidity approach to selected tumors even inside the skull or brain.

2.5. Benefits of ESS

The overall goal of sinus surgery is to improve the drainage pathway of the sinuses. By opening the natural drainage pathway of the diseased sinus, the frequency, duration and severity of infections should be reduced. Sinus surgery is not without risk, but it does have major benefits. Sinus issues left uncorrected may lead to abscess formation, permanent loss of sense of smell vision, or even death. Benefits of sinus surgery include asthma relief, polyps and fungus removal and less recurrence of sinus infections.

Although there are patients who have mechanical obstruction due to their particular anatomy, many patients have an intrinsic problem with the lining (mucous membrane) of their nose and sinuses. While the patients with mechanical obstruction, will receive the maximal benefit from surgery, the benefit for patients with mucous membrane disease is also tangible because the larger opening created during surgery will allow better drainage and more medication and rinses to get into the sinuses and help treat the diseased lining.

One of the most important benefits of surgery is the ability to deliver medications (e.g. sprays, rinses, nebulized drugs) to the lining of your sinuses after they have been accessed. Therefore, surgery is an adjunct to, not a replacement for, proper medical management. It is important to note, however, that if you are one of the patients who have diseased mucous membranes or form nasal polyps, no amount of surgery can change this fact. So although surgery plays a role in managing the disease, it may not cure sinus disease with polyps or other types of chronic inflammation. Therefore, it should be emphasized that surgery is one of the multiple steps in managing the disease.

2.6. Possible risks and complications related to functional endoscopic sinus surgery

Extreme care is required with this surgery due to the proximity of the sinuses to the eyes, optic nerves, brain and internal carotid arteries. However, these serious risks are rare occurrences and there are many potential benefits from a well-performed endoscopic sinus surgery with appropriate indications. All surgical procedures have risks and complications namely:

1. Bleeding from the nose in the days following the operation

2. Infection
3. Injury to the nasolacrimal duct or sac
4. Need for frequent post-surgical visits for cleaning
5. CSF leak
6. Impaired taste and/or smell (usually temporary)

2.7. CT navigation

Computed tomography (CT) navigation is a tool that may be used by surgeons to better correlate surgical anatomy with pre-operative CT imaging. A computer is used to identify the 3-dimensional location of a probe tip placed within the patient's nose or sinuses.

Definitive proof that CT navigation improves outcomes and decreases complications is lacking. A Swedish study of 212 patients undergoing sphenoethmoidectomy published in 2008 concluded that the clinical success of the procedure was similar with or without the use of CT navigation, and that the rate of complications might be slightly reduced.[27]

3. Endoscopic facelift (forehead lift, brow lift, midface lift)

As humans age, lines and wrinkles naturally form on the forehead due to constant muscle movement, making one look older than he/she would like. Additionally, those horizontal lines across the forehead, or vertical lines between the brows, can cause one to look angry, stressed, or simply unpleasant and unapproachable. Fortunately, with the help of endoscopic surgery, one can achieve a fresh-faced, smooth, youthful appearance.

3.1. Technique

In preparation for a classic forehead lift, the hair is tied back with rubber bands in front and behind the incision area. An incision is usually made across the top of the head, just behind the hairline. Forehead skin is gently lifted and portions of facial muscle and excess skin are removed. The incision is then closed with stitches or clips. The result of a forehead lift is a younger, more rested look (Figure 4).

In an endoscopic forehead lift, the muscles and tissues that cause the furrowing or drooping are removed or altered to smooth the forehead, raise the eyebrows and minimize frown lines. Surgeons may use the conventional surgical method, in which the incision is hidden just behind the hairline; or it may be performed with the use of an endoscope. Both techniques yield similar results, smoother forehead skin and a more animated appearance.

Low, heavy "V" shaped eyebrows create a tired, older, masculine, unfriendly appearance. Opening up the eyes and brows and smoothing the forehead is both powerful and subtle. Patients look more awake, fresh, healthy and youthful. Forehead surgery is normally done in combination with an eye lift (blepharoplasty) for best results.

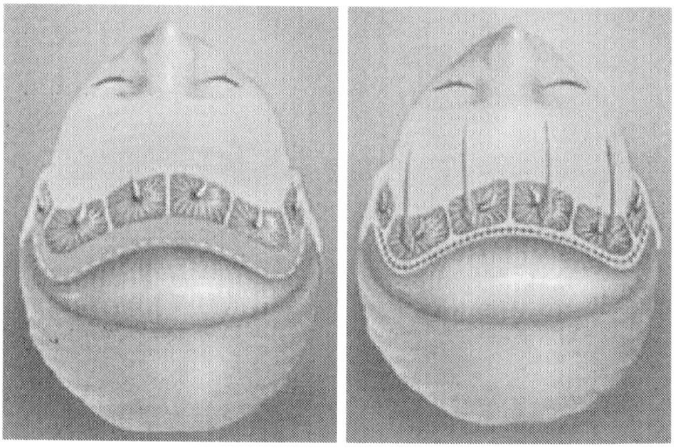

Figure 4. Classic forehead lift incision

Before the operation, motivations and demands of the patients must be analyzed. A careful study of the upper facial region and its relations with the rest of the face should be made. A preoperative assessment is normally conducted as required. The anesthesiologist will be seen in consultation at the latest 48 hours before surgery. No medication containing aspirin should be taken within 10 days prior to surgery. Smoking cessation is strongly recommended at least one month before and one month after surgery. An antiseptic shampoo should be used the night before and / or in the morning. It is essential to fast (not eat or drink) 6 hours before surgery.

3.2. Type of anesthesia

Two methods are possible:

- Local anesthesia deepened by intravenous tranquilizer
- General anesthesia

The choice between these different techniques will be the result of a discussion between patient, surgeon and the anesthesiologist.

Hospitalization is short. The admission is in the morning (or even the day before in the afternoon) and the discharge is permitted either in the evening or the day after the operation.

3.3. Technique of endoscopic forehead and eyebrow lift

Each surgeon adopts his/her own technique that he/she adapts to in each case in order to obtain the best results. However, some common basic principles are as follows:

Incisions are between 5 and 10 mm long, are three to five in number and are placed in the scalp, a few centimeters behind the forehead hairline. One of them will allow the passage of the endoscope connected to a mini video camera, the other giving way to the different instruments specifically adapted to endoscopic surgery. The path of these incisions is of course the future location of scars, which are therefore virtually invisible since they are very short and hidden in the hair. Detachment includes the temples and facial bones (Figures 5 and 6).

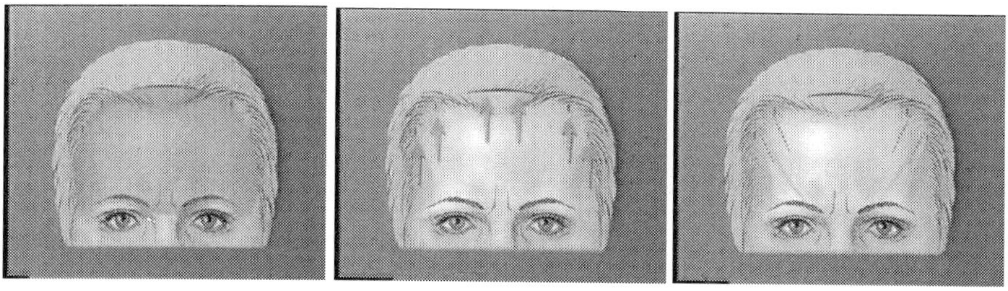

Figure 5. Incision sites for endoscopic forehead (brow) lift surgery

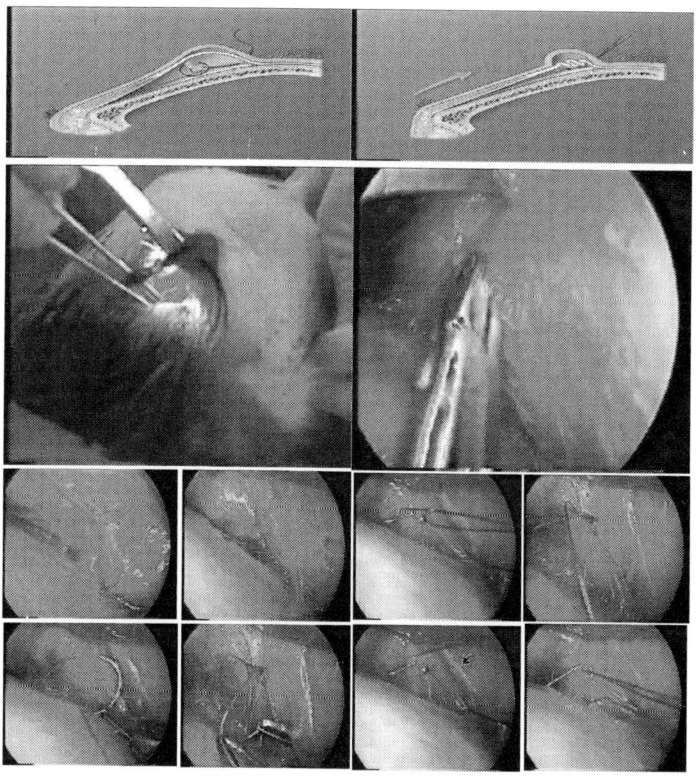

Figure 6. Dissection and suturing during endoscopic surgery

Replacement: Loose tissue will be retightened to soften the "crow's feet", move the tail of the eyebrows upward, and above all the cheek and fat under the eyes that had accumulated over the nasolabial folds will be held in position by deep fixation.

Sutures: The small incisions are closed, often with skin staples that are easily removed or with buried absorbable sutures.

Depending on the surgeon, the extent of improvements and the possible need for additional procedures, the intervention may take 2 to 3 hours. Possibly some discomfort with a feeling of tension on the temples and cheek may occur. The postoperative course is mainly marked by the appearance of edema (swelling) and ecchymosis (bruising) the size and duration of which is highly variable from one individual to another. The dressing should be removed between the 1st and 3rd days. Staples are removed between the 8th and 15th day. The stigma of the intervention will diminish gradually, allowing the return to normal social and professional life after a few more days (10-20 days depending on the magnitude of the surgery). Some numbness of the operated area, possibly some itching on the skull, may be observed during the first weeks. They gradually disappear. A delay of 3 to 6 months is necessary to assess the final outcome. This is the time for all of the edema to be reabsorbed and for the tissues to regain their flexibility. In most cases, intervention results in improvement and significant rejuvenation of the upper face, with an attenuation of nasolabial folds, padding the area under the eyes and cheeks (with disappearance of the "valley tears") and a decrease of the lower eyelid height.

The results are generally durable, although the aging process is not stopped by the intervention, the benefit of the lift will be present many years after.

3.4. Ideal candidates

Most patients opting for lifting are aged between 40 and 50 years, when brow lines and eyelids begin to sag noticeably and wrinkles or creases begin to appear along the forehead. Heredity sometimes causes these problems for people in their 20s and 30s, in which case a brow lift can help. Anyone considering this procedure should have a thorough understanding of what it can and cannot accomplish. After an in-depth discussion, some decide that a brow lift performed in conjunction with other procedures (e.g. a facelift (rhytidectomy) or eyelid surgery (**blepharoplasty**) will provide the best results

3.5. Facelift complications

All surgical procedures carry some uncertainty and risk. Even in the best hands, complications do occur. Fortunately, these are usually treatable. Patients vary in their anatomy, physical reaction to surgery, anesthesia, and healing capabilities, so that the outcome is never completely predictable. Surgeons know from experience that two operations in different patients, done almost exactly the same way, may have very different outcomes. Even operations on two sides of the same face or body can have different outcomes, particularly in terms of discomfort, bruising and swelling. Patients are often surprised at this.

It is best if patients anticipate having a complication, and if they do not that is a bonus. There is a well-known phrase in surgery: "The only way to avoid complications is by not operating."

http://dx.doi.org/10.5772/59160

Experienced surgeons, particularly toward the end of their careers, are often very candid and admit that they've seen just about every complication in their practice over the years. It is important for the patient and doctor to have a mutual trustful relationship to manage complications when they develop.

A complication rate of 1% is commonly quoted. It seems small, only one in a hundred, and perhaps this is a rate that is comfortable from a psychological standpoint, an event that sometimes happens to other people. But it should not be too reassuring, even if it is correct. If patients encounter a complication, it's 100 percent as far as they are concerned. They have to understand that it could happen to them. They should have the surgery only if they can tolerate the risks.

Facelift risks and complications may include:

1. Excessive scarring, bleeding, hematoma, infection, skin necrosis, facial weakness or paralysis caused by facial nerve injury, asymmetry, numbness, burning or cold sensations, facial pain, skin contour irregularities, skin discoloration, swelling, hair loss along the incision lines or elsewhere and corneal injury.
2. Corneal injury. It is imperative that the corneas be protected from drying out. Normally, at night, the cornea is protected by the closed eyelids. However, after surgery, the eyelids may not close completely, due to swelling or weakness of the orbicularis muscle that encircles the eyelids. Incomplete eyelid closure places the cornea at risk. Until eyelid function returns, it is imperative that the corneas be kept from drying out with the use of lubricating ointment and eye drops.
3. Earlobe deformity ("pixie ear") is an unnaturally tethered ear. The earlobe is pulled down by the facelift scar. Usually this results from too much skin removal around the ear, so that there is tension on the skin closure, pulling down on the earlobe. Experienced plastic surgeons avoid any skin tension in the area of the earlobe to prevent such a complication of surgery.
4. The "lateral sweep," is an unnatural, operated-on appearance that can happen after facelifts that draw back on the skin of the lateral face, while leaving the vertical descent of the cheek and jowl untreated. The skin form may form horizontal folds. It is not a harmonious or pleasing appearance.
5. Another post-surgical problem is "joker's lines," unnatural lines of tension that extend from the corners of the mouth to the ears. Both problems may be prevented, and treated, with a deep-plane facelift that incorporates a cheek lift.
6. Tragal deformity: flattening of the tragus (the small bump just in front of the ear canal) may be avoided by using a pre-tragal incision, which is my preference. The tragus is a unique structure that is very difficult to recreate.
7. Nerve damage may concern some sensory branches and then be responsible for certain insensitivity and itching of the forehead and scalp that eventually subside after a few months. A paralysis of the frontal branch is much rarer and, fortunately, is only temporary in most cases described.

8. General dissatisfaction with the cosmetic results, possibility of revision surgery, depression or emotional mood changes may also develop.

3.6. Preoperative instructions

Before undergoing brow lift surgery, we must provide pre-operative instructions; these may include:

1. Stopping smoking four weeks before surgery

2. Stop taking certain medications, herbs, and vitamins (including those that thin the blood) two weeks before surgery

3. Purchase all supplies that will be needed during recovery, including pain medication, bandages, and groceries, before the day of surgery

4. Not eating or drinking anything after midnight the day of surgery

5. Not wearing make-up, contact lenses, or jewelry on the day of surgery

6. A family member or friend should drive the patient home.

3.7. Benefits of brow lift surgery

All men and women over the age of 40 see signs of aging in the face. The forehead is usually one of the first places where lines and wrinkles appear due to excessive muscle movement. Fortunately, brow lift surgery can do away with a number of cosmetic flaws on the upper third portion of the face. The many benefits of brow lift surgery include: Increase confidence with enhanced appearance, rejuvenated appearance, alleviation of tension in the forehead muscles, causes minimal side effects, fast recovery, excellent, long-lasting results (up to 10 years or more), incisions are well hidden and scarring is minimal, natural-looking results and few potential risks or complications.

4. Endoscopic midface lift

An endoscopic mid-facelift, also known as the anti-gravity lift, is a surgical procedure able to provide a natural, more youthful and refreshed appearance to the face by repositioning sagging cheeks, softening smile lines, reducing lower eye hollowness, elevating the corners of the lips, and restoring cheek fullness.

4.1. Best candidates

The best candidate for an endoscopic mid-facelift is a physically healthy man or woman who has realistic expectations and is interested in improving the appearance of sagging or sunken cheeks, smile lines, lower eye hollowness, and sagging corners of the lips. The procedure is ideal for patients in their late thirties to early sixties.

4.2. Technique

After anesthesia is administered, tiny incisions are placed inconspicuously within the hairline at the temple and inside of the mouth. An endoscope is inserted into the incisions to help guide the surgeon as he or she elevates the fat pads of the cheeks as well as the deeper tissues. The incisions are then closed with sutures (Figure 7).

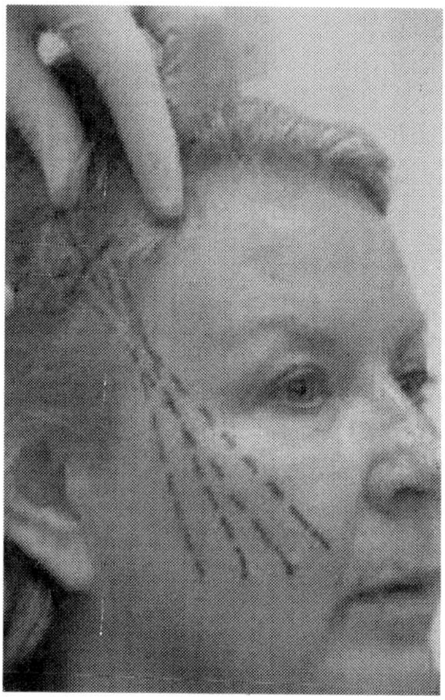

Figure 7. Schematic endoscopic midface lift. Tiny incisions are inconspicuously placed within the hairline at the temple and inside of the mouth, thus allowing for no visible scarring. There is no visible scarring after an endoscopic mid-facelift as very tiny incisions are inconspicuously placed inside of the mouth and within the hairline at the temple.

After an endoscopic mid-facelift, patients typically experience minimal discomfort which can easily be controlled with pain medication. Swelling and bruising may occur and typically fades within a few weeks. The head should be elevated for the first few days to help minimize swelling. Stitches are typically removed within seven days. Patients can typically return to work within a week after an endoscopic mid-facelift. As with all types of surgery there are potential complications that can occur with an endoscopic mid-facelift.

5. Endoscopic repair of facial fracture

Endoscopy is not a new concept; it is however, relatively new to the field of craniomaxillofacial surgery. Surgeons weigh the risk of an operation and its approach against the benefits of preventing complications, and recommend surgery based on this analysis. In general, if a procedure has a lower risk of complications, it is more widely applied. Endoscopic techniques may provide lower rates of complications and higher acceptance rates in patients, and therefore, they may be more widely employed. Because these techniques are very detailed and have a steep "learning curve," surgeons should be patient in their evaluation and use.

5.1. Frontal sinus fracture repair

Fractures of the frontal sinus and orbit are relatively common in facial trauma patients (5 to 15% of all maxillofacial traumas).[28]-[31] Although a significant percentage of these fractures can be managed non-operatively, operative intervention is often required to avoid late complications. Frontal sinus fracture is commonly treated via an endoscope. If the fracture is a simple type that places a small depression on the forehead, it is very amenable to endoscopic techniques. Frontal sinus fractures essentially come in four types.

The first type is anterior table fracture only, which is perfect for endoscopic technique because these fractures are the easiest to treat and the most conspicuous. The fragments must be evaluated with anatomic precision. The bony fragments may be reduced in situ or, more likely, removed, plated, and replaced either through a scalp or a brow incision.

The second (most common) fracture type is fracture of the anterior and posterior tables. Because a large amount of energy is required to cause this type of fracture, patients are often comatose or require c-spine precautions and wound care until open reduction and internal fixation (ORIF) can be done. These fractures are often associated with CSF leakage and need not only facial and sinus surgery, but also dural repairs and brain surgery. Patients often require cranialization of the sinus and cannot be treated with endoscopic techniques.

The third type of fracture is fracture of the posterior table itself. These fractures are rare, but when they occur they require a craniotomy for repair.

The fourth type of fracture is one that disrupts the ducts. If the duct is damaged, the patient would benefit from some procedure to defunctionalize the sinus. This could be cranialization (if a craniotomy is required) or obliterations with bone or fat.

An illustration detailing the incisions for endoscopic repair of anterior table frontal sinus fractures can be seen in Figure 8.

5.2. Orbital fractures

Orbital fractures are common and typically occur as blow-out fractures (BOF). BOF fractures are fractures that result in trauma directly over the orbital rim and floor. These fractures are not associated with the typical zygomaticomaxillary complex fractures. Medial orbital fractures are treated similarly to floor fractures except that these require more extensive knowledge of intranasal anatomy. To undertake the endoscopic repair, you must be aware of endoscopic skull base anatomy and be comfortable taking or medializing the middle turbinate and taking the uncinate process and ethmoid bulla down. Medial wall fractures are essentially an extended ethmoidectomy and treated via placement of an alloplastic sheet.

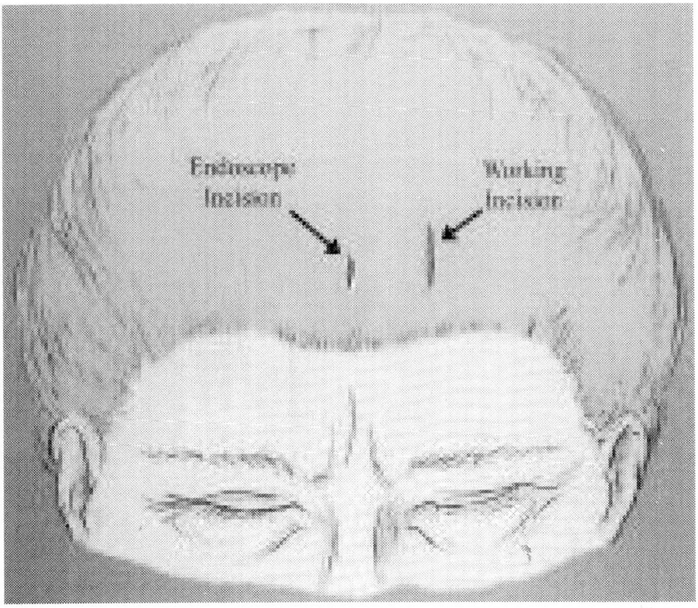

Figure 8. Illustration of incisions used for endoscopic repair of anterior table frontal sinus fractures. The working incision is in line with the fracture. The endoscope incision is just medial to the working incision.

The instrumentation is virtually identical. These techniques were first used for endoscopic subcondylar repair [28]-[30] and are now also used for transantral orbital floor reconstruction, zygomatic arch and frontal sinus repair. Subcondylar fractures are difficult to treat openly in even the best of circumstances and seeing and treating the condyle in its native position has numerous advantages. Once this use became more common, other facial fractures began to be examined from an endoscopic perspective.

Some of the more typical complications of orbital fractures are diplopia from muscle entrapment, visual loss, and exophthalmoses from volume expansion into the surrounding sinus leading to pseudoptosis. The typical complications from frontal sinus injuries are much less common but much more significant when encountered. These include frontal contour irregularities, spinal fluid leak (predisposing to meningitis), ocular complications including vision loss and blindness and late complications i.e. mucoceles (Figure 9).

Traditionally, external transorbital approaches have been used in the repair of blowout fracture (BOF) of the orbit. External approaches generally require either a medial canthal incision, a subciliary incision, or a transconjunctival incision, depending on the location, extent and complexity of the fracture. External repairs with transorbital incisions have known complications that include external scars, ectropion and a frequent need for alloplastic materials to support the fractured wall.[32]

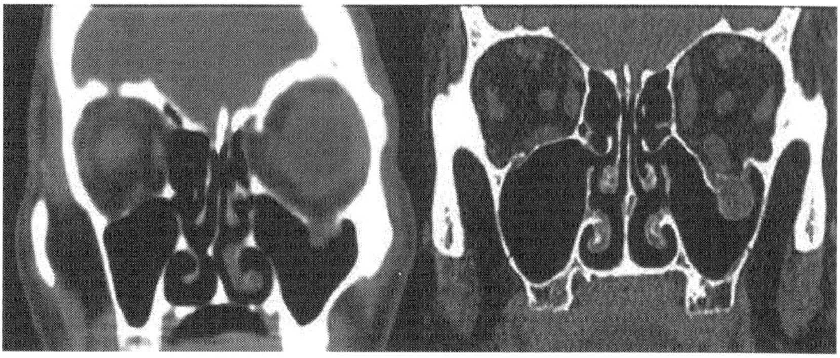

Figure 9. Coronal CT views of left orbital blow-out fracture

Endoscopic repair of BOF of the orbit has been reported to provide surgeons with several advantages over conventional external repair. [32]-[42]

First, it provides excellent visualization of the medial and inferior walls of the orbit, which enables safe removal of bony fragments and clear anatomic reduction of fractures. Second, the use of intraocular alloplastic implants, commonly used with external repairs, can be avoided or minimized.

Third, endoscopy virtually eliminates the risk of significantly visible facial scarring and eyelid complications, reported with transorbital incisions. Fourth, endoscopic surgery can be performed under local anesthesia, which makes intra-operative evaluation of ocular movements and diplopia possible.

When the anterior maxillary wall is fractured, Medpor is used to support the orbital floor; an endoscope enables clear identification of the bony shelves so that the implant can be placed safely and with adequate support (Figures 10 and 11).

No specific major disadvantages have been reported for endoscopic repair of BOF.[42], [43] One potential difficulty with transantral repair of inferior BOF is in the fabrication and maintenance of a balloon that conforms to the shape of the orbital floor to support the reduced orbital tissue. Under usual circumstances, the balloon is removed three to four weeks after surgery.

In medial BOF, the balloon can be removed early if the fracture is small or if only those bony fragments that might interfere with ocular muscle function are removed. In inferior BOF, the balloon can be removed early when a trapdoor type fracture is reduced with the bony fragment intact or when the fracture site is supported by a large bony fragment or implant. Usually, the balloon packing that supports the medial wall can be removed earlier than a balloon catheter that supports the inferior wall because the inferior wall must be rigid enough to support the orbit against gravity. Failure of diplopia to improve after adequate repositioning of orbital tissue is not an infrequent outcome after surgery for BOF.[42], [45] There are a few explanations for residual diplopia even after adequate surgery.

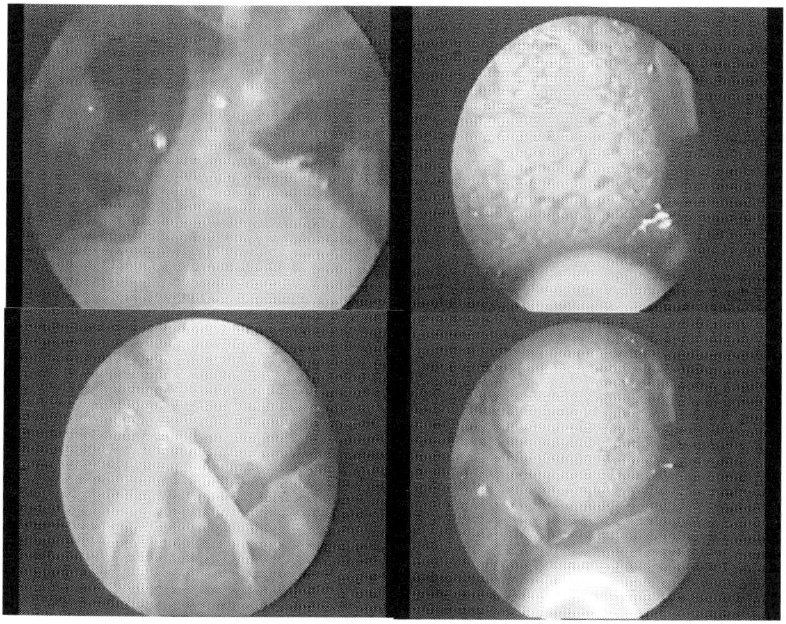

Figure 10. endoscopic repair of orbital floor fracture via alloplastic material

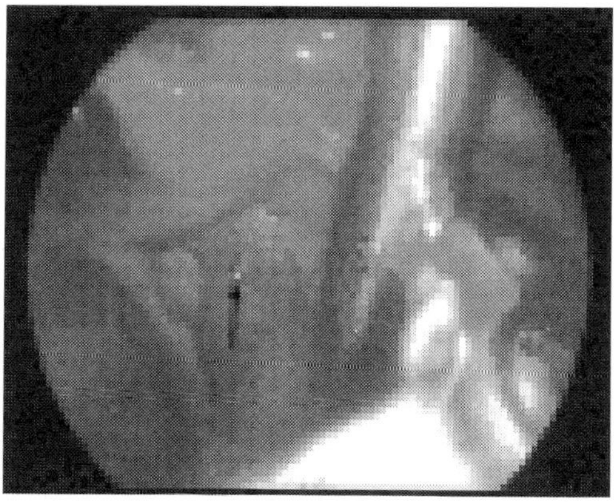

Figure 11. Medpor with the screw placed as a handle (arrow). Medpor in place to hold periorbital fat above the floor defect.

- The first possible explanation is that entrapment, contusion, or hematoma of ocular muscle by fractured
- Second, there may be an undetected, persistent palsy of the oculomotor nerve. [45],[46]

- Third, altered globe position may occur.

Exophthalmos of greater than 2 mm is another indication for surgery, mostly for cosmetic reasons.

Endoscopic repair of orbital blowout fractures represents an innovative and highly successful and safe alternative to external repairs.

Early applications for endoscopic treatment of facial trauma include subcondylar fractures of the mandible, [47]-[50] orbital blow-out fractures, [51]-[56] frontal sinus fractures, [57]-[58] and zygomatic fractures. [57]-[58]

Advantages of endoscopic repair include the following: More accurate fracture visualization, small external incisions, reduced soft tissue dissection, potential for visualization around corners and reduced duration of hospital stay.

Disadvantages of endoscopic repair include the following: Need for delicate instrumentation, moderate learning curve for the techniques, narrow field of view and limited ability for bimanual instrumentation without an assistant.

Indications for endoscopic repair are generally related to fracture location, size, degree of comminution, and the surgeon's ability. Some of the techniques described herein are still under development, and surgeons contemplating the use of these techniques must determine if institutional review board approval is necessary.

6. Endoscope-assisted transoral reduction and internal fixation of mandibular condylar process fractures

Owing to the risk of facial nerve damage and the creation of visible scars, surgical treatment of condylar mandible fractures using an extraoral approach remains controversial. The transoral endoscopically assisted approach of condylar fractures has been reported to avoid these complications. **Kokemueller** studied closed treatment of mandibular condylar neck fractures by endosurgical treatments. Treatment options may yield acceptable results for displaced condylar neck fractures. Especially in patients with severe malocclusion directly after trauma, endoscope-assisted transoral open reduction and fixation seems to be the appropriate treatment for prevention of occlusal disturbances.[59], [60]

The treatment of condylar mandible fractures with a minimal invasive endoscopically assisted technique is reliable and may offer advantages for selected cases, particularly concerning the lower occurrence of facial nerve damage.[61] In the treatment of condylar injuries, the endoscope is not only an aid; it alters the treatment philosophy, from the conservative MMF to anatomic repair. Each surgeon will have to decide on his or her indications for endoscopic repair, and indeed this may depend heavily on his or her experience and patient preference. The authors feel that anatomic reduction and fixation are the best ways to restore preinjury facial aesthetics and mandibular dynamics and to prevent late sequelae of internal derange-

http://dx.doi.org/10.5772/59160

ment. Thus, nowadays surgeons strongly advocate endoscopic repair of adult condylar neck and subcondylar fractures that demonstrate severe displacement or dislocation.

7. Summary

The use of endoscopes has become one of many standard methods for treatment of fractures within the head and neck. As the boundaries of endoscopic surgery expand further, patients will receive the benefits of shorter incisions, less pain and earlier recovery. And, as the surgeons become more and more facile with the instruments, more indications for this type of repair are justified, and more patients ultimately benefit from less invasive surgery. Traditional lid incisions may lead to rates as high as 5 to 10% of lid malposition, which is quite high, considering that the fractures in themselves have a very low rate of complications. Initial reports on transantral approaches were met with some skepticism, but new endoscopic techniques are much easier to perform and interest in this technique has re-emerged. The main advantages of these endoscopic techniques for the orbital fractures are: no skin incisions, easy visualization of the defect, and direct view of the posterior ledge. Despite all these benefits, endosurgery requires training experience and skill of the surgeon.

Author details

Gholamreza Shirani[1], Shiva Solahaye Kahnamouii[2*] and
Mohammad Hosein Kalantar Motamedi[3]

*Address all correspondence to: shiva.kahnamouii@gmail.com

1 Department of Oral and Maxillofacial Surgery, Tehran University of Medical Sciences, Tehran, Iran

2 Department of Oral and Maxillofacial Surgery, Neuroscience Research Center, Drug Applied Research Center, Stem Cell Research Center, Cardiovascular Research Center, Tehran University of Medical Sciences, Tehran, Iran

3 Trauma Research Center, Baqiyatallah University of Medical Sciences and Azad University of Medical Sciences, Tehran, Iran

References

[1] Bernard D. The origins of minimally invasive surgery. Outpatient Surg. 2006:6–7.

[2] Johnson G W, Christ J E. The endoscope breast augmentation: transumbilical insertion of saline-filled breast implants. Plast Reconstr Surg. 1993; 92:801–808.

[3] Guyuron B. Endoscopic forehead rejuvenation: I. Limitations, flaws, and rewards. Plast Reconstr Surg. 2006; 117:1121–1133.

[4] Iglesias M, Bravo L, Chavez-Muñoz C, Barajas-Olivas A. Endoscopic abdominoplasty an alternative approach. Ann Plast Surg. 2006; 57:489–494.

[5] Momeni A, Padron N T, Bannasch H, Borges J, Stark G B. Endoscopic transmaxillary subpectoral augmentation mammaplasty: a safe and predictable procedure. J Plast Reconstr Aesthet Surg. 2006; 59:1076–1081.

[6] Serra-Renom J M, Guisantes E, Yoon T, Benito-Ruiz J. Endoscopic breast reconstruction with intraoperative complete tissue expansion and partial detachment of the pectoralis muscle. Ann Plast Surg. 2007; 58:126–130.

[7] Chen SHT, Gedebou T, Chen PHH. The endoscope as an adjunct to correction of nipple inversion deformity. Plast Reconstr Surg. 2007; 119:1178–1182.

[8] Hallock G G. Endoscope-assisted suction extraction of lipomas. Ann Plast Surg. 1995; 34:32–34.

[9] Huang MHS, Cohen S R, Burstein F D, Simms C A. Endoscopic pediatric plastic surgery. Ann Plast Surg. 1997; 38:1–8.

[10] Hallock G G. An endoscopic technique for decompressive fasciotomy. Ann Plast Surg. 1999; 43:668–670.

[11] Hallock G G. Tendon-graft harvest using endoscopic guidance. Plast Reconstr Surg. 1996; 97:1057–1061.

[12] Hallock G G, Rice D C. An endoscopic subcutaneous dissector for obtaining vein grafts. Ann Plast Surg. 1998; 41:595–599.

[13] Hallock G G. Endoscopic retrieval of the sural nerve. J Reconstr Microsurg. 1995; 11:347–350.

[14] Lin C H, Mardini S, Levin S L, Lin Y T, Yeh J T. Endoscopically assisted sural nerve harvest for upper extremity posttaumatic nerve defects: an evaluation of functional outcomes. Plast Reconstr Surg. 2007; 119:616–626.

[15] Swain B. Transaxillary endoscopic release of restricting bands in congenital muscular torticollis—a novel technique. J Plast Reconstr Aesthet Surg. 2007; 60:95–98.

[16] Lee C H, Lee C, Trabulsy P P. Endoscopic-assisted repair of a Malar fracture. Ann Plast Surg. 1996; 37:184–186.

[17] Serra JMR, Benito J R, Monner J, Zayeulas J, Parraga A. Tissue expansion with endoscopy. Ann Plast Surg. 1997; 38:101–108.

[18] Toranto J D, Yu D, Cederna P S. Endoscopic versus open tissue expander placement: is less invasive better? Plast Reconstr Surg. 2007; 119:894–906.

[19] Hallock G G. Adipofascial flap harvest using endoscopic assistance. Ann Plast Surg. 1997; 38:649–652.

[20] Miller M J, Robb G L. Endoscopic technique for free flap harvesting. Clin Plast Surg. 1995; 22:755–773.

[21] Hallock G G. Minimally invasive harvest of the gracilis muscle. Plast Reconstr Surg. 1999; 104:801–805.

[22] Saltz R. Endoscopic harvest of the omental and jejunal free flaps. ClinPlast Surg. 1995; 22:747–754.

[23] Katz R D, Taylor J A, Rosson G D, Brown P R, Singh N K. Robotics in plastic and reconstructive surgery: use of a telemanipulator slave robot to perform microvascular anastomoses. J ReconstrMicrosurg. 2006; 22:53–57.

[24] Gulamhuseinwala N, Rose V. An alternative device for illuminated retraction in augmentation mammaplasty. J Plast Reconstr Aesthet Surg. 2007; 60:101–110.

[25] Kennedy DW (Oct 1985). "Functional endoscopic sinus surgery. Technique". Arch Otolaryngol 111 (10): 643–9.

[26] Stammberger H, Posawetz W (1990). "Functional endoscopic sinus surgery. Concept, indications and results of the Messerklinger technique". European Archives of Oto-rhino-laryngology 247 (2): 63–76.

[27] Khalil H, Nunez DA (2006). "Functional Endoscopic Surgery for Chronic Rhinosinusitis". Cochrane Database of Systematic Reviews (3): CD004458.

[28] Holy CE, Ellison JM, Schneider C, Levine HL (2014). Medical Devices 7: 83–9.

[29] Tschopp, Kurt; Esther G. Thomaser (14 May 2008). "Outcome of functional endonasal sinus surgery with and without CT-navigation". Rhinology 46 (2): 116–120.

[30] Zingg M, Chowdhury K, Ladrach K, et al. Treatment of 813 zygomalateral orbital complex fractures. Arch Otolaryngol Head Neck Surg 1991; 117:611–20.

[31] Appling WD, Patrinely JR, Salzer TA. Transconjunctival approach vs. subciliary skin-muscle flap approach for orbital fracture repair. Arch Otolaryngol Head Neck Surg 1993; 119:1000 –7. (Grade B).

[32] Mullins JB, Holds JB, Branham GH, et al. Complications of the transconjunctival approach: a review of 400 cases. Arch Otolaryngol Head Neck Surg 1997; 123:385– 8. (Grade C).

[33] Yamaguchi N, Arai S, Mitani H, et al. Endoscopic endonasal techniques of the blow-out fracture of the medial orbital wall. OperTechniq Otolaryngol Head Neck Surg 1991; 2:269 –74. (Grade C).

[34] Michel O. Medial orbital wall fracture: results of minimally invasive endoscopically controlled endonasal surgical technique. Laryngorhinootologie 1993; 72:450–4. (Grade C).

[35] Jin HR, Shin SO, Choo MJ, et al. Endonasal endoscopic reduction of blowout fractures of the medial orbital wall. J Oral Maxillofac Surg 2000; 58:847–51.

[36] Rhee JS, Lynch J, Loehrl TA. Intranasal endoscopy-assisted repair of medial orbital wall fractures. Arch Facial Plast Surg 2000; 2:269 –73.

[37] Lee MJ, Kang YS, Yang JY, et al. Endoscopic transnasal approach for the treatment of medial orbital blow-out fracture: a technique for controlling the fractured wall with a balloon catheter and Merocel. Plast Reconstr Surg 2002; 110:417–26.

[38] Saunders CJ, Whetzel TP, Stokes RB, et al. Transantral endoscopic orbital floor exploration: a cadaver and clinical study. Plast Reconstr Surg 1997; 100:575– 81.

[39] Ikeda K, Suzuki H, Oshima T, et al. Endoscopic endonasal repair of orbital floor fracture. Arch Otolaryngol Head Neck Surg 1999; 125: 59–63.

[40] Chen CT, Chen YR. Endoscopically assisted repair of orbital floor fractures. Plast Reconstr Surg 2001; 108:2011– 8.

[41] Persons BL, Wong GB. Transantral endoscopic orbital floor repair using resorbable plate. J Craniofac Surg 2002; 13:483– 8.

[42] Strong EB, Kim KK, Diaz RC. Endoscopic approach to orbital blowout fracture. Otolaryngol Head Neck Surg 2004; 131:683–95.

[43] Dulley B, Fells P. Long-term follow up of orbital blowout fracture with or without surgery. Mod Probl Ophthalmol 1970;19:467–70

[44] Lyon DB, Newman SA. Evidence of direct damage to extraocular muscles as a cause of diplopia following orbital trauma. Ophthal Plast Reconstr Surg 1989; 5:81–91.

[45] Thering HR, Bogart JN. Blowout fracture of the medial orbital wall with entrapment of the medial rectus muscle. Plast Reconstr Surg 1979; 63:848 –52.

[46] Wojno TH. The incidence of extraocular muscle and cranial nerve palsy in orbital floor blow-out fractures. Ophthalmology 1987; 94: 682–7.

[47] Linder T E, Simmen D, Stool S E. Revolutionary inventions in the 20th century: the history of endoscopy. Arch Otolaryngol Head Neck Surg. 1997; 123:1161–1163.

[48] Eaves F F, III, Price C. Equipment and instrumentation. In: In: Bostwick J III, Eaves FF III, Nahai F, editor. Endoscopic Plastic Surgery. Vol. 23 St. Louis: Quality Medical Publishing; 1995.

[49] Lee C, Mueller R V, Lee K, Mathes S J. Endoscopic subcondylar fracture repair: functional, aesthetic, and radiographic outcomes. Plast Reconstr Surg. 1998; 102(5):1434–1443. Discussion 1444–1445.

[50] Manolidis S, Hollier L H., Jr Management of frontal sinus fractures. Plast Reconstr Surg. 2007; 120(suppl 2):32S–48S.

[51] Mackenzie D J, Arora B, Hansen J. Orbital floor repair with titanium mesh screen. J Craniomaxillofac Trauma. 1999; 5(3):9–16. Discussion 17–18.

[52] Zingg M, Chowdhury K, Lädrach K, Vuillemin T, Sutter F, Raveh J. Treatment of 813 zygoma-lateral orbital complex fractures. New aspects. Arch Otolaryngol Head Neck Surg. 1991; 117(6):611–629.

[53] Munro I R, Fearon J A. The coronal incision revisited. Plast Reconstr Surg. 1994; 93:185–187.

[54] Wolfe S A. The influence of Paul Tessier on our current treatment of facial trauma, both in primary care and in the management of late sequelae. Clin Plast Surg. 1997; 24:515–518.

[55] Walter W L. Early surgical repair of blowout fracture of the orbital floor by using the transantral approach. South Med J. 1972; 65(10):1229–1243.

[56] Strong E B, Kim K K, Diaz R C. Endoscopic approach to orbital blowout fracture repair. Otolaryngol Head Neck Surg. 2004; 131(5):683–695.

[57] Strong E B, Buchalter G M, Moulthrop T H. Endoscopic repair of isolated anterior table frontal sinus fractures. Arch Facial Plast Surg. 2003; 5(6):514–521.

[58] Cummings C W, Schuller D E, Thomas J R, Robbins K T, Harker L A. Otolaryngology: Head and Neck Surgery. Philadelphia: Mosby; 2004.

[59] Lesley WS. Endosurgical repair of an iatrogenic facial arteriovenous fistula due to percutaneous trigeminal balloon rhizotomy. J Neurosurg Sci. 2007 Dec; 51(4):177-80.

[60] Kokemueller H, Konstantinovic VS, Barth EL, Goldhahn S, von See C, Tavassol F, Essig H, Gellrich NC Endoscope-assisted transoral reduction and internal fixation versus closed treatment of mandibular condylar process fractures--a prospective double-center study. J Oral Maxillofac Surg. 2012 Feb; 70(2):384-95.

[61] Schmelzeisen R, Cienfuegos-Monroy R, Schön R, Chen C, Cunningham L, Goldhahn S. Patient Benefit From Endoscopically Assisted Fixation of Condylar Neck Fractures —A Randomized Controlled Trial Journal of Oral and Maxillofacial Surgery 2009; 67: 1:147–158.

Section 10

Bone grafting and Regenerative Techniques for Implant Surgery

Chapter 23

Regenerative Techniques in Oral and Maxillofacial Bone Grafting

Arash Khojasteh, Mohammad Esmaeelinejad and
Farzad Aghdashi

Additional information is available at the end of the chapter

http://dx.doi.org/10.5772/59236

1. Introduction

The art and science of reconstruction of maxillofacial bony defects is a field of interest for most of maxillofacial surgeons due to its importance and prerequisite role for other surgical procedures. Despite significant improvements during last decades in this field, challenge still exists to determine which type of reconstruction techniques and materials is the treatment of choice. Although dental implants are considered as a standard and effective treatment to restore dental defects nowadays, lack of adequate bone quantity is a pitfall for dental implant reconstruction procedures. Grafting techniques have a long history in the literature with different donor sources and technical innovations and improvements. These methods are the most common techniques in bone reconstruction yet, but in the era of bioengineering, new alternative horizons lie ahead.

Regenerative techniques for maxillofacial hard tissue reconstruction like other tissue engineering procedures is based on three principle elements; stem cells, scaffolds, and growth factors. The balanced scenario of bone induction and conduction is a critical issue in every bone regeneration procedure [1].

Current approaches used in clinical circumstances to reconstruct bony defects include different bone grafting methods, such as autologous bone grafts, allografts, bone-graft substitutes, distraction osteogenesis, and guided bone regeneration.

Bone-graft substitutes have been developed to be used as scaffolds to promote cell migration, proliferation and differentiation for bone regeneration without need to violate other tissue from a donor site [2.[

Distraction osteogenesis and guided bone regeneration are brilliant concepts which work basically by modifying normal bone healing process. Soft callous enlarging guidance is the key element in distraction osteogenesis and space maintaining for relatively slow growing hard tissue is the fundamental of guided bone regeneration techniques. This chapter introduces methods of bone reconstruction and regeneration in oral and maxillofacial surgery. Indeed the knowledge of exact indications and advantages of each method is invaluable for the surgeon.

2. Anatomy of the skeleton

The fundamental bony skeleton of the jaws consist of a mandible and two maxillary bones. Because of the functional aspect of these structures and their atrophic changes during aging, anatomical features have specific importance to distinguish defects and determine the proper treatment plan. The quantity and quality of bone in the alveolar process and adjacent structures are the key elements of this issue. The anatomical knowledge of these structures is also a determinant factor when using them as donor sites for reconstruction.

The alveolar bone of mandible and maxilla is a functional bony process which harbors teeth in a dentate human. After tooth loss, this bony structure loses its dimensions both vertically and horizontally [3]. After atrophic sequences, the maxillary alveolar arch diameter decreases, despite the fact that the mandibular alveolar arch enlarges in diameter and a pseudo-class III relation may appear in severe atrophic alveolar ridges (Figure 1).

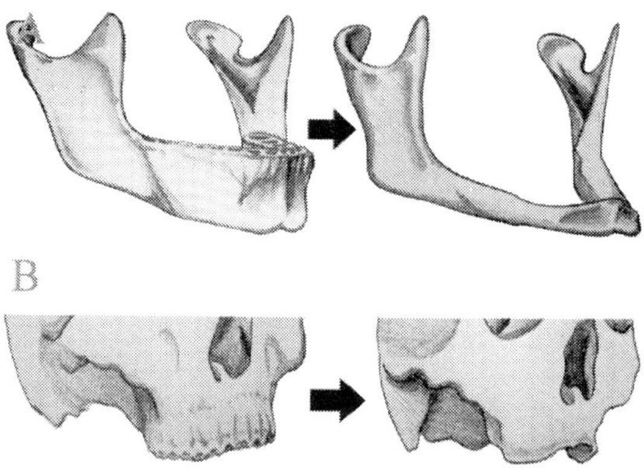

Figure 1. A, The atrophic changes of mandible. B, The atrophic changes of maxilla.

The quality of edentulous alveolar bone is classified to D1, D2, D3 and D4 based on cortical bone thickness and density of trabecular bone respectively.

D1 demonstrates the thickest cortical bone and the most dense trabecular part and is usually located in anterior mandible;

http://dx.doi.org/10.5772/59236

D4 demonstrates a large volume of low density trabecular bone and thin cortices and is located mainly in posterior maxilla.

D2 and D3 with intermediate characteristics are located in posterior mandible and anterior maxilla respectively [4].

The maxillary tuberosity is located in the posterior maxillary bone on each side and contains low density D4 bone and attached to the pterygoid plates at the pterygomaxillary junction. It is located next to important anatomical structures- the pterygomaxillary fissure and pterygo-palatine fossa.

The maxillary sinus is a pyramidal cavity in each maxilla with a broad base medially and an apex laterally. Its size varies depending on the patient's age and presence of teeth. During the lifetime the sinus enlarges continuously and at the age about 12, the floor of the sinus is almost at the level of the nasal floor. Maxillary posterior teeth loss and sinus pneumatization are responsible for decreasing bone volume in this area.

The mandible is the largest bone of the face and generally consists of thicker cortical bone compared to the maxilla. The anterior border of ramus as runs toward the mandibular body creates external oblique ridges bilaterally. The mandibular canal begins from the mandibular foramen at the middle medial surface of ramus horizontally and vertically and ends at the mental foramen on the buccal surface of the mandibular body near the apices of the premolar teeth on both sides. The least distance from the mandibular canal to the buccal cortex is in the distal part of the mandibular first molars. The canal course through the mandible usually makes a loop near the mental foramen with about a 3 mm diameter. The neurovascular bundle travels through this canal to supply sensation and blood to the mandibular teeth and some part of the chin.

The buccal fat pads or Bichat's fat are located lateral to the buccinator muscles bilaterally and consist of four parts; body, temporal, buccal, and pterygoid extensions. Buccal fat pads are supplied by the temporal and transverse facial arteries. The buccal fat pads are very useful structures in reconstruction of oral defects [5, 6].

3. Recipient site classification and defect analysis

The importance of alveolar bone defect analysis and classification is to determine the best regenerative treatment for each specific defect. This is more obvious when an evidence-based decision is made according to all data presented in the literature. Parameters which can describe alveolar bony defects are:

- Anatomic position of defect in the jaws (mandible/maxilla, anterior/posterior)
- Dimensions of the defect
- Morphology of the defect
- Type of reconstruction (vertical/horizontal)

- Relation of augmentation and defect region (internal; inside the contour and external, outside the ridge contour)
- Defect base width and number of residual bony walls surrounding the defect

Anterior and posterior parts of the mandible and maxilla have different bone qualities; hence they have different regenerative capacities [7]. The length of the defect affects the degree of vascularization. In vertical defects with no sufficient width to accept implants, the augmentation procedure becomes complicated because both dimensions require restoration [8]. It has been suggested that a wide bony defect base has greater capacity for bone regeneration compared to a narrow base defect [7]. The number of surrounding bony walls around the defect is mentioned in the literature as stabilization for the initial blood clot [8].

Different classifications to describe alveolar ridge defects have been documented [9-11]. Seibert et al. classified the defects of the alveolar ridge based on dimension in which the resorption had occurred: horizontal defects (class I, 33%), vertical defects (class II, 3%) and the most common variant mixed horizontal and vertical defects (class III, 56%) [10].

Some similar classifications were suggested by other investigators according to the morphology of the alveolar bone defects. A classification published by Wang and Al-Shammari, the defects were subdivided in: horizontal, vertical, and combined [12]. Each group was further classified based on the amount of the deficiency.Studer (1996) documented the first quantitative classification of alveolar defects based on predicting need to reconstruct deficiencies, with classes defined as < 3 mm, 3–6 mm and > 6 mm [8].

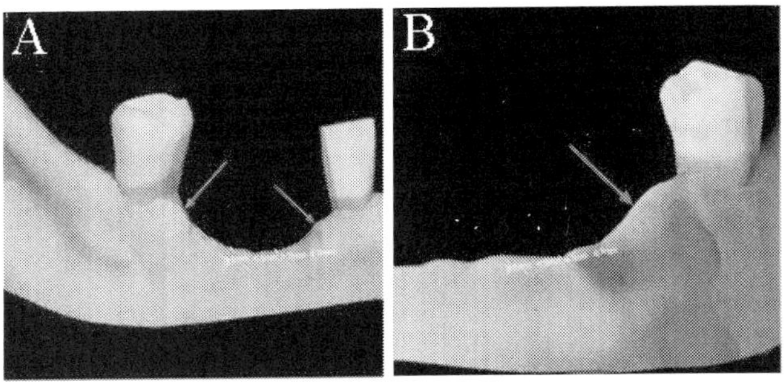

Figure 2. A, Interdental partial edentulism. Class A: two-wall defect. The arrows show the defect walls. B, Free end partial edentulism. Class B: one-wall defect (arrow).

The Cologne classification of alveolar ridge defects uses orientation of the defect (horizontal, vertical, combined and sinus area) reconstruction needs associated with the defect (small: < 4 mm, medium: 4-8 mm large: > 8 mm) [8].Khojasteh et al. in 2013 in a literature review stressed the clinical importance of recipient site characteristics for vertical ridge augmentation concluded that information regarding the characteristics of the initial vertical defect is not comprehensively incorporated in most of the studies [8]. They proposed a classification with regard to the number of surrounding bony walls (A: Two-wall defects, B: One-wall defects, C:

A defect with no surrounding walls) and width of defect base (I: A bony defect with a base width of 5 mm or more, II: A bony defect with a base width of 3 mm or more, but less than 5 mm, III: A bony defect with a base width less than 3 mm, (Figure 2).

4. Donor sites in oral and maxillofacial surgery

Various donor sites to harvest free bone grafts are used in oral and maxillofacial surgeries. Each site has its own indications, advantages and disadvantages. Ideally, the surgeons prefer to harvest bone from a site that is close to the recipient site to operate in one surgical site and avoid making more skin scars. In reality, the quality and quantity of bone sometimes necessitates grafting from other sites.

5. Bone harvesting from intraoral donor sites

5.1. The chin

Cortical or corticocancellous block graft in sizes up to 4 cm can be harvested from the mandibular symphysis area intraorally (Figure 3). The mandibular symphysis as a donor site has been documented to provide sufficient bone to reconstruct alveolar ridge defects 4-6 mm in horizontal and up to 4 mm in vertical dimensions and can cover a span up to 3 teeth in length [13]. The available block graft may be harvested from this site is 10 mm (height) 15 mm (width), 6 mm (thickness), with an average volume of 860 cc [14]. The symphysis can provide over 50% larger graft volume in comparison to the lateral ramus region [15]. The typical symphysis corticocancellous bone graft consists of 65% cortical bone and 36% cancellous bone [14]. Because of slow resorption rate of chin grafts, it can also be used as an onlay graft for facial defects.

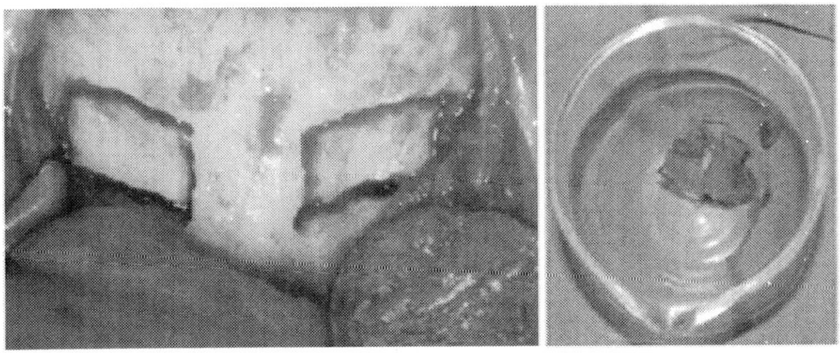

Figure 3. Block bone graft harvested from the mandibular symphysis

5.2. Lateral ramus

The mandibular lateral ramus or retro-molar region is advocated for corticocancellous bone harvesting with approximately 100% cortical composition (Figure 4).

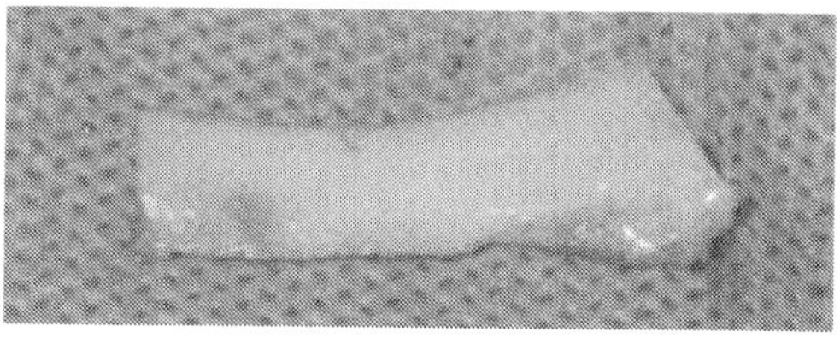

Figure 4. Block bone graft harvested from mandibular lateral ramus area.

A buccal shelf block graft can provide sufficient bone to reconstruct alveolar defects 2-3 teeth in length. Horizontal and vertical defects up to 3 to 4 mm can be augmented from this donor site [16, 17]. The maximum dimensions of ramus cortical bone blocks are 4mm (thickness) 15 mm width and 35 mm in length depending on the regional anatomy. The clinical access, position of the inferior alveolar canal, molar teeth, and width of the posterior mandible are factors limiting the amount of possible graft that may be harvested [16, 17]. The morbidity of this region has been reported lower than the mandibular symphysis region [15].

5.3. Maxillary tuberosity

Among intra-oral donor sites, the maxillary tuberosity typically provides a smaller amount of bone (Figure 5).

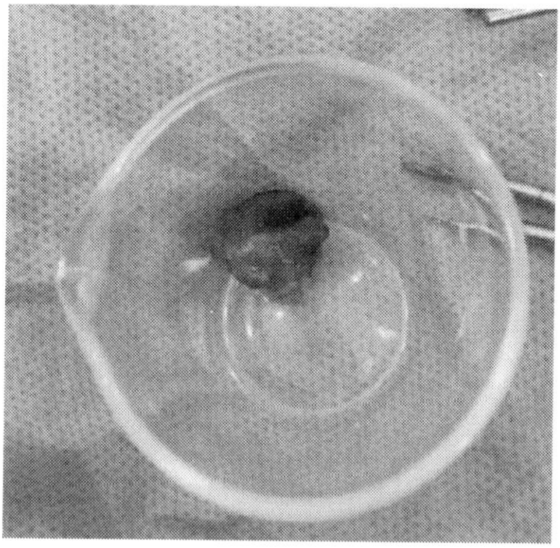

Figure 5. Block bone graft harvested from the maxillary tuberosity.

http://dx.doi.org/10.5772/59236

This region is usually used for harvesting cancellous bone to fill defects and for sinus lifting procedures. Existence of the 3rd molar in this site decreases the available bone for harvesting. Other anatomical limitations for using this site include: the maxillary sinus, pterygoid plates and the greater palatine canal.

5.4. Anterior palate

This area is used as a donor site usually for anterior maxillary reconstruction, especially when an impacted canine is imbedded in this region (Figure 6).

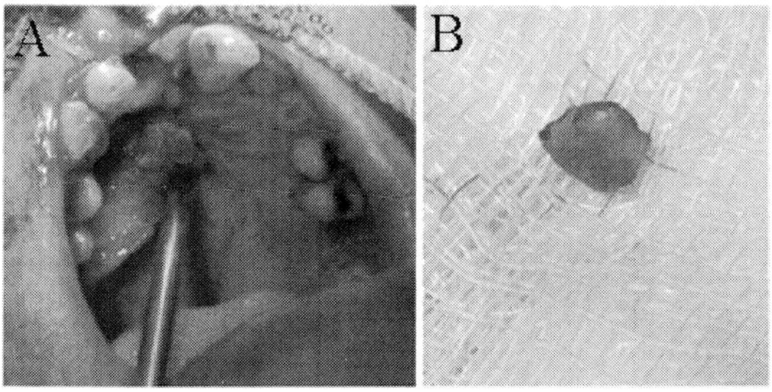

Figure 6. A, palatal flap is retracted and the donor site for harvesting palatal bone graft is exposed. B, block bone graft harvested from the anterior palate.

The corticocancellous block, cancellous or crescent-shaped grafts can be harvested from this site. The average amount of bone in this area in dentate patients is 2 cc and 2.4 in edentulous patients [18].

6. Other intraoral sources

Maxilla buttress or zygomatic processes of maxilla, anterior nasal spine and bone exostosis also have been documented as donor sites. These areas provide little bone and are prefer choices for adjacent recipient sites or in combination with other bone substitutes.

7. Bone grafting with extra oral donor sites

7.1. Iliac crest

The iliac crestal bone is the most common extra-oral donor site for bone grafts. It may be harvested vascularized, non-vascularized, cortical, cancellous or corticocancellous in different shapes and in large sizes (Figure 7).

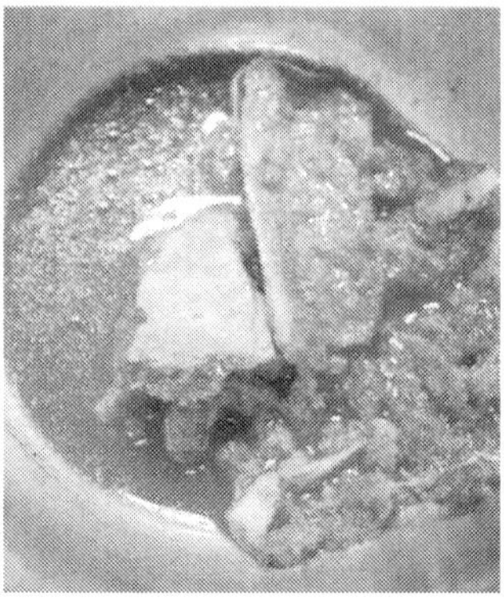

Figure 7. Iliac bone graft harvested to reconstruct the mandible.

The location of the iliac crest permits the surgeons to harvest bone graft and operate simultaneously to save operating time. A full-thickness iliac crest bone graft consists of two thick cortices with sufficient amount of cancellous bone in between and can restore the thickness and height of mandibular bone efficiently. The graft shows a good success rate, and dental implant insertion is possible in this type of bone graft [19, 20]. Mandibular continuity defects treated with free iliac bone grafting are documented with about a 70% success rate [21]. The rate of successful union is decreased significantly where the defect is longer than 6 cm [21, 22]. The posterior iliac crest also can be used as a donor site. Morbidity rate for anterior iliac crest bone grafts is more than posterior iliac site (23% and 2% respectively) [23].

Complications. Postoperative pain, iliac fractures, gate disturbances, hematoma, herniation of abdominal contents, vascular injury, nerve injury, unsightly contour defects along the iliac crest and growth disturbances in young ages [24].

7.2. Calvarial graft

The calvarium is a popular cortical bone grafting site basically for its mechanical features and very slow resorption rate [24]. It is suggested for facial augmentation, orbital roof and floor reconstruction, and covering midface defects rather than alveolar defects. Typically, the outer cortex is used as a cortical plate graft (Figure 8), although a full-thickness or inner cortex graft may be used.

The skull growth continues to the age of 8 and become thicker until the age of 20 years. The thickest portion is located at the parietal region. This donor site can provide 8 by 10 cm of bone [25]. Thickness of the calvarial bone is highly variable so preoperative radiographs help the surgeon to harvest bone safely [25]. It should keep in mind that dura is tightly adherent to the inner cortex and can easily be injured if the inner cortex is aimed to be harvested. Also various vascular structures are located just under the bone at different sites, like the superior sagittal sinus in the midline. The inner and outer cortices may merge together in inferior and lateral portions. Other anatomic structures, such as transcortical emissary veins, subcortical vessels,

http://dx.doi.org/10.5772/59236

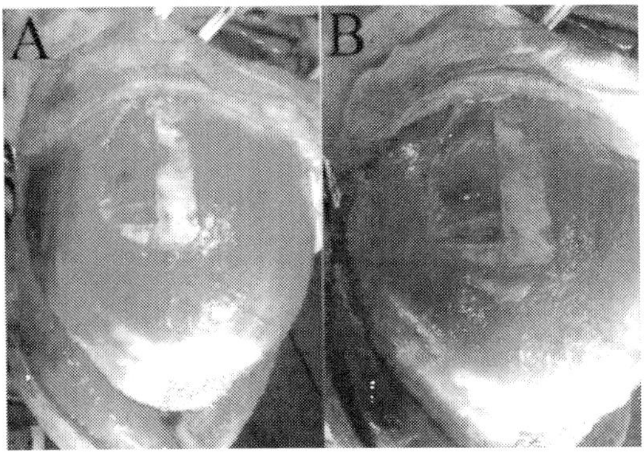

Figure 8. Calvarial bone graft harvesting approach. A, The scalp is retracted and calvarium is exposed. B, The osteotomy site is visible.

and aberrant arachnoid plexuses are also at risk and should be considered in the surgical procedures [25]. Temproparietal regions can be used to harvest more curved grafts and straight grafts can be harvested from occipital or frontal regions.

Complications. Contour deformity at the donor site and grafting bone fracture in harvesting are the most common complications. Dural exposure or rupture is another complication but is not common. Intracranial hemorrhage due to this type of graft harvesting has been reported.

7.3. Tibial graft

The anterior surface of the tibial plateau is mentioned as a donor site for cortical or corticocancellous bone grafts. Proper mechanical features of the tibial cortex seem to be useful in augmentation of atrophic alveolar ridges for implant insertion or facial bone defect reconstruction. Up to 40 cc cancellous bone can be harvested from the tibia (Figure 9).

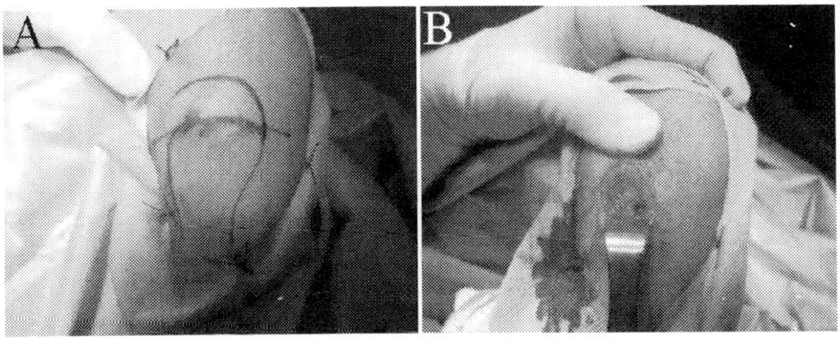

Figure 9. Tibial bone graft harvesting approach. A, the donor site is indicated before making the incision. B, the flap is retracted and bone graft is harvested using a curette.

The most common approach for this purpose is laterally at Gerdy's tubercle [26].

7.4. Rib graft

Free rib bone was one of the first autogenous bone grafts used for reconstruction of mandibular defects. Osseous or osseochondral grafts can be harvested from fifth to seventh ribs. Although costochondral grafts remain popular for the treatment of mandibular ramus and condylar defects, the quality and quantity of rib bone make it less popular for jaw defect reconstruction nowadays [27].

Complications. Postoperative chest wall pain, pleural injury leading to pneumothorax, and overgrowth of the graft [27, 28].

8. Reconstruction techniques

Different reconstruction techniques have been known and well documented for bony defects in the oral and maxillofacial area. Distraction osteogenesis and guided bone regeneration techniques, grafting procedures and especially autogenous bone grafting still are the treatments of choice in most alveolar bony defects. Soft tissue consideration and management should be borne in mind for successful stable results.

8.1. Bone grafting

"Any implanted material that promotes bone healing" is defined as a bone graft [24]. Ideally it must be: osteoconductive, osteoinductive and osteogenic.

An osteoconductive capacity means allowing or directing the new bone to form within the material structure.

An osteoinductive capacity describes supplying recruitment and/or differentiation factors for bone-forming cells by the grafting material.

An osteogenic graft material provides induced or inducible bone-forming cells.

Bone grafts are used not only for a defect facilitating healing but also for contour augmentations. For this purpose more attention is directed towards the amount and rate of graft resorption. Graft incorporation is proportional to amount of graft resistance to resorption [24].

Bone grafts can be classified as:

Autografts (transferring bone in one human(,

Allografts (transferring inter-humans), and

Xenografts (transferring from other species, synthetic materials and any combination of them).

Autografts can be cancellous, cortical, corticocancellous, vascularized bone or aspirated bone marrow. The main advantage of autogenous bone is retention of at least some osteogenic cells without triggering the immune system. On the other hand donor site morbidity and limited amount are basic disadvantages. Ideally, the bone graft should be incorporated into the recipient bed; the space that the bone graft occupies should finally become viable bone with physiological remodeling mechanisms. Many factors are involved in the incorporation process namely the graft type, graft bed (recipient site), and interface in between. Graft related factors including the type of graft, porosity and mechanism of incorporation. Recipient site viability and vascularity are very important in any autogenous grafting procedures. Graft incorporation has been summarized by Bauer and Muschler in five steps [24[

1. Hematoma formation, release of bone inducing factors and cellular recruitment
2. Inflammation and development of fibrovascular tissue, connecting the graft to the adjacent bone
3. Vascular invasion of the graft
4. Focal resorption of the graft by recruited osteoclasts
5. New bone formation, union between the graft and the surrounding bone, and graft remodeling

Graft stabilization is other critical issue in bone graft incorporation and vascularization. Instability leads to bone resorption and infection. Cancellous bone grafts can be packed in defect cavities. In these cases more graft material transfer, leads to more vital cells and increase in osteogenesis. Cortical or corticocancellous block grafts should be stabilized using fixation devices.

8.2. Bone Grafting with intra oral donor sites (localized bone augmentation)

8.2.1. Symphysis block harvesting

There are three basic approaches to access the mandibular symphysis for bone graft harvesting: 1) sulcular, 2) attached gingiva, or 3) vestibular. The advantages of sulcular and attached gingiva approaches are reductions in wound dehiscence and bleeding compared to the vestibular approach. Use of the sulcular approach is not advocated in pre-existing periodontal diseases or crowns. The vestibular approach is done through the mucosa 5 to 10 mm below the mucogingival junction; first by partial thickness dissection apically for 3mm to maintain 3mm of periosteum and mentalis muscle fibers on the bone side, which will be used to reattach the muscle fiber [29]. Below this level a full thickness incision is made and full thickness flap reflection is used. Careful attention must be paid to prevent trans-section of the mental nerve at the distal extent of the incision bilaterally (Figure 10).

It is suggested that at least 5 mm bone is maintain below the teeth apices, inferior border and bilaterally anterior to mental foramina. When a large bone block is needed, the anterior most portion of the symphysis the mental protuberance must be retained. If it is necessary to harvest two graft blocks from each side, leaving a 3mm midline connection to maintain support for the chin profile is necessary [30].The block graft can be osteotomized by a rotary bur, reciprocating saw, or piezo instrument. Using rotary burs has disadvantages of losing some amount of bone in comparison to two other methods. Osteotomies should enter the inter-cortical layer, giving close attention not violate the lingual cortex. A fine osteotome or chisel can be used to

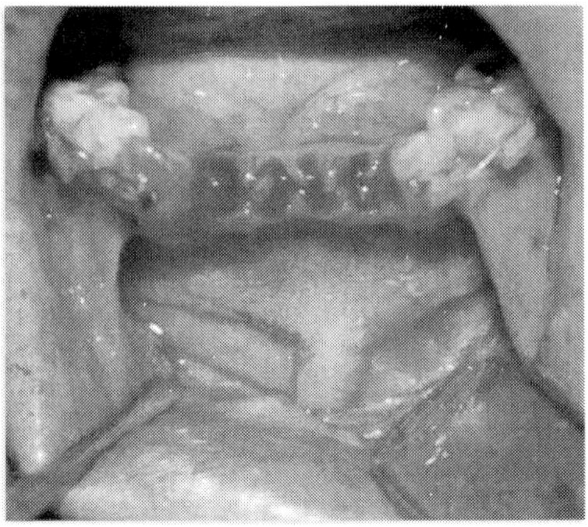

Figure 10. Full mucoperiosteal flap retracted to expose the donor site for harvesting symphyseal bone. Two osteotomy sites are determined on both sides and 3mm bone is maintained in between to support the chin profile.

reflect block bone graft from its bed. After block removal a hemostatic agent can be used in the donor site. Some clinicians prefer to fill the donor site with Freeze Dried Bone Allograft (FDBA), especially when a large block has been harvested. In the vestibular approach, when closing, a resorbable suture is first used to attach the mentalis muscle to the 3mm periosteal muscle layer left on the bone side.

8.2.2. Lateral ramus block harvesting

The approach to harvest bone graft from the lateral ramus can proceed two different ways: 1) Vestibular or 2) Sulcular. The vestibular approach has access through the area through vestibular incision on external oblique ridge. Advantage of this approach is lack of disturbing the periodontium of the adjacent teeth. The indication of sulcular approach is when recipient site is located nearby. The distal extent of the incision should not be more than occlusal plane to minimize the risk of facial nerve damage, bleeding and exposing buccal fat. Osteotomy is suggested to be performed in a defined sequence; superior cut, then anterior, then posterior and finally inferior cut (Figure 11).

The superior cut length and thickness is important. This cut is usually made approximately 4 mm medial to the external oblique ridge but can be performed up to 6 mm depending on the regional anatomy. It may be extended anteriorly to the distal area of the first molar, depending on the anatomy. The anterior and posterior vertical cuts are made in parallel to the predicted length and width of the bone graft block, and are limited by anatomic position of the mandibular canal, which determines the harvesting block width. Complete cortical penetration of inferior osteotomy cut is avoided due to its proximity to the mandibular canal in many cases. An osteotome or a chisel can be used to remove the bone graft from its bed avoiding penetrating excessively to damage mandibular canal. Closing the incision usually is done without applying any graft or hemostatic agent.

http://dx.doi.org/10.5772/59236

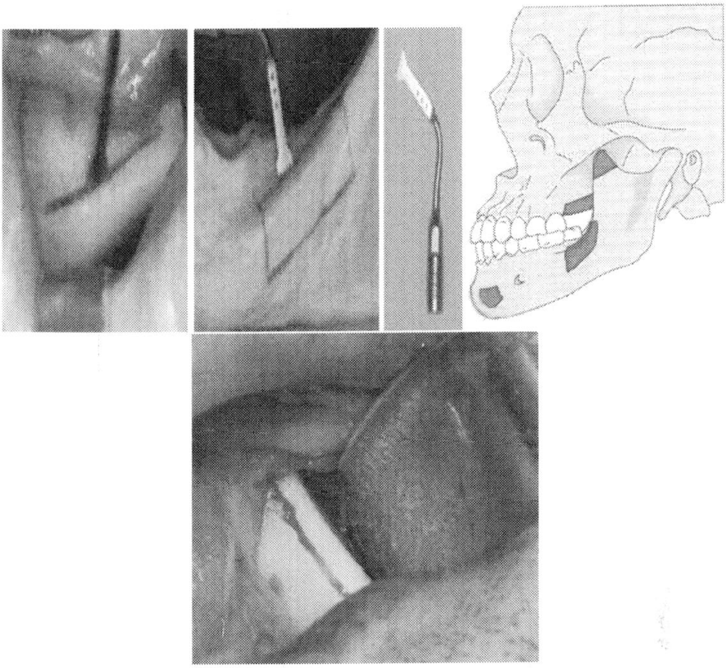

Figure 11. Intraoral approach to harvest the lateral ramus bone block. The osteotomy line of the superior cut is seen.

8.3. Anterior iliac crest bone grafting

Anterior iliac crest bone grafts are common used grafts not only in maxillofacial surgery but also in orthopedic surgery. The iliac crest is almost subcutaneous and cortical or corticocancellous grafts in different shapes and size can be taken from this region simply and safety. The *anterior superior iliac spine (ASIS),* is easily palpable which is located in the most anterior and superior portion of the crest. Posteriorly along the crest of the ilium in the widest portion is the iliac tubercle. The incision starts 2 cm posterior to ASIS and continues up to 8 cm along the crest. The neural branches, which are in risk of damage, are iliohypogastric, subcostal branches and lateral femoral cutaneous nerves. Retracting the skin medially and avoiding extending the incision posteriorly are suggested to decrease this risk. Dissecting laterally and violating iliotibial fascia is not recommended. Harvesting bone from iliac crest can be performed via different approaches including using a trephine device, monocortically and bicortically with different techniques (Figure 12).

Usually monocortical bone blocks are harvested from the medial surface with osteotomes or a saw. In young ages, the border portion of the iliac crest consists of chondral structure which should be bypassed in the harvesting procedure. Closing the donor site is done in three layers, and a vacuum drain usually is placed. Minor complications of this bone graft harvesting included superficial infections, superficial seromas, and minor hemato-

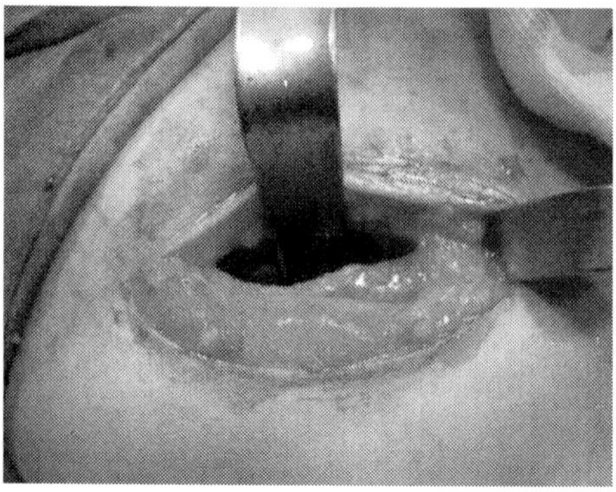

Figure 12. Iliac bone graft harvesting procedure.

mas. Major complications are herniation of abdominal contents, vascular injuries, deep infections at the donor site, neurologic injuries, deep hematoma formation requiring surgical drainage, and iliac fractures [31].

8.4. Placing the bone graft into the recipient site

A moist environment with saline is suggested as a reservoir for the autogenous bone graft. Cortical or corticocancellous block grafts can be adjusted for recipient site with burs, saws or discs. The block should be prepared so that when placed in the recipient site it does not rock and fits snuggly and is in intimate contact with the underlying host bone bed. Fixation of the block graft is a principle issue. Screws and plates are devices, which can be used to achieve sufficient stability. Applying two screws is recommended and using the lag screw technique is suggested. The recipient bed and block graft may be penetrated to facilitate vascular ingrowths. Applying particulate bone graft around the bone block is usually advocated to maintain space for more osteogenesis. The graft structure is then covered with a barrier membrane to prevent soft tissue ingrowth into the integrating new bone especially when particulate materials are added. Tension free closure of the grafted site is critical to success.

8.5. Anatomic repositioning

8.5.1. Distraction osteogenesis

Distraction osteogenesis (DO) is a contemporary method that has been used in oral and maxillofacial defects. DO is a method to generate new bone by gradual separation of bone segments. In this procedure a distractor device is placed on two sides of an osteotomy site (Figure 13).

After a latency period the device is gradually activated and makes a gap between two bone segments. The new immature bone is generated between these two segments in the created gap. Then the device will not be activated for a period to give the new bone a time to mineralize

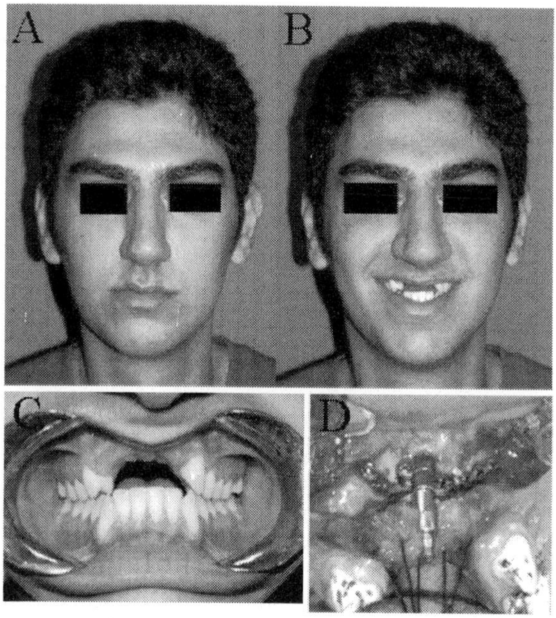

Figure 13. A. Patient with premaxillary deficiency. B. The patient has lost his anterior incisal teeth due to an anterior maxillary defect. C. Intra-oral view of the premaxilla defect. D. DO device is inserted in the surgery phase.

and turn into mature bone. This is called the consolidation phase and is usually twice the activation period. After the consolidation period the device is removed. During the activation period the surrounding soft tissue grows simultaneously with the bone formation (Figure 14). This is why the DO is also called distraction histogenesis. DO devices are divided into two groups of intraoral and extraoral types each of which have certain indications.

Indications. DO was generally used in orthopedics years before being used in maxillofacial surgery. The most popular indication of DO is in hemifacial or hemimandibular microsomia. Actually DO was used in a case of hemicraniofacial microsomia successfully for the first time by McCarthy et al. in 1992 [32]. The most important indication of DO is in syndromes associated with congenital anomalies like cerebral palsy, hemifacial microsomia, Treacher–Collins syndrome, Pierre–Robin sequence, Nager syndrome and others. Investigations have shown the successful results of DO in such cases [33].

DO in vertical dimension is another important indication. Although new methods of bone grafting like fibular microvascular graft have been broadly used in these defects sometimes their use is restricted by the large size of the defect. In these large defects DO is a better technique to regenerate new bone and reconstruct the defect [34]. Sometimes the combination of microvascularized grafts with DO procedure is an ideal technique to reconstruct large defects especially defects caused by resection of pathologic lesions [7].

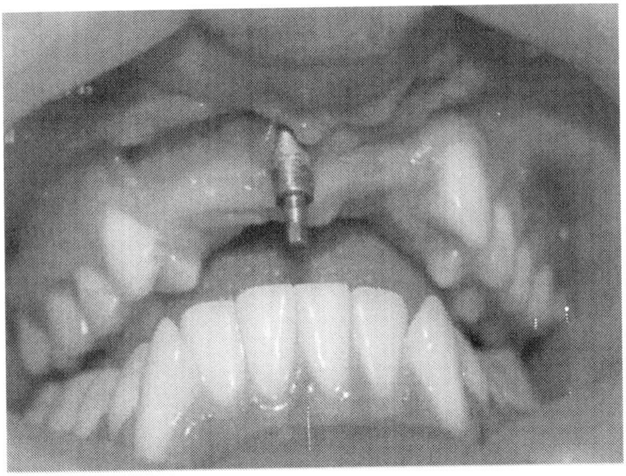

Figure 14. Inserted DO device is shown to generate new bone for reconstruction of the maxilla. The distractor device has been activated for months. The alveolar bone height has increased.

DO in transverse dimension is an interesting method being used in patients with arch constriction or an alveolar cleft. Reviews of the clinical studies about the use of DO in maxillary hypoplasia in patients with cleft lip and palate have shown the benefits of this technique as an alternative to orthognathic surgeries [35]. The important advantage of DO in these patients is unchanged or better velopharyngeal function. This method can be used in the mixed dentition period which is an advantage of this procedure comparing to orthognathic surgery procedures.

DO has been recently used in patients with midface hypoplasia in craniosynostosis like Crouzon, Apert, and Pfeiffer syndromes. Several investigations have evaluated this technique and compared it to LeFort III osteotomy [36, 37]. Although LeFort III osteotomy has been widely used to correct the maxillary retrusion, it is not possible to advance the midface a large amount. Lefort III-DO technique has been suggested in patients with great discrepancy; however trials have shown higher relapse of this method compared to the usual LeFort III osteotomy procedure. The advantage of LeFort III-DO technique is the lower risk for severe complications like cerebrospinal fluid leakage, meningitis, and infection.

Advantages. Simultaneous distraction of the soft tissue is a great advantage of this technique. The quality or quantity of the soft tissue bed makes the results of bone grafting unpredictable and reduces the success of the bone graft. In most cases DO obviates the need for bone grafting in the future. Morbidity of a donor site is also eliminated. The process of inserting and removing the device is less extensive as well.

Disadvantages.DO is a technique sensitive procedure and should be performed by an expert surgeon. The quality of the device is an important factor in success rate of the DO results. Loosening of the screws and displacement of the device may occur in some cases. DO procedures consist of two operations: one for insertion of the device and a second surgery to remove it. Sometimes a third surgery is needed in the future to achieve the perfect outcome especially when DO has been performed in a young patient. Unpredictable outcomes or malocclusion are inadvertent results. Motor and sensory nerve dysfunction is an untoward complication of DO. This complication is especially seen in DO of the mandible which may lead to permanent or transient weakness of marginal branch of facial nerve or hypoesthesia of inferior alveolar nerve. Scar formation and infection should be considered a more usual complication of DO.

8.6. Nerve repositioning

Rehabilitation of edentulous patients is often complicated and requires special consideration. In edentulous patients with atrophic bone above the mandibular canal is insufficient; repositioning the inferior alveolar nerve (IAN) is a treatment option. This treatment is done if the overall bone height is enough to place implant fixtures, but the IAN interferes with this procedure. Repositioning of IAN is done to move the nerve from the canal placing it in a new position (outside the bone).

Nerve lateralization is a procedure in which the IAN is exposed and retracted laterally while the surgeon is inserting the fixtures. Then the nerve is left to fall back against the inserted fixtures or the lateral cortex. In nerve transposition technique the IAN, mental nerve and incisive nerve are exposed by corticotomy of the bone surrounding the mental foramen. Then the IAN is transected from its junction with the incisive nerve. In this way the nerve is freed and its retraction is much easier. The IAN is replaced posteriorly after cutting the incisive nerve. The surgeon is able to install the implant fixture after distalization of the IAN (Figure 15).

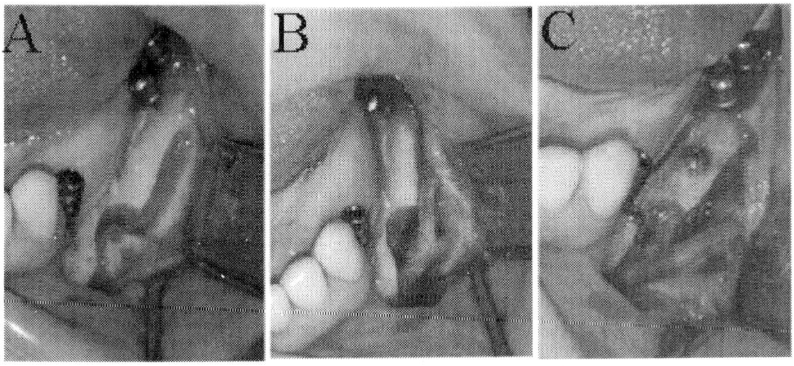

Figure 15. A, Nerve lateralization in an atrophic mandible to eliminate the nerve interfering with implant surgery. B, The IAN is transposed from the mandibular canal to make space for installation the implants. C, Simultaneous implant installation is also possible in this technique.

Indications. The actual indication of IAN transposition or lateralization is in atrophic posterior mandible where remaining bone above the mandibular canal is less than 10 mm [38,39]. There is no actual contraindication of IAN transposition reported in the literature.

Advantages. The risk of damage to IAN during the installation of fixtures is reduced by retracting and repositioning the nerve. The surgeon is able to use a longer fixture which may engage the inferior cortex of the mandible. The fixtures have more stability due to their bicortical insertion. This procedure is performed simultaneously with implant fixture installation with or without bone grafting.

Disadvantages. The risk of damage to the IAN is a prominent disadvantage of nerve transpositioning; Traction on the nerve usually causes temporary sensory loss [40]. Mandibular fracture, implant loss, hemorrhage, and osteomyelitis are other possible complications in long implant installation, associated with the transposition and lateralization of the IAN [38, 41, 42].

9. Guided bone regeneration (GBR)

The treatment and rehabilitation of edentulism with dental implants has become a routine treatment modality in contemporary dental practice. Nevertheless, tooth loss is frequently associated with subsequent bone loss, often resulting in inadequate bone dimensions for ideal dental implant placement. Alveolar ridge resorption in partially and totally edentulous patients may interfere with the safe and correct positioning and placement of implants. When ridge resorption occurs, bone augmentation is essential to guarantee adequate bone volume, to provide patients with proper inter-arch dimensions, and to insure a satisfactory aesthetic result.

9.1. Classic GBR

Guided bone regeneration (GBR) is an important concept concerning restoration of deficient alveolar sites (e.g., an extraction site or deficient alveolar ridge) for implant placement. GBR uses an occlusive membrane interface between gingiva and the alveolar bone tissue to promote osteogenic tissue regeneration. The occlusive membrane acts as a barrier when placed into the surgical site, preventing connective and epithelial tissue migration into the defect. Progenitor cells located in the adjacent alveolar bone or blood are then able to recolonize the root area and differentiate into a new osteogenic tissue with the formation of new bone.

The strategy to isolate the bone defect with a material that will function as a physical barrier to avoid gingival cell invasion led to the development of GBR membranes. These membranes need to exhibit: (1) biocompatibility to allow integration with the host tissues without eliciting inflammatory responses, (2) proper degradation profile to match those of new tissue formation, (3) adequate mechanical and physical properties to allow its placement in vivo, and (4) sufficient sustained strength to avoid the membrane collapse and perform their barrier function. GBR membranes are divided into two groups, nonresorbable and resorbable, according to their degradation characteristics.

Indications. The most popular application of GBR is in dehiscence and fenestration type defects with simultaneous implant placement (Figure 16).

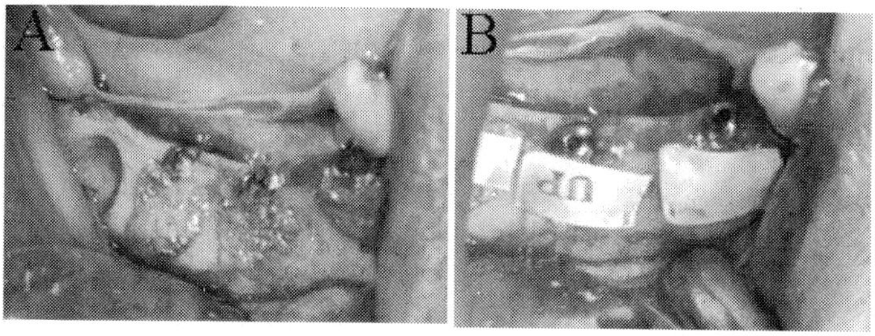

Figure 16. A, GBR is an efficient technique in correcting the dehiscence bone defects around implants. B, Exposed threads of the fixtures are covered by bone materials and a membrane to promote the osteogenic cells to generate new bone according to the guided regeneration concept.

The exposed threads of implants may be covered by bone materials and a membrane to prevent migration of the epithelial and connective tissue cells to the surgical site. So the osteogenic cells have the opportunity to migrate into the defect site and promote new bone formation. The bony dehiscence after installation of fixtures can be treated successfully by using GBR technique [43].

The other indication for GBR is an atrophic ridge either before or during implant surgery. The important consideration in reconstruction of ridge atrophy is appropriate case selection. Based on a general guide it is suggested to perform GBR procedure in A1, A2 or B1 defects of Khojasteh et al. classification. Application of GBR technique in these defects is associated with high implant survival rates [8]. Studies on installation of implants simultaneously with GBR showed a survival rate of 92.2% in horizontal defects. Others have reported the success rate of implants after the GBR procedure (non-simultaneous implant placement) reported 100% success in horizontal defects. The mean bone augmentation in these defects was 3.31 mm [43].

Advantages. GBR allows for the re-growth of the bone and the tissue. GBR is a relatively easy and predictable method which can be used under local anesthesia for small defects. In large defects due to trauma or resection of tumors the combination of this technique with bone grafting is an appropriate procedure for bone augmentation [43.[

Disadvantages. As the procedure takes approximately six months to heal completely, the likelihood of failure is higher if the patient does not take appropriate care. Apart from this, the success is also defect specific as the chances of success may be smaller if the condition is severe [44].

The patient can contribute to the success of the procedure by maintaining good plaque control, nonsmoking, anti-infective therapy, and systemic health maintenance.

9.2. Cortical tenting (Osteogenic GBR)

A usual limitation in reconstruction of the oral and maxillofacial region is the resorption of bone grafts due to contraction of overlying soft tissue. Excessive bone grafting is not always the ideal technique to compensate for resorption. We are not able to harvest a large amount of graft in all cases. Sometimes the defect size is larger than the harvested bone graft. In some cases we prefer to harvest the bone graft from an intra-oral recipient site rather than an extra-oral site because of its morbidity. The *cortical tenting technique* has been suggested as an alternative method.

Cortical tenting is a reconstruction method in which a block bone graft together with bone substitutes are used to augment the horizontal and vertical deficiencies [45]. The first step in this method is to harvest an appropriate block graft for the recipient site. There are several intraoral sites to harvest a block graft; however the ideal graft should be prepared after weighing the advantages and disadvantages. The lateral ramus of the mandible is a popular donor site and is used in most studies [46-48]. The cortical nature of this bone graft is the reason for its high resistance to resorption, although prolong neovascularization and the risk of damage to IAN are important disadvantages of this block graft [46, 49]. The other useful donor sites are maxillary tuberosity and chin. A retrospective study by Khojasteh et al. showed that the greatest vertical bone gain was in the defects where tuberosity was used as a block graft [46]. The simplicity of bone harvest and lower risk for nerve damage are other advantages of this donor site.

After preparing a block graft it must be adapted to the recipient site and fixed properly with a gap from the surface of the defect (Figure 17A). Then bone materials are used to fill the gaps (Figure 17B).

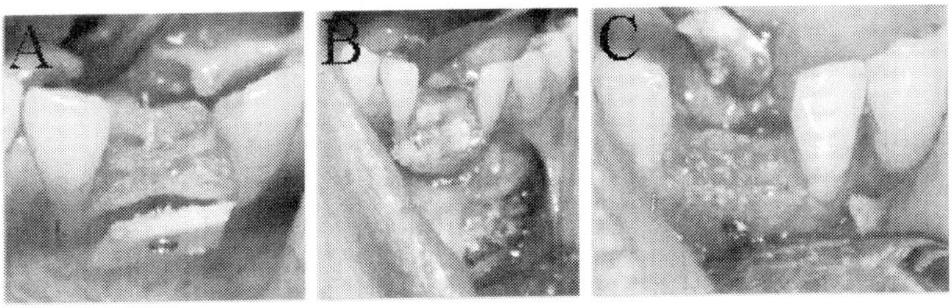

Figure 17. A, An anterior mandible defect after retracting the soft tissue flap. Lateral ramus bone block is harvested as a block graft and fixed with micro-screws with a gap from the buccal surface. B, The gap between the bone graft and alveolar bone is filled with bone materials. C, The defect has filled with new generated bone after 20 weeks.

The bone substitute could also be used to cover the bone block. With this technique we anticipate the bone resorption and prevent this complication by tenting the periosteum [50]. Then a membrane is used to cover the site. The soft tissue flap is sutured last (Figure 18).

Indications. This technique is most useful in horizontal defects of the anterior maxilla. After extracting the maxillary incisors a saucer-shaped defect may present in the premaxilla. This kind of defect could be properly corrected with the tenting technique [46, 50]. This method is also applicable in atrophic posterior mandibles [45]. Three-dimensional reconstruction with this technique is possible in atrophic ridges [51].

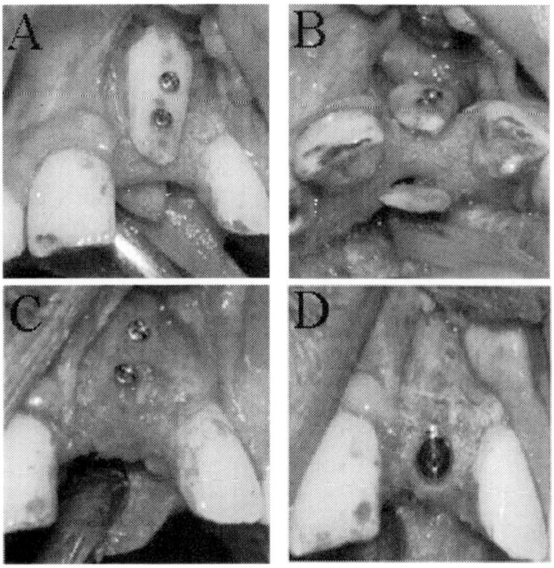

Figure 18. A, The defect of anterior maxilla is obvious after retracting the soft tissue flap. B, Lateral ramus bone block is harvested as a block graft and fixed with micro-screws. C, The surgical site is ready for implant surgery after 20 weeks. D, The deficiency is corrected and installation of the implant was performed without any problems.

Advantages. This technique decreases the patient's morbidity and is relatively simpler than other procedures. This procedure can be performed under local anesthesia. The bone particulates in the tenting technique promote the vascularization in the graft and improve bone regeneration and remodeling [52.[

Disadvantages. The tenting technique is not suitable in most combined horizontal and vertical defects. This method is not suitable for large defects resulting from severe trauma or resection of pathologic lesions. Complications including hematoma and nerve damage due to bone harvesting from chin and lateral of mandibular ramus respectively are some other disadvantages of this procedure. Inflammation, infection, graft exposure, and graft failure are other complications mentioned in the literature [46].

9.3. GBR in combination with onlay bone graft (OBG)

Reconstruction of combined defects with representation of both horizontal and vertical bone deficiencies requires specific consideration. Decision- making in rehabilitation of these kinds of defects involves the patient's preferences, defect size, and cost considerations [53].Combination of GBR and OBG is an appropriate technique in reconstruction of small combined defects before implant surgery. By applying this procedure the surgeon is able to use longer and wider implants, increasing the surface area resulting in a higher survival rate. In this technique a block bone graft is harvested and fixed in the defect area usually for vertical augmentation followed by using classic GBR procedure to restore the remaining defects (Figure 19).

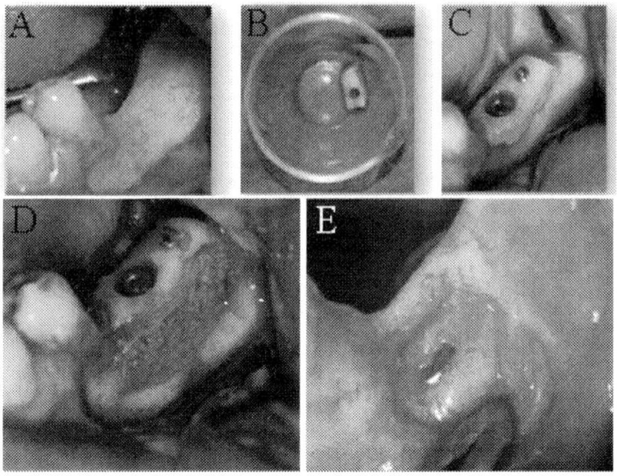

Figure 19. A, The atrophic ridge of posterior mandible is selected as the recipient site. B, Lateral ramus bone graft is harvested as an OBG. C, The OBG is fixed to augment the defect vertically. D, Bone materials are used to reconstruct the horizontal defect by GBR procedure. E, The surgical site is ready for insertion of implant fixtures.

Approximately after 6 months the surgical site is ready to install the implant fixtures. The average bone gain presented in the literature is 4.3 mm after performing this procedure [43].

Indications. This procedure is suitable for small to moderate defects in partial edentulous patients. This technique is usually indicated in combined defects to reconstruct horizontal and vertical defects. The common indication of this technique is in the anterior maxilla.

Advantages. This procedure can be performed under local anesthesia. This technique removes the need for harvesting extraoral bone grafts and reduces discomfort of the patient.

Disadvantages. This technique is not for large defects. The high failure rate of this technique in posterior of mandible is one of the major drawbacks of this technique [54].

10. Regenerative cell therapy

Although the autograft is accepted as the gold standard for the treatment of bone defects, some drawbacks of autogenous bone grafts such as limited graft accessibility, prolonged operation time and donor site morbidity as well as high costs, continue to drive the quest for development of alternative methods for bone regeneration and repair. Three new strategies are recently undergoing investigation:

Stem cell therapy; the transplantation of cultured osteogenic cells from host tissues like bone marrow.

Protein therapy; the application of osteoinductive growth factors in various reconstruction techniques.

Gene therapy; the transduction of genes encoding cytokines with osteogenic capacity into cells at the repair sites.

Bone engineering techniques consist of three main components: cell, growth factor, and carrier. Osteogenic cells are responsible for the generation of new bone. Without existing cells with osteogenic potential no new bone would be produced and no defect would be reconstructed. The proteins with osteoinductive potential known as growth factors are the second factor needed for reconstruction of defects. These growth factors are responsible for enhancement of new bone formation by affecting the cells which play a role in bone healing. The application of cultured cells or growth factors without any scaffold is almost impossible. Choosing the right scaffold for delivery of the cells and growth factors and acting as mesh for new bone formation is a significant issue in bone engineering.

11. Growth factors in bone regeneration

Protein therapy has demonstrated the most practical promise, mainly incorporating osteoinductive morphogens. Several osteoinductive cytokines have been suggested and investigated in the literature including bone morphogenetic proteins (BMPs), vascular endothelial growth factor (VEGF), platelet derived growth factor (PDGF), and transforming growth factor beta (TGF-β). Bone morphogenetic proteins have the most experimental and practical potential. Some studies however have shown the efficacy of other growth factors on bone reconstruction[55]. Synergic effects of two or more growth factors have been evaluated in some studies [56, 57].

Bone morphogenic proteins (BMPs). BMP is a large family of growth factors released naturally from different human tissues and acts in regenerating bone and cartilage tissue. The efficacy of BMP has been evaluated in several investigations [58-60]. After producing recombinant human BMP (rhBMP) the use of this cytokine became more popular in clinical studies. BMP can be applied in the surgical site by a carrier namely absorbable collagen sponge (ACS) or poly lactic glycolic acid (PLGA). The positive influence of BMP on bone regeneration in defects of the oral and maxillofacial area has been shown in most studies [55].

Platelet-derived growth factor (PDGF). PDGF promotes new bone formation. This facilitating bone regeneration factor is suggested to be used in maxillofacial defects where bone grafting is needed [61, 62]. PDGF improves the new bone formation by three main methods including mitogenesis, angiogenesis macrophage activation. The major role of PDGF is in differentiation of pre-osteoblasts to osteoblasts and proliferation of mesenchymal stem cells (MSCs). The usual carrier for PDGF has a mineral part in most investigations [55].

Vascular endothelial growth factor (VEGF). VEGF is an angiogenic factor which usually is released in response to hypoxia or tissue damage. VEGF has been used in different studies with both polymeric scaffolds and ceramic carriers [63, 64]. This growth factor is sometimes applied in combination with other promoting factors like BMP and PDGF to improve it's the regenerative features [65-67]. Despite all the important roles of VEGF investigated and presented in the literature most studies showed that this growth factor is less inductive than BMP in bone regeneration [55.[

Basic fibroblast growth factor (bFGF). bFGF is an important growth factor in wound healing, formation of granulation tissue and remodeling [68]. Several studies evaluated the effect of bFGF in bone regeneration; however its role is not as important as other factors like BMP [55].

Transforming growth factor beta (TGF-β). TGF-β is a group of proteins released from several tissues including macrophages and plays an important role in healing. The bone regenerative features of rhTGF- β1, rhTGF-β2, and TGF-β3 have been evaluated in different investigations. The usual carrier for the delivery of this growth factor in these studies is a gelatinous matrix. Some of these researches have shown the positive influence of this growth factor in bone regeneration [55].

Indications. The most common usage of growth factors is in implant surgery. The defects created during the procedure or post-operative bone dehiscences may be corrected with the application of growth factors. **Advantages.** Growth factors are presented as an alternative for bone grafts in reconstruction of maxillofacial defects. These proteins reduce the morbidity of the patients by removing the need of harvesting bone grafts. These factors are responsible for the major events in regeneration including angiogenesis, cell differentiation, mitogenesis, and bone formation [69]. Furthermore the combination of these proteins with bone grafts promotes the generation of new bone and facilitates healing of the defects.

Disadvantages. The high costs of producing growth factors are the major limitations for using these materials in humans. Production of recombinant growth factors as rhBMP and rhPDGF requires a period of time and high costs [70]. Application of growth factures is very technique sensitive and the clinician should be an expert in this procedure. Choosing a slow releasing scaffold is still a challenge among surgeons to use with the growth factor as a carrier. The appropriate dosage and useful concentration of these proteins in bone regeneration is another controversial issue which should be resolved. The excess amount of growth factor or wrong application of them may lead to ectopic bone formation and result in insufficient correction of the deficiencies.

12. Carriers in bone regeneration

Biomaterial carriers are needed for delivery and sustained release of growth factors. The application of growth factors without a proper carrier is very hard and their handling is almost impossible. There is no universal carrier for this purpose. Several biomaterial carriers have been suggested to be effective in delivery of certain growth factors and accelerate bone formation. The osteoconductive ability of the scaffold should be considered in choosing the right carrier for the purpose. The advantages and disadvantages of usual growth factor carriers are presented in Table 1.

http://dx.doi.org/10.5772/59236

Biomaterial carrier	Preparation technique	Advantages	Disadvantages
PLGA	solvent casting/ particulate leaching	Control over porosity, pore sizes and Crystallinity; high porosity	Residual solvents; limited mechanical properties
ACS	Freeze drying method	Facilitates surgical implantation and retention of the growth factor at the treatment site; hemostasis	Low porosity and low mechanical strength
HA	Particle aggregated scaffold	High mechanical strength	Brittleness, low fracture strength, and high density
NBM	Production methods of cadavers' bone	High porosity and interconnectivity	Potential host reaction, limited supply, excessive resorption, and potential disease transmission
DBM	demineralization process on allogenic bone	High porosity	Limited particle sizes range
β-TCP	Ceramic-based injectable scaffold	Facilitate early revascularization And accelerate bone regeneration; serves as a rich source for calcium and phosphorus	Brittleness, low fracture strength, and high density

PLGA,Polylactic co-glycolic acid; ACS, Absorbable collagen sponge; HA, Hydroxyapatite; NBM, Natural bone matrix; DBM, Demineralized bone matrix; β-TCP, Beta tri-calcium phosphate.

Table 1. The pros and cons of most common scaffolds

13. Cell therapy

13.1. MSCs harvesting sources

Cell therapy is a new technique in reconstruction of bone deficiencies presented as an alternative for bone grafting. The self-renewal ability and the capability of differentiating to osteogenic cells have made the stem cells a popular source in regeneration of bone defects. Several tissues have been suggested as the source of stem cells including fat, umbilical cord blood, lung, liver, skin, periosteum, and skeletal muscle [71]. Recently dental pulp was used as a new origin for extracting stem cells for regenerative purposes [72]. The usual source of MSCs in each study and various models is different. According to the literature the most common origin to harvest the MSCs in rat models is human bone marrow-derived mesenchymal stem cells (hBMSCs) usually extracted from femur or tibia [73-75]. The most common source in harvesting MSCs to regenerate the bone defects in rabbit and dog models as well as human studies is the iliac bone [71]. By considering the reduced differentiation potential of MSCs harvested from bone marrow investigators have attempted to find new sources of MSCs. Birth associated tissues like umbilical cord and dental pulp as well as adipose tissue are new sources that have been found to contain MSCs [76].

13.2. MSCs culture and differentiation protocol

MSCs as a compartment of various cell populations are aspirated from the selected origin like the iliac crest or buccal fat pad. The aspirated cells are cultured in a medium with Dulbecco's modified Eagle's medium (DMEM) and fetal bovine serum (FBS) for 3 h in a 37 degrees 5% CO2 incubator. Then the non-adherent cells are discarded after three hours and adherent cells are washed with phosphate-buffered saline (PBS) and fresh medium is replaced. The culture is treated with 0.5 ml of 0.25% trypsin containing 0.02% ethylene-diamine-tetra-acetic acid (EDTA) for 2 min at room temperature when the primary culture is confluent. A purified population of MSCs can be obtained 3 weeks after the initiation of culture [77]. The third generation of the cells is usually used in the studies (Figure 20) [78, 79]

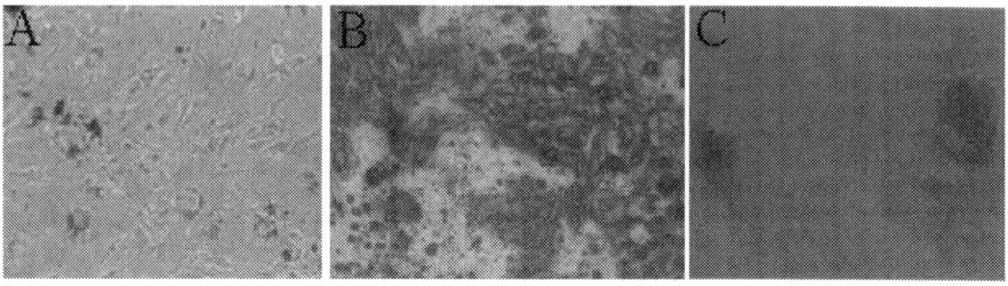

Figure 20. A, Proliferation of MSCs under light microscopy. B, Alizarin red staining for evaluating differentiation of MSCs to osteoprogenitor cells. Mineralization of the extracellular matrix is visualized by this staining technique. C, Oil red staining of MSCs, depicted adipogenic differentiation.

13.3. MSCs culture on scaffolds

Several investigations have evaluated the efficacy of stem cell regenerative ability on animals [78-82]. The stem cells should be implanted on an appropriate scaffold before delivery to the surgical site. According to the literature TCP is an efficient carrier for the stem cells to be loaded on and transplanted to the surgical site [71, 80, 81]. After preparation the choice carrier for reconstruction purpose it should be immerged into the medium impregnated with the MSCs. The MSCs should be implanted on the scaffold after 2 hours in 37ºC. Scanning electron microscope (SEM) is a useful assay to evaluate the presence of MSCs on the scaffold (Figure 21). Tripoding adherence of MSCs on the scaffold can be assessed under SEM [78].

13.4. Current trends in MSCs application in bone regeneration

Presentation MSCs as a novel regenerative technique in reconstructing bone defects provoked lots of investigators to evaluate the efficacy of MSCs application in oral and maxillofacial areas. Omitting the need for bone harvesting from a donor site and reducing the patient morbidity by application of MSCs in bone reconstruction promises a bright future for researchers around the world. Comparing the application of MSCs in bone regeneration to the control groups which bone materials were used has shown the increase of new bone formation. Implantation of MSCs together with bone minerals improves the regeneration of bone defects by delivery

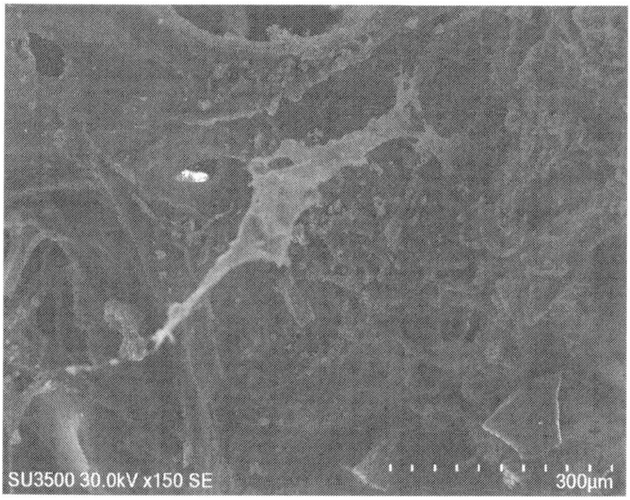

Figure 21. SEM Evaluation of MSCs (×50). SEM analysis shows lodging of the cells within the pores of the scaffold.

of the cells responsible for synthesizing new bone directly to the defect site [80]. Experimental studies on rat models have shown that the maximum bone formation was 2.53 mm in the β-TCP/MSC group 6 weeks after the surgery [79]. Histomorphometric analysis of the rabbit experiments at 6 and 12 weeks post-operation has demonstrated significantly higher bone formation in the group which MSCs were applied in combination with PRGF and nano-HA [78]. Histological analysis of rabbit models in other investigations demonstrated that the mean amount of vertical bone was higher in the MSCs group than the control group (2.09 mm versus 1.03 mm) after two months [82]. Choosing the appropriate scaffold for delivery of MSCs is important to gain the highest rate of new bone formation. The different studies on dog mandibles have indicated the importance of scaffolds on bone formation [61, 80, 81]. Jafarian et al. showed that six weeks after delivering dog BMSCs with biphasic scaffold (HA/TCP) or NBBM (Bio-Oss) in a through-and-through 10-mm mandibular defect, new bone formation was 65.78% and 50.31%, respectively [80]. Histomorphometric analysis in Khojasteh et al. study showed that after 8 weeks of the scaffold implantation (polycaprolactone-tricalcium phosphate (PCL-TCP)) higher amount of lamellar bone was generated more on the test side (48.63%) than control side (17.27%) [81]. Khojasteh et al. in another study applied MSCs with recombinant platelet derived growth factor (rh-PDGF) in mandibular defects in dogs; however the result showed only 21.52% new bone formation [61].

Nowadays the major concern about the application of MSCs in bone defect reconstruction is its effectiveness and delivery technique in human cases. Application of MSCs in sinus floor lifting in posterior atrophic maxilla has been assessed in human trials and reports. Several organic and inorganic materials have been suggested for sinus augmentation in the literature. MSCs seeded on an appropriate scaffold are new regenerative techniques advocated for this procedure. High mean percentage of new generated bone in these studies may indicate the important inductive potential of MSCs [83]. Alveolar cleft of maxilla is another recipient site for applying MSCs instead of autografts to reduce morbidity. Some authors have shown successful results of using MSCs in alveolar clefts [84] whilst some others did not [85]. The amount of new bone formation may be insufficient for reconstruction of clefts; however it is usually enough for orthodontic tooth movements [85]. The combination of MSCs and a growth factor may increase their inductive and regenerative potential; however the results were not satisfactory yet [86].

Indications. Alveolar clefts are examples of the maxillofacial defects which cell therapy may be useful [85, 86]. Cell therapy is also indicated in augmentation of the sinus floor [83].

Advantages. It avoids the drawbacks of bone grafting like donor site morbidity. The stem cells are able to differentiate to different cell linings based on the combined growth factor. By extracting the cells from the own patient autologous transplantation is possible and no immune-suppressive therapy is necessary.

Disadvantages. Accessibility and the requirement for a large amount of cells are the main disadvantages of cell therapy as well as expenditure of time and money to provide the adequate cells for regeneration in large defects. The genetic damage occurrence of adult stem cells is a possibility in old patients. Embryonic stem cells have the risk of rejection and uncontrolled proliferation (turning into a teratoma).

14. Summary

Bone regeneration and anatomical bone reconstruction in defects of oral and maxillofacial region have been always a critical and controversial issue. There are lots of regenerative techniques suggested to be effective in oral and maxillofacial defects; however no one can absolutely choose the best efficient procedure. The quantity and quality of the regenerated bone is another aspect of defect reconstruction which should be highly considered. Although several regenerative procedures can be used in a certain defect, the regenerated bone may not be functional all the time.

Author details

Arash Khojasteh[1], Mohammad Esmaeelinejad[2*] and Farzad Aghdashi[2]

*Address all correspondence to: esmaeelnejad@gmail.com

1 Department of Oral and Maxillofacial Surgery, Dental Faculty, Shahid Beheshti University of Medical Sciences, Tehran, Iran

2 Department of Oral and Maxillofacial Surgery, Dental Faculty, Shahid Beheshti University of Medical Sciences, Tehran, Iran

References

[1] Jimi E, Hirata S, Osawa K, Terashita M, Kitamura C, Fukushima H. The current and future therapies of bone regeneration to repair bone defects. Int J Dent. 2012;2012:148261.

[2] Dimitriou R, Jones E, McGonagle D, Giannoudis PV. Bone regeneration: current concepts and future directions. BMC Med. 2011;9:66.

[3] Chen ST, Buser D. Clinical and esthetic outcomes of implants placed in postextraction sites. Int J Oral Maxillofac Implants. 2009;24 Suppl:186-217.

[4] Trisi P, Rao W. Bone classification: clinical-histomorphometric comparison. Clin Oral Implants Res. 1999;10(1):1-7.

[5] Hassani A, Khojasteh A, Alikhasi M. Repair of the perforated sinus membrane with buccal fat pad during sinus augmentation. J Oral Implantol. 2008;34(6):330-3.

[6] Khojasteh A, Mohajerani H, Momen-Heravi F, Kazemi M, Alikhasi M. Sandwich bone graft covered with buccal fat pad in severely atrophied edentulous maxilla: a clinical report. J Oral Implantol. 2011;37(3):361-6.

[7] Behnia H, Homayoun S, Qaranizade K, Morad G, Khojasteh A. Multidisciplinary reconstruction of a palatomaxillary defect with nonvascularized fibula bone graft and distraction osteogenesis. J Craniofac Surg. 2013;24(2):e186-90.

[8] Khojasteh A, Morad G, Behnia H. Clinical importance of recipient site characteristics for vertical ridge augmentation: a systematic review of literature and proposal of a classification. J Oral Implantol. 2013;39(3):386-98.

[9] Cawood JI, Howell RA. A classification of the edentulous jaws. Int J Oral Maxillofac Surg. 1988;17(4):232-6.

[10] Seibert JS. Reconstruction of deformed, partially edentulous ridges, using full thickness onlay grafts. Part II. Prosthetic/periodontal interrelationships. Compend Contin Educ Dent. 1983;4(6):549-62.

[11] Tinti C, Parma-Benfenati S, Polizzi G. Vertical ridge augmentation: what is the limit? Int J Periodontics Restorative Dent. 1996;16(3):220-9.

[12] Wang HL, Al-Shammari K. HVC ridge deficiency classification: a therapeutically oriented classification. Int J Periodontics Restorative Dent. 2002;22(4):335-43.

[13] Pikos MA. Mandibular block autografts for alveolar ridge augmentation. Atlas Oral Maxillofac Surg Clin North Am. 2005;13(2):91-107.

[14] Neiva RF, Gapski R, Wang HL. Morphometric analysis of implant-related anatomy in Caucasian skulls. J Periodontol. 2004;75(8):1061-7.

[15] Misch CM. Comparison of intraoral donor sites for onlay grafting prior to implant placement. Int J Oral Maxillofac Implants. 1997;12(6):767-76.

[16] Pikos MA. Block autografts for localized ridge augmentation: Part I. The posterior maxilla. Implant Dent. 1999;8(3):279-85.

[17] Pikos MA. Block autografts for localized ridge augmentation: Part II. The posterior mandible. Implant Dent. 2000;9(1):67-75.

[18] Hassani A, Khojasteh A, Shamsabad AN. The anterior palate as a donor site in maxillofacial bone grafting: a quantitative anatomic study. J Oral Maxillofac Surg. 2005;63(8):1196-200.

[19] Sekine J, Sano K, Ikeda H, Inokuchi T. Rehabilitation by means of osseointegrated implants in oral cancer patients with about four to six years follow-up. J Oral Rehabil. 2006;33(3):170-4.

[20] Guven O. Rehabilitation of severely atrophied mandible using free iliac crest bone grafts and dental implants: report of two cases. J Oral Implantol. 2007;33(3):122-6.

[21] Pogrel MA, Podlesh S, Anthony JP, Alexander J. A comparison of vascularized and nonvascularized bone grafts for reconstruction of mandibular continuity defects. J Oral Maxillofac Surg. 1997;55(11):1200-6.

[22] Foster RD, Anthony JP, Sharma A, Pogrel MA. Vascularized bone flaps versus nonvascularized bone grafts for mandibular reconstruction: an outcome analysis of primary bony union and endosseous implant success. Head Neck. 1999;21(1):66-71.

[23] Ahlmann E, Patzakis M, Roidis N, Shepherd L, Holtom P. Comparison of anterior and posterior iliac crest bone grafts in terms of harvest-site morbidity and functional outcomes. J Bone Joint Surg Am. 2002;84-a(5):716-20.

[24] Bauer TW, Muschler GF. Bone graft materials. An overview of the basic science. Clin Orthop Relat Res. 2000(371):10-27.

[25] Pensler J, McCarthy JG. The calvarial donor site: an anatomic study in cadavers. Plast Reconstr Surg. 1985;75(5):648-51.

[26] Ko EC, Chang CM, Chang P, Kao CC, Chen KJ, Wu IF, et al. Tibial Cancellous Bone Grafting in Jaw Reconstruction: 10 Years of Experience in Taiwan. Clin Implant Dent Relat Res. 2013.

[27] Saeed NR, van Eeden SP, Hensher R, Kent JN. Re: follow up of mandibular costochondral grafts after release of ankylosis of the temporomandibular joints. Br J Oral Maxillofac Surg. 2007;45(1):91.

[28] Peltomaki T, Isotupa K. The costochondral graft: a solution or a source of facial asymmetry in growing children. A case report. Proc Finn Dent Soc. 1991;87(1):167-76.

[29] Gapski R, Wang HL, Misch CE. Management of incision design in symphysis graft procedures: a review of the literature. J Oral Implantol. 2001;27(3):134-42.

[30] Toscano N, Shumaker N, Holtzclaw D. The art of block grafting: a review of the surgical protocol for reconstruction of alveolar ridge deficiency. J Implant Adv Clin Dent. 2010;2:45-66.

[31] Arrington ED, Smith WJ, Chambers HG, Bucknell AL, Davino NA. Complications of iliac crest bone graft harvesting. Clin Orthop Relat Res. 1996(329):300-9.

[32] McCarthy JG, Schreiber J, Karp N, Thorne CH, Grayson BH. Lengthening the human mandible by gradual distraction. Plast Reconstr Surg. 1992;89(1):1-8; discussion 9-10.

[33] Chopra S, Enepekides DJ. The role of distraction osteogenesis in mandibular reconstruction. Curr Opin Otolaryngol Head Neck Surg. 2007;15(4):197-201.

[34] Kunkel M, Wahlmann U, Reichert TE, Wegener J, Wagner W. Reconstruction of mandibular defects following tumor ablation by vertical distraction osteogenesis using intraosseous distraction devices. Clin Oral Implants Res. 2005;16(1):89-97.

[35] Scolozzi P. Distraction osteogenesis in the management of severe maxillary hypoplasia in cleft lip and palate patients. J Craniofac Surg. 2008;19(5):1199-214.

[36] Nout E, Cesteleyn LL, van der Wal KG, van Adrichem LN, Mathijssen IM, Wolvius EB. Advancement of the midface, from conventional Le Fort III osteotomy to Le Fort III distraction: review of the literature. Int J Oral Maxillofac Surg. 2008;37(9):781-9.

[37] Saltaji H, Altalibi M, Major MP, Al-Nuaimi MH, Tabbaa S, Major PW, et al. Le Fort III distraction osteogenesis versus conventional Le Fort III osteotomy in correction of syndromic midfacial hypoplasia: a systematic review. J Oral Maxillofac Surg. 2014;72(5):959-72.

[38] Luna AH, Passeri LA, de Moraes M, Moreira RW. Endosseous implant placement in conjunction with inferior alveolar nerve transposition: a report of an unusual complication and surgical management. Int J Oral Maxillofac Implants. 2008;23(1):133-6.

[39] Gasparini G, Boniello R, Saponaro G. Long term follow-up in inferior alveolar nerve transposition: our experience. 2014;2014:170602.

[40] Yaghmaei M, Mashhadiabbas F, Shahabi S, Zafarbakhsh A, Yaghmaei S, Khojasteh A. Histologic evaluation of inferior alveolar lymphatics: an anatomic study. Oral Surg Oral Med Oral Pathol Oral Radiol Endod. 2011;112(5):564-7.

[41] Babbush CA. Transpositioning and repositioning the inferior alveolar and mental nerves in conjunction with endosteal implant reconstruction. Periodontology 2000. 1998;17(1):183-90.

[42] Misch C. Implantes dentais contemporâneos: Elsevier Brasil; 2011.

[43] Milinkovic I, Cordaro L. Are there specific indications for the different alveolar bone augmentation procedures for implant placement? A systematic review. Int J Oral Maxillofac Surg. 2014;43(5):606-25.

[44] Linde A, Alberius P, Dahlin C, Bjurstam K, Sundin Y. Osteopromotion: a soft-tissue exclusion principle using a membrane for bone healing and bone neogenesis. J Periodontol. 1993;64(11 Suppl):1116-28.

[45] Morad G, Khojasteh A. Cortical tenting technique versus onlay layered technique for vertical augmentation of atrophic posterior mandibles: a split-mouth pilot study. Implant Dent. 2013;22(6):566-71.

[46] Khojasteh A, Behnia H, Shayesteh YS, Morad G, Alikhasi M. Localized bone augmentation with cortical bone blocks tented over different particulate bone substitutes: a retrospective study. Int J Oral Maxillofac Implants. 2012;27(6):1481-93.

[47] Roccuzzo M, Ramieri G, Bunino M, Berrone S. Autogenous bone graft alone or associated with titanium mesh for vertical alveolar ridge augmentation: a controlled clinical trial. Clin Oral Implants Res. 2007;18(3):286-94.

[48] Roccuzzo M, Ramieri G, Spada MC, Bianchi SD, Berrone S. Vertical alveolar ridge augmentation by means of a titanium mesh and autogenous bone grafts. Clin Oral Implants Res. 2004;15(1):73-81.

[49] Hwang KG, Shim KS, Yang SM, Park CJ. Partial-thickness cortical bone graft from the mandibular ramus: a non-invasive harvesting technique. J Periodontol. 2008;79(5):941-4.

[50] Le B, Burstein J, Sedghizadeh PP. Cortical tenting grafting technique in the severely atrophic alveolar ridge for implant site preparation. Implant Dent. 2008;17(1):40-50.

[51] Khoury F, Khoury C. Mandibular bone block grafts: diagnosis, instrumentation, harvesting techniques and surgical procedures. Bone Augmentation in Oral Implantology New Malden, United Kingdom: Quintessence publishing Co, Ltd. 2007:169-83.

[52] Louis PJ, Gutta R, Said-Al-Naief N, Bartolucci AA. Reconstruction of the maxilla and mandible with particulate bone graft and titanium mesh for implant placement. J Oral Maxillofac Surg. 2008;66(2):235-45.

[53] Pommer B, Zechner W, Watzek G, Palmer R. To graft or not to graft? Evidence-based guide to decision making in oral bone graft surgery. Bone Grafting. 2012:1-25.

[54] Nissan J, Ghelfan O, Mardinger O, Calderon S, Chaushu G. Efficacy of cancellous block allograft augmentation prior to implant placement in the posterior atrophic mandible. Clin Implant Dent Relat Res. 2011;13(4):279-85.

[55] Khojasteh A, Behnia H, Naghdi N, Esmaeelinejad M, Alikhassy Z, Stevens M. Effects of different growth factors and carriers on bone regeneration: a systematic review. Oral Surg Oral Med Oral Pathol Oral Radiol. 2013;116(6):e405-23.

[56] Kanczler JM, Ginty PJ, White L, Clarke NM, Howdle SM, Shakesheff KM, et al. The effect of the delivery of vascular endothelial growth factor and bone morphogenic protein-2 to osteoprogenitor cell populations on bone formation. Biomaterials. 2010;31(6):1242-50.

[57] Young S, Patel ZS, Kretlow JD, Murphy MB, Mountziaris PM, Baggett LS, et al. Dose effect of dual delivery of vascular endothelial growth factor and bone morphogenetic protein-2 on bone regeneration in a rat critical-size defect model. Tissue Eng Part A. 2009;15(9):2347-62.

[58] Carstens MH, Chin M, Li XJ. In situ osteogenesis: regeneration of 10-cm mandibular defect in porcine model using recombinant human bone morphogenetic protein-2 (rhBMP-2) and Helistat absorbable collagen sponge. J Craniofac Surg. 2005;16(6): 1033-42.

[59] Jovanovic SA, Hunt DR, Bernard GW, Spiekermann H, Wozney JM, Wikesjo UM. Bone reconstruction following implantation of rhBMP-2 and guided bone regeneration in canine alveolar ridge defects. Clin Oral Implants Res. 2007;18(2):224-30.

[60] Wikesjo UM, Qahash M, Thomson RC, Cook AD, Rohrer MD, Wozney JM, et al. rhBMP-2 significantly enhances guided bone regeneration. Clin Oral Implants Res. 2004;15(2):194-204.

[61] Khojasteh A, Dashti SG, Dehghan MM, Behnia H, Abbasnia P, Morad G. The osteoregenerative effects of platelet-derived growth factor BB cotransplanted with mesenchymal stem cells, loaded on freeze-dried mineral bone block: A pilot study in dog mandible. J Biomed Mater Res B Appl Biomater. 2014.

[62] Schwarz F, Ferrari D, Podolsky L, Mihatovic I, Becker J. Initial pattern of angiogenesis and bone formation following lateral ridge augmentation using rhPDGF and guided bone regeneration: an immunohistochemical study in dogs. Clin Oral Implants Res. 2010;21(1):90-9.

[63] Yonamine Y, Matsuyama T, Sonomura T, Takeuchi H, Furuichi Y, Uemura M, et al. Effectable application of vascular endothelial growth factor to critical sized rat calvaria defects. Oral Surg Oral Med Oral Pathol Oral Radiol Endod. 2010;109(2):225-31.

[64] Wernike E, Montjovent MO, Liu Y, Wismeijer D, Hunziker EB, Siebenrock KA, et al. VEGF incorporated into calcium phosphate ceramics promotes vascularisation and bone formation in vivo. Eur Cell Mater. 2010;19:30-40.

[65] De la Riva B, Sanchez E, Hernandez A, Reyes R, Tamimi F, Lopez-Cabarcos E, et al. Local controlled release of VEGF and PDGF from a combined brushite-chitosan system enhances bone regeneration. J Control Release. 2010;143(1):45-52.

[66] Luo T, Zhang W, Shi B, Cheng X, Zhang Y. Enhanced bone regeneration around dental implant with bone morphogenetic protein 2 gene and vascular endothelial growth factor protein delivery. Clin Oral Implants Res. 2012;23(4):467-73.

[67] Samee M, Kasugai S, Kondo H, Ohya K, Shimokawa H, Kuroda S. Bone morphogenetic protein-2 (BMP-2) and vascular endothelial growth factor (VEGF) transfection to human periosteal cells enhances osteoblast differentiation and bone formation. J Pharmacol Sci. 2008;108(1):18-31.

[68] Esmaeelinejad M, Bayat M. Effect of low-level laser therapy on the release of interleukin-6 and basic fibroblast growth factor from cultured human skin fibroblasts in normal and high glucose mediums. J Cosmet Laser Ther. 2013;15(6):310-7.

[69] Lee K, Silva EA, Mooney DJ. Growth factor delivery-based tissue engineering: general approaches and a review of recent developments. J R Soc Interface. 2011;8(55): 153-70.

[70] Demain AL, Vaishnav P. Production of recombinant proteins by microbes and higher organisms. Biotechnology Advances. 2009;27(3):297-306.

[71] Khojasteh A, Behnia H, Dashti SG, Stevens M. Current trends in mesenchymal stem cell application in bone augmentation: a review of the literature. J Oral Maxillofac Surg. 2012;70(4):972-82.

[72] Morad G, Kheiri L, Khojasteh A. Dental pulp stem cells for in vivo bone regeneration: a systematic review of literature. Arch Oral Biol. 2013;58(12):1818-27.

[73] Akita S, Fukui M, Nakagawa H, Fujii T, Akino K. Cranial bone defect healing is accelerated by mesenchymal stem cells induced by coadministration of bone morphogenetic protein-2 and basic fibroblast growth factor. Wound Repair Regen. 2004;12(2):252-9.

[74] Kim J, Kim IS, Cho TH, Lee KB, Hwang SJ, Tae G, et al. Bone regeneration using hyaluronic acid-based hydrogel with bone morphogenic protein-2 and human mesenchymal stem cells. Biomaterials. 2007;28(10):1830-7.

[75] Yoon E, Dhar S, Chun DE, Gharibjanian NA, Evans GR. In vivo osteogenic potential of human adipose-derived stem cells/poly lactide-co-glycolic acid constructs for bone regeneration in a rat critical-sized calvarial defect model. Tissue Eng. 2007;13(3): 619-27.

[76] Zomorodian E, Baghaban Eslaminejad M. Mesenchymal stem cells as a potent cell source for bone regeneration. Stem Cells Int. 2012;2012:980353.

[77] Grassel S, Stockl S, Jenei-Lanzl Z. Isolation, culture, and osteogenic/chondrogenic differentiation of bone marrow-derived mesenchymal stem cells. Methods Mol Biol. 2012;879:203-67.

[78] Behnia H, Khojasteh A, Kiani MT, Khoshzaban A, Mashhadi Abbas F, Bashtar M, et al. Bone regeneration with a combination of nanocrystalline hydroxyapatite silica gel, platelet-rich growth factor, and mesenchymal stem cells: a histologic study in rabbit calvaria. Oral Surg Oral Med Oral Pathol Oral Radiol. 2013;115(2):e7-15.

[79] Khojasteh A, Eslaminejad MB, Nazarian H. Mesenchymal stem cells enhance bone regeneration in rat calvarial critical size defects more than platelete-rich plasma. Oral Surg Oral Med Oral Pathol Oral Radiol Endod. 2008;106(3):356-62; discussion 63.

[80] Jafarian M, Eslaminejad MB, Khojasteh A, Mashhadi Abbas F, Dehghan MM, Hassanizadeh R, et al. Marrow-derived mesenchymal stem cells-directed bone regeneration in the dog mandible: a comparison between biphasic calcium phosphate and natural bone mineral. Oral Surg Oral Med Oral Pathol Oral Radiol Endod. 2008;105(5):e14-24.

[81] Khojasteh A, Behnia H, Hosseini FS, Dehghan MM, Abbasnia P, Abbas FM. The effect of PCL-TCP scaffold loaded with mesenchymal stem cells on vertical bone augmentation in dog mandible: a preliminary report. J Biomed Mater Res B Appl Biomater. 2013;101(5):848-54.

[82] Khojasteh A, Eslaminejad MB, Nazarian H, Morad G, Dashti SG, Behnia H, et al. Vertical bone augmentation with simultaneous implant placement using particulate mineralized bone and mesenchymal stem cells: a preliminary study in rabbit. J Oral Implantol. 2013;39(1):3-13.

[83] Shayesteh YS, Khojasteh A, Soleimani M, Alikhasi M, Khoshzaban A, Ahmadbeigi N. Sinus augmentation using human mesenchymal stem cells loaded into a beta-tricalcium phosphate/hydroxyapatite scaffold. Oral Surg Oral Med Oral Pathol Oral Radiol Endod. 2008;106(2):203-9.

[84] Pradel W, Tausche E, Gollogly J, Lauer G. Spontaneous tooth eruption after alveolar cleft osteoplasty using tissue-engineered bone: a case report. Oral Surg Oral Med Oral Pathol Oral Radiol Endod. 2008;105(4):440-4.

[85] Behnia H, Khojasteh A, Soleimani M, Tehranchi A, Khoshzaban A, Keshel SH, et al. Secondary repair of alveolar clefts using human mesenchymal stem cells. Oral Surg Oral Med Oral Pathol Oral Radiol Endod. 2009;108(2):e1-6.

[86] Behnia H, Khojasteh A, Soleimani M, Tehranchi A, Atashi A. Repair of alveolar cleft defect with mesenchymal stem cells and platelet derived growth factors: a preliminary report. J Craniomaxillofac Surg. 2012;40(1):2-7.

Chapter 24

Facial Augmentation with Implants

Farzin Sarkarat, Behnam Bohluli and
Roozbeh Kahali

Additional information is available at the end of the chapter

http://dx.doi.org/10.5772/59188

1. Introduction

The public's demand for facial beauty has increased over time. Different cosmetic procedures have been introduced to meet this demand. The essentials of facial cosmetic surgery are: 1- Volume replacement and 2- Facial augmentation. Better aesthetic results have been achieved by using less invasive surgical techniques including lifting procedures, injectable fillers, autologous fat transfer, and facial implants.

The malar eminence and chin are the most common facial sites augmented via implants. Autologous tissues have been the gold standard for facial augmentation for years; but today alloplastic materials are more commonly used.

Drawbacks of autogenous grafting include: donor site morbidity, limited availability, limited moldability, and unpredictable resorption [1].An ideal alloplastic implant must be made out of a material that has low bioactivity or toxicity. It must also be stable and biocompatible [2]. An understanding of these qualities is needed to prevent complications or to treat them should they occur.

2. The aging process

One of the primary advancements in cosmetic facial surgery has been the realization of volume loss in aging and volume replacement via cosmetic surgery [3-6]. The abundance of midfacial volume is one of the main reasons that makes a person look young, which means having the right amount of fat in the right areas of the face. The loss or shift of this fat is a main contributor to facial aging [7]. Loss of volume and volume shift occur in all regions of the face and neck and are the reasons for aged appearance [5, 6].The youthful midface has voluminous and superiorly positioned malar fat pads. The malar fat pad is a triangular structure with its base against the nasolabial fold and its apex over the malar region. Due to actinic skin changes as well as gravity, fat atrophy, and deep connective tissue laxity, the malar fat pads lose volume and descend lower into the face with age. The sum of these aging changes frequently yields a hollow midface.

3. Treatment

There are a wide variety of procedures for achieving volume replacement and facial augmentation including lifting procedures [7, 8], injectable fillers [9-11], autologous fat transfer [12, 13], and facial implants [14, 15]. Facial implants are an optimum for most patients. The main advantage is that they are a permanent option when compared with fillers; and they are available in many anatomical shapes and sizes. They are easily placed, the recovery is minimal, and they have a low complication rate.

Autogenous bone and cartilage have been used to repair traumatic, congenital, and surgical defects of the face. The increased morbidity of the donor site, limited supply, resorption, and migration contributed to decrease in their use. Gold, silver, paraffin, and ivory fell out of favor because of their tissue incompatibility and lack of malleability. Polymeric silicone, polyamide mesh, expanded polytetrafluoroethylene, and high-density polyethylene, replaced the previous materials because of their increased malleability and biocompatibility [16].

The midface is the area in which facial implants are more commonly used. Implants in the nasojugal crease are used to correct tear trough deformity. Nasal implants are not widely used, but can be used to correct defects caused by rhinoplasty. Malar and submalar implants (Figure 1) are the most commonly used implants in the midface [17].

The lower face is another area where facial implants are frequently used. Chin implants (Figure 2) are one of the most common facial implants performed by cosmetic surgeons [18]. Volume restoration, in addition to the re-suspension and removal of excess tissue, remains the current goal of aesthetic surgery. Facial implants play a major role in volume restoration.

4. Implant types

Facial implants are categorized according to their site (malar, submalar, paranasal, chin, etc.). They can also be prefabricated, anatomical or custom-made. Facial implants are available in many shapes and sizes. The submalar implant is best described as an implant that restores the volume the patient has lost with age. This is in contrast to malar augmentation, which generally changes a patient's appearance while augmenting volume. Volume is lost in the malar region but is significantly less than the volume lost in the submalar region. Smaller implants generally restore a former appearance, whereas larger implants change the patient's appearance. The submalar zone is the area of maximum midface atrophy in most patients. Most female patients

http://dx.doi.org/10.5772/59188

are treated with a small submalar implant. The medium implant is most frequently used in the male patient. If the patient is looking for replacement of atrophic losses that occur with aging, the smaller implant is preferable. A larger implant is reserved for the patient who desires to not only replace volume that has been lost but also augment an appearance that was previously unsatisfactory to the patient. Microgenia is effectively addressed with chin augmentation [19, 20]. The placement of an extended alloplastic anatomic chin implant is a simple, safe, and easily performed procedure. The patient's appearance is enhanced by restoring the chin and cervico-mental region [21, 22]. Most patients with a mild to moderately deficient chin are well treated with an alloplastic implant [19]. In patients with severe microgenia, a chin implant combined with soft tissue filling and tension restoration is most effective.

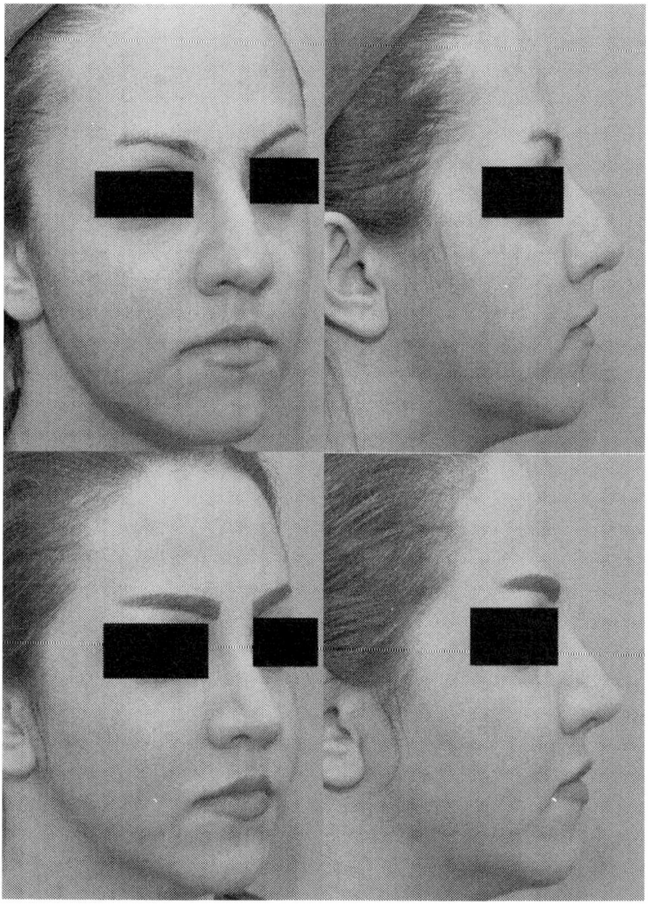

Figure 1. Malar augmentation with facial implant. Above: Before. Below: After.

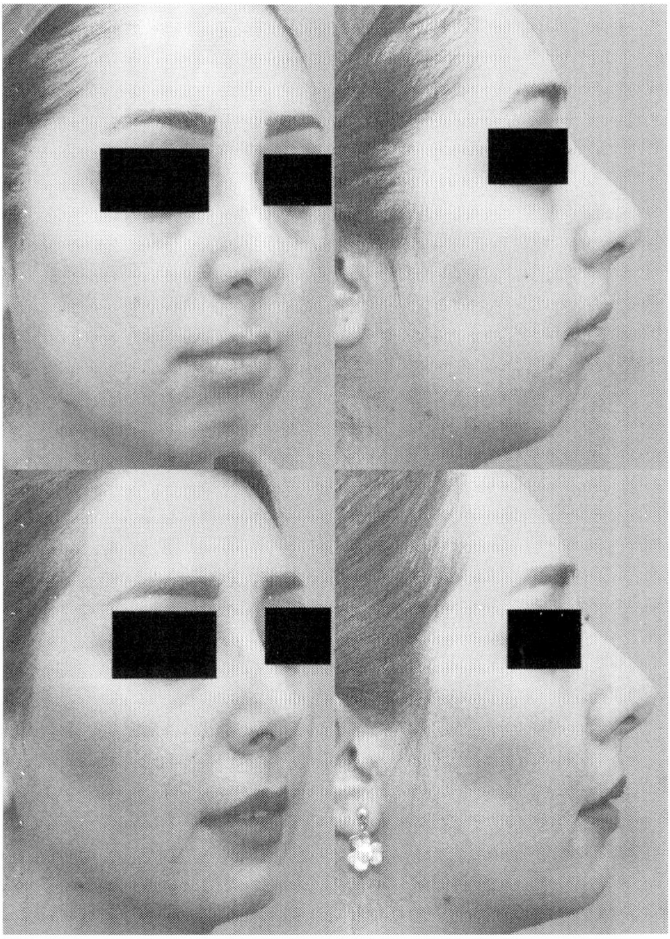

Figure 2. Chin augmentation with facial implant, Above: Before, Below: After.

Facial implants are made of various materials. It is crucial that the surgeon be familiar with these materials and their advantages and disadvantages.

4.1. Metal implants

Cobalt chromium alloys, stainless steel, gold, and titanium have been used as facial implants. The corrosive characteristics of metals placed in the body limited their use. Stainless steel was used in the plating of skeletal fractures of the face. Titanium has largely replaced stainless steel and cobalt-chromium alloys as the metal of choice because of its strength, low tissue reactivity, reduced artifact on CT, safety during MRI studies and its corrosive resistance over time [23].

Its use is generally limited to dental implants and facial skeletal plating for maxillofacial trauma [1, 24, and 25].

4.2. Silicone implants

Silicone implants have been used for years. Polydimethylsiloxane is nonporous implant with smooth contours. Its pliable nature and resistance to high temperatures used in sterilization make it the most versatile facial implant. It also can be easily carved and shaped. Polydimethylsiloxane becomes encapsulated in a mild chronic inflammatory process. Because no links are formed between the polydimethylsiloxane and its fibrous tissue envelope, they are more prone to displacement, persistent seromas and a tendency toward extrusion [26-29].

4.3. Polyester fiber

Polyester fiber is comprised of nonabsorbable strands of polyethylene terephthalate which is a porous material, allowing tissue ingrowth and subsequent implant stability. The excellent tensile strength, durability, biocompatibility, and flexibility of polyester fiber have led to its use in facial implants. Infection rates are lowered with antibiotic impregnation [30, 31]. Its disadvantages are the surgical time required to prepare the mesh with folding and suturing and inflammatory reactions most commonly seen after facial trauma [32].

4.4. Polyamide mesh

Polyamide mesh is an organopolymer related to nylon. It has the advantage of flexibility, ease of molding and allowing tissue ingrowth into the implant which is related to the implant stability. Polyamide mesh creates an intense foreign body response and chronic inflammation. Hydrolytic degradation has been noted to occur after implantation, leading to loss of volume [33].

4.5. High-density polyethylene

High-density polyethylene (HDPE) which is more commonly known as "Medpor" (Prex Surgical, Inc., College Park, Georgia), is a stable, porous and extremely inert implant with minimal foreign body reactions which does not degrade over time. It is malleable when heated but otherwise has a lack of pliability. Although the large average pore size encourages fibrous tissue ingrowth, leading to firm attachment and high stability [34, 35], but fibrous ingrowth does not guarantee stability of HDPE implants against bone and may require additional fixation.

4.6. Polymethylmethacrylate

Polymethylmethacrylate (PMMA) has high strength and rigidity for bony reconstruction of the face. It has been used to repair orbital, malar, and cranial defects [36-38]. PMMA is available as a powder consisting of polymer and catalyst and a liquid form of the monomer. When mixed, an exothermic reaction occurs. The heat generated by the reaction has led to untoward events in orthopedic surgery, although such complications have not been reported in craniofacial reconstruction. PMMA is well tolerated without significant inflammatory foreign body reactions. Being able to create customized implants unique to each patient's needs is one of its main advantages.

4.7. Expanded polytetrafluoroethylene

ePTFE known as "Gore-Tex" (W.L.Gore and Associates, Flagstaff, AZ), is a fibrillated polymer of polytetrafluoroethylene, with pores between the fibrils averaging 22 microns in diameter which allows limited soft tissue ingrowth while creating only a mild chronic inflammatory response, providing early stabilization and permitting removal when necessary [39]. ePTFE is spongy in consistency, inert, and does not change shape or resorb with time. It also has been found to be non-carcinogenic and is rarely allergenic [28, 40]. Because ePTFE is hydrophobic, it does not absorb antibiotic solutions [41].

4.8. Hydroxyapatite

Calcium hydroxyapatite is mixed in a fashion similar to methylmethacrylate to form a cement that can be contoured to each individual patient's needs. Because it forms the synthetic, inorganic constituent of bone, it can induce osseointegration. Mixing does not result in an exothermic reaction. It is now used more commonly as an injectable implant.

5. Implant selection

The surgeon must be able to make a decision regarding the selection of an implant based on chemical composition, physical structure, and planned site for application. Characteristics of an ideal implant include biocompatibility, chemical inertness, lack of elicitation of foreign body or hypersensitivity reaction, non-carcinogenicity, and ease of shaping and carving [42].

Common implant materials include expanded PTFE, methyl methacrylate, porous polyethylene, and silicone rubber. Porous polyethylene and silicone rubber implants are the most commonly used. Silicone rubber implants can be easily trimmed, being flexible, conform well to underlying anatomy and become well encapsulated. They can be easily be removed or replaced if necessary.

The structure of porous polyethylene implants allows better tissue integration, but this can also be extremely problematic when attempting to remove or replace an implant. Significant tissue injury, defects or implant fragmentation can occur with removal.

Most patients, as they age, lose volume in the submalar region. The submalar area includes the hollow area of the infraorbital, anterolateral maxillary region, and canine fossa regions. Most of these patients have a hollow submalar region. They usually have adequate and well-defined zygomatico-malar esthetics and adequately projected cheekbones. These patients are best treated with only submalar augmentation, as their problem is loss of submalar volume.

The second type of common facial esthetic deficiency found is in patients who have adequate submalar and anterior maxillary projection but deficient cheekbones and hypoplasia of the zygomatico-malar regions. These patients are best treated with a malar implant.

The third type of common midfacial aging change is seen in a patient who has submalar deficiency in addition to need of more zygomatico-malar augmentation. These patients need both submalar and malar augmentation. These patients are well treated with the combined submalar shell implant. This implant is designed to augment the submalar region as well as a portion of the zygomatico-malar region.

Careful examination and thorough analysis aid in coming to a decision about what size of implant to use to achieve the desired effect [43]. Clinical photography serves as a powerful tool. A similar approach is applied to the chin and prejowl complex. This approach helps determine what type of implant to use.

Fewer surface imperfections allow greater resilience against degradation by mechanical forces [44]. This advantage must be balanced with the increased possibility of migration as compared with porous implants. The implant should not create a severe immune response, one that may harm the host or damage the implant. Synthetic implants stimulate inflammatory response with acute and chronic phases [45]. Significant immunogenicity can result in degradation or rejection of the implant. Bacteria are capable of implant invasion when pore size decreases. Implants with pore sizes between 1 and 50 microns may be more susceptible to infection than materials with larger pores, because they do not permit tissue granulation and delivery of host inflammatory cells to mount an adequate immune response.

6. Implant placement

6.1. Malar and submalar augmentation

The placement of midfacial implants is a simple surgical procedure for experienced maxillofacial surgeons. The implants are always placed in the subperiosteal plane. With the exception of the infraorbital neurovascular bundle, there is little vulnerable anatomy in the midface region, when dissecting in the subperiosteal plane. The implants can also be placed concomitantly with other esthetic or orthognathic procedures.

With the patient in the sitting position, the atrophic submalar area is marked and the zygomatic arch is outlined. The patient is prepared and draped. Several approaches to the malar and submalar region exist including subciliary, transconjunctival, and intraoral. The intraoral approach if preferred. The procedure is begun by injecting about 5 mL of 2% lidocaine with 1:100,000 epinephrine in the subperiosteal plane along the anterior maxilla, malar region, and the anterior zygomatic arch region. An incision is made just below the maxillary vestibule, approximately 1 cm above the canine tooth (Figure 3). The mucosa and soft tissues are incised in the canine fossa region and through the periosteum. Subperiosteal dissection is performed (Figure 4).

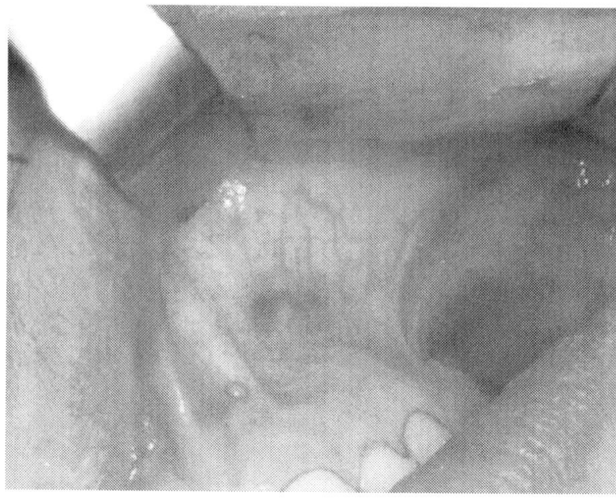

Figure 3. Intraoral approach for malar implant placement

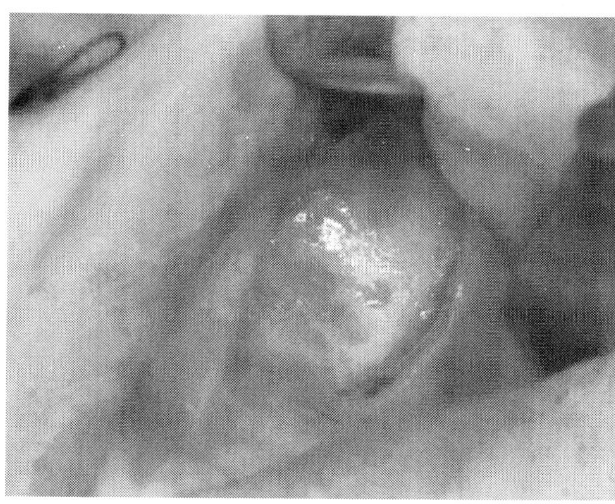

Figure 4. Subperiosteal dissection for malar implant placement

The borders of this dissection pocket are the lateral portion of the inferior orbital rim, superiorly, the zygomatic arch superolaterally and the masseteric fascia laterally. The buccal fat pad must be avoided. The extent of the dissection is dictated by the shape and size of the implant. The combined submalar and shell implants require more dissection over the malar and zygomatic regions. The dissected pocket should be just slightly larger than the actual implant size. As the subperiosteal dissection is begun in the anterior maxillary region, it is important

http://dx.doi.org/10.5772/59188

to protect the infraorbital neurovascular bundle. After the anterior maxilla is dissected, the periosteal elevator is angled and the remainder of the dissection is primarily in an oblique vector over the malar region and extends over the anterior portion of the zygomatic arch. After the implant pocket is dissected, the area is checked for hemostasis (Figure 5). The pocket is then irrigated with antibiotic solution (300 mg of clindamycin and or gentamicin mixed with 30 mL of sterile water) and the implant is placed. The implants are also soaked in antibiotic solution. This is especially important for porous implants (Figure 6).

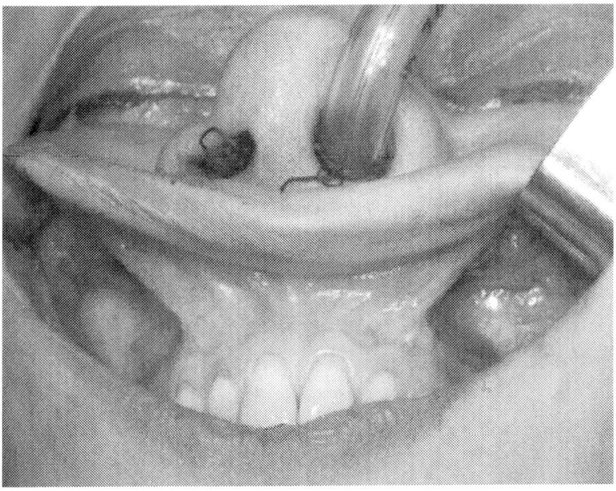

Figure 5. The subperiosteal pocket is checked for hemostasis

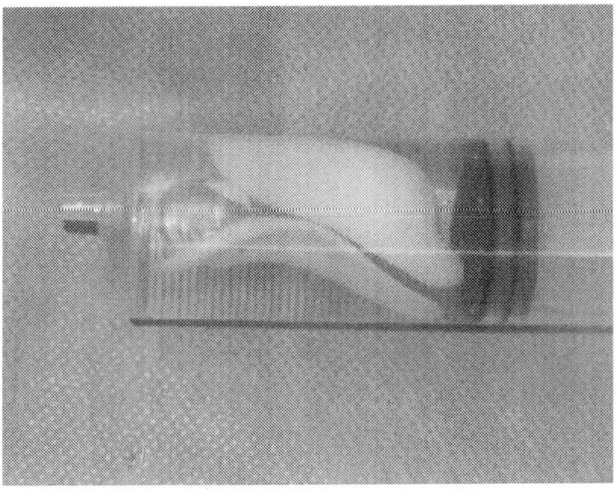

Figure 6. The implants are also soaked in Gentamicin solution

A well-conforming implant in a tight pocket does not generally need fixation. If the pocket is considerably larger than the implant and there is increased mobility of the implant, a single fixation screw can be placed. The fixation screw is best placed in the thicker bone of the buttress area (Figure 7). Finally, the incision is closed with interrupted 4-0 absorbable suture (Figure 8).

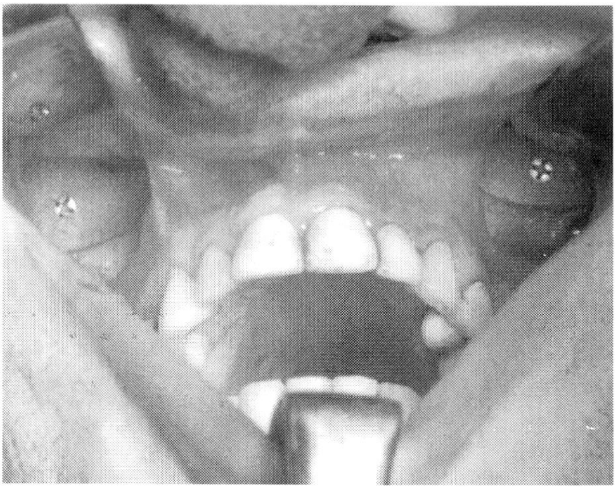

Figure 7. Implant fixation

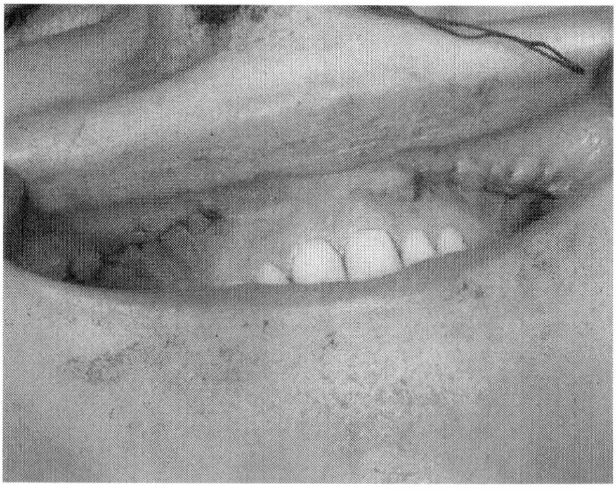

Figure 8. Incision closureChin augmentation

http://dx.doi.org/10.5772/59188

There are two main approaches to chin augmentation; one with an intraoral incision, and one with an incision in the submental crease. The main advantage of the intraoral incision is the avoidance of an external scar. The submental incision is preferred because the external scar is well camouflaged in the submental crease and there is no need to divide the mentalis muscle.

A 2-cm incision is made in the submental crease centered about the midline. Sharp and blunt dissection is used to reach the periosteum of the lower edge of the mandible in the midline. A sharp incision is made through the periosteum laterally. A subperiosteal dissection is performed to create a pocket for the implant. Dissection laterally should be performed as close to the mandibular border as possible to avoid injuring the mental nerve. After the implant is inserted a stabilizing stitch or screws may be used. The incision is then closed in two layers.

When using an intra-oral approach, a 2 to 3-cm incision is made in the mandibular labial sulcus about 10 to 15-mm away from mucogingival junction (Figure 9). Then the mentalis muscle and periosteum are transected and a subperiosteal dissection is performed (Figure 10). Care must be taken not to injure the mental nerve.

The implant is inserted over the chin bone and screws are used for fixation (Figures 11 and 12). Then the mentalis muscle portions are aligned and sutured together. The mucosa is closed with absorbable sutures.

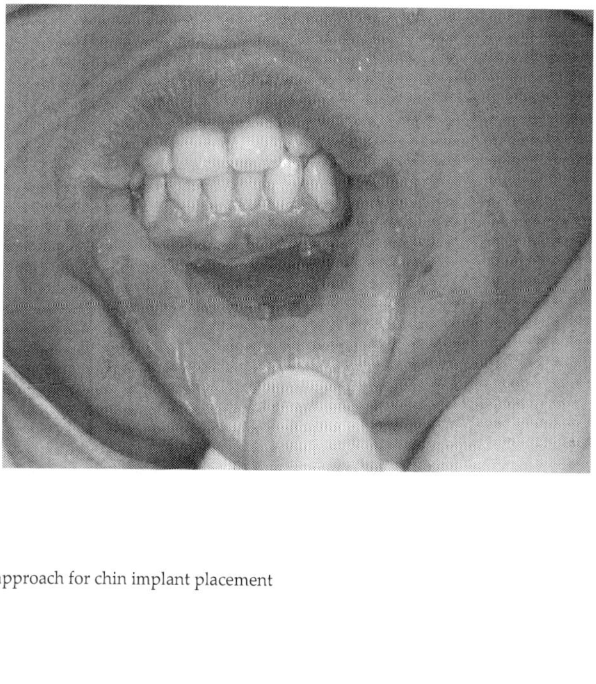

Figure 9. Intra-oral approach for chin implant placement

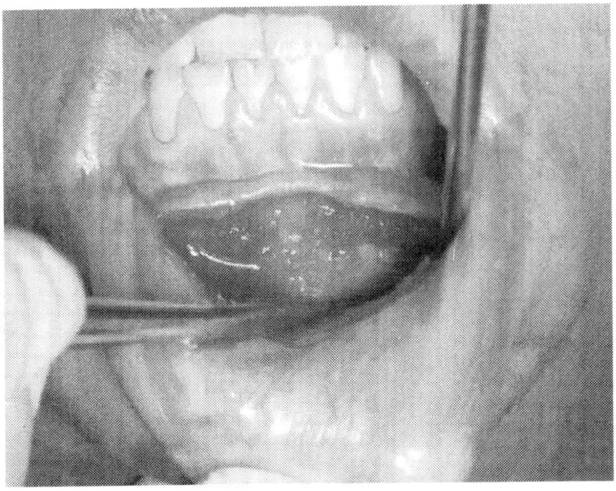

Figure 10. Subperiosteal dissection for chin implant placement

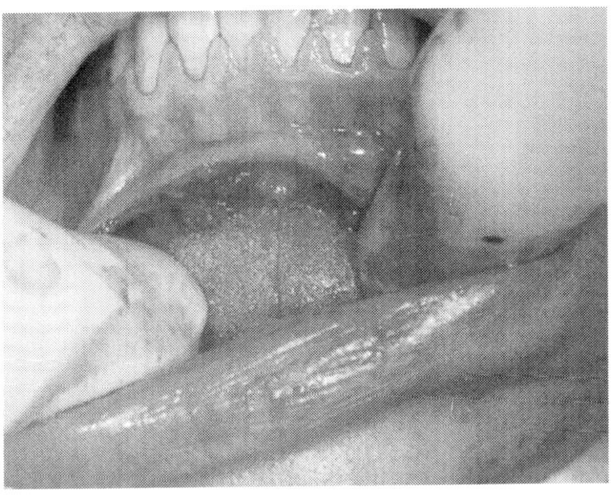

Figure 11. Implant placement

http://dx.doi.org/10.5772/59188

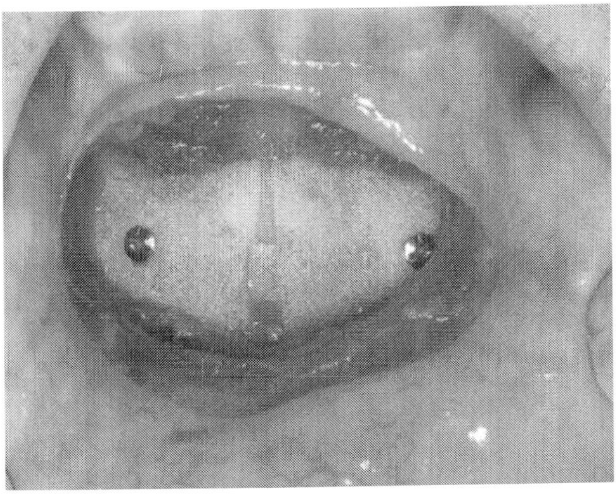

Figure 12. Implant fixation

7. Postoperative sequelae

The patient must be warned that during the first 1 to 2 weeks he or she will experience abnormal animation when smiling and talking. The tissue dissection violates the orbicularis oris and lip elevator muscles, which heal uneventfully with the return of normal animation. Significant edema is not uncommon, especially with larger implants and in the early postoperative period. Cold packs and steroids are routinely used. Severe swelling may indicate hematoma formation and, if necessary it must be drained. This can usually be done by opening the incision and suctioning the blood or clot from under or around the implant without compromising the result. Minor hematomas will usually heal uneventfully without treatment. Occasionally, subconjunctival or periorbital ecchymosis is seen but remains a rare occurrence and heals uneventfully.

8. Post operative care

No dressings are required and the postoperative care includes analgesics, antibiotics, and steroids if desired. The patient is instructed to avoid significant talking and animation for the first 48 hours and is asked to follow a liquid or soft diet for the same period. Ice packs are used for the first 24 hours.

9. Complications

9.1. Improper selection or placement

Improper placement of the implant is the most common complication followed by improper implant selection. The implant should be slightly smaller than the desired increase in fullness. Selecting too large an implant will lead to excessive soft tissue tension, which could lead to ischemia, necrosis, or extrusion. Placement of malar implants too laterally can cause the eyes to look too close together. Placement of the implants too medially and inferiorly will give a chipmunk look or appearance.

9.2. Neuropraxia

Neuropraxia can occur from impingement of the nerve by a large implant, migration or improper placement of the implant, a traction injury, a thermal injury, or a direct traumatic injury from dissection. Most patients regain sensation and function within three weeks. Dissection for Malar implants involves elevating tissue around the infraorbital nerve. Weakness of the zygomaticus, orbicularis oculi, or the frontalis muscles can be induced by disturbance of the temporofrontal branch of the facial nerve while dissecting posteriorly over the middle third of the zygomatic arch. Straying from the subperiosteal plane predisposes to dissection into the parotid and facial nerve branches and facial musculature. During dissection of the chin, it is important to avoid the mental nerve, which is approximately underneath the area of the premolars intraorally. The marginal mandibular branch of the facial nerve, which supplies muscles of the lower lip and chin, is above the periosteum over the inferior border of the mandible. A severe traction injury or perforation of the periosteum can injure the marginal mandibular branch of the facial nerve.

9.3. Edema and ecchymosis

The majority of postoperative edema and ecchymosis resolves in two weeks, but edema can persist for 6 months and even up to a year [46]. Implant fixation is important because excessive continuing movement can cause tissue injury, chronic inflammation, and suboptimal soft tissue acceptance with prolonged edema. This could also be due to a nonspecific immune reaction to the implant material.

9.4. Hematoma and seroma

Abnormal fluid collection can be the result of inadequate hemostasis, over-dissection, traumatic handling of the tissues, dead space around or underneath the implant or elevated blood pressure. Hematomas and seromas encourage the growth of bacterial contamination potentiating cellulitis and infection. They can result in excessive fibrosis producing soft tissue defects. Smaller hematomas (<5 cc) resolve without treatment in 10–14 days. Large hematomas need to be recognized and evacuated with the implant removed as necessary. Seromas usually present around 2 weeks after surgery. Presence of liquefied hematomas or seromas 2 to 4 weeks postoperatively may be drained percutaneously [47].

http://dx.doi.org/10.5772/59188

9.5. Infection

Implants can be contaminated by hematogenous, contiguous spread, or direct inoculation. Foreign bodies have been shown to reduce the number of bacteria required to produce an infection by 104 to 106 power [48]. Chemical composition, surface roughness, surface configuration, and hydrophobicity influence the potential for implant contamination. Hydrophilic materials are more resistant to adhesion than hydrophobic materials. Scalfani and colleagues found that PTFE with an average pore size of 22 microns became infected at lower inoculum counts and sooner than polyethylene with a pore size of 150 microns [48]. Most infections in the early postoperative time period are more likely to occur with porous implants because of increased surface area, irregularity, and surface energy, which facilitates bacterial adherence. Infections that occur years after surgery are most probably caused by hematogenous spread or direct violation of the implant capsule with bacterial seeding like an injection. Late malar implant infections have been associated with dental injections as reported by Cohen and Kawamoto [49].

S. aureus is the main pathogen and is usually susceptible to penicillin or cephalosporin. A better chance of eradicating the infection with antibiotics and drainage is possible with nonporous implants. In the presence of a purulent infection, the implant should be removed and scrubbed and sterilized to remove the biofilm. In addition, debridement and copious irrigation of the implant pocket and a prolonged postoperative antibiotic course are necessary. If rapid improvement does not occur and the implant needs to be removed, it should not be replaced for 6–8 weeks to allow for resolution of the infection and inflammation [50].

9.6. Migration and contour changes

Migration is usually the result of over dissection, improper implant size selection and lack of fixation. Supraperiosteal placement can predispose the implant to mobility especially without adequate fixation. Anatomic implants have decreased the potential for migration, rotation, and displacement. Delayed contour changes have been reported in association with silastic implants. This is thought to be associated with capsular contracture around the implant in addition to calcification of the capsule itself.

9.7. Extrusion

Adequate soft tissue bulk with good quality tissue for coverage of the implant and tension-free correct plane insertion are critical to preventing implant extrusion. Decreased tissue perfusion causes wound healing problems. Highly scarred and thinned tissues tend to atrophy over time and are at a higher risk for postoperative infection, exposure, and extrusion [35]. Excessive tension is a result of placing too large an implant in a small pocket. In addition to tension free closure, subperiosteal placement helps prevent exposure.

9.8. Palpability

This can be the result of improper implant size selection, improper contour selection, improper positioning, improper fixation or capsular contracture. Thin overlying tissue and supraperiosteal placement of the implant predispose to palpability.

9.9. Lip dysfunction

Altered lip function occurs because dissection can interfere with the muscles responsible for smiling mimetics. Other factors include edema, interposition of a solid implant which stretches the muscles of the midface, or interference with the facial nerve during dissection over the zygomatic arch. The edema can cause dysfunction in the muscles of the lips resembling facial nerve dysfunction. When dysfunction is due to muscle displacement, it usually takes 1–3 months for the muscles to reattach and the capsule to become soft and distensible.

9.10. Bone resorption

Bone erosion under alloplastic implants was a significant problem with early implants. It was often attributed to foreign body reaction between the implant and the bone or to pressure from the mentalis muscle against the implant. Improper implant positioning, pressure due to an oversized implant, subperiosteal placement and hardness of the implant were also considered.

The resorption from anatomic malar and chin implants is minimal and self-limiting. Bone erosion occurs less with anatomic extended implants because of greater distribution of the pressure forces over a broader anatomic area. Resorption appears to occur in the first 12 months after placement but can appear radiographically as soon as 2 months. Labial incompetence and hyperactive mentalis lead to pressure and migration of the implant superiorly onto the thinner bone of the alveolus, which predisposes to resorption. When severe resorption is present, the implant must be removed.

9.11. Postoperative asymmetry

Asymmetry is more likely to be noticed in malar implants. It is usually caused by initial malposition or by creation of asymmetric bilaterally dissected spaces. It can also be the result of unrecognized preoperative skeletal or soft tissue deficiencies. It is important to point out preexisting asymmetry before treatment selection. Although major asymmetries require a second surgery, minor asymmetries have a natural tendency to adjust and correct themselves over a 6-month postoperative period as healing progresses and the tissue around the implant relaxes and softens.

10. Summary

Loss of volume and volume shift occur in all regions of the face and neck and contribute to the aged appearance. Volume replacement and contour augmentation of the face are the essentials of facial cosmetic surgery. The development of less invasive volume replacement procedures has been an evolution in achieving better aesthetic results. These procedures include lifting procedures, injectable fillers, autologous fat transfer, and facial implants.

Facial volume augmentation by using facial implants is a very safe procedure that is used widely for facial rejuvenation which can be used concomitantly with other rejuvenation

http://dx.doi.org/10.5772/59188

procedures. It is crucial for the cosmetic surgeons to be familiar with various implant materials and their advantages and disadvantages.

Author details

Farzin Sarkarat*, Behnam Bohluli and Roozbeh Kahali

*Address all correspondence to: sarkarat@hotmail.com

Department of Oral and Maxillofacial Surgery, Bouali Hospital, Islamic Azad University of Medical Sciences, Tehran, Iran

References

[1] Sclafani AP, Romo T. Biology and chemistry of facial implants. Facial Plast Surg 2000;16(1):3–6.

[2] Eppley B. Alloplastic implantation. Plast Reconstr Surg 1999;104(6):1761–85.

[3] Terino EO. The art of alloplastic facial contouring. St. Louis (MO): Mosby; 2000.

[4] Terino EO. Facial contouring with alloplastic implants: aesthetic surgery that creates three dimensions. Facial Plast Surg 1999;7:55–83.

[5] Constantinides MS, Doud-Galli SK, Miller PJ, et al. Malar, submalar, midfacial implants. Facial Plast Surg 2000;16:35–44.

[6] Terino EO. Alloplastic facial contouring by zonal principles of skeletal anatomy. Clin Plast Surg 1992;19:487.

[7] Niamtu J: The adjustable vector deep plane midface lift. Atlas Oral Maxillofac Surg Clin North Am 12:199, 2004

[8] Watson S, Niamtu J, Cunningham L: Endoscopic midface lift, *in* Atlas of Oral and Maxillofacial Surgery Clinics of North America. Philadelphia, PA, WB Saunders, 2003, pp 145-155

[9] Niamtu J: The use of Restylane in cosmetic facial surgery. J Oral Maxillofac Surg 64:317, 2006

[10] Niamtu J: Minimally invasive cosmetic surgery, *in* Oral and Maxillofacial Surgery Clinics of North America. Vol 17. Philadelphia, PA, Saunders, 2005, pp 17-27

[11] Steinsapir KD, Steinsapir SM: Deep-fill hyaluronic acid for the temporary treatment of the Naso-jugal groove: A report of 303 consecutive treatments. Ophthal Plast Reconstr Surg 22:344, 2006

[12] Little JW: Applications of the classic dermal fat graft in primary and secondary facial rejuvenation. Plast Reconstr Surg 109:788, 2002

[13] Obagi S: Autologous fat augmentation for addressing facial volume loss. Oral Maxillofac Surg Clin North Am 17:99, 2005

[14] Roy D, Mangat DS: Facial implants. Dermatol Clin 23:541, 2005

[15] Binder WJ, Azizzadeh B, Binder WJ: Malar and submalar augmentation. Facial Plast Surg Clin North Am 16:11, 2008

[16] Quatela VC, Sabini P. Synthetic implants. In: Papel ID, editor. Facial plastic and reconstructive surgery. New York7 Thieme Medical Publishing; 2002. p. 61– 72.

[17] Silver WE. Malar augmentation. Facial Plast Surg 1992; 8:133– 9.

[18] Romo III T, Baskin JZ, Sclafani AP. Augmentation of the cheeks, chin and pre-jowl sulcus, and nasolabial folds. Facial Plast Surg 2001;17:67–78.

[19] Zide BM, Pfeifer TM, Longaker MT. Chin surgery: I. Augmentation—the allures and the alerts. Plast Reconstr Surg 1999;104:1843.

[20] Tardy ME, Thomas JR, Brown RJ. Facial aesthetic surgery. St. Louis (MO): Mosby; 1995.

[21] Auger TA, Turley PK. The female soft tissue profile as presented in fashion magazines during the 1900's. A photographic analysis. Intern J Adult Orthodon Orthognath Surg 1999;14:7–18.

[22] Perrett DI, May KA, Yoshodawa S. Facial shape and judgements of female attractiveness. Nature 1994; 368:239–42.

[23] Morehead JM, Holt GR. Soft-tissue response to synthetic biomaterials. Otolaryngol Clin North Am 1994;27(1):195–201.

[24] Albrektsson T, Branemark PI, Jacobsson M, et al. Present clinical applications of osseointegrated percutaneous implants. Plast Reconstr Surg 1987;79(5):721–31.

[25] Branemark PI, Albrektsson T. Titanium implants permanently penetrating human skin. Scand J Plast Reconstr Surg 1982;16(1):17–21.

[26] Wilson J, Merwin GE. Biomaterials for facial bone augmentation: comparative studies. J Biomed Mater Res 1988;22(A2 Suppl):159–77.

[27] Davis PK, Jones SM. The complications of silastic implants. Experience with 137 consecutive cases. Br J Plast Surg 1971;24(4):405–11.

[28] Silver FH, Maas CS. Biology of synthetic facial implant materials. Facial Plast Surg Clin North Am 1994;2:241–53.

[29] Morrison AD, Sanderson RC, Moos KF. The use of Silastic as an orbital implant for reconstruction of orbital wall defects: review of 311 cases treated over 20 years. J Oral Maxillofac Surg 1995;53(4):412–7.

[30] Gross EJ, Hamilton MM, Ackermann K, et al. Mersilene mesh chin augmentation. A 14-year experience. Arch Facial Plast Surg 1999;1(3): 183–9 [discussion: 190].

[31] McCollough EG, Hom DB, Weigel MT, et al. Augmentation mentoplasty using Mersilene mesh. Arch Otolaryngol Head Neck Surg 1990; 116(10):1154–8.

[32] Choe KS, Stucki-McCormick SU. Chin augmentation. Facial Plast Surg 2000;16(1):45–54.

[33] Costantino PD, Friedman CD, Lane A. Synthetic biomaterials in facial plastic and reconstructive surgery. Facial Plast Surg 1993;9(1):1–15.

[34] Spector M, Flemming WR, Sauer BW. Early tissue infiltrate in porous polyethylene implants into bone: a scanning electron microscope study. J Biomed Mater Res 1975;9(5):537–42.

[35] Wellisz T, Kanel G, Anooshian RV. Characteristics of the tissue response to MEDPOR porous polyethylene implants in the human facial skeleton. J Long Term Eff Med Implants 1993;3(3):223–35.

[36] Gladstone HB, McDermott MW, Cooke DD. Implants for cranioplasty. Otolaryngol Clin North Am 1995;28(2):381–400.

[37] van Gool AV. Preformed polymethylmethacrylate cranioplasties: report of 45 cases. J Maxillofac Surg 1985;13(1):2–8.

[38] Abrahams IW. Repair of orbital floor defects with premolded plastic implant. Arch Ophthalmol 1966;75(4):510–2 %R 10.1001/archopht.75.4.510.

[39] Maas CS, Gnepp DR, Bumpous J. Expanded polytetrafluoroethylene (Gore-Tex soft-tissue patch) in facial augmentation. Arch Otolaryngol Head Neck Surg 1993;119(9): 1008–14.

[40] Levine B, Berman WE. The current status of expanded polytetrafluoroethylene (Gore-Tex) in facial plastic surgery. Ear Nose Throat J 1995; 74(10):681–2, 684.

[41] Mole B. The use of Gore-Tex implants in aesthetic surgery of the face. Plast Reconstr Surg 1992;90(2):200–6.

[42] Scales J, Winter G. Clinical considerations in the choice of materials for orthopedic internal devices. J Biomed Mater Res 1975;9:167–76.

[43] Terino EO. Alloplastic facial contouring: surgery of the fourth plane. Aesthetic Plast Surg 1992;16:195– 212.

[44] Bapna MS, Lautenschlager EP, Moser JB. The influences of electrical potential and surface finish on the fatigue life of surgical implant materials. J Biomed Mater Res 1975;9(6):611–21.

[45] Donald PJ. Cartilage grafting in facial reconstruction with special consideration of irradiated grafts. Laryngoscope 1986;96(7):786–807.

[46] Terino EO. Chin and malar augmentation. In: Complications and problems in aesthetic plastic surgery. New York: NY; 1992. Ch 6.

[47] Yarmechuck MJ. Infraorbital rim augmentation. Plast Reconstr Surg 2001;107(6): 1585–92.

[48] Sclafani AP, Thomas JR, Cox AJ, et al. Clinical and histologic response of subcutaneous expanded polytetraflouroethylene and porous high density polyethylene implants to acute and early infection. Arch Otolaryngol Head Neck Surg 1997;123: 328–36.

[49] Cohen SR, Kawamoto HK. Infection of proplast malar implants following dental injections. Plast Reconstr Surg 1992;89(6):1148–51.

[50] Louis PJ, Cuzalina LA. Alloplastic augmentation of the face. Atlas Oral Maxillofac Surg Clin North Am 2000; 8(2):127–91.

Chapter 25

Management of Bone Grafting Complications in Advanced Implant Surgery

Mehdi Sezavar, Vahid Mesgarzadeh,
Shahrouz Shafayifard and M. Reza Soleimanpour

Additional information is available at the end of the chapter

http://dx.doi.org/10.5772/59967

1. Introduction

1.1. The perfect bone graft

In spite of the fact that the bone materials that are currently being used are not absolutely perfect,the bone graft material of choice must have 2 mandatory features:

1. Immunologically neutral
2. Physiologically safe

In an immunological point of view, the graft should neither be rejected nor be contaminated to transmit microbial diseases. The graft should be biologically compatible, preferably resorbed after formation of new bone, though supplying a scaffold and sustaining mechanical stability for new bone regeneration. In a physiological point of view, a perfect bone graft substance should support the host osteogenically,osteoinductively and osteoconductively.

2. Biosafety of bone grafting material

Contagious substances should be absent in an ideal biocompatible bone grafting material. Carbonate, Calcium phosphate and Sulfate bone graft materials are typically biocompatible with no risk of being rejected by the host. Virus, Prion and bacterial contamination of bone grafting materials are not of our concern in autogenous or alloplastic bone grafts. The prevalence of HIV infection in freeze-dried bone and demineralized freeze-dried bone allografts has been reported to be 1 in 8,000,000 and 1 in 2.800.000 respectively. The prevalence of bovine spongiform encephalopathy transmission with bovine xenograft reckoned to be less than that of being hit by lightning.

Thus, the risk of disease transmission from an allograft or xenograft is almost zero as long as the disinfection/sterilization protocols are followed by manufacturers. The world health organization affirmed that bone is classified as type IV (no transmission) for prion diseases. Therefore all currently available bone graft materials are secure and reliable concerning disease transmission potential.

3. Bone grafting drawbacks

3.1. Preservation of the alveolar socket

Socket preservation procedure serves to maintain the alveolar bone existing volume including height and width by delivering graft materials into the alveolar socket after extraction and to enhance new bone formation inside the socket. Various techniques and materials have been applied and so far they have shown favorable results. Complications may either be caused by surgical procedures or treatment planning. Excessive amounts of graft should be avoided. Graft materials should gently be compacted keeping adequate between its particles to allow revascularization and penetration of proteins and growth factors. Furthermore the flap design has to be considered regarding the augmentation site specially in critical sites such as esthetic zone. Park and Wang introduced the mucogingival pouch flap design to preserve the papilla,improve graft retention and reduce exposure of the membrane. However in case that the interdental space is less than 6mm, the mucogingival pouch flap may threaten the overall blood supply of the flap caused by the vertical releasing incision. Thus wise treatment planning is needed to avoid possible complications. Disappearance and contamination of the grafts placed inside the dental socket may be expectable. Membranes used for GBR also strengthen the risk of exposure and infection. Froum evaluated the healing of sockets underwent preservation using hydroxyapatite and nonabsorbable inorganic bovine bone mineral covered by either ePTFE membrane or acellular dermal matrix allograft. Having not adequately covered the socket with soft tissue, 1 of 8 sockets covered by acellular dermal matrix and 6 of 8 sockets covered by ePTFE exhibited exposure of membranes which consequently led to early removal of the membranes because of potential infection. Reduction of facial facial keratinized tissue followed by primary closure itself can be considered as a complication. Though this can be avoided by wise treatment planning and allowing the socket to heal for 6 to 8 weeks in advance before grafting. Recently formed keratinized tissue growing over the dental socket will provide adequate coverage without giving away the facial width.

3.2. Guided bone regeneration or ridge augmentation

Guided bone regeneration (GBR) was proved to be effective in regenerating new bone on alveolar ridges with atrophies both vertically and horizontally accompanied with membranes. Much the same as onlay bone graft which also acts as a space maintainer, GBR may serve similar complications related to the use of onlay grafts. Furthermore, GBR may also include the use of membrane and sometimes microscrews. Thus, complications that pertain to GBR may vary such as membrane exposure, microscrew exposure and infection. Critical inflammatory reactions have also been recorded. The prevalence of flap sloughing associated with nonabsorbable membranes was high. Exposure of fixation screw or membrane may often lead to local inflammations accompanied with decreased new bone formation. There have been arguments over the significance of early membrane exposure on regenerative outcome of guided tissue regeneration and GBR operations. Several studies have reported that the responses were better when the membranes remained submerged while some other studies cast doubt on this issue.

3.3. Monocortical onlay grafts

Complications with regard to ridge augmentation using the onlay bone grafts mainly include infection, opening of the incision line, bone fracture, Nerve malfunction, rupture of mucosa over the implant, loss of portion of the bone graft, dehiscence of the wound and graft movement. While the most common complication is the incision line opening that leads to contamination of graft, delay in vascularization and loss of graft material, the most deleterious outcome on survival of implants in the augmentation site is related to wound dehiscence.The prevalence of unintentional skin/mucosa perforation was 5.2% for mandible as augmentation site with onlay bone graft and the incidence for infection occurred in 1 of the 11 patients(9.1%) that resulted in partial loss of graft. Infection of the graft can be caused by endogenous bacteria, deprived aseptic surgical technique or inadequacy of primary closure. Antibiotics were used to prevent bacterial infection and to enhance collagen formation. However it was found that tetracycline arrests the bone formation chelating calcium at the graft. Thus, other antibiotics such as penicillin or clindamycin have been suggested.

3.4. Sinus lifting

Sinus lifting procedure is performed when there is insufficient height for implant placement by lifting the Schneiderian membrane apically with bone grafting materials at the posterior maxillary edentulous ridge. Perforation of the Schneiderian membrane, opening of the incision line, sinusitis, formation of cysts, misplacement of graft particles and mucosal dehiscence are complications with regard to sinus lift procedures. Perforation of sinus membrane can either be pre existing or be caused by tearing during the operation and its prevalence has been reported ranging from 10% to 34%. Sinus perforation can be managed using an absorbable membrane. Pathologic conditions affiliated with paranasal sinuses are very prevalent. More than 31 million people around the world suffer from sinusitis each year. The infection of sinus may potentially cause critical complications such as sinusitis, orbital cellulitis, meningitis, cavernous sinus thrombosis and osteomyelitis. The incidence of acute sinusitis is reported to be around 3%. Moreover sinusitis may result in more complicated situations. Loss of bone graft particles and sequestrae is not prevalent but possible. Failure of Branemark implants at the grafted sites after a mean period of 32 months was 6.7%. A comprehensive pre operative assessment is important to detect any existing pathologic condition in maxillary sinus. This surely can reduce the risk of mucus and bacterial infection in the surgical field and compromising bone healing. Moreover due to vicinity of the maxillary sinus to vital structures such as brain, cavernous sinus, etc, post-operative complications can be critical and life threatening.

4. Etiologies related with bone grafting complications

4.1. Technique associated

Precautions have to be taken while harvesting bone from the ramus when the inferior cut is below the inferior alveolar canal. Elevation of the bone graft should be avoided unless assured that the nerve is not attached to the inside surface of the bone graft. As the thickest area of the ramus is 12.23 mm and the thinnest area is 2.35mm, the thickness of bone graft will not be homogenous. About 60% of the inferor alveolar canals were reported to be notched to the inner surface of the mandibular cortical plate or the third molar root surface. Thus it is recommended that whie performing the osteotomy, after 2 mm of penetration great care be taken with the surgical bur short before reaching cancellous bone to avoid damaging the inferior alveolar nerve. The mean thickness of the lateral cortical wall of the maxillary sinus has been reported to be 0.91±0.43 mm. Cautious removal of the bone with surgical bur while performing the sinus lift procedure is crucial in preservation of sinus membrane integrity. A recently developed piezoelectric ultrasonic surgical device(piezotome, Acteon, Bordeaux, France) presents an alternative way to safely remove hard tissue keeping the soft tissue intact,is an effective tool for sinus lift procedures as well as harvesting autogenous bone from the ramus. Attaching an onlay bone graft to the host site can affect revascularization of a graft. A loose graft may develop nonunion and become compressed and encapsulated. To ensure close adaptation, the fixation screws should be tightened. Contamination is usually an outcome of poor infection control during the surgery. Rinsing with chlorhexidine before surgery is recommended before the surgery on order to reduce the risk of infection. A study showed that infections were more prevalent when using nonresorbable membranes for GBR comparing with the use of bioabsorbable membranes over a bovine bone xenograft. A suitable membrane and proper membrane removal timing may be effective in reduction of the risk of infection. To prevent exposure of membrane or fixation microscrews, tension free flap is mandatory.

4.2. Anatomy related

Ramus

Complications with regard to harvesting bone from the ramus may include damage to the nerve, opening of the incision line, fracture of the mandible and trismus. The prevalence of nerve damage caused by harvesting autogenous bone from the ramus is far less comparing to that of the mandibular symphysis. Buccal nerve damage followed by incision along the external oblique ridge is expectable. Nevertheless rarely are any reports present with regard to the incidence of buccal mucosa sensory loss and patients do not often pay attention to the change. On the contrary in this procedure, the potential of injuring the inferior alveolar nerve is of great consideration. A great understanding of the local normal anatomy is required to prevent such complications. Trismus may also be experienced by the patient underwent bone harvesting from the ramus area because of the masseter muscle retraction. But the symptom is not permanent. Furthermore, other complications related to ramus harvesting procedure may consist of third molar involvement and mandibular fracture ; though not reported.

Mandibular symphysis

Associated with mandibular symphysis/chin graft, complications such as insufficient bone regeneration, altered sensation, nerve damage, pulp necrosis, vascular damage, opening of the incision line and bone fracture may occur. Incomplete bone regeneration was found more prevalent in old patients. Nevertheless, it was reported that the change in profile was not obvious. Change in sensation of mandibular anterior incisors after loss of support of the mentalis muscle was reported. The manifestation of dullness usually resolved within 6 months. A high incidence of anterior mandibular incisors pulp necrosis was reported. Negative pulpal reaction and canal obliteration may be caused by damage to pulp vasculature. There have been reports on prevalence of nonvital teeth after genioplasty or subapical osteotomy. An effective preventive way is to keep about 4 to 5 mm clearance from the root apices and avoidance of harvesting bone close to them. Patients should also be informed about possible disturbances that may occur in the function of the inferior alveolar nerve which may last longer than 12 months. Damage to incisal branch of the inferior alveolar nerve is expectable if the graft is harvested too deep into the cancellous bone. Similarly mental nerve damage may occur if the graft is harvested too distally. Fracture and posterior displacement of the lingual cortical plate of the anterior mandible was reported as a specific complication which occurred during the healing phase but not at the time of surgery. On the whole, careful measurement and assessment before the surgery are required to avoid facing most of the complications.

Maxillary tuberosity

Precaution has to be taken with regard to the adjacent anatomical elements such as the maxillary sinus, pterygoid plates, proximal teeth and the greater palatine canal when using the maxillary tuberosity as harvesting site. Although rare, oral-antral communication may occur when harvesting bone which can be closed using the buccal fat flap as coverage, antibiotics and decongestants. Bleeding and tethering of the lateral and medial pterygoid muscles has been reported to be a potential complication when the tuberosity was fractured.

4.3. Patient related

Systemic issues affecting bone grafting include smoking, diabetes, alcoholism, radiation, osteoporosis and medication.

4.3.1. Bisphosphonates

An inorganic analog of pyrophosphate, Bisphosphonate has recently been used to treat osteoporosis or bone metastatic malignancies by reduction of osteoclastic differentiation and induction of osteoclastic apoptosis. Bisphosphonate lets remodeling spaces be filled with new bone by its anti-osteoclastic effect and as a result, abates the prevalence of fractures and also increases the bone strength. Nevertheless, it was also found that not only does the bisphosphonate suppress bone turnover but also interacts with micro-damage repair mechanism of bone. The accumulation of the micro-damage reduces the strength of the bone resistance against traumas. Furthermore, another drawback of the bisphophonate is that it decreases vascularity in regenerative connective tissue. It was found that IV use of bisphosphonate in metastatic malignancies may contribute to osteonecrosis of the jaw. However the relationship between osteonecrosis and use of bisphosphonate has not yet been recognized. Bisphosphonate related osteonecrosis appears to be multifactorial. The susceptibility of osteonecrosis in patients underwent IV bisphosphonate therapy for cancer was four times more than others. For patients who receive IV bisphosphonate, aggressive dental procedures should be avoided due to risk of jaw osteonecrosis. With insufficient research documents, guided regeneration and bone grafts should be applied with great caution (see Dental management of patients receiving oral bisphosphonate therapy, expert panel recommendations, report of the council on scientific affairs, ADA, June 2006)as reduced integrity of the bone and decreased vascularity may have negative drawbacks on grafted site. The incidence of osteonecrosis caused by oral administration of bisphosphonate is considered to be very low among the most common alendronates prescribed. Thus, patients underwent IV bisphophonate therapy are contraindicated for advanced surgical operations. This includes but not limited to implant placement, dental extraction and periodontal procedures. Latterly, suggested that dentist should discuss the risks, benefits and alternative treatments with the patients underwent bisphosphonate therapy before any surgical procedures. Before starting the treatment, the discussion and the patient informed approval should be documented.

4.3.2. *Smoking*

Almost 75% of the patients referred to periodontists were either current tobacco users or claimed previous use of tobacco. It was reported that smoking has negative effects on revascularization of the bone regenerative treatments such as bone grafting, majorly because of its vasoconstriction effect on arteries. Retardation of graft integration is caused as a consequent of decreased blood supply. The rate of infection caused by smoking-induced change in oral flora is 2 to 3 times more in smokers contributing to negative effects on complications of periodontal procedures, including bone grafting. Levin and Schwartz-Arad reported that nicotine, carbon monoxide and hydrogen cynide from smoking are possible risk factors that result in weakened wound healing. This consequently threatens the success of bone grafting and implant surgeries. Notwithstanding the cigarettes smoked, a patient with a smoking history, presented higher rate of failure of implants placed in grafted maxillary sinus. Smoking has negative influences on onlay grafts. While nonsmokers presented only 23.1% rate of complications in monocortical onlay grafts,smokers had a 50% rate. Nevertheless no relations were found in this article between sinus lift procedure complications and smoking tendency. Surprisingly failure rate in maxillary bone was 1.6 times more than that of mandible undergoing the same periodontal procedure showing that the maxilla was more prone to negative reactions of tobacco. Furthermore bone grafting procedures are negatively affected by use of tobacco with bone loss of 4 times as much as in nonsmokers. Such bone loss was majorly a consequent of estrogens suppression caused by over expression of interleukin-1, interleukin-6 and tumor necrotising factor(TNF)-α. Quitting smoking has been shown to decrease the progression of periodontal diseases and contribute the healing process of the bone graft.

4.3.3. *Diabetes*

Diabetes is able to enhance expression of TNF-α which has been blamed to be responsible for apoptosis of osteoblasts and their precursors. This enhanced apoptosis is considered to be influential to the bone healing process. cellular malfunctions such as prolonged infiltration of inflammatory cells, decreased production of growth factors and cell synthesis and increased proteolytic activities are all assumed to be blamed for delayed healing and failure of bone grafts. Osteopenia and delayed bone healing are both characteristics of diabetic bone disease. Moreover, recurrent nonenzymatic protein glycation contributes to formation of advanced glycation end product(AGE) that can be accumulated in different tissues such as bone. Further alveolar bone loss can occur followed by accumulation of AGE.

4.3.4. Radiation

Osteopenia may be experienced, after one yearin mature patients underwent head and neck radiotherapy. Osteoblasts activities may be diminished by radiation and results in decrease of bone matrix. Moreover, following long-term vascular damage caused by radiotherapy, osteonecrosis might happen. Due to poor blood supply and superficial location of mandible, most cases of head and neck radionecrosis were found in that area. Weakened areas of the bone are more susceptible to fracture. However, Despite the drawbacks mentioned above, one study reported that bone grafting in radiated bone tissues showed a survival rate of 89%. Another study reported that the prevalence of post-radiotherapy operative complications was 42%, while bone grafting procedures in nonirradiated sites had a 28% complication rate.

4.3.5. Alcoholism

The use of alcohol is shown to have adverse impact on intraoral bone grafting operations by increasing osteoclast activities and weakening oseoblast proliferation. An animal study reported that alcoholic beverages caused considerable delay in reparative process of alveolus. Another study demonstrated that use of ethanol led to suppression of bone turnover and provoked bone resorption. Other negative effects on bone grafting procedures attributed to the use of alcohol may be ascribed to possible direct toxic effect of ethanol in periodontal structures and other elements in oropharynx. Even a higher rate of complication in surgical procedures of the mandible was presented by patients consuming large amounts of alcohol when combined with other predisposing factors such as poor nutrition. Thus, it has been suggested that quitting ethanol consumption should be applied a few weeks before aggressive dental operations to minimize complications.

5. Complications of autogenous bone grafting

The use of autogenous bone graft with dental implants was originally discussed by Branemark.

5.1. Maxillary tuberosity bone graft

The major complication with maxillary tuberosity graft harvesting is oroantral communication. Grafts may be harvested with a chisel or rongeurs. The chisel edge should be kept slightly superficial to the maxilla to shave off pieces of tuberosity bone and prevent inadvertent sinus communication.

5.2. Mandibular symphysis bone graft

A CT scan or panoramic radiograph is used to evaluate the available bone at this donor site. Lateral cephalometric radiograph can be useful to determine the anteroposterior dimension of the anterior mandible. A vestibular incision is made in the mucosa between the cuspid teeth. Limiting the distal extent of the incision will reduce the risk of mental nerve injury. The mandibular symphysis is associated with a higher incidence of postoperative complications. Incidence of temporary mental nerve paresthesia for symphysis graft patients is usually low. Ptosis of the chin has not occurred and can be prevented by avoiding complete degloving of the mandible.

5.3. Mandibular ramus

The limits of the ramus area are dictated by clinical access. After graft preparation, the donor site is not augmented with bone substitutes because the inferior alveolar nerve may be exposed and irritated by the graft particles. The potential for damage to the IAN, as opposed to its peripheral mental branches is of greater concern with the ramus graft technique. Patients may experience trismus following surgery and should be placed on postoperative glucocorticoids and NSAIDs medications to help reduce dysfunction.

5.4. Tibia

There has been a low reported incidence of significant complications with this procedure. Complications may include hematoma formation, wound dehiscence, infection and fracture. The patient should avoid strenuous exercise for 4 to 6 weeks. Although quite rare most cases of tibia fracture are due to a bony access too low on the leg.

5.5. Ilium

The grafting of larger areas of bone deficiency often requires bone harvesting from the ilium. The crestal incision is made about 2cm below the anterior superior iliac spine and extending caudally 4 to 5 cm. Care is taken not to cut through the external oblique or gluteal muscles during this incision because this increases postoperative discomfort and slows ambulation. All bleeding from the marrow is controlled with small amounts of bone wax or collagen hemostatic. The patient is advised to avoid any lifting or twisting for the next 6 weeks to preclude hip fracture. The use of a pain pump with long acting local anesthetics has dramatically reduced the level of postoperative pain from the hip area.

5.6. Rib graft

The preferred donor ribs are the fourth and fifth ribs. The fifth rib is superior to the fourth in growing female patients. A major complication in rib harvesting is pleural perforation. In this case a chest tube catheter is inserted in to the area of pleural compromise to a length of approximately 1 to 2 cm; with the red rubber catheter in position, a purse string suture is placed to fix the tube which should be attached to a chest tube bottle. For small perforations the anesthesiologist provides positive pressure and maintains this position while a surgical knot is tightened. All patients having costochondral or rib harvests require a postoperative chest radiograph performed and clinical inspection for pneumothorax. If a pneumothorax is noted a chest tube may be placed.

5.7. Cranial bone

Cranial bone just superior and posterior to the temporal crest is generally quite thick and accidental full thickness harvest and or dural perforation is minimized. An incision is made beginning 1cm inferior to superior temporal line to avoid main arterial trunks of the superficial temporal and posterior auricular arteries thus reducing bleeding; the parietal bone, which is flat and also quite thick as compared with other areas of the cranium.

5.8. Grafting recipient sites

The bone graft should have intimate contact with underlying host bone. Following harvest, the bone graft may be stored in sterile saline. The graft is mortised into position and fixated to the ridge with screws. Complete flap coverage and tension free closure is essential to the successful incorporation of the bone graft. After the periosteal releasing incision is made, the flap is gently stretched to assess closure without tension. Although it is important that the flap margins are well approximated, the sutures should not be pulled too tightly or ischemia will occur. It is imperative that the graft is immobilized during healing postoperatively. The patient should continue antibiotic therapy for at least 1 week. Smoking has been associated with a high rate of wound dehiscence and graft failure. Cholorhexidine rinsing is used for oral hygiene until the sutures are removed.

6. Complications of inferior alveolar nerve repositioning

Nerve mobilization procedures are precise methods that require clinical experience, knowledge of anatomy, and the ability to intervene in the event of potential accidents and/or complications. [1] In the last few years, IAN repositioning has been used widely as an alternative to short implants or bone grafts for osseointegrated implant placement in the posterior mandible of patients who do not have sufficient bone height for conventional treatment. Among the advantages of IAN repositioning is the option to use standard implants with bicortical anchorage, increasing primary stability, which is essential in the osseointegration process. Osseointegrated implants placed in combination with IAN repositioning present a lower risk of bone loss than short implants when both are placed in similar circumstances. [2] For clinical situations with less than the minimum height for short implants (5 mm), IAN repositioning is the technique indicated. [3] This procedure also increases the resistance to occlusal forces and promotes a good proportion between implant and prosthesis. [4] Compared to the option of performing a graft to allow placement of standard implants, in addition to the lower cost, IAN repositioning can be performed under local anesthetic, does not require a donor site, and has a lower morbidity rate. [5, 6]

IAN repositioning also presents many disadvantages. The technique does not recover the alveolar ridge anatomy and temporarily weakens the mandible. Mandibular fractures associated with endosseous implants have been documented and are generally related to high levels of resorption in edentulous mandibles. Also, nerve mobilization leads to many factors that can increase the occurrence of fractures. [7, 9] A large portion of the buccal cortex is removed, reducing the structural integrity of a region that is under constant stress during chewing. [8] In addition to that, sites that have been prepared and subsequently abandoned due to bad angulation or insufficient initial stability are areas of bone fragility susceptible to fracture. [7] Poor nutrition as a consequence of blood perfusion changes associated with this nerve mobilization can also be a cause of fracture. [10] Another disadvantage of IAN repositioning is the risk of nerve damage. The duration and degree of neurosensory disturbance has been related directly to the amount of compression and tension applied to the nerve during the procedure, [11] or to chronic distension/compression of the nerve after the surgery. [12] Hypoesthesia, paresthesia, and hyperesthesia are the most common complications. [13]

The success rate of the lateralization procedure, regarding the osseointegration process, varies from 93.8% to 100%, and thus both patients and surgeons believe this to be a safe procedure; however, a small percentage of patients will have nerve damage for the rest of their lives. [14] Concerning the use of materials as barriers between the implant and nerve, there is controversy in the literature, because while some authors consider the use of resorbable membranes to be helpful, [4] others have observed faster healing of the bone wound without barriers, followed by the restoration of the mandibular canal. [15] One advancement is the utilization of piezoelectric devices, which allow the surgeon to perform the osteotomy without damaging soft tissue, because piezoelectric devices only affect mineralized tissues. In vitro tests have shown a lower risk of injury when piezoelectric devices are used compared to conventional rotary devices. [16]

7. Complications of sinus lifting

A variety of complications can happen during and after sinus lifting. As all the other surgical techniques, this procedure is prone to all common complications of oral surgery but in this chapter we will focus on complications of this procedure.

7.1. Membrane perforations

The most common complication during sinus graft surgery is tearing of the sinus membrane. Causes of this condition include: Pre-existing perforations, tearing during scoring of the lateral wall window, existing or previous pathologic condition, and elevating of the membrane from the bony walls. This complications occurs about 10% to 34% of thc time. The perforation of the sinus membrane should be sealed to prevent contamination of the graft from the mucus and the contents of the sinus and to prevent the graft materials from extruding into the sinus proper. The surgical correction of a perforation is initiated by elevating the sinus mucosal regions distal from the opening. Once the tissues are elevated away from the opening, the membrane elevation with a sinus curette should approach the tear from all sides so that the torn region may be elevated without increasing the opening size. The antral membrane elevation technique decreases the overall size of the antrum, thus folding the membrane over itself and resulting in closure of the perforation.

If the sinus membrane tear is larger than 6 mm and cannot be closed off with the circumelevation approach, then a resorbable collagen membrane, but of a longer resorption cycle, may be used to seal the opening. The remaining sinus mucosa is first elevated as described previously. A piece of collagen matrix is to cut to cover sinus tear opening and overlap the margins more than 5 millimeters. Because no antibiotic is used on the collagen to make this procedure easier to perform, additional antibiotic is added to the graft material. Once the opening is sealed, the sinus graft procedure maybe completed in the routine fashion. A sinus perforation may cause an increased risk of short-term complications. A torn membrane may increase the risk of bacterial penetration into the graft material. Furthermore, mucus may violate the graft influencing the amount of bone formation. Drip of the graft material into the sinus proper may occur as a result of torn membrane, travel to and through the ostium and either be abolished through the nose or block the ostium and prevent normal sinus drainage. Ostium obstruction is also possible from swelling of the membrane related to the surgery. These conditions increase the risk of infection. However, despite these potential complications, the risk of infection is low (less than 5%)

7.2. Antral septa

Antral septa are the most common osseous anatomical variant seen in the maxillary sinus. Sinus septa may create added difficulty at the time of surgery. Maxillary septa can prevent adequate access and visualization to the sinus floor; therefore inadequate or incomplete sinus grafting is possible. These dense projections complicate the surgery in several ways. After scoring the lateral-access window in the usual fashion, the lateral-access window may not fracture and rotate into its medial position. The strut reinforcement is also more likely to tear the membrane during the releasing of the access window.

7.3. Management of septa based on location

The septa maybe in the anterior, middle, or distal partof the antrum. When the septum is found in the anterior section, the lateral access window is divided into sections: one in front of the septa and another distal to the structure. This permits the release of each section of the lateral wall after tapping with a blunt instrument. The elevation of each released section permits investigation into the exact location of the septa and to continue the mucosal elevation.

When the strut is located in the middle region of the sinus, it is more difficult to make two separate access windows within the direct vision of the surgeon. As a result, one access window is made in front of the septa. The sinus curette then proceeds up the anterior aspect of the web, towards its apex. The curette then slides toward the lateral wall and above the septum apex. The curette may slide over the crest of septum approximately 1 to 2 mm. A firm pulling action fractures the apex of the septum. Once the septum is separated off the floor, the curette may proceed more distal along the floor and walls.

When the septum is in the posterior compartment of the sinus, it is often distal to the last implant site. When this occurs, the posterior septum is treated through the posterior wall of the sinus.

8. Short-term postoperative complications

8.1. Incision line opening

Incision line opening is uncommon for this procedure because the crestal incision is in attached gingiva and at least 5 mm away from the lateral access window. Incision line opening occurs more commonly when lateral augmentation is performed at the same time as sinus graft surgery, or when implants are placed over above the residual crest and covered with the soft tissue. It may also occur when a soft tissue-supported prosthesis compresses the surgical area during function before suture removal. The consequences of the incision line opening are delayed healing, leaking of the graft material into the oral cavity, and increased risk of infection. However, if the incision line failure is not related to the lateral onlay graft and is only on the crest of the ridge and away from the sinus access window, then the posterior crestal area is allowed to heal by secondary intention. If incision line opening includes a portion of nonresorbable membrane, then the membrane should be cleaned at least twice daily with oral rinses of chlorhexidine. If the incision line does not close after two months, then a surgical procedure should reenter the site, expand the tissues, remove the bone regeneration membrane, and reapproximate the tissue.

8.2. Nerve impairment

In severely atrophic maxillas, the infra orbital neurovascular structures exiting the foramen may be close to the intraoral residual ridge and should be avoided when performing sinus graft procedures to minimize possible nerve impairment.

8.3. Acute maxillary sinus rhinosinusitis

Acute postoperative sinusitis occurs as a complication in approximately 3% to 20% of sinus graft procedures, and it represents the most common short term complication. Most often the infection begins more than 1 week after surgery.

Radiographic evaluation of acute rhinosinustis is both expensive and often inaccurate. As such, a patient history for acute sinusitis is a benefit and is diagnostic when two or more of the following factors are present: (1)facial congestion or fullness, (2)nasal obstruction or blockage, (3)nasal discharge, (4)purulence or discolored postnasal discharge, (5)facial pain or pressure, (6)hyposomia or anosomia, (7)purulence in the nares on physical examination, (8)fever, (9)headache, (10)halitosis, (11)dental pain, (12)cough, (13)ear pain.

Previous studies and treatment modalities used amoxicillin as the first drug of choice. However, with the increasing prevalence of penicillinase and beta-lactamase producing strains of haemaphilus influenza and moraxells catarrhalis, along with penicillin-resistant strains of streptococcus pneumonia, other alternative antibiotic drugs should be selected. If symptoms are not alleviated with antibiotic and decongestant medications, then possible referral to the patient's physician or otolaryngologist is warranted.

8.4. Overfilling the sinus

The maximum length requirement of an implant with adequate surface of design is rarely more than 15 mm, and as a result, the goal of the initial sinus graft is to obtain at least 16mm of vertical bone from the crest of ridge. Overfilling the sinus can result in blockage of the ostium, especially if membrane inflammation or the presence of a thickened sinus mucosa exists. The majority of sinus graft overfills do not have postoperative complications. If, however, a postoperative sinus infection occurs without initial resolution, re-entry and removal of a portion of the graft and changing the antibiotic protocol may be appropriate. [17, 18]

Author details

Mehdi Sezavar*, Vahid Mesgarzadeh, Shahrouz Shafayifard and M. Reza Soleimanpour

*Address all correspondence to: m_s7605@yahoo.com

Department of Oral and Maxillofacial Surgery,Islamic Azad University,Dental branch, Tehran, Iran

References

[1] Babbush CA. Transpositioning and repositioning the inferior alveolar and mental nerves in conjunction with endosteal implant reconstruction. Periodontology 1998;17: 183–90.

[2] Vasco MA, Hecke MB, Bezzon OL. Analysis of short implants and lateralization of the inferior alveolar nerve with 2-stage dental implants by finite element method. J CraniofacSurg 2011;22:2064–71.

[3] Fernandez Dıaz J.O., Naval Gıas L. Rehabilitation of edentulous posterior atrophic mandible: inferior alveolar nerve lateralization by piezotome and immediate implant placement. Int J Oral MaxillofacSurg 2013;42:521–6.

[4] Sethi A. Inferior alveolar nerve repositioning in implant dentistry: a preliminary report. Int J Periodontics Restorative Dent 1995;15: 474–81.

[5] Rosenquist B. Fixture placement posterior to the mental foramen with transpositioning of the inferior alveolar nerve. Int J Oral Maxillofac Implants 1992;7:45–50.

[6] Dario LJ, English Jr R. Achieving implant reconstruction through bilateral mandibular nerve repositioning. J Am Dent Assoc 1994;125:305–9.

[7] Luna AH, Passeri LA, de Moraes M, Moreira RW. Endosseous implant placement in conjunction with inferior alveolar nerve trans-position: a report of an unusual complication and surgical management. Int J Oral Max-illofac Implants 2008;23:133–6.

[8] Karlis V, Bae RD, Glickman RS. Mandibular fracture as a complication of inferior alveolar nerve transposition and placement of endosseous implants: a case report. Implant Dent 2003;12:211–6.

[9] Kan JY, Lozada JL, Boyne PJ, Goodacre CJ, Rungcharassaeng K. Mandibular fracture after endosseous implant placement in con-junction with inferior alveolar nerve transposition: a patient treatment report. Int J Oral Maxillofac Implants 1997;12: 655–9.

[10] Bradley JC. The clinical significance of age changes in the vascular supply to the mandible. Int J Oral Surg 1981;10(Suppl. 1):71–6..

[11] Robinson PP. Observations on the recovery of sensation following inferior alveolar nerve injuries. Br J Oral MaxillofacSurg 1988;26:177–89.

[12] Nocini PF, De Santis D, Fracasso E, Zanette G. Clinical and electrophysiological assessment of inferior alveolar nerve function after lateral nerve transposition. Clin Oral Implants Res 1999;10:120–30.

[13] Sandstedt P, Sorensen S. Neurosensory disturbances of the trigeminal nerve: a long-term follow-up of traumatic injuries. J Oral MaxillofacSurg 1995;53:498–505.

[14] Hirsch JM, Bra°nemark PI. Fixture stability and nerve function after transposition and lateralization of the inferior alveolar nerve and fixture installation. Br J Oral MaxillofacSurg 1995;33:276–81.

[15] Yoshimoto M, Watanabe IS, Martins MT, Salles MB, Ten Eyck GR, Coelho PG. Microstructural and ultrastructural assessment of inferior alveolar nerve damage following nerve lateralization and implant placement: an experimental study in rabbits. Int J Oral Maxillofac Implants 2009; 24:859–65.

[16] Metzger MC, Bormann KH, Schoen R, Gell-rich NC, Schmelzeisen R. Inferior alveolar nerve transposition—an in vitro comparison between piezosurgery and conventional bur use. J Oral Implantol 2006;32:19–25

[17] Misch CE: Contemporary implant dentistry, 2008,third edition

[18] Lindhe J: Clinical periodontology and implant dentistry,2008, fifth edition

[19] Fonseca Raymond.J; Oral and Maxillofacial Surgery; 2009; Vol 1 Second Ed

[20] Epker Bruce; Dentofacial Deformities: Integrated Orthodontic and surgical correction; Volume III

Section 11

Basic and VSP- CAD/CAM Craniomaxillofacial Reconstruction

Chapter 26

Reconstruction of Facial Hair Bearing Areas in the Male Patient

Shahram Nazerani

Additional information is available at the end of the chapter

http://dx.doi.org/10.5772/59191

1. Introduction

Hair bearing regions of the face have been the hallmarks of Manhood through the ages and the defects of these regions are psychologically traumatizing and sometimes demeaning for the male patients in several cultures. The reconstruction of these areas is very difficult due to scarcity of donor areas and the available donors such as scalp have anatomically different hair morphology and the hair follicles' proximity is quite different from the face, on the other hand the facial skin thickness and texture is another matter of concern making a "look alike" reconstruction almost impossible. In this chapter we will try to address this difficult reconstruction challenge.

1.1. Terminology

In humans, usually only pubescent or adult males are able to grow beards. [1, 2]

The Beard or Barba is defined as:

1. The hair on a man's chins, cheeks, and throat.
2. A hairy or hair like growth such as that on or near the face of certain mammals.

Moustache or Mustache refers to:

1. The unshaved growth of hair above the upper lip and sometimes down the sides of the mouth, especially when grown and groomed.
2. Something similar to the grown and groomed hair above the human upper lip

1.2. Historical background [3]

Throughout the course of history, societal attitudes towards male beards have varied depending on factors such as prevailing cultural-religious traditions and the fashion trends. Some religions (such as Islam and Sikhism and Judaism) have always considered a full beard to be absolutely essential for all males able to grow one. [4]

1.2.1. Ancient Egypt [3]

The highest ranking Ancient Egyptians grew hair on their chins which was often dyed or hennaed (reddish brown) and sometimes plaited with interwoven gold thread. A metal false beard, or postiche, which was a sign of sovereignty, was worn by queens and kings. This was held in place by a ribbon tied over the head and attached to a gold chin strap, a fashion existing from about 3000 to 1580 BC. [5] Mesopotamian civilizations (Sumerian, Assyrians, Babylonians, Chaldeans and Medians) devoted great care to oiling and dressing their beards, using tongs and curling irons to create elaborate ringlets and tiered patterns.

1.2.2. Ancient Iran [3]

The Iranians (Persians) were fond of long beards (Figure 1), and almost all the Iranian kings had a beard. In Travels by Adam Olearius, a King of Iran commands his steward's head to be cut off, and on its being brought to him, remarks, "what a pity it was, that a man possessing such fine mustachios, should have been executed." Men in the Achaemenid era wore long beards, with warriors adorning theirs with jewelry. Men also commonly wore beards during the Safavid and Qajar eras. [6]

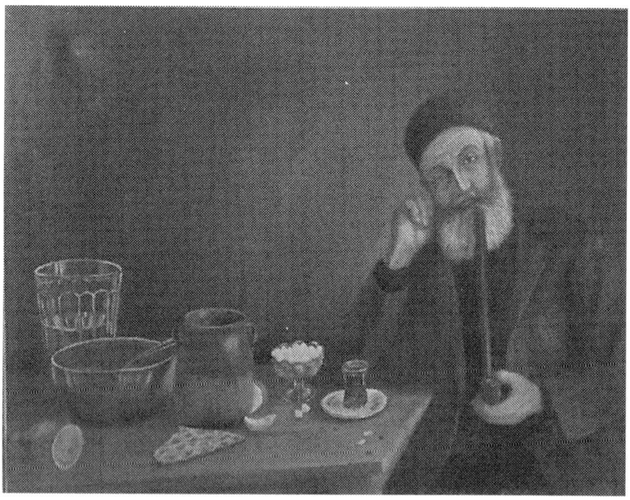

Figure 1. A 19th century painting of an Old Persian man after lunch, note the full beard.

http://dx.doi.org/10.5772/59191

1.2.3. Ancient Macedonia [3]

At the time of Alexander the Great the custom of smooth shaving was introduced. [7, 8] Reportedly, Alexander ordered his soldiers to be clean-shaven, fearing that their beards would serve as handles for their enemies to grab and to hold the soldier as he was killed. The practice of shaving spread from the Macedonians, whose kings are represented on coins, etc. with smooth faces, throughout the whole known world of the Macedonian Empire (Figure 2).

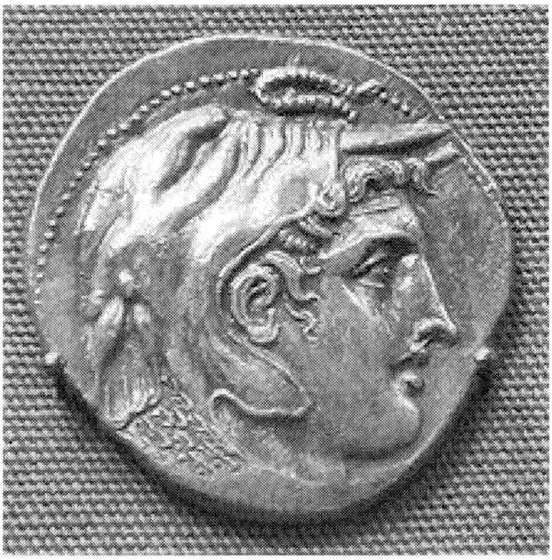

Figure 2. A coin depicting a cleanly shaven Alexander the Great.

Laws were passed against it, without effect, at Rhodes and Byzantium; and even Aristotle conformed to the new custom, unlike the other philosophers, who retained the beard as a badge of their profession. A man with a beard after the Macedonian period implied a philosopher, and there are many allusions to this custom of the later philosophers in such proverbs as: "The beard does not make the sage." [9]

1.2.4. Ancient Rome 3

Shaving seems to have not been known to the Romans during their early history (under the Kings of Rome and the early Republic). Pliny tells us that Ticinius was the first who brought a barber to Rome, which was in the 454th year from the founding of the city (that is, around 299 BC). Scipio Africanus was apparently the first among the Romans who shaved his beard. However, after that point, shaving seems to have caught on very quickly, and soon almost all Roman men were clean-shaven; being clean-shaven became a sign of being Roman and not Greek. Only in the later times of the Republic did the Roman youth begin shaving their beards only partially, trimming it into an ornamental form; prepubescent boys oiled their chins in hopes of forcing premature growth of a beard. [10]

1.2.5. The middle ages [3]

In the middle ages, the beard had still an important role, figure 3 depicts the picture of El Cid or " The Mister" in Arabic. (Figure 3). [11]

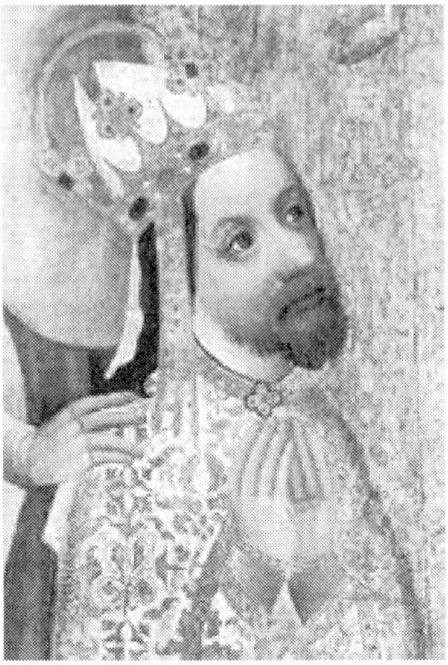

Figure 3. Charles IV, Holy Roman Emperor.

While most noblemen and knights were bearded, the Catholic clergy were generally required to be clean-shaven. This was understood as a symbol of their celibacy. By the early 20th century beards began a slow decline in popularity. Although retained by some prominent figures who were young men in the Victorian period (like Sigmund Freud), most men who retained facial hair during the 1920s and 1930s limited themselves to a moustache or a goatee (such as with Marcel Proust, Albert Einstein, Vladimir Lenin, Leon Trotsky, Adolf Hitler, and Joseph Stalin). In America, meanwhile, popular movies portrayed heroes with clean-shaven faces and "crew cuts". Concurrently, the psychological mass marketing of companies like Gillette popularize short hair and clean shaven faces as the only acceptable style for decades to come. Those who grow beards are frequently either old, Central Europeans, members of a religious sect that require it or those who are in academia.

1.3. Modern prohibition of beards [3]

Professional airline pilots are required to be clean shaven to facilitate a tight seal with auxiliary oxygen masks. Similarly, firefighters may also be prohibited from full beards to obtain a proper seal with equipment. This restriction is also fairly common in the oil and gas industry for the same reason in locations where hydrogen sulfide gas is a common danger. Other jobs may prohibit beards as necessary to wear masks or respirators. [12] Isezaki city in Gunma, Japan,

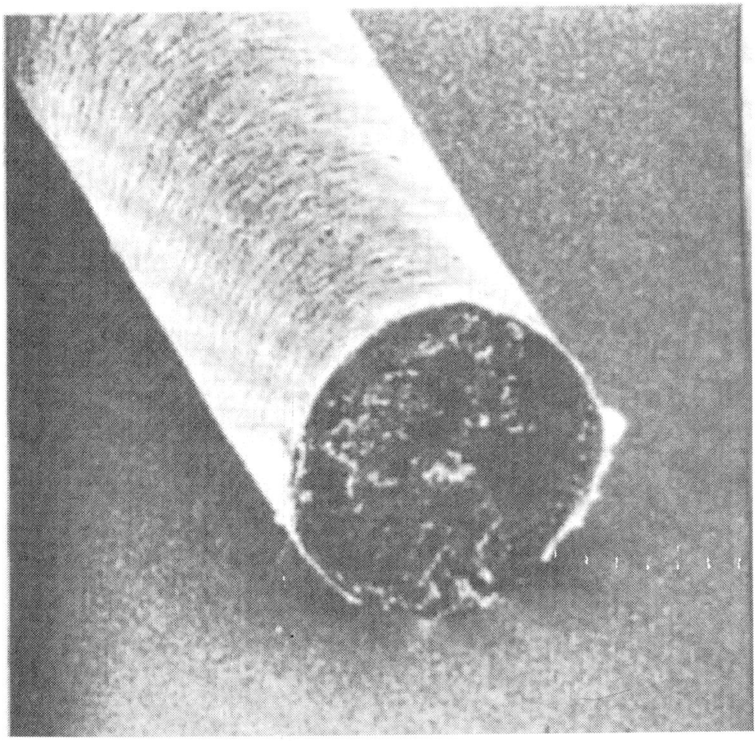

Figure 4. An Asian scalp hair, note the roundness of the hair, reprinted by permission of The Society of Cosmetic Chemists

decided to ban beards for male municipal employees on May 19, 2010. [13] Brigham Young University generally requires its students and employees to be clean-shaven. However, Brigham Young himself was often seen with a beard. [14]

2. Anatomy and physiology of facial hair

Human hair has been categorized into three ethnic groups according to distinguishable characteristics: Asian, Caucasian, and African hair. These ethnic groupings show distinct characteristics in hair density, diameter, shape, mechanical properties and composition. [15]

The hair follicle itself determines the appearance of the hair. The typical hair follicle of Asian hair is round (Figures 4 and 5), whereas those of Caucasians and Africans are ovoid and elliptical, respectively. [16]

The shape of the hair follicle is thus believed to contribute to the appearance and the geometry of the hair. Asian hair has a circular geometry, African hair has an elliptical shape, and hair of

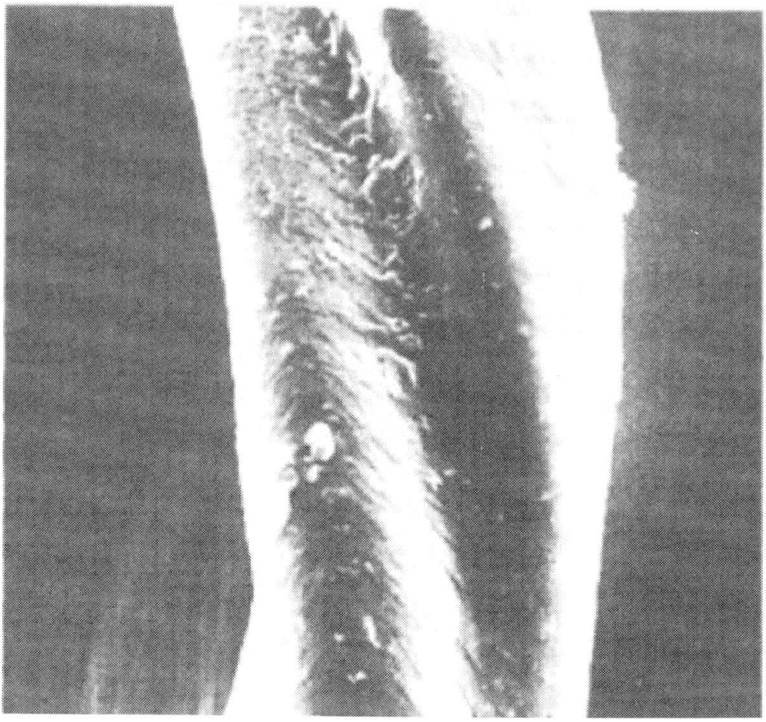

Figure 5. Asian beard hair, note the different contour of the beard hair from scalp hair, reprinted by permission of The Society of Cosmetic Chemists

Caucasians is of an intermediate shape. The chemical and protein composition of hair does not vary across ethnic groups, and there is no difference in the keratin types. However, African hair generally has less tensile strength and breaks more easily.

3. The units of the face

The face consists of 6 major aesthetic units comprised of: forehead, eye/eyebrow, nose, lips, chin, and cheek. These aesthetic units can be subdivided into additional anatomical subunits. For example, the nose can be divided into nasal tip, dorsum, columella, soft-tissue triangles, sidewalls, and nasal alar regions. Correct orientation of planned incisions next to these mobile functional and aesthetic facial structures is important to avoid distortion when closing wounds.

In this chapter we focus on the hair bearing units of the male face which are designated as the mustache and beard namely units 4c, d, 5a, b, 7 and some part of unit 9 in the neck (Figures 7 and 8).

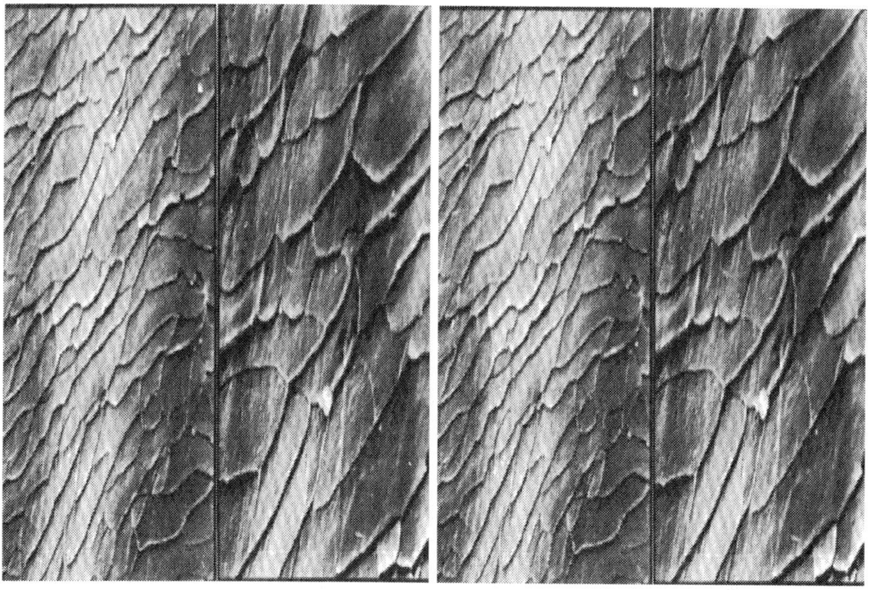

Figure 6. Comparison of the cuticular patterns of scalp and beard hair, reprinted by permission of The Society of Cosmetic Chemists

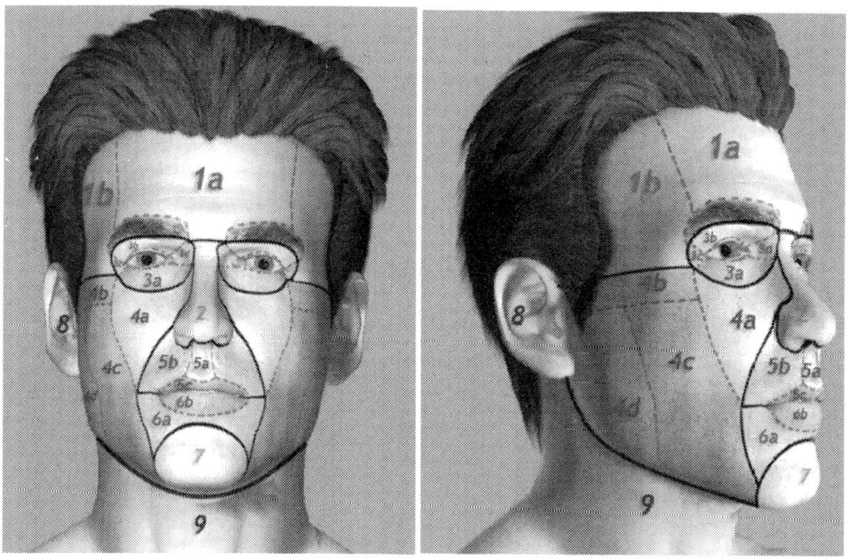

Figure 7. The human face units, used by permission of author Davide Brunelli M.D, www.med-ars.it

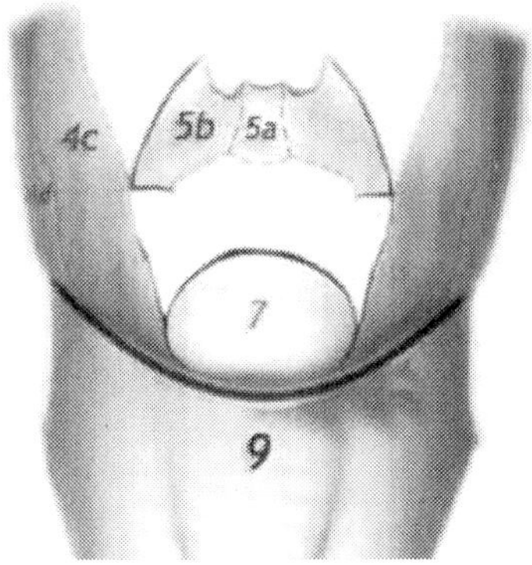

Figure 8. The hair bearing units in the male face, used by permission of author Davide Brunelli M.D, www.med-ars.it

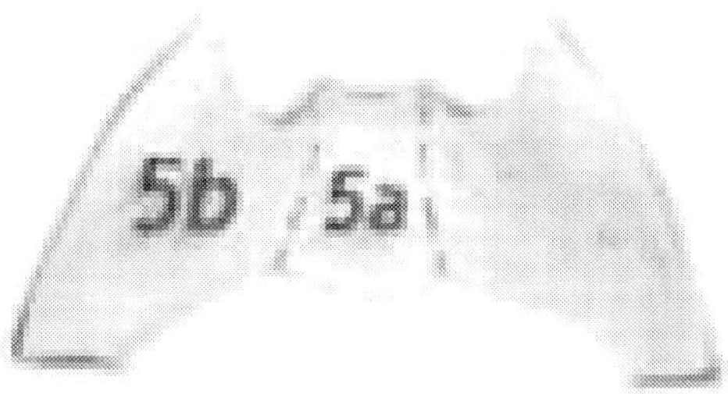

Figure 9. The mustache unit, used by permission of the author Davide Brunelli M.D, www.med-ars.it

3.1. The Mustache

Loss of the mustache in the male patient causes cosmetic and psychological problems. The mustache also has the ability to cover the perioral scars and defects and is favored by the patients with scars around the mouth and upper lip such as cleft lip patients (Figure 9).

Full thickness defects of the units 5a and b or upper lip area in addition to esthetically unappealing elicit the functional problems such as drooling, speech disorders and poor oral hygiene, the partial thickness defects are more of an esthetic nature with asymmetrical structure.

The two potential sources of hair-bearing skin are the bearded face, neck and the scalp. The texture, hair bearing quality, and color match make local beard skin on the face a preferable donor site, but this is possible only for relatively small defects; otherwise, the resulting scar at the donor site is unacceptable. In these cases, local advancement or V-Y advancement flaps are

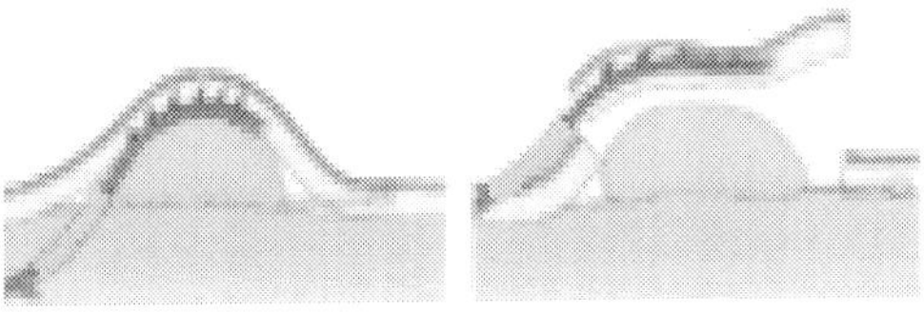

Figure 10. Flap prefabrication stages, vascular pedicle transferred under the skin paddle and the pedicle is wrapped by either Gore-Tex or silicone and a tissue expander is inserted for expansion, after proper expansion the flap is transferred as a free or island flap. The prelaminated flap can then be transferred to reconstruct the mustache or beard area. [23] Distant pedicled scalp flaps such as the extended midline forehead flap, transposition or island scalp flap, and bipedicle visor flap are other viable options.

used. Tissue expansion of this hair-bearing region to increase the surface area of the bearded face with Abbe and submental flaps have been described to bring hair-bearing tissue to the upper lip from the lower lip and bearded face and vice versa. [17] However, one must note the difference in hair distribution in the upper and lower lips when planning this flap.

The submental island flap reported by Martin et al is another source of hair bearing tissue with acceptable donor scar. [18]

The hair follicle match of the submental area is excellent and the follicle orientation is also correct, this flap can be transferred as a bipedicle type with limited arc of rotation and several other flap types reported by Tsur and Hyakusoku. [19]-[22]

The main drawback of submental flap is the need for several revision procedures, which have the potential risk of Alopecia due to too much thinning of the flap or damaging the vascular supply of the flap. [17, 22]

The flap prelamination is another option, in this technique a vascular pedicle is transposed under a random pattern flap and after maturation this composite tissue is transferred, it has some drawbacks such as the need for microvascular expertise and the potential risk of peripheral flap failure. (Figure 10)

3.2. Beard and Sideburns

The male bearded region can be subdivided into a preauricular zone, which includes the sideburn and the buccomandibular zone (Figure 11).

The sideburn is an important anatomical structure determining the boundary between the head and the face and providing an aesthetic reference for balanced facial symmetry. The normal sideburn dimensions have been well described by Giraldo. [24] The sideburn shape is largely rectangular or trapezoidal. According to Juri, the most frequent causes for absence of the sideburn are trauma, burns, surgery, and infection. [25] Small defects within or involving the sideburn can be reconstructed with a single V-Y flap, opposing V-Y flaps, extended V-Y flaps, or double extended V-Y flaps. V-Y flaps are designed within hair-bearing regions and non–hair-bearing regions according to the characteristics of the tissue to be replaced. Additional options for sideburn reconstruction include a scalp transposition flap. Larger defects

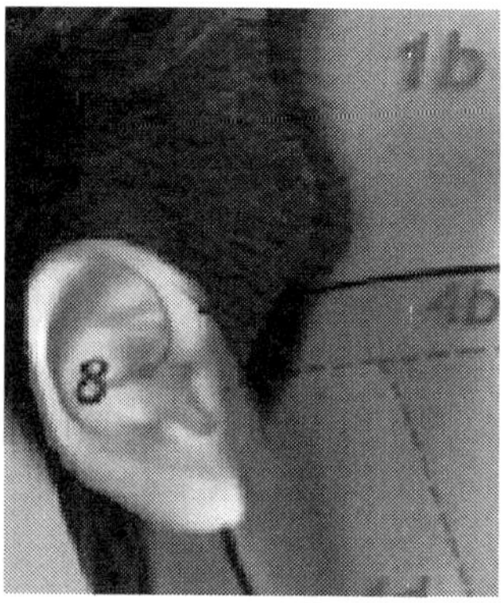

Figure 11. The side burn area, used by permission of author Davide Brunelli M.D, www.med-ars.it

including the sideburn and adjacent cheek or beard region can be reconstructed with a combination of any of these three primary options: the scalp transposition flap, the cervicofacial advancement flap, or the pedicled submental flap.

4. Cheek reconstruction

The cheek provides abundant subcutaneous tissue, which is mobile and has a perfect color match. Because of the laxity of the cheek, adjacent undermining and primary closure can be used to reconstruct many defects. Flaps can be designed within this tissue with minimal distortion to surrounding facial features and minimal dead space (Figure 12).

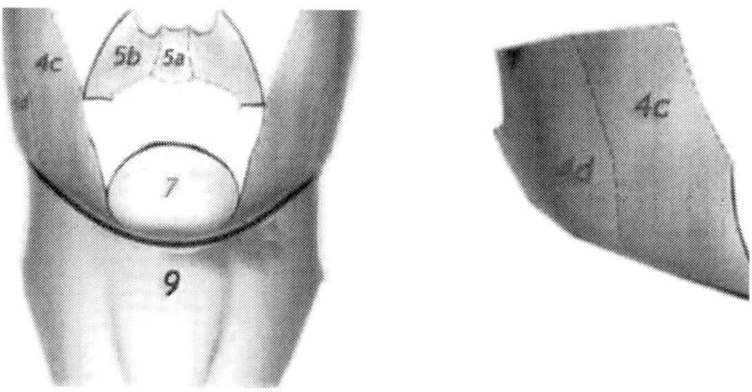

Figure 12. The cheek unit with subdivision of c and d, used by permission of author Davide Brunelli M.D, www.med-ars.it

In females the face has almost no hair so the reconstruction can begin at a younger age and more donor sites are available than the male patients. In the female neck skin can be expanded and be used to cover the chin and even cheek defects (Figure 13 - 15).

http://dx.doi.org/10.5772/59191

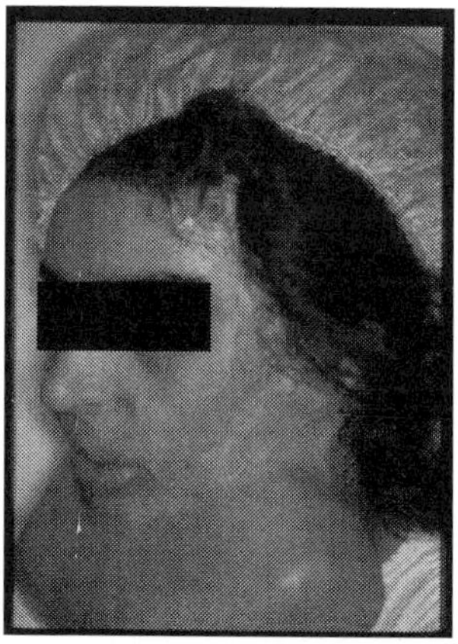

Figure 13. Bilateral cheek scars, expanded neck skin via tissue expander

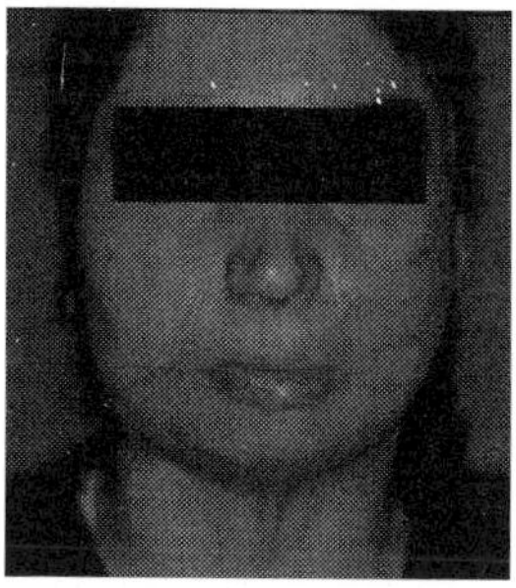

Figure 14. Frontal view of the scar after 5 years

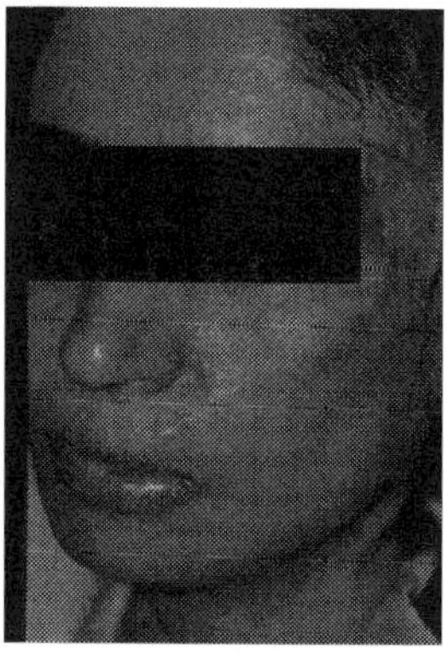

Figure 15. Result 8 years postoperatively

In the male child or adolescent, a facial skin defect reconstruction is completely different from females because transferring a hair bearing flap in a child is unsightly and the definite reconstruction of the facial hair bearing areas must be postponed until the patient has grown hair (Figures 16 and 17).

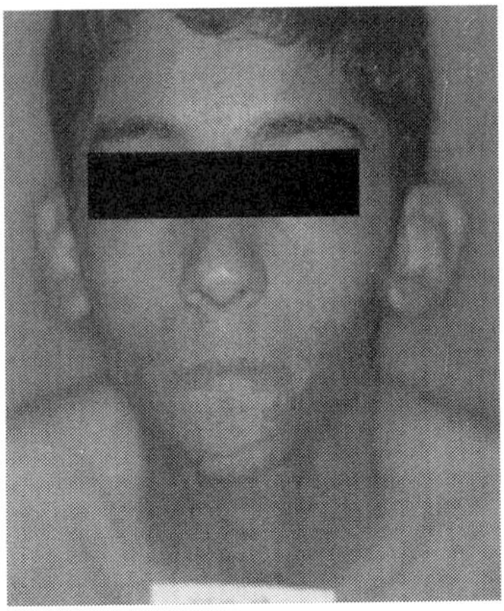

Figure 16. A 14-year-old male patient with a unit 4 scar

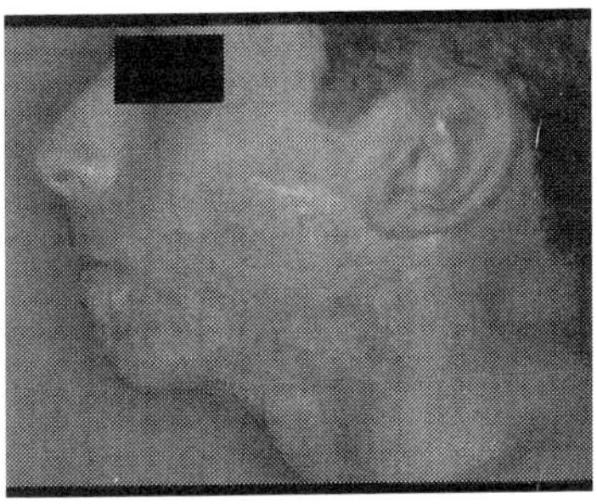

Figure 17. Lateral view of the same patient

5. Neck reconstruction

Zone 9 is the neck area contiguous with the chin and if the facial hair is present there is no need to reconstruct this area with hair bearing flaps, in these instances the patient can cover the neck scar with a beard.

6. Available donor sites

6.1. Submental island flap

6.1.1. Anatomy

The submental island flap is a fasciocutaneous flap that includes a rhomboid area of skin, subcutaneous tissue, and platysma located below the inferior border of the mandible (Figure 18). This flap was first reported by Martin et al. [26]

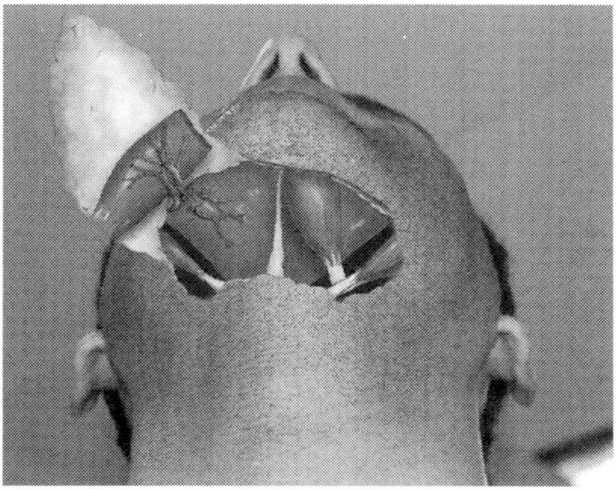

Figure 18. The submental flap raised on its vascular pedicle

Injection studies into the submental artery have found that it can supply a large skin paddle, as large as 10 _16 cm, reaching from one angle of the mandible to the contralateral angle. [27] Although this horizontal dimension includes an area supplied by bilateral submental arteries, the entire flap can be perfused by one side. Practically speaking, the anteroposterior dimension of the skin flap that can be harvested is limited by the ability to achieve primary closure, which depends on the patient's skin laxity and age, which can be estimated by marking out the desired anteroposterior dimension of the flap and attempting to pinch the marks together with forceps.

The locations of the perforator vessels connecting the submental artery to the subdermal plexus (which perfuses the areas listed above) are variable. This flap has a shorter pedicle compared to scalp flaps, is rather thick and arch of rotation or pivot point is short; in the young the donor site scar becomes hypertrophic and in view.

6.2. Expanded scalp

The expanded scalp has two benefits namely thinning the density of the hair follicles and also a thinner skin brought in to the defect. These flaps can be transferred as pedicle flaps or free flaps. [28, 29] The expanded flap can be covered by the scalp hair is not very noticeable until late in expansion (Figure 19).

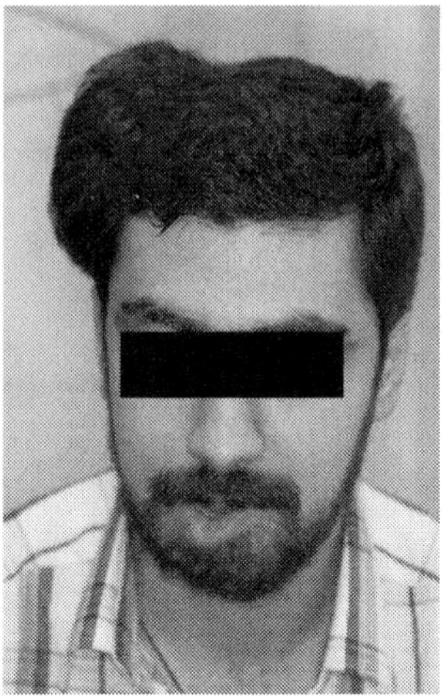

Figure 19. The expander is in place; the patients usually grow hair on the opposite side of the expansion area to compensate.

6.3. Visor flap

The frontal visor flap first described by Leon Dufourmental in 1919 has stood the test of time; and with tissue expansion to overcome the donor site morbidity it is the only solution in bilateral facial defects in the male patient. [30] The scalp visor flap has an excellent blood supply, guaranteed by its double pedicle with the two superficial temporal arteries.

6.4. Adjacent skin reconstruction, expanded and non-expanded

In small defects it is possible to expand the adjacent skin and reconstruct the defect by the "same skin".

6.5. Hair transplantation

Another option for reconstruction of facial hair is Hair Transplantation; there are different techniques of hair transplantation, each with their inherent advantages and disadvantages. The most common and known hair transplantation method is the so-called 'strip' method. [31]

A strip of skin containing hair follicles is removed, cut into grafts and implanted in the recipient area. In the past years, new methods have developed of which the most promising is the follicle unit extraction (FUE). [32] With this method, whole follicle units are extracted one by one and

http://dx.doi.org/10.5772/59191

implanted one by one into the recipient area. Although the FUE method is more patient friendly and leaves only tiny scars compared with the strip method, which leaves visible linear scars at the donor area, the major disadvantage of both methods is that the extracted hair follicles are removed and the source of potential grafts will be consumed in time. The only way to preserve a significant part of the donor hair follicles could be partial FUE. This idea is not unrealistic and is supported by different experiments [33] Reynolds found that, although the dermal papillae of humans cannot induce new hair growth, the sheath of the lower part of the hair follicle can.

The main drawback of hair transplantation is the esthetic result; in a full thickness facial scar with depressed and discolored skin with poor vascularity the result might not be very satisfactory.

Hair transplantation can be very useful in small and patchy hair bearing area defects or as an adjunct operation in the remaining hairless scar.

7. Algorithm of treatment

In the female patient the final reconstruction can be done at any time but the male patient's reconstruction should be postponed until the facial hair has grown because a bearded face in a child is not socially acceptable and a non-hair bearing reconstruction of the face in these patients, although reported in the literature, might lead to dissatisfaction in later years.

Although at some point during the treatment of the patients we have combined all the treatment modalities such as covering a flap scar with hair transplantation or combining expansion with adjacent tissue VY or Z plasty I propose an algorithm of treatment based on the face units. There are generally four types of hair bearing area defects:

Type 1 is a partial unit defect

Type 2 is total unit defect

Type 3 is bilateral or multiple unit defects with two subtypes type 3a: multiple unit and 3b: bilateral

Type 4 is isolated unit 9 defect

7.1. Type 1 defect

For partial unit defects (Figures 20 to 22), the treatment modalities available are:

1. Defect resection and primary repair
2. Local tissue expansion and reconstruction
3. Hair transplantation

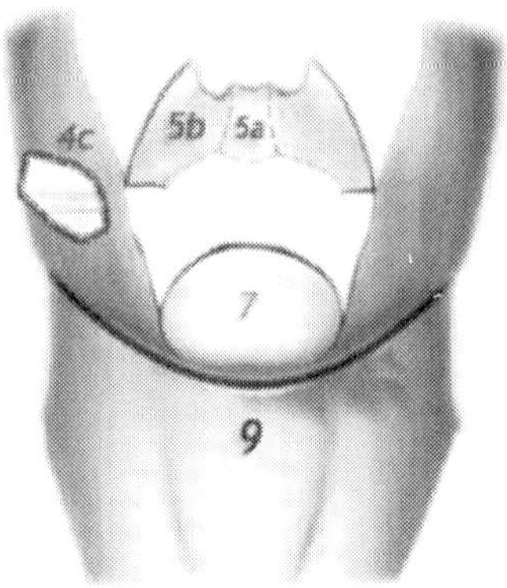

Figure 20. A partial unit defect can be anywhere on the face, used by permission of author Davide Brunelli M.D, www.med-ars.it

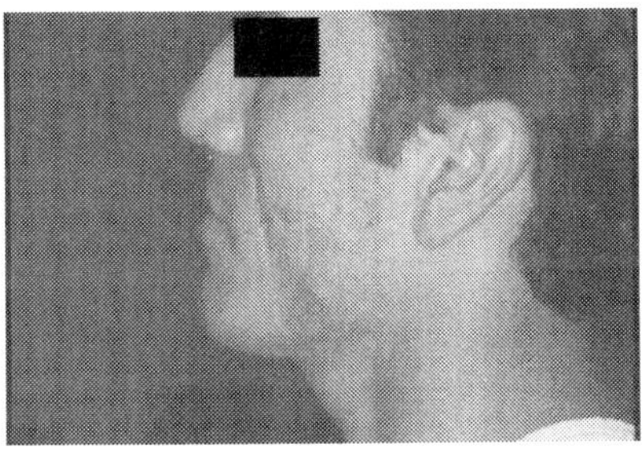

Figure 21. A type one defect of unit 4

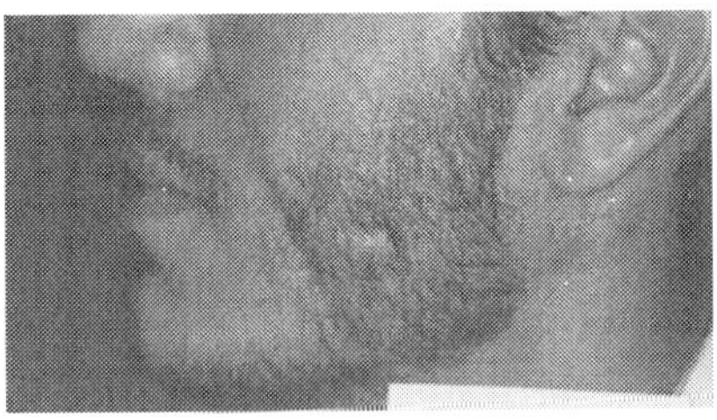

Figure 22. After resection and repair and one stage hair transplantation. Some areas need more transplantation

7.2. Type 2 defect

Total unit defects which can be either unit 4 or 5 (Figures 23 to 34).

The reconstruction options are :

1. Expanded scalp
2. Expanded submental flap

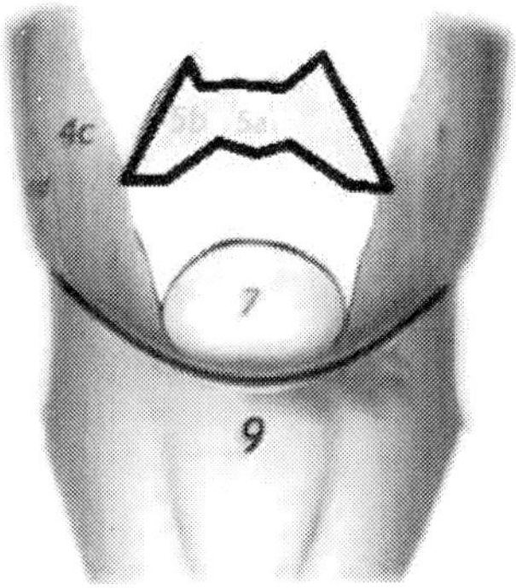

Figure 23. Unit 5 defects, used by permission of author Davide Brunelli M.D, www.med-ars.it

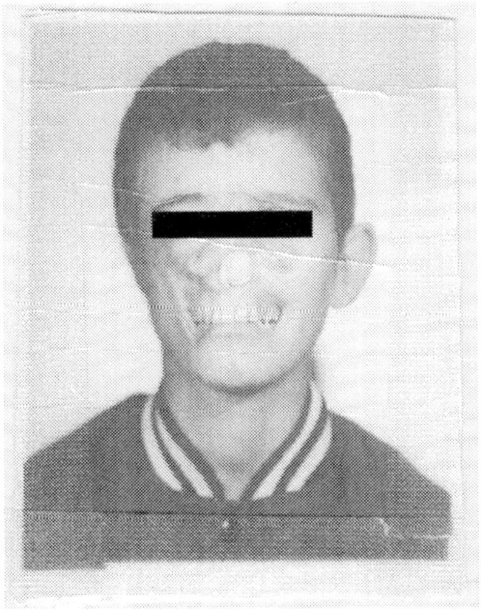

Figure 24. A unit five defect 20 years after reconstruction by an expanded scalp visor flap

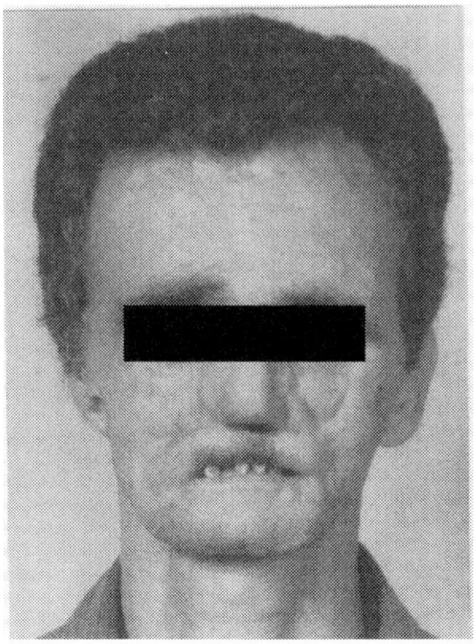

Figure 25. A unit five defect 20 years after reconstruction by an expanded scalp visor flap

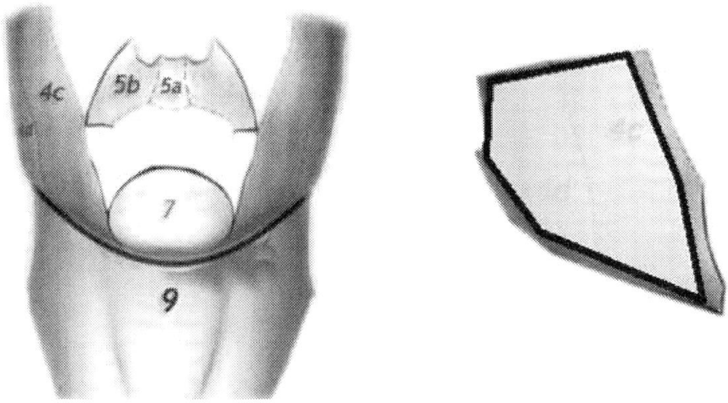

Figure 26. Unit 4 defect, used by permission of author Davide Brunelli M.D, www.med-ars.it

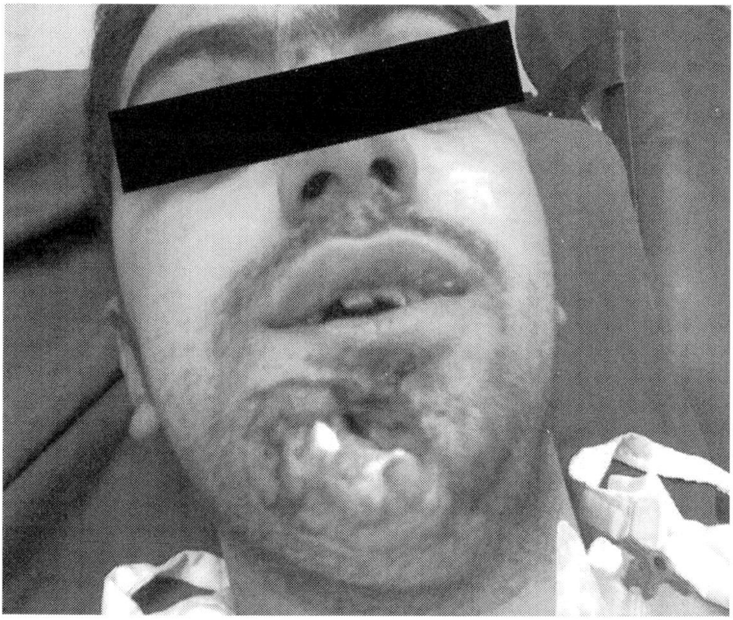

Figure 27. Unit 7 full thickness defect

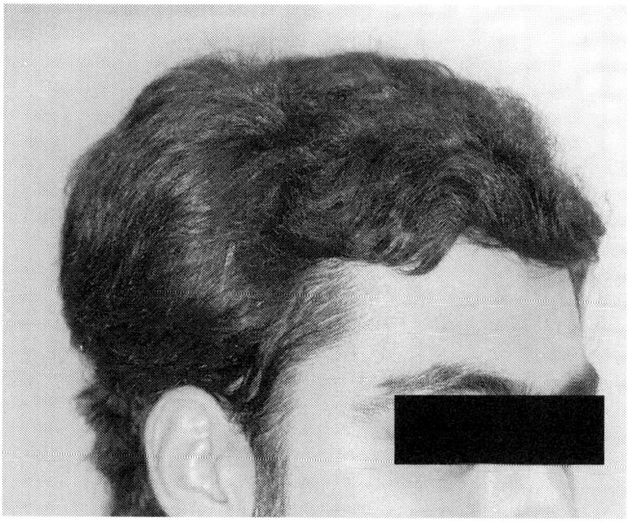

Figure 28. The expanded scalp flap

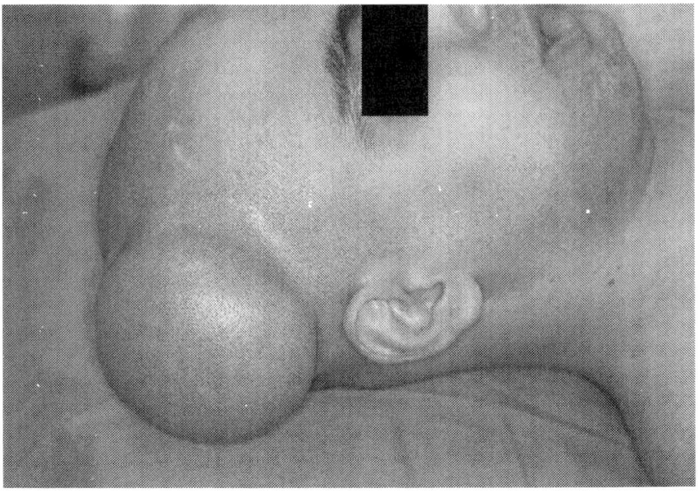

Figure 29. Expansion is complete.

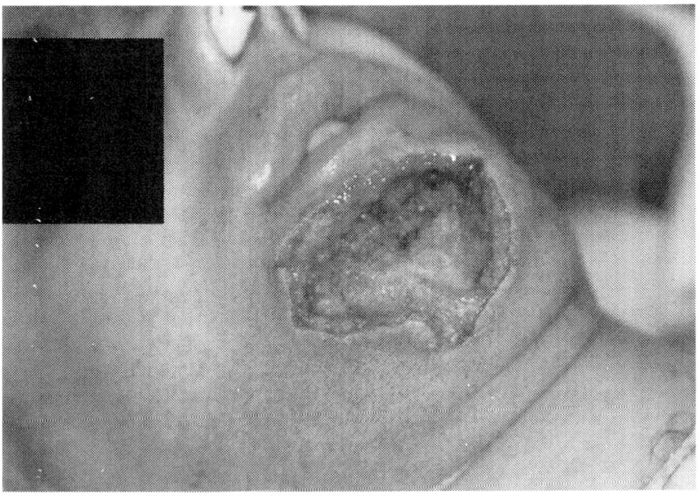

Figure 30. The defect after resection of scar tissues

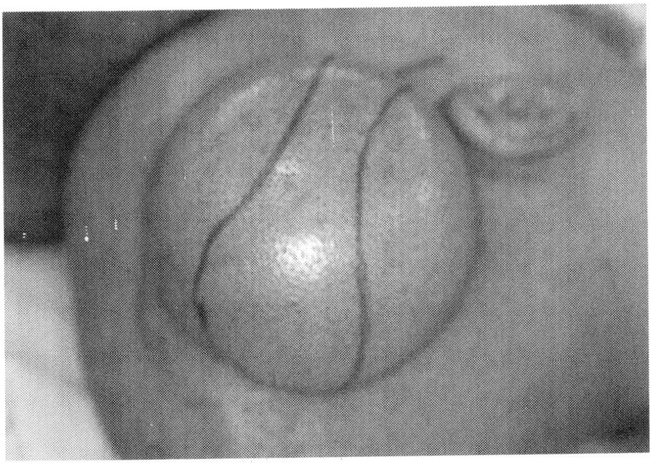

Figure 31. Outline of the flap design is over the highest expanded area to bring a less dense follicle area to the recipient site.

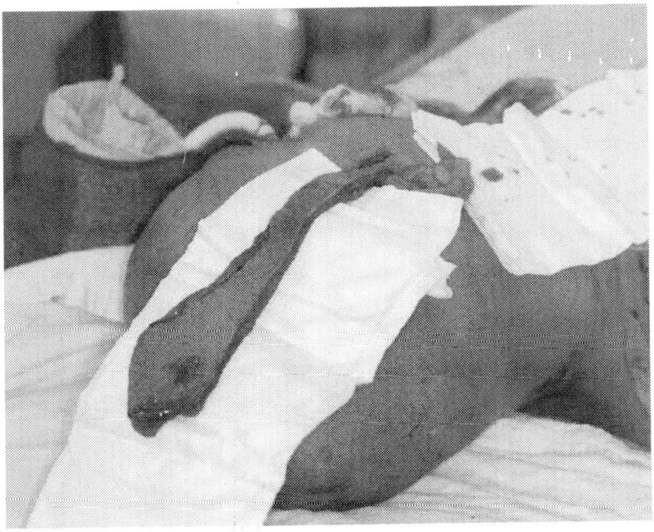

Figure 32. The flap is elevated on the superficial temporal vessels as a pedicle flap

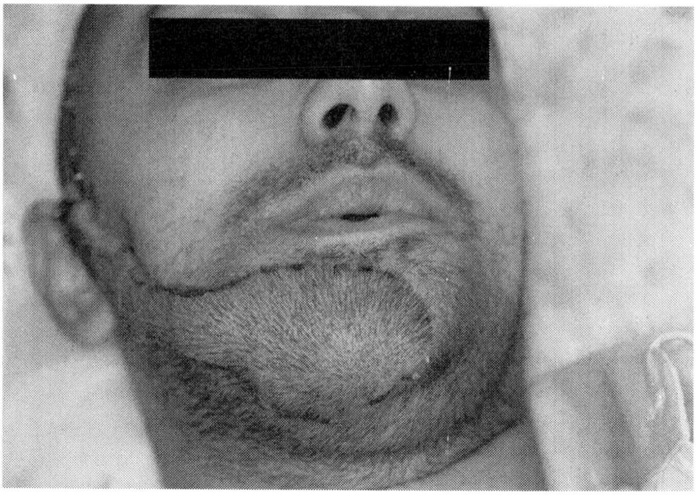

Figure 33. The flap covers the defect completely. Note the pedicle lying over the face.

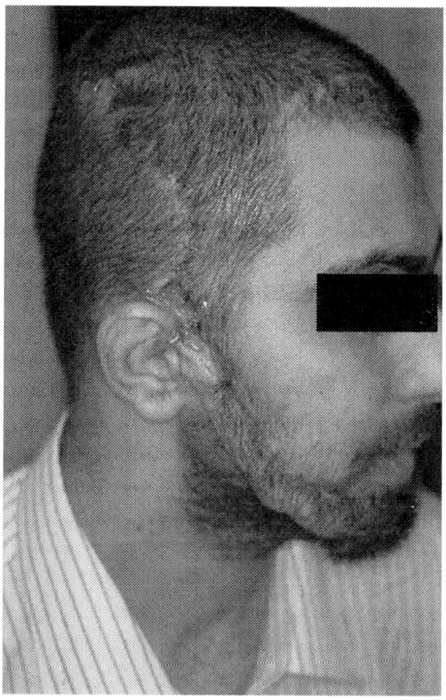

Figure 34. The flap pedicle ready to be severed and returned to its original place.

http://dx.doi.org/10.5772/59191

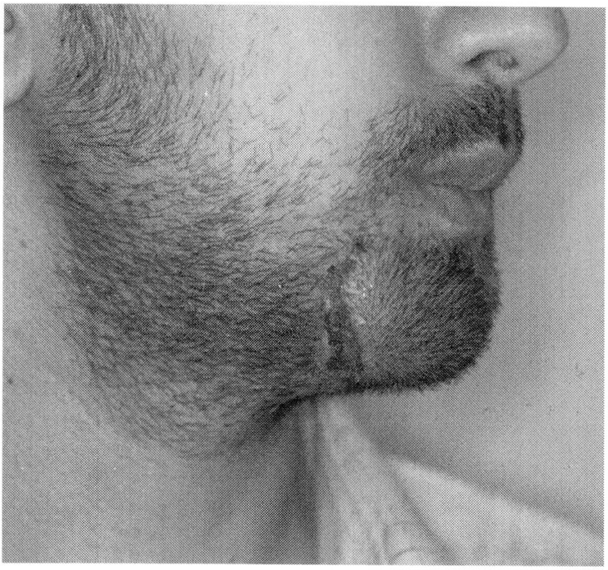

Figure 35. The flap after severance

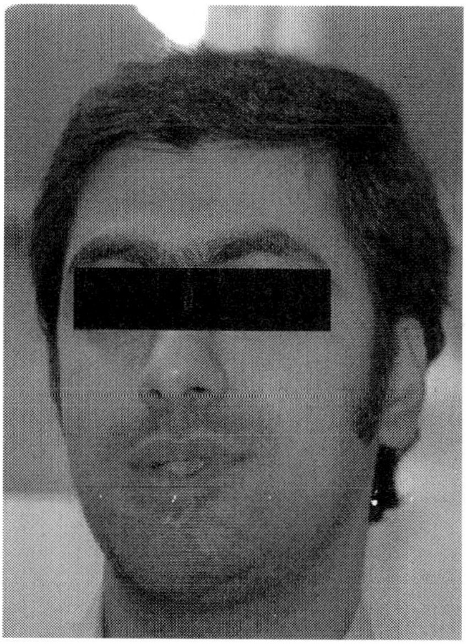

Figure 36. The patient 5 years after the last operation.

7.3. Type 3 defect

Bilateral unit defects or multiple unit defects may be best treated via an expanded Visor flap (Figures 35 to 45).

Type 3a

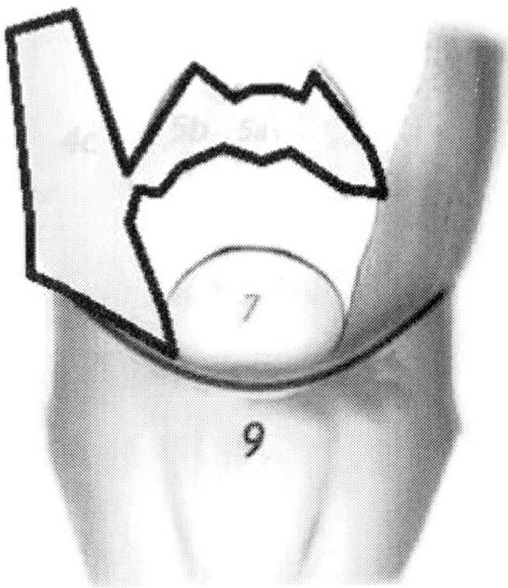

Figure 37. Type 3a defect, bilateral involvement of units or combined units, used by permission of author Davide Brunelli M.D, www.med-ars.it

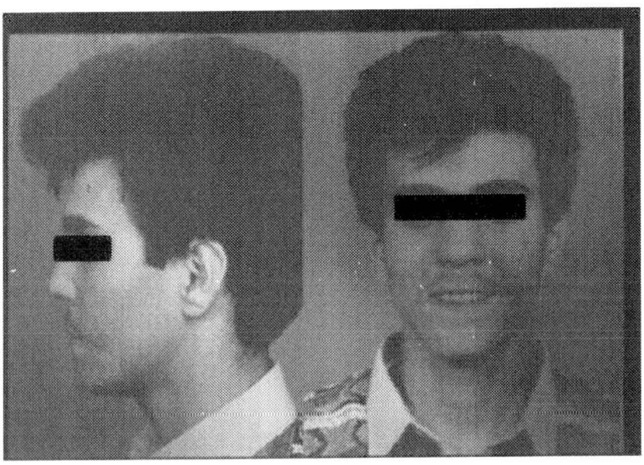

Figure 38. A bilateral unit 4 and 7 defect

http://dx.doi.org/10.5772/59191

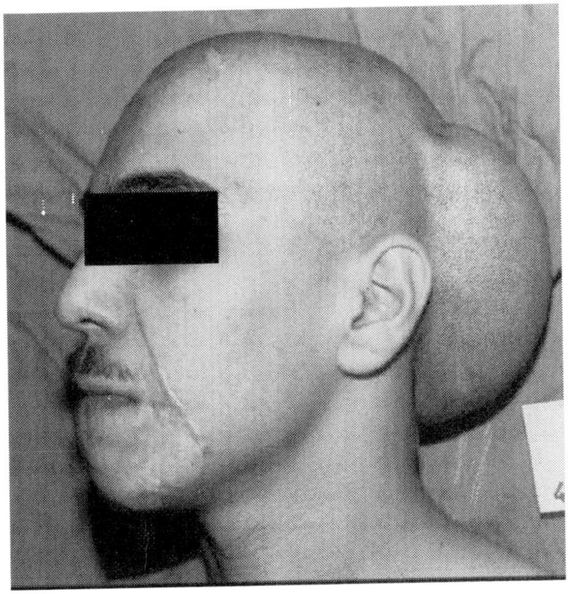

Figure 39. The expanded occipital flap

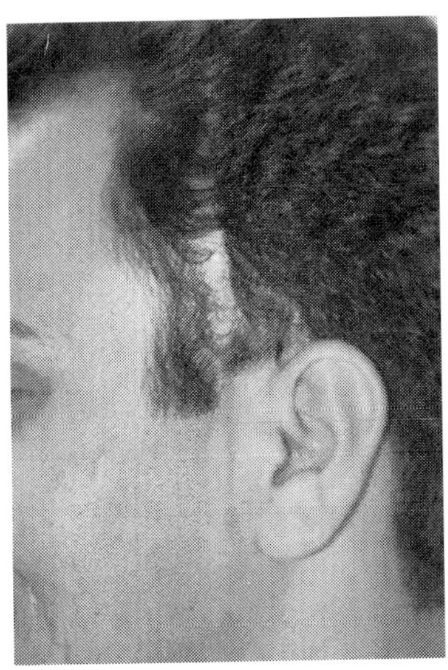

Figure 40. The flap is transferred on the temporal pedicle

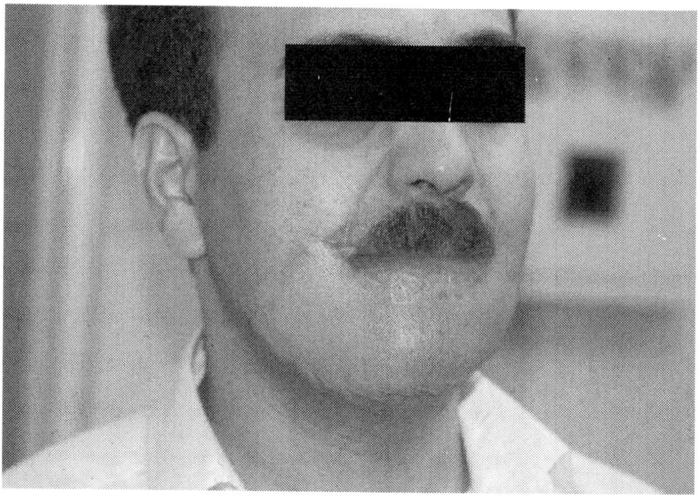

Figure 41. Ten years after the operation

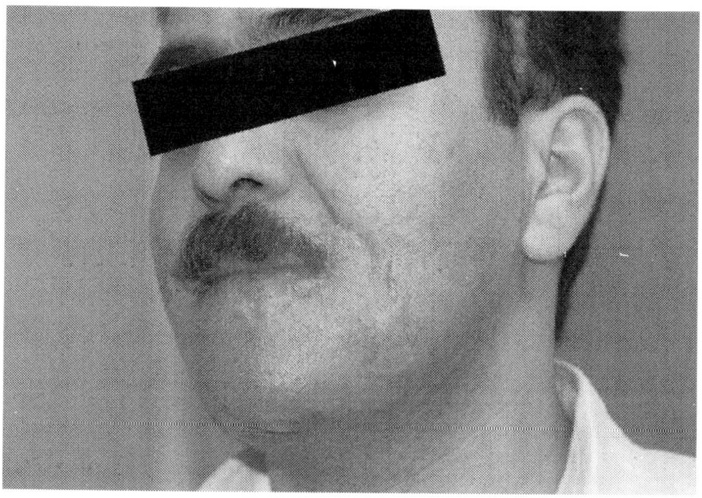

Figure 42. Another view with small Z- plasties to cover the scar

http://dx.doi.org/10.5772/59191

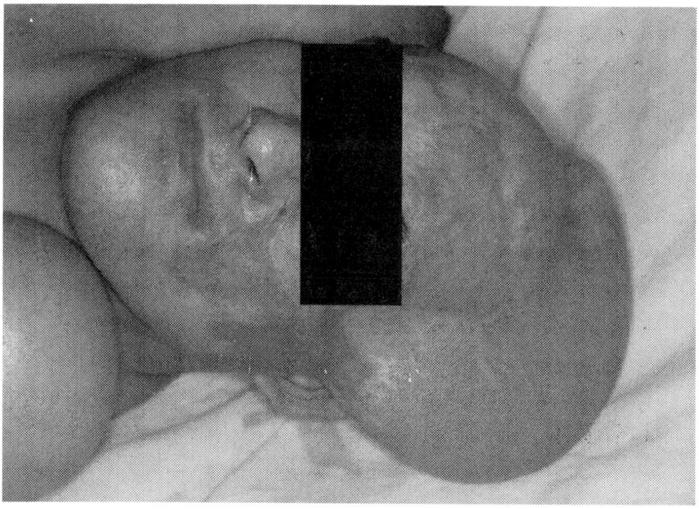

Figure 43. Type 3a : multiple unit with sideburn involvement; units 4 and 5 partial defects with expansion in place

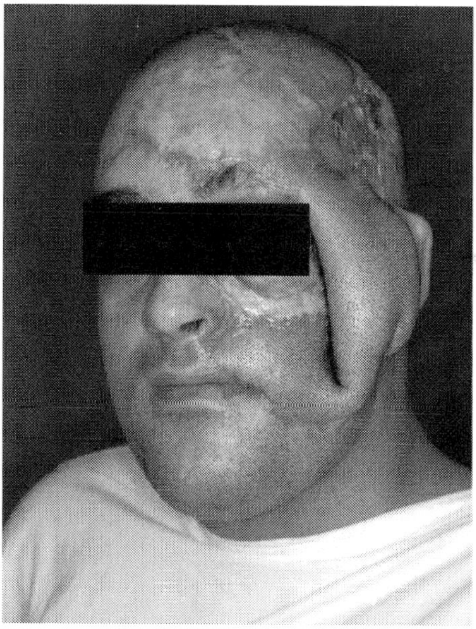

Figure 44. Expanded supraclavicular skin for forehead coverage and expanded scalp for reconstruction of multiple units.

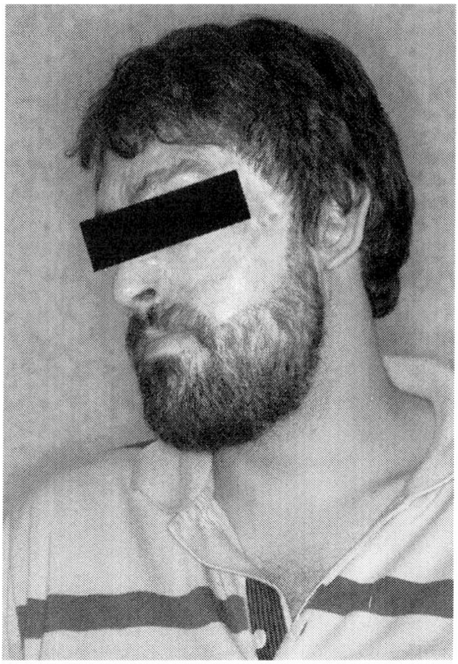

Figure 45. The result after two years

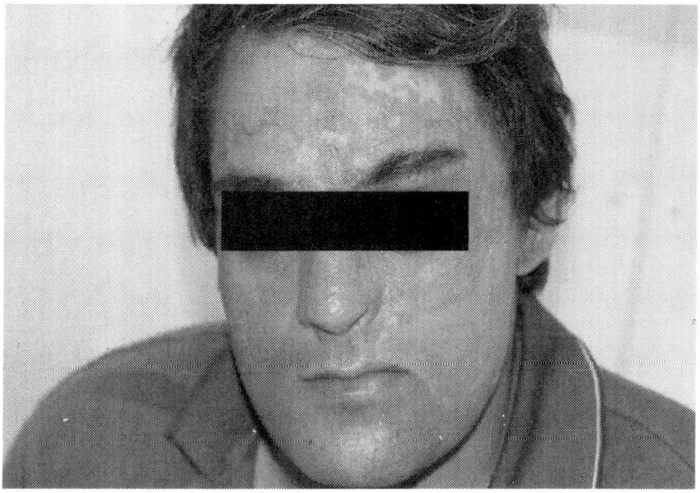

Figure 46. Ten years after operation

http://dx.doi.org/10.5772/59191

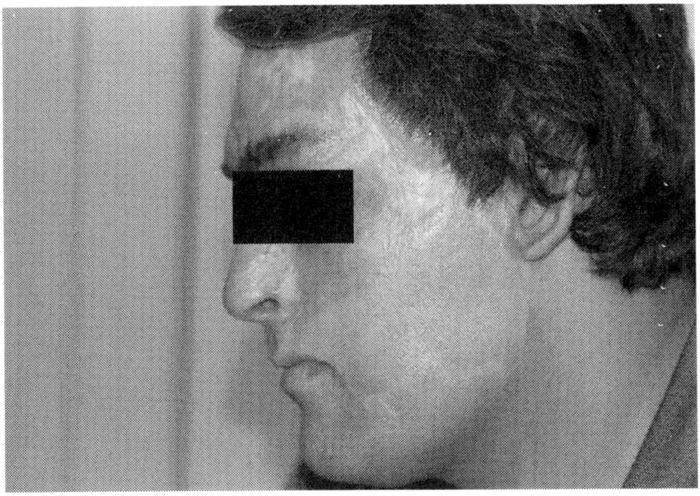

Figure 47. Another view of the patient with Z- plasties to cover the scar

Type 3b

Bilateral near total defects (Figures 46 to 49)

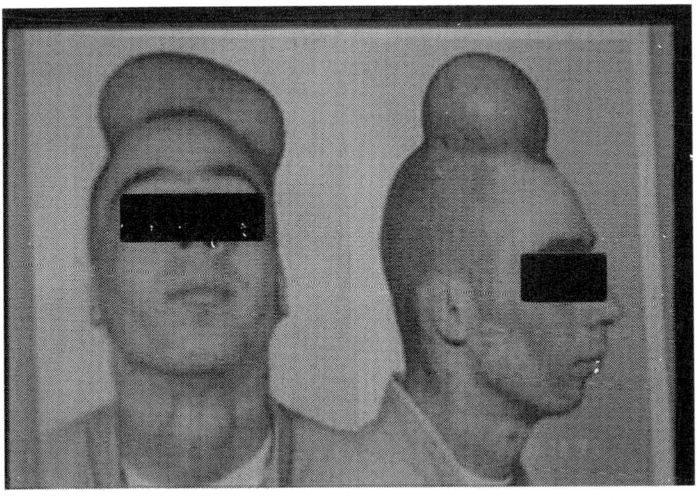

Figure 48. Bilateral unit 4 and 9 involvement with expansion in place.

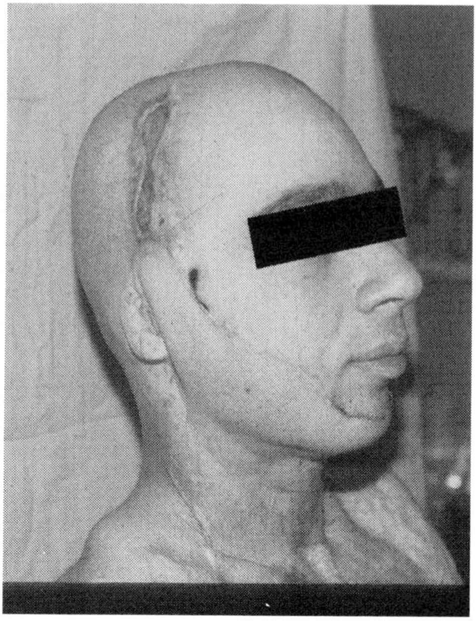

Figure 49. The flap in place

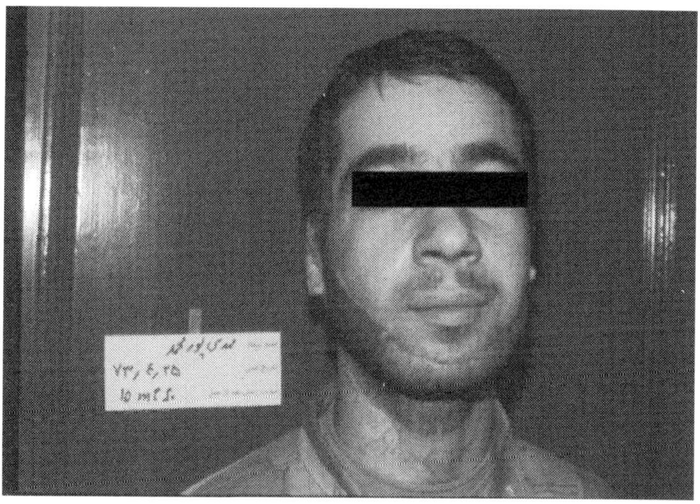

Figure 50. The result after two years.

http://dx.doi.org/10.5772/59191

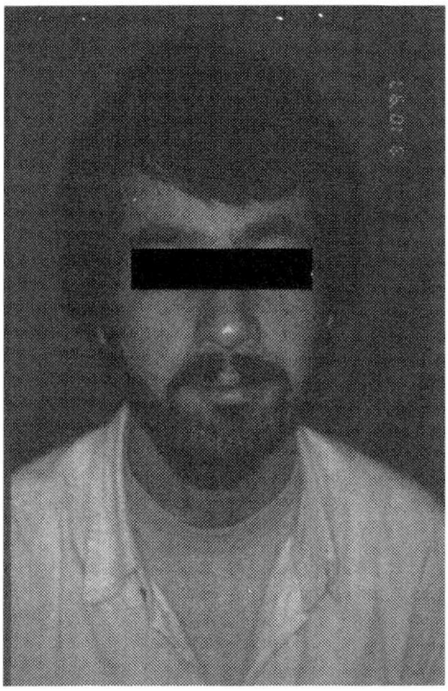

Figure 51. Ten years after the operation.

7.4. Type 4 defect

7.4.1. Isolated unit 9 defects

These defects are unique in that although they bear hair they can be reconstructed with non-hair bearing flaps especially when unit 4 is intact. The beard will cover the scar of this area (Figures 52 - 55)

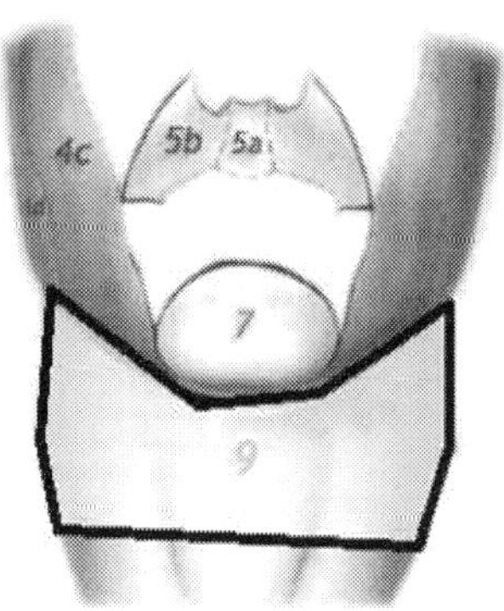

Figure 52. Isolated unit 9 defects can be reconstructed with non-hair bearing flaps

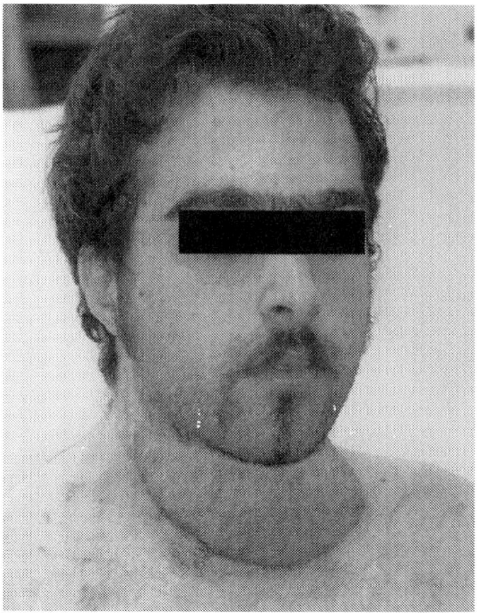

Figure 53. An isolated unit 9 defect reconstructed by an expanded trapezius flap, the anterior trunk was involved in the scar.

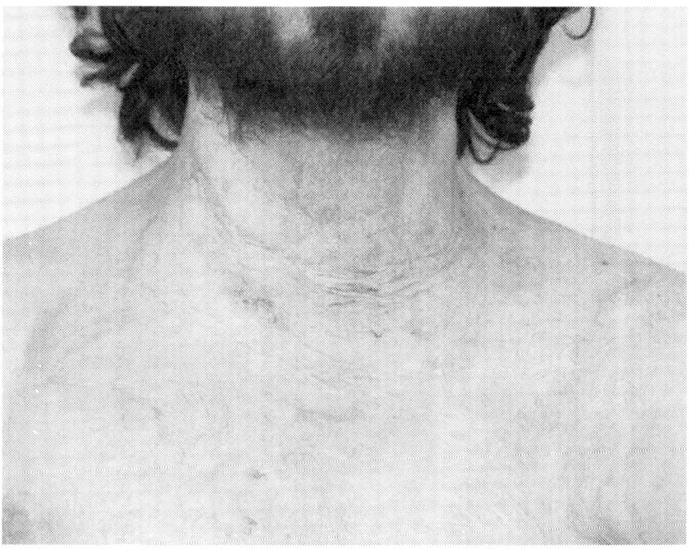

Figure 54. The flap after defatting, note the hair which was present before defatting has become very thin after defatting or transfer.

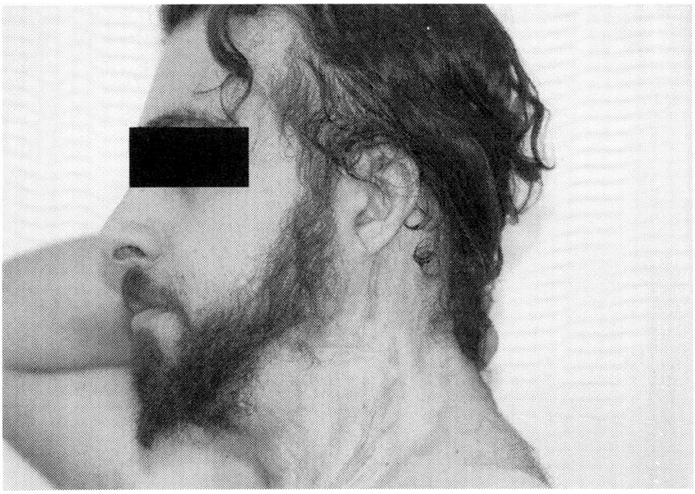

Figure 55. The end result after 7 years, the flap is hidden behind the beard.

8. Summary

Facial hair bearing area reconstruction is one of the most demanding reconstructive procedures and the options available are not an exact match. The facial region recognition and available donors are the prerequisites for the reconstructive surgeon treating these difficult conditions.

Author details

Shahram Nazerani*

Address all correspondence to: Snazeranimd@gamil.com

Dept. of Surgery, Firuzgar Medical Center, Iran University of Medical Sciences, Tehran, Iran

References

[1] Darwin, Charles (2004). The Descent Of Man And Selection In Relation To Sex. Kessinger Publishing. p. 554.

[2] Randall VA (2008). "Androgens and hair growth". Dermatol Ther 21 (5): 314–28.

[3] Sahih Bukhari, Book 72, Hadith #780 Allah's Apostle, salallahu aleihi wa sallam/ peace and blessings of Allah be upon him, said, "Cut the moustaches short and leave the beard (as it is)."

[4] Zokon Yisrael KiHilchso, http://holmininternational613.com/books/ BEARD_JEWISH_LAW-E.pdf

[5] Sherrow, Victoria (2006). Encyclopedia of Hair: A Cultural History. Greenwood Publishing Group. p. 59.

[6] The Oxford Handbook of Iranian History, PP300

[7] Helen Bunkin, Randall Williams: Beards, Beards, Beards (Hunter & Cyr, 2000)

[8] Chrysippus ap. Athen. xiii. 565 a

[9] Ancient Greek: πωγωνοτροφία φιλόσοφον οὐ ποιεῖ. De Is. et Osir. 3 (cited by Peck)

[10] Petron. 75, 10 (cited by Peck)

[11] Corpus Christianorum, Continuatio Mediaevalis LXII, Apologiae duae: Gozechini epistola ad Walcherum; Burchardi, ut videtur, Abbatis Bellevallis Apologia de Barbis. Edited by R.B.C. Huygens, with an introduction on beards in the Middle Ages by Giles Constable. Turnholti 1985

[12] Citing Lucian's Demonax 13, Cynicus 1 - John Sellars (1988). The art of living: the Stoics on the nature and function of philosophy. Burlington, VT: Ashgate Publishing Limited

[13] "Gunma bureaucrats get beard ban | The Japan Times Online". Search.japantimes.co.jp. 2010-05-20. Retrieved 2011-11-24.

[14] Job Bulletin". Agency.governmentjobs.com. 2013-03-22. Retrieved 2014-02-26

[15] Franbourg A, Hallegot P, Baltenneck F, et al. Current research on ethnic hair. J Am Acad Dermatol 2003; 48(6):S115–9

[16] Tolgyesi E, Coble F., Fang S., Kairinen E.O., A comparative study of beard and scalp hair. J Soc Cosmet Chemists, 1982; 34, 361-382

[17] Zhang B, Wang JG, Chen WL, et al. Reverse facialsubmental artery island flap for reconstruction of oropharyngeal defects following middle and advanced-stage carcinoma ablation. Br J Oral Maxillofac Surg 2011;49:194–7

[18] Koshima I, Inagawa K, Urushibara K, et al. Combined submental flap with toe web for reconstruction of the lip with oral commissure. Br J Plast Surg 2000; 53:616–9

[19] Yilmaz M, Menderes A, Barutc¸u A. Submental artery island flap for reconstruction of the lower and mid face. Ann Plast Surg 1997;39:30–5.

[20] Zhang B, Wang JG, Chen WL, et al. Reverse facialsubmental artery island flap for reconstruction of oropharyngeal defects following middle and advanced-stage carcinoma ablation. Br J Oral Maxillofac Surg 2011;49:194–7.

[21] Wang WH, Hwang TZ, Chang CH, et al. Reconstruction of pharyngeal defects with a submental island flap after hypopharyngeal carcinoma ablation. ORL J Otorhinolaryngol Relat Spec 2012;74:304–9.

[22] Abboud O, Shedid D, Ayad T. Reconstruction of the prevertebral space with a submental flap: a novel application. J Plast Reconstr Aesthet Surg 2013; 66(12):1763–5.

[23] a textbook of advanced Oral and Maxillofacial surgery, chapter 18, p. 516

[24] Giraldo F1, González C, Garnica I, Ferrón M, Rus JA. A Sideburn reconstruction with an expanded supraauricular trapezoidal flap, Plast Reconstr Surg. 1997 Jul;100(1): 257-61.

[25] Juri J, Juri C, Colnago A. The surgical treatment of temporal and sideburn alopecia. Br J Plast Surg. 1981 Apr;34(2):186-93

[26] Martin D, Baudet J, Mondie JM, et al. The submental island skin flap. A surgical protocol. Prospects of use. Ann Chir Plast Esthet 1990;35:480–4

[27] Faltaous AA, Yetman RJ. The submental artery flap: an anatomic study. Plast Reconstr Surg 1996; 97:56–60 [discussion: 61–2

[28] Expanded tubed flap in scalp reconstruction: a modern option in an old technique. Caleffi E, Fasano D, Bocchi A, Papadia F. Plast Reconstr Surg. 1988 Dec;82(6):1075-8 Microvascular transplantation of expanded free scalp flaps between identical twins.

[29] Valauri FA, Buncke HJ, Alpert BS, Lineaweaver WC, Argenta LC. Plast Reconstr Surg. 1990 Mar;85(3):432-6

[30] Dufourmentael L. Essai de reconstruction totale u massif maxillaire inferieur. Reconstr Maxillofacial 1919:3:141-156

[31] Bisaccia E, Scarborough D. Hair transplant by incisional strip harvesting. J Dermatol Surg Oncol 1994;20(7):443–8

[32] Rassman WR, Bernstein RM, McClellan R, Jones R, Worton E, Uyttendaele H. Follicular unit extraction: minimally invasive surgery for hair transplantation. Dermatol Surg 2002;28((August) 8):720–8

[33] Gurlek A, Alaybeyoglu N, Demir CY, Aydogan H, Bilen BT, Ozturk A. Aesthetic reconstruction of large scalp defects by sequential tissue expansion without interval. Aesthetic Plast Surg 2004;28((July–August) 4):245–50

[34] Kim JC, Choi YC. Regrowth of grafted human scalphair after removal of the bulb. Dermatol Surg 1995;21(4):312–3.

Chapter 27

Basics of Microvascular Reconstruction of Maxillomandibular Defects

Reza Tabrizi and Barbad Zamiri

Additional information is available at the end of the chapter

http://dx.doi.org/10.5772/59303

1. Introduction

Effective reconstruction following ablative surgery of maxillomandibular defects requires the provision for adequate oral lining, skin, and replacement of missing bone; in some situations, restitution of function of the temporomandibular joint also requires reconstruction-preferably achieved in one stage. Conventional replacement of bone defects usually involves the use of autogenous cancellous bone grafts from either the iliac crest or ribs after provision of adequate skin cover by pedicled axial-pattern skin flaps such as a pectoralis major flap.[1]

Early reconstructive efforts with nonvascularized bone grafts were plagued by a high incidence of postoperative complications and poor long-term outcomes. [2] Inadequate local blood supply due to poorly vascularized flaps or irradiation resulted in rapid resorption of the grafts. The advent of techniques in which composite flaps containing skin and bone together with their own independent blood supply transferred either as pedicled osteocutaneous flaps or free osteocutaneous flaps has revolutionized the concepts of head and neck reconstruction.[1] Early postoperative complications decreased even in the setting of postoperative radiation; and expectations for successful oral rehabilitation, including placement of osseointegrated implants, rose markedly.[2]

1.1. History

The first vascular anastomosis was introduced by J.B. Murphy in 1892; and Alexis Carrel made an end to end anastomosis by using a three-stay suture technique. [3] The first anastomosis in a dog was performed by Krizek. [4] Following him, the first free flap was published in 1971. [3]

2. Assessment of maxillomandibular defects

Each defect is individualized according to the missing component. In the maxillomandibular area the size of soft tissue as well as bone defect, the underlying etiology (cancer, trauma, and infection), anatomic location, aesthetic visibility, associated functional disabilities and the availability of a local and or distant donor site should be evaluated. [5] Compatibility of the donor tissue with the area being reconstructed should be considered with regard to skin color, texture, thickness of soft tissue, bone quantity and quality and also shape of the bone component to restore the mandible and maxilla; further restoration with dental implants can be done. It has been shown that any mandibular defect greater than 6.0 cm is prone to failure and thus free flaps in these defects are indicated.[6] Restoration of stable retentive dentition is a prerequisite to a successful functional oral rehabilitation. This is best achieved with endosseous implants, capable of supporting a stable dental prosthesis, placed directly into vascularized bone flaps at the time of mandibular reconstruction The iliac crest is the most consistently implantable donor site, followed by the scapula, fibula, and radius (with 83%, 78%, 67%, and 21% of sections from each donor site satisfying the criteria for implantability respectively). Consistent regional differences in implantability were encountered at each donor site except the scapula. [7] In a cadaver study, the dimensions of bone available for implant placement from the iliac crest, scapula, fibula, and radius osseous flaps were measured. The iliac crest and fibula flaps had bone dimensions consistently adequate for implant placement. Bone availability for the safe placement of implants into the scapula flap was found in the majority of specimens. The radius flap group had the highest number of specimens that were inadequate for implant placement. [8] Another study demonstrated that nearly all of the iliac crests had adequate dimensions for the positioning of four 10 mm implants. In 63% of the scapulae, it

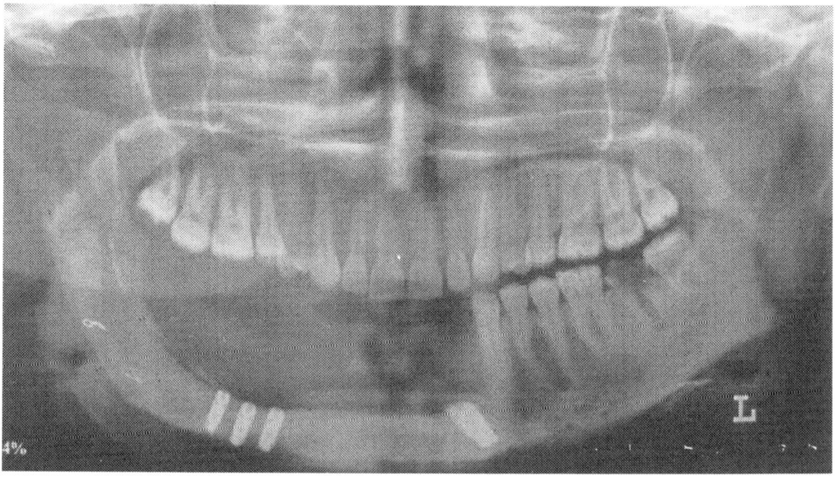

Figure 1. Four implants placed after a fibula flap graft.

was also possible to place four 10 mm implants. In the case of the scapula, half of the female subjects lacked enough available bone for the insertion of four 10 mm implants because of their inadequate width. Bone density and cortical thickness were found to be similar in the iliac crest and scapula. Age and side do not have an important influence on cortical bone dimensions and density. In contrast to the iliac crest, the lateral margin of the scapula astonishingly showed increasing values for bone density and increasing thickness of the cortex. Analogical advanced biological age works in conformity with the scapula flap (Figure 1). [9]

3. Microvascular composite tissue transplantation

In the maxillomandibular area, surgeons encounter soft and hard tissue defects due to ablation of cancer or severe destructive trauma. After introducing the ability to repair vessels less than 2 mm in diameter, microvascular transplantation found its place in reconstruction surgery. A microvascular composite transplantation was defined as a composite flap (soft and hard tissue with their associated blood supply) which is removed from a part of the body and anastomosed to the recipient site vessels. It has been shown that a reliable anastomosis can be achieved with an external lumen diameter of 0.5 to 2mm with a patency rate of 95%. [10]

The frequency of using various free flaps is different according to defect site, the surgeon's experience and condition of the patient. In a retrospective study, flap donor sites included radial forearm (n = 183), fibula (n = 145), rectus abdominis (n = 38), subscapular system (n = 28), iliac crest (n = 5), and a jejunal flap. Age, sex, diagnosis, comorbidities, tumor stage, defect site, primary vs. secondary reconstruction, and history of surgery, radiation therapy, or chemotherapy were considered for choosing a flap. [11]

4. Common microvascular flaps in the maxillomandibular region

Radical cancer ablative surgery and severe traumatic injury can result in complicated defects in the maxillomandibular area which need a complex reconstruction plane. In a small or simple defect, it may be appreciated that the defect is restored with a regional flap. However, microvascular reconstruction of large defects with hard and soft tissue deficiency is a standard approach. The primary use of the free muscle or musculocutaneous flap in the maxillomandibular area consist of provision of tissue bulk for a large defect, coverage of vital structures, provision of skin for the face and mucosa for intraoral lining.[12] Furthermore, a composite osteocutaneous flap provides a skeletal framework to restore function.[12]

5. Radial forearm flap

As the radial forearm flap was originally developed in China, it is often named the China flap. [13] Primarily this flap was introduced as a large flap incorporating most of the circumference of the forearm and was applied as a free flap to cover burns contractures, mainly in the head and neck. [14] The radial forearm flap is a good flap for intraoral reconstruction, offering thin, pliable predominantly hairless skin to replace oral mucosa. The vascularity of the area allows considerable variation in the design of this fasciocutaneous flap and offers the possibility of including bone as an osteocutaneous flap. Furthermore, the vascular anatomy of the flap simplifies the technical aspects of free tissue transfer. Based on ten clinical cases the design of the flap is described and its versatility in differing clinical situations is illustrated. [15] The rich vascularity of the flap results in rapid healing and minimizes wound healing complications, and there is a potential for sensory reinnervation. The flap can be harvested at the same time of tumor surgery. [13]

The radial forearm flap has mostly been used to reconstruct the oral floor, tongue and the maxilla [16] (Figure 2). The osteocutaneous radial flap is robust, reliable, and relatively simple to harvest, which will ensure that it remains one of the established reconstructive options in most maxillofacial units. Many surgeons prefer to use a limited number of trusted flaps, and these qualities will ensure that in the intermediate future most surgical trainees will continue to be shown the fasciocutaneous radial flap as both the basic training flap and the established option for reconstruction. Evidence from observational clinical studies and one randomized clinical trial indicates that there is increasing support for the use of the evolutionary technique of suprafascial dissection to minimize morbidity at the donor site. The suprafascial donor site may be repaired with either a meshed or unmeshed partial-thickness skin graft, or a fenestrated full-thickness skin graft, with good rates of successful healing. The application of a negative pressure dressing to the wound seems to facilitate the healing of all types of skin grafts. The subfascial donor site, however, remains more prone to complications. It may be helpful to position the donor site of the flap more proximally, but this has not been proven. These refinements probably produce the best outcomes that can currently be achieved, given the inherent flaws of the radial donor site.[17] Evidence based on clinical observational studies and biomechanical studies supports the routine or selective use of prophylactic internal fixation to strengthen the radial osteocutaneous donor site. This allows safe harvesting of the maximum volume of available bone, up to half of the circumference, with minimal risk of fracture or long term complications. The incidence of fracture with the plate placed either anteriorly or posteriorly is equally low, but the anterior position is technically easier and probably less likely to cause additional morbidity. The introduction of prophylactic internal fixation consolidates the role of the osteocutaneous radial flap for repair of defects that require a relatively small volume of bone and an appreciable area of thin soft tissue, particularly when a long vascular pedicle is desirable. This includes low level defects of the maxilla, some defects of the mandible and niche reconstructions, such as the orbital rim. The radial forearm flap remains useful as a first choice when there is appreciable peripheral vascular disease, when there are other serious coexisting medical conditions, when it is the preferred choice of the patient for functional reasons such as mobility of the lower limb or hip or when it is a salvage flap used when other reconstructive options have been exhausted. [18]

http://dx.doi.org/10.5772/59303

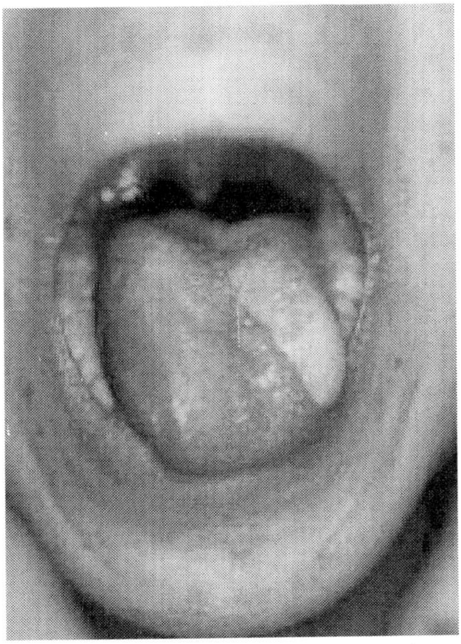

Figure 2. A radial forearm flap used to reconstruction of tongue after hemiglossectomy.

5.1. Flap anatomy

The radial artery branches from the brachial artery near the antecubital fossa and courses deep between the flexor carpi radialis and brachioradialis muscles in the proximal forearm. The artery emerges from this muscle approximately 7 cm cephalic to the wrist crease to enter the subcutaneous tissue.[19] Nine fasciocutaneous branches from the radial artery supply the skin of the forearm, four in the proximal forearm arising between the brachio-radialis and pronator teres muscles and nine in the distal forearm arising between the brachioradialis and flexor carpi radialis muscles.[14] Venus drainage is through either the venae comitante that accompany the radial artery or the much larger superficial venous drainage system via the cephalic vein. The cephalic vein courses subcutaneously on the radial side of the wrist near the superficial radial nerve. The vein goes cephalically supramedially toward the antecubital fossa. Several branches of the superficial radial nerve are found cephalad to the anatomical snuffbox in intimate relation to the cephalic vein. Saving of this nerve is important to maintain sensation over the radial aspect and the index finger. [19]

5.2. Flap component

This is a true septocutaneous flap with a main vessel lying in the septum, giving perforators superficially to supply the fascia, fat and skin and deeper branches to supply underlying tendons, muscles, nerves and bone.[14] The Allen test is noninvasive and reliably detects circulation problems by evaluation of arterial inflow in the presence of one functioning artery. Edgar V. Allen first introduced the test in 1929 as a non-invasive assessment of hand circulation in patients with thromboangiitis obliterans. The test was modified in the 1950s to assess the ulnar artery before cannulation of the radial artery. A similar method is used today to detect the ulnar artery inflow before harvesting the radial forearm flap. [19] The nondominant arm is usually selected for flap harvest. The design and position of the skin island in the volar forearm depend on several factors, including the desire to include the superficial venous drainage system and specific functional and cosmetic requirements at the recipient site. [19] It is usually projected over the course of the radial artery and one of the subcutaneous veins. The paddle is frequently outlined over the distal radius to obtain a vascular pedicle of greatest length (Figure 3). [13]

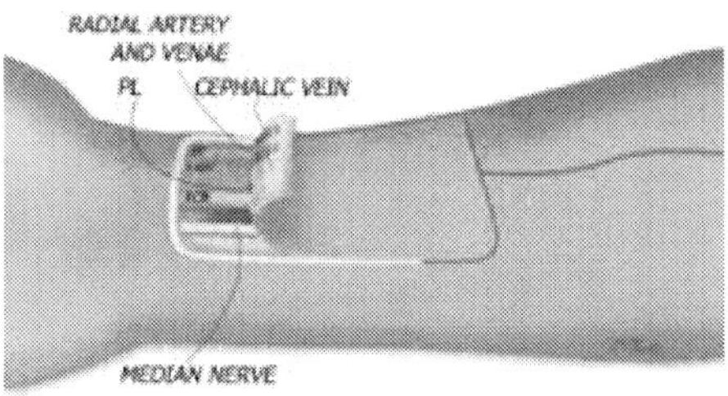

Figure 3. A radial forearm flap

5.3. Flap dimensions

The skin part of the flap commonly has 12 cm length (range 4-30 cm) and 5 cm width (range 4-15 cm) and 1 cm thickness (range 0.5-2cm). The bone part of the flap has 10 cm length (range 6-14 cm) and 1 cm width (range 0.7-1.5 cm) and 1 cm thickness (range 0.7-1.5 cm).[14]

5.4. A common radial forearm flap harvesting technique

A tourniquet is placed. The skin island is outlined over the distal forearm, including the radial artery and cephalic vein, and the flap edges are incised. The incision is extended deeply to include the deep fascia, except along the proximal edge, where the superficial veins and nerves are in the immediate subcutaneous tissue plane. The radial artery is exposed and temporarily closed to assess the adequacy of the circulation to the hand through the ulnar artery. The flap is raised from the ulnar and radial sides. It is necessary to include the deep fascia but saving the final peritenon. [19] Where bone is to be included in the lateral intermuscular septum, the periosteum of the radius must be preserved. Available bone extends from the insertion of the pronator teres to the distal styloid where there is no muscle attachment on the radial border. This provides a length of about 10-12 cm. Dissection can be performed as described, but, at the radial border of palmaris longus, the plane is deepened to expose the flexor pollicis longus and pronator quadratus.

5.5. Complications

A major problem with radial forearm flap relates to its donor site and the effect on function and aesthetics (Figure 4). Injury to the superficial radial nerve results in numbness over the anatomic snuffbox and radial side of the thumb and index finger. A devastating complication is vascular problems of the hand because of inadequate blood supply by the ulnar artery. It has been shown that a significant functional forearm and wrist range-of-motion morbidity associated with the harvest of a radial forearm fasciocutaneous free flap may occur in the early postoperative period. [20]

The radial forearm free flap results in measurable quantitative changes in hand function and limited changes in patient perception. [21]

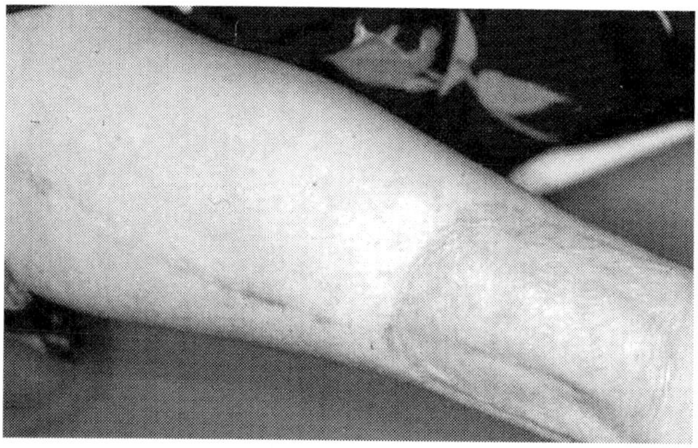

Figure 4. A severe scar of the donor site after a radial forearm flap

5.6. Radial forearm flap updates

The radial forearm flap has been used for reconstruction of palatal defects and for total lower lip reconstruction.[22, 23] It is suggested to use a full-thickness skin graft from the neck to cover the radial forearm free flap donor site in patients undergoing neck dissection and microvascular reconstruction for ablative head and neck oncologic surgery. The primary advantage is avoiding a third surgical site. Complications were comparable to those using Full-thickness Skin Grafting from other harvest sites. Importantly, cross-contamination from the head and neck with the forearm was not a problem. [24] The pre-operative application of topical tissue expansion tapes produces measurable changes in skin biomechanical properties. The location of this change on the dorsal forearm is consistent with the method of tape application. This increase in skin pliability may account for the improved rate of primary donor site closure reported using this technique. [25] AlloDerm with split-thickness skin graft has been used to cover the donor site after radial forearm flaps. Results demonstrated thicker coverage of the forearm defect, with minimal donor site morbidity and superior cosmetic results. [26]

6. Fibula flap

The fibula bone is most commonly used in oral and maxillofacial reconstruction following benign or malignant jaw tumor ablation Hidalgo, in 1989, reported the first mandibular reconstruction using a vascularized fibula free flap. [27]. It has several advantages over other bones, including being the longest bone with lengths up to 25 cm, having bicortical structures that can support osseointegrated dental implants, having a large caliber and long vascular pedicles which provide easier anastomosis, and having thin and pliable skin paddles as well as available muscular cuffs around the fibula which can be used for reconstructing the various soft tissue defects (Figures 5 and 6). The morbidity at the donor site is also low and the operation time is reduced because of a two-team approach.

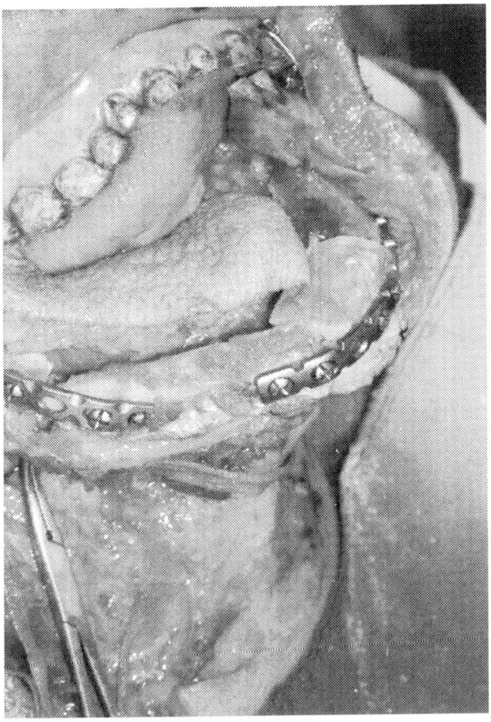

Figure 5. A composite fibula flap used to restore the hemimandible and the oral floor.

http://dx.doi.org/10.5772/59303

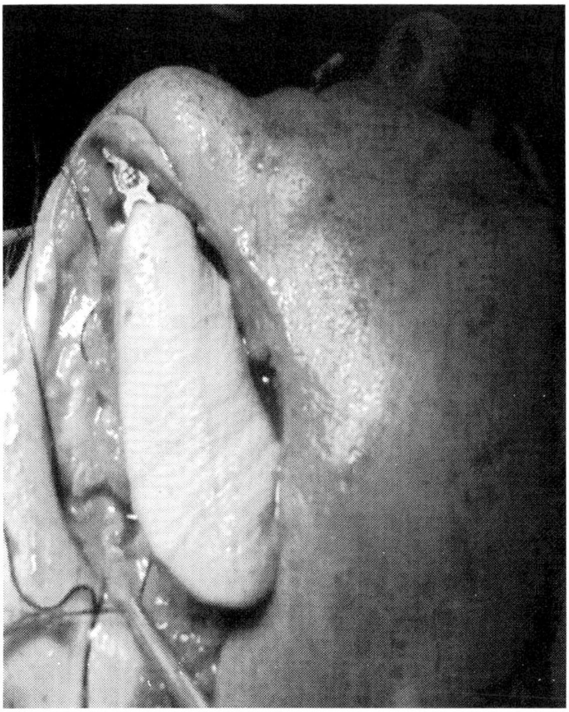

Figure 6. A composite fibula flap for reconstruction of the hemimandible and soft tissue defect on the face.

6.1. Flap anatomy

The arterial supply of the fibula flap is the peroneal artery. The peroneal artery branches from the posterior tibial artery just proximal to the head of the fibula. The external diameter of the peroneal artery is 1.5-2.5 mm. The pedicle length varies and may be quite long if a large segment of the proximal part of the bone is resected. The skin over the lateral leg is also nourished by the peroneal artery via septocutaneous vessels that course posterior to the fibula to enter the posterior crural intermuscular septum. [19] Venous drainage of the flap is primarily by venae comitante (two) of the peroneal artery. The venae comitante often merge to form a single large vein near the posterior tibial artery. Sensory innervation to the corresponding lateral leg skin is mostly supplied by the lateral sural nerve. It can be detected under microscopic view. It is possible to enclose the lateral sural nerve with the fibula flap to improve function of recipient site (Figure 7). [28]

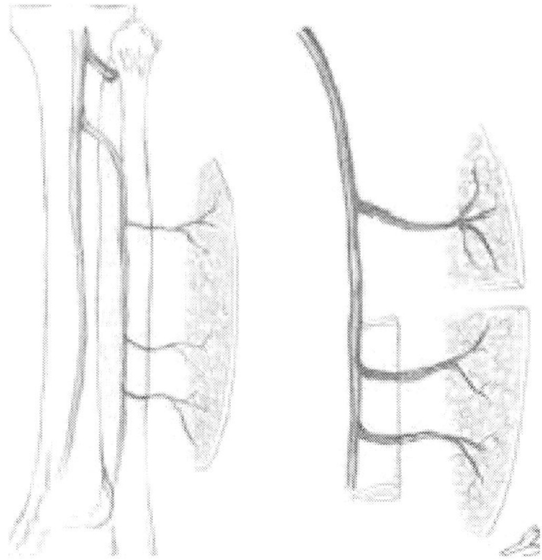

Figure 7. Anatomy of a free fibula flap

6.2. Flap component

The fibula flap is harvested as a bone flap and may consist of muscles (soleus or flexor hallucis longus), overlying fascia and/or skin (Figure 8). [28]

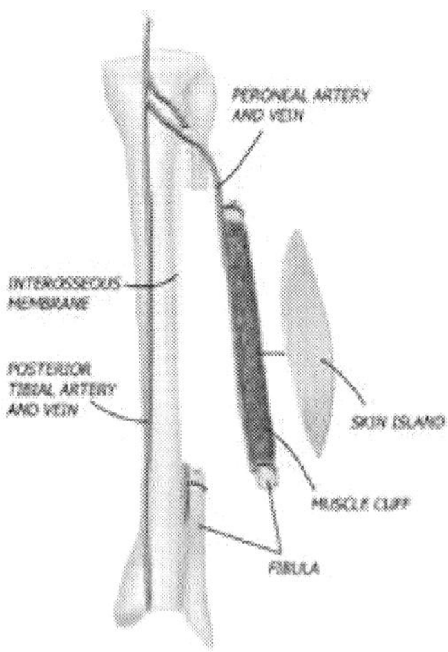

Figure 8. Components of a fibula flap

6.3. Flap dimensions

The skin paddle length can be 12 cm and its width can be 6 cm. The bony part length is 16 cm (range 6-26 cm) and its thickness 2 cm.

6.4. A common fibula flap harvesting technique

A tourniquet is placed on the thigh and the knee is partially flexed for access to the postero-lateral leg. Firstly, the fibula bone outline and a skin paddle (if it is included in the flap) are marked on the skin. Then an incision is made on the anterior outline. Dissection proceeds anterior to the posterior intramuscular septum, through which fasciocutaneous perforators run. The common peroneal nerve which runs below the level of the head of the fibula is identified and preserved with the peroneal muscles of the anterior surface of the fibula, reflecting the peroneus longus and brevis muscles. The anterior intermuscular septum is incised to gain access to the anterior part. Dissection is extended through the extensor digitorum and extensor hallucis longus. After access to the fibula bone, the maximum length of the bone is included with proximal osteotomy 6 cm inferior to the fibular head and distal osteotomy 8 cm superior to the lateral malleolus (Figure 9).[28]

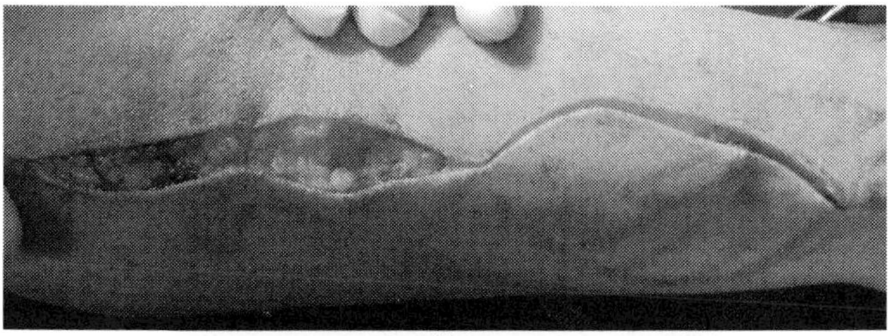

(a)

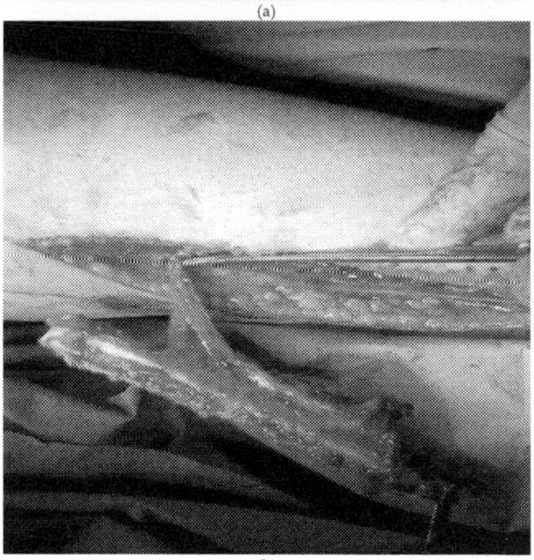

(b)

Figure 9. (a): The outline of a fibula flap with a skin paddle. (b): A fibula flap harvest. Note its vascular pedicle.

6.5. Complications

The most feared potential donor site complication in fibula flap transfer is foot ischemia secondary to the sacrifice of the peroneal artery. In the most common situation, terminal branches of the peroneal artery arise at the level of the ankle, and the blood supply to the foot is provided by the anterior and posterior tibia arteries. In patients with atherosclerosis of the anterior or posterior tibial vessels, collaterals from the peroneal artery may provide a significant contribution to pedal circulation. The majority of patients with peripheral vascular disease of the lower extremities are easily identified on the basis of history and physical examination. However, there is another group of patients with congenital vascular anomalies for whom the peroneal artery provides a significant contribution to the foot circulation. This subpopulation of patients present a unique difficulty when performing a preoperative evaluation in anticipation of performing a fibula free flap, because they may have a normal history and physical examination.[29] In general, the patient perception of donor-site morbidity is low. Complaints however, were frequently mentioned, including pain (60 percent), dysesthesia (50 percent), a feeling of ankle instability (30 percent), and inability to run (20 percent). Gait analyses revealed that patients walked at a lower preferred velocity, compared with control subjects. Furthermore, it was demonstrated that significant increases in the coefficients of variation of stride time during walking under visual and cognitive loads and during walking at a velocity higher than the preferred compared with normal walking.[30] Noticeable limitation and discomfort in ankle function and range of motion with aggressive physical activity may result after fibula harvest, particularly if tibiofibular fusion is performed.[28] Commonly the bone flap may tolerate venous thrombosis for up to 24 hours because of spontaneous bleeding from the medullary canal before the artery undergoes thrombosis, but venous drainage of the skin paddle must be managed by reoperation.[28]

6.6. Fibula flap updates

Proximal peroneal perforator in the dual-skin paddle configuration of fibula free flap has been used to reconstruct composite oral defects. The proximal peroneal perforator was found to be anatomically reliable and clinically useful in composite oral cavity reconstruction. [31] The free fibula flap has been reported to be an appropriate option for mandibular reconstruction in bisphosphonate-related osteonecrosis of the jaws. [32] The keys for gaining maximum success in a fibula flap include:

1. Harvesting the distal fibula when recipient vessels are distant
2. Flap selection based on the anatomy of perforators
3. Use of the skin paddle for postoperative flap monitoring
4. Protection of the flap's soft-tissue cuff
5. Preventing venous thrombosis which is essential to reduce flap complications
6. Aligning fibular struts and protecting the vascular pedicle when the double-barrel technique is used

http://dx.doi.org/10.5772/59303

7. Minimizing the gap between the double-barrel struts and implementing a long-term follow-up of dental implants

8. Selecting osteosynthesis materials

9. Mastering the learning curve and clinical competence in microvascular reconstruction. [33]

It has been shown that function can reliably be reestablished after segmental mandibulectomy and condylectomy reconstructed with a vascularized fibula flap whose distal end is not precisely contoured or actively seated in the glenoid fossa, as a valid alternative to condylar reconstruction. [34] Skin paddle harvesting is a factor that influences the operation time and patient satisfaction of fibula free flap surgery. An increase in body mass index is related to an increase in donor-site morbidity after fibula free flap transfer. [27]

7. Deep circumflex iliac artery flap

For large oromandibular defects such as subtotal glossectomy with anterior mandibulectomy the options for reconstruction are limited. The composite fibular flap will not easily provide the mass of soft tissue required or the mobility to set it in. A scapular free flap can supply the tissue needed in a chimerical fashion but without the quality or length of bone, and it requires the patient to be turned. Two free flaps can be used such as a fibular with an anterolateral thigh flap, but this lengthens the operating time, and increases morbidity and complications.

A deep circumflex iliac artery flap **(DCIA)** flap is a good single flap option in these circumstances. [35] DCIA flap, a composite osteomusculocutaneous flap of the iliac crest, abdominal wall musculature and overlying skin, has evolved significantly during the previous 30 years since its inception in the late 1970s. With an increasingly reported role for a range of facial, lower limb, and upper limb reconstructions, its most widespread utility has been for hemimandibular defect reconstruction. Furthermore, the iliac crest has long been used for these various bony reconstructions, its versatility as a composite flap has largely been limited by an understanding of the finer vascular anatomy of the region. Initial attempts to harvest the iliac crest flap using the superficial circumflex iliac artery as its vascular supply in 1978 met with less than ideal results. Although greater success was achieved with the DCIA pedicle flap after the landmark report by Taylor and Townsend in 1979, detailing the DCIA as the main blood supply to the iliac crest, a lack of familiarity with the DCIA perforators in these early studies limited the use of the DCIA flap as a composite flap. [36]

7.1. Flap anatomy

Vessel branches supplying the flap are the ascending branch, which supplies the internal oblique muscle, nutrient endosteal perforators, and periosteal contributions to the iliac crest, and musculocutaneous perforators which supply the overlying skin. The dominant blood supply to the iliac crest flap is provided by deep circumflex iliac (DCIA) artery (length=9 cm and diameter=2.8 mm). The DCIA generally arises deep to the inguinal ligament from the femoral artery or the external iliac artery deep to the inguinal ligament or less frequently from the external iliac artery superior to the inguinal ligament. Venous drainage of the flap is to the deep circumflex iliac vein. This flap does not have a motor reinnervation. Sensory nerve comes from T12 (Figure 10). [37]

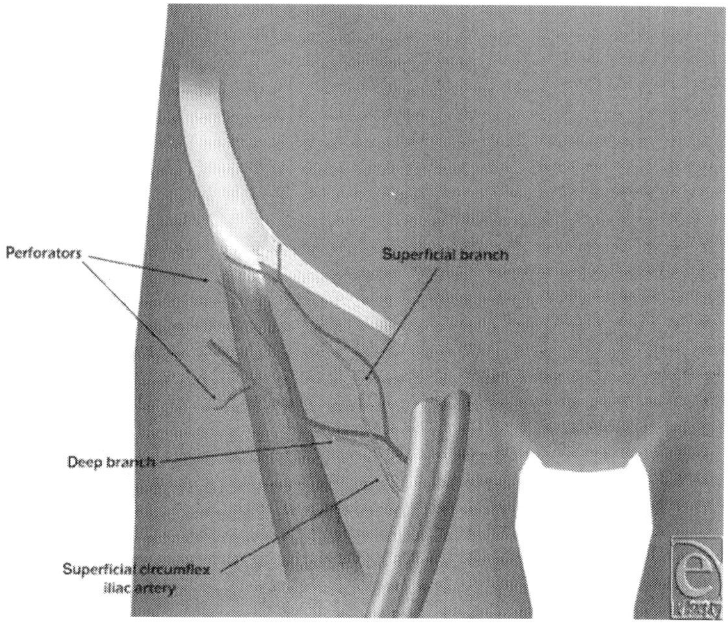

Figure 10. Anatomy of the DCIA flap

7.2. Flap components

The iliac crest flap provides for a great many options in flap composition. It may be harvested as a bone-only or a composite flap, which may include muscle, fascia, fat and skin.

7.3. Flap dimensions

Skin island length commonly is 15 cm and its width 8-10 cm with variable thicknesses. The bony part length is commonly 7 cm and its height 4 cm with 1 cm thickness.

7.4. A common deep circumflex iliac artery flap harvesting technique

An incision is first made 2 cm above the mid-point of the line between the anterior superior iliac spine and the pubic tubercle to identify the origin of the deep circumflex iliac artery; dissection is performed following the course of the deep circumflex artery. Around the anterior superior iliac spine, one can find the ascending branch arise to enter the abdominal muscula-

http://dx.doi.org/10.5772/59303

ture, which is dissected free as a backup vessel. The insertion of the abdominal musculature to the inner lip of the iliac bone is detached, with a small muscular cuff preserved between the deep circumflex artery and the iliac crest to protect the minute osteomusculocutaneous branches entering the inner cortex. After detachment of the abdominal musculature along the superior edge of the iliac crest is performed for about 6.5 cm, the deep circumflex artery can be found to sweep medially upward into the abdominal musculature, ending as a musculocutaneous perforator, nourishing the overlying skin. Meticulous dissection is performed to isolate the vascular pedicle from the abdominal musculature; the skin paddle is centered on the perforator with the previous incision along the iliac crest as the inferolateral margin of the cutaneous flap; finally the flap is harvested to the actual need. [38]

7.5. Complications

Bulky skin paddle may result in poor cosmetic or functional outcomes. A hernia or abdominal contour deformity can occur in 10% of patients. [37] Postoperative sequelae include injury to the lateral femoral cutaneous and ilioinguinal nerves, which can produce unpleasant dysesthesia or anesthesia. [13] The incidence of gait disturbance and chronic hip pain after the flap harvesting may be greatly decreased by preserving the anterior superior iliac spine and using unicortical bone flap.

7.6. Deep circumflex iliac artery flap updates

A free vascularized iliac bone flap based on superficial circumflex iliac perforators (SCIPs) has been introduced. Compared with a conventional iliac bone flap, which is based on deep circumflex iliac vessels, this flap is less invasive, less bulky and can include a reliable skin island. In addition, an SCIP-deep inferior epigastric perforator (DIEP) bipedicle soft--tissue flap has been developed, which can contribute to safe transfer of larger DIEP flaps.[39] An anatomical study described variations in DCIA flap. The origin of the DCIA was 5.30 ± 6.22 mm (mean ± SD) superior to the inguinal ligament, and the DCIV was 4.75 ± 3.14 mm medial to the origin of the DCIA. The length of the DCIA from its origin to the level of the anterior superior iliac spine was 59.35 ± 9.06 mm, and the vertical distance between the anterior superior iliac spine and DCIA was 18.50 ± 3.82 mm. With regard to the branching pattern of the ascending branch, most cases (n = 18, 90%) exhibited 1 origin and 2 branches, and the remaining 2 cases (10%) had 2 origins and 2 branches. The distance from the DCIA origin to the branch point in cases exhibiting 1 origin and 2 branches was 36.83 ± 16.10 mm. [40]

8. Scapular flap

The scapular region is an excellent source of cutaneous, fascial, muscular, osteomuscular-cutaneous free or pedicled flaps based on the subscapular artery and its branches. In 1978, the scapular free flap was introduced by Sajio. The flap was based on the circumflex scapular vessels. These vessels supply the vast thoracodorsal fascial network of the back, which provide an abundant tissue source beyond the flap margin. The scapular osteocutaneous free flap has been used mostly in reconstruction of craniomaxillofacial defects, including the orbit, the maxilla and palatal defects. [13] Scapular bone provides thin bone for restoring orbital floor defects in conjunction with malar regions, orbital rim and alveolar defects.

8.1. Flap anatomy

The subscapular artery gives rise to the circumflex scapular artery supplying the scapular and parascapular skin. The superficial branch of the circumflex scapular artery reaches the subcutaneous tissue at the level of the triangular space. At this point it provides several branches. The main two branches are the horizontal and vertical ones. [41] Venae comitante of the horizontal and vertical branches of the circumflex scapular vein are the venous drainages of the flap. The horizontal and vertical branches drain into the circumflex scapular vein, then the subscapular vein and finally the axillary vein. The third, fourth and fifth intercostal nerves through lateral and posterior branches provide sensory innervation of this region. There is no motor nerve involvement in this procedure (Figure 11).

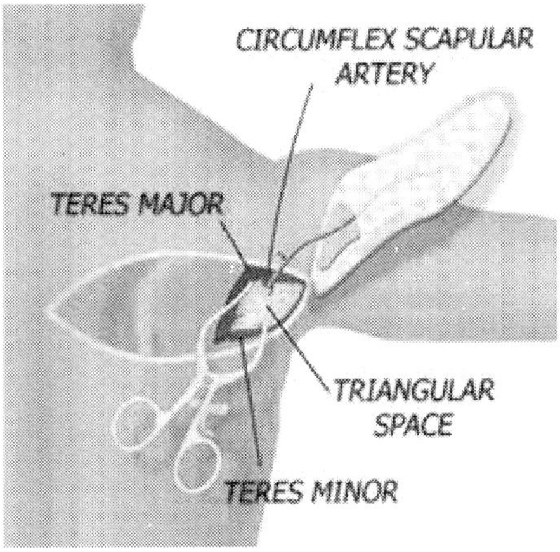

Figure 11. Anatomy of the scapular flap.

8.2. Flap components

This is a skin and subcutaneous flap which may include bone, fascia and muscle. These flaps are extremely reliable with a consistent vascular pedicle of good length and large caliber. The color of the back skin may provide a better match for head and neck reconstruction.

8.3. Flap dimensions

Skin island length is 18-20 cm with 7-8 cm width and 2 cm thickness. The bone length is about 10-14 cm with 2-3 cm width and 1.5-3 cm thickness.

http://dx.doi.org/10.5772/59303

8.4. A common scapular flap harvesting technique

The site of flap incision is infiltrated with lidocaine with2% epinephrine. The outline of skin paddle is marked. It is important to mark the location of the flap on the patient's back relative to flap size, and to mark the orientation relative to the pedicle and its branches. An incision is made from the posterior border of the deltoid muscle 3 cm lateral and parallel to the lateral border of the scapula, ending approximately at the angle. The dissection of the cutaneous flap is extended medially in a plane just superficial to the deep muscular fascia of the infraspinatus muscle. The thoracodorsal fascia is preserved during dissection. The circumflex vessels arise sharply over the lateral edge of the scapula and are just superficial to the facial base of dissection. [13] The lateral scapular bone flap and the branches to the bone from the pedicle are carefully dissected and preserved in the triangular space. An incision is made 2 to 3 cm medial to the bone edge through the muscles on the scapula inferior to the bone. If a bipedicle bone flap is desired with 2 vascular sources on the same pedicle, in this situation the angular branch from thoracodorsal vessel should be included in the flap design. The donor site is closed primarily, with the use of appropriate drain placement and the patient is turned to the supine position (Figure 12).

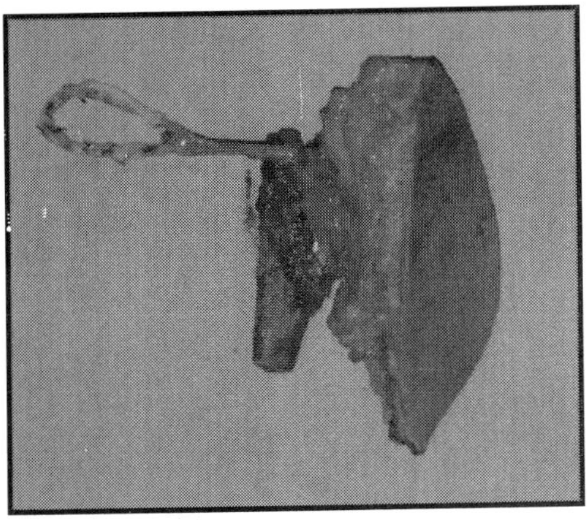

Figure 12. A skin paddle of the scapular flap.

8.5. Complications

Extended scapular flap loss is a major problem because a large area remains uncovered. Closure of the donor site under tension will result scar dehiscence and an unsightly result.

8.6. Scapular flap updates

The scapular tip free flap (STFF) has been used in reconstruction of mandibular defects. Low morbidity, early ambulation time, possibility of simultaneous harvesting with the tumor resection and large musculocutaneous paddles in the chimerical version of the flap are advantages of the STFF. This makes it a good choice in elderly patients, when other bone containing free flaps are not indicated because of the related morbidity, when other flaps are not available or when wide composite defects are approached.[42] Fibular and scapular osseous free flaps for oromandibular reconstruction were compared based on a patient-centered approach to flap selection. Results demonstrated the free fibula flaps and subscapular flaps are complementary options for oromandibular reconstruction. The fibular free flaps are ideal for younger patients, extended defects, multiple osteotomies, and limited soft-tissue requirements. The subscapular system free flaps are excellent options for (1) elderly patients; (2) those with significant comorbidities, such as peripheral vascular disease; and (3) mandible defects associated with complex soft-tissue requirements.[43] For immediate mandibular reconstruction, a scapular flap provides short-term results equivalent to those with a fibular flap but with less donor-site morbidity. The major drawbacks of the fibular flap include prolonged healing of the donor site and the delayed mobilization of patients. Although our first choice of vascularized bone graft is the fibular flap, the scapular flap is an alternative for those patients, especially elderly patients, in whom fibula harvest can result in significant morbidity. [44] Minimally invasive harvesting techniques may reduce potential donor-site morbidity. A reverse-flow scapular osteocutaneous flap has been introduced for head and neck reconstruction. The distal end of the thoracodorsal artery and subscapular vein were used in this type of the flap. There has been no report on endoscopically assisted harvesting of the scapular adipofascial flap. [45, 46]

Author details

Reza Tabrizi[1*] and Barbad Zamiri[2]

*Address all correspondence to: tabmed@gmail.com

1 Assistant Professor, Department of Oral and Maxillofacial Surgery, Shahid Beheshti University of Medical Sciences School of Dentistry, Shiraz, Iran

2 Associated Professor, Department of Oral and Maxillofacial Surgery, Shiraz University of Medical Sciences School of Dentistry, Shiraz, Iran

References

[1] Jones, N.F. and B.C. Sommerlad, Reconstruction of the zygoma, temporo-mandibular joint and mandible using a compound pectoralis major osteo-muscular flap. Br J Plast Surg, 1983. 36(4): p. 491-7.

[2] Hidalgo, D.A., A.L. Pusic, and F.-C. Wei, Free-flap mandibular reconstruction: a 10-year follow-up study. Plastic and reconstructive surgery, 2002. 110(2): p. 438-449.

[3] Fu-Chan Wei, S.S., Principle and Techniques of microvascular surgery. Plastic surgery. Saunders-Elsevier 2006. 1: p. 507-538.

[4] Krizek, T.J., et al., Experimental transplantation of composite grafts by microsurgical vascular anastomoses. Plastic and reconstructive surgery, 1965. 36(5): p. 538-546.

[5] Jason A.Spector, J.P.L., cutaneos defects :Flaps,Grafts,and Expansion. Current Therapy in plastic surgery,Saunders,Elsevier, 2006: p. 11-21.

[6] Nandra, B. The Maximum length of free bone grafts for Mandibular reconstruction-Are bone grafts greater then 6.0 cm more susceptible to infection and exposure? in 2014 Annual Meeting. 2014. Aaoms.

[7] Moscoso, J.F., et al., Vascularized bone flaps in oromandibular reconstruction: a comparative anatomic study of bone stock from various donor sites to assess suitability for enosseous dental implants. Archives of Otolaryngology–Head & Neck Surgery, 1994. 120(1): p. 36-43.

[8] Frodel, J.L., et al., Osseointegrated implants: a comparative study of bone thickness in four vascularized bone flaps. Plastic and reconstructive surgery, 1993. 92(3): p. 449-455.

[9] Beckers, A., et al., Comparative densitometric study of iliac crest and scapula bone in relation to osseous integrated dental implants in microvascular mandibular reconstruction. Journal of Cranio-Maxillofacial Surgery, 1998. 26(2): p. 75-83.

[10] Disa, J.J., et al., Simplifying microvascular head and neck reconstruction: a rational approach to donor site selection. Annals of plastic surgery, 2001. 47(4): p. 385-389.

[11] Suh, J.D., et al., Analysis of outcome and complications in 400 cases of microvascular head and neck reconstruction. Archives of Otolaryngology–Head & Neck Surgery, 2004. 130(8): p. 962-966.

[12] Mathes JS, H.S., Flap classification and application. Plastic surgery. Saunders-Elsevier, 2006. 1: p. 365-481.

[13] Quershy FA, P.M., Reconstruction of the maxillomandibular cancer patient. Fonseca oral and maxillofacial surgery,Saunders, 2000. 7: p. 361-444.

[14] S.Souter, D., Radial forarm flap. Flaps and reconstruction surgery,Saunders-Elsevier, 2009(25): p. 321-338.

[15] Soutar, D., et al., The radial forearm flap: a versatile method for intra-oral reconstruction. British Journal of Plastic Surgery, 1983. 36(1): p. 1-8.

[16] Santamaria, E., M. Granados, and J.L. Barrera-Franco, Radial forearm free tissue transfer for head and neck reconstruction: versatility and reliability of a single donor site. Microsurgery, 2000. 20(4): p. 195-201.

[17] Avery, C., Review of the radial free flap: is it still evolving, or is it facing extinction? Part one: soft-tissue radial flap. British Journal of Oral and Maxillofacial Surgery, 2010. 48(4): p. 245-252.

[18] Avery, C., Review of the radial free flap: still evolving or facing extinction? Part two: osteocutaneous radial free flap. British Journal of Oral and Maxillofacial Surgery, 2010. 48(4): p. 253-260.

[19] Dolan, R., Microvascular surgery. Lore and Medina, An atlas of head and neck surgery,Saunders-El, 2005: p. 1417-1470.

[20] Skoner, J.M., et al., Short-Term Functional Donor Site Morbidity After Radial Forearm Fasciocutaneous Free Flap Harvest. The Laryngoscope, 2003. 113(12): p. 2091-2094.

[21] Sardesai, M.G., et al., Donor-site morbidity following radial forearm free tissue transfer in head and neck surgery. Journal of otolaryngology-head & neck surgery= Le Journal d'oto-rhino-laryngologie et de chirurgie cervico-faciale, 2008. 37(3): p. 411-416.

[22] Ahuja, R.B., P. Chatterjee, and P. Shrivastava, A novel route for placing free flap pedicle from a palatal defect. Indian journal of plastic surgery: official publication of the Association of Plastic Surgeons of India, 2014. 47(2): p. 249.

[23] Silberstein, E., et al., Total Lip Reconstruction with Tendinofasciocutaneous Radial Forearm Flap. The Scientific World Journal, 2014. 2014.

[24] Hanna, T.C., W.S. McKenzie, and J.D. Holmes, Full-Thickness Skin Graft from the Neck for Coverage of the Radial Forearm Free Flap Donor Site. Journal of Oral and Maxillofacial Surgery, 2014.

[25] Chung, J., et al., The effect of topically applied tissue expanders on radial forearm skin pliability: a prospective self-controlled study. Journal of Otolaryngology-Head & Neck Surgery, 2014. 43(1): p. 8.

[26] Wester, J.L., et al., AlloDerm with split-thickness skin graft for coverage of the forearm free flap donor site. Otolaryngology--Head and Neck Surgery, 2014. 150(1): p. 47-52.

[27] Vittayakittipong, P., Donor-site morbidity after fibula free flap transfer: a comparison of subjective evaluation using a visual analogue scale and point evaluation system. International journal of oral and maxillofacial surgery, 2013. 42(8): p. 956-961.

[28] Christopher J.Salgado, S.L.M., Samir Mardani,Fu-chan Wei, Fibula flap. 1th edition ed. 2009: Saunders,Elesiever 439-455.

[29] Blackwell, K.E., Donor site evaluation for fibula free flap transfer. American journal of otolaryngology, 1998. 19(2): p. 89-95.

[30] Bodde, E.W., et al., Donor-site morbidity after free vascularized autogenous fibular transfer: subjective and quantitative analyses. Plastic and reconstructive surgery, 2003. 111(7): p. 2237-2242.

[31] Potter, J.K., et al., Proximal Peroneal Perforator in Dual–Skin Paddle Configuration of Fibula Free Flap for Composite Oral Reconstruction. Plastic and reconstructive surgery, 2014. 133(6): p. 1485-1492.

[32] Spinelli, G., et al., Microsurgical Reconstruction After Bisphosphonate-Related Osteonecrosis of the Jaw: Our Experience With Fibula Free Flap. Journal of Craniofacial Surgery, 2014. 25(3): p. 788-792.

[33] Pitak-Arnnop, P., et al., Fibular flap for mandibular reconstruction: Are there old tricks for an old dog? Revue de stomatologie, de chirurgie maxillo-faciale et de chirurgie orale, 2013. 114(1): p. 15-18.

[34] Chao, J.W., et al., Oral Rehabilitation Outcomes After Free Fibula Reconstruction of the Mandible Without Condylar Restoration. Journal of Craniofacial Surgery, 2014. 25(2): p. 415-417.

[35] Bisase, B., et al., The deep circumflex iliac artery perforator flap (DCIAP)—A reconstructive option for the large composite oro-mandibular cutaneous defect. British Journal of Oral and Maxillofacial Surgery, 2013. 51(8): p. 962-964.

[36] Ting, J., et al., Developments in image-guided deep circumflex iliac artery flap harvest: a step-by-step guide and literature review. Journal of oral and maxillofacial surgery: 2014. 72(1): p. 186-197.

[37] Elisabeth K.Beahm, M.M., Hanasono,Saleh Shenaq, Flaps and reconstruction surgery,Iliac Flap. 2009: Saunders,Elesiever 339-357.

[38] Zheng, H.-P., et al., Modified deep iliac circumflex osteocutaneous flap for extremity reconstruction: Anatomical study and clinical application. Journal of Plastic, Reconstructive & Aesthetic Surgery, 2013. 66(9): p. 1256-1262.

[39] Iida, T., et al., A free vascularized iliac bone flap based on superficial circumflex iliac perforators for head and neck reconstruction. Journal of Plastic, Reconstructive & Aesthetic Surgery, 2013. 66(11): p. 1596-1599.

[40] Kim, H.-S., et al., Anatomical basis of the deep circumflex iliac artery flap. Journal of Craniofacial Surgery, 2013. 24(2): p. 605-609.

[41] Claudio Angrigiani, J.P., Marcelo MackFarlane Fapls and reconstruction surgery,Scapular and parascapular flap. 2009: Saunders,Elsevier. 271-285.

[42] Bianchi, B., et al., Reconstruction of mandibular defects using the scapular tip free flap. Microsurgery, 2014.

[43] Dowthwaite, S.A., et al., Comparison of fibular and scapular osseous free flaps for oromandibular reconstruction: a patient-centered approach to flap selection. JAMA Otolaryngology–Head & Neck Surgery, 2013. 139(3): p. 285-292.

[44] Fujiki, M., et al., A comparison of perioperative complications following transfer of fibular and scapular flaps for immediate mandibular reconstruction. Journal of Plastic, Reconstructive & Aesthetic Surgery, 2013. 66(3): p. 372-375.

[45] Al-Benna, S., J.J. Kirkpatrick, and I. Taggart, Minimally Invasive Harvesting of Adipofascial Scapular Flaps. Annals of plastic surgery, 2014. 72: p. 666-669.

[46] Zevallos, J.P. and M.L. Urken, Reverse-flow scapular osteocutaneous flap for head and neck reconstruction. Head & neck, 2013. 35(6): p. E171-E174.

Chapter 28

Reconstruction of the Face Following Cancer Ablation

Ata Garajei, Ali Arabkheradmand,
Mohammad Hosein Kalantar Motamedi,
Alex E. Pazoki and Ashkan Rashad

Additional information is available at the end of the chapter

http://dx.doi.org/10.5772/59746

1. Introduction

Following ablation of a tumor that is the primary lesion or metastatic tissue, facial reconstruction is needed to restore and replace both hard and soft tissue losses. Ideally, reconstruction should strive to restore the maxillofacial form, quality of tissues, oral competence, and oral cavity functions, allowing the patient to return and adapt to society. Each area to be reconstructed must be considered individually to define the characteristics needed to provide the structural bed for total functional return. To focus on the reconstructive approaches and goals, an anatomic list should be compiled that includes:

1. Structures that are missing and their function,
2. Structures that are present but with compromised blood supply and/or function, and
3. Structures that are present and working well [1].

In general, goals of the reconstructive surgeon revolve around the restoration of functions, including normal deglutition with tongue and pharyngeal components; adequate oral competence; adequate mandibular mobility for functional mastication, with complete dental rehabilitation; airway support and patency after a tracheotomy to allow decannulation; fluent speech function paralleling deglutition; protective sensory function, especially sensations of the tongue, corneal blink reflexes, and trigeminal facial sensory nerves; and overall movement of the head and neck region, including shoulder lift and the muscles of the face [2]. As with all aspects of life, form usually follows function. Special attention must be paid to the preoperative facial aesthetic units that can be redefined, such as the mandibular symphysis, angle of the jaw, malar regions, nose, and teeth. The end result is a patient who is able to return to a normal lifestyle, engaging in routine activities of family life, work, and society. Reconstructive principles have been formulated to increase the predictability of successful surgery. They include the use of a team approach to decrease operative time by synchronous resection and flap preparation; avoidance of multiple flaps and vein grafts whenever possible; minimizing of flap ischemia by shaping the flap while still vascularized; and slight overcorrection of the soft tissue deficiency with well-vascularized soft tissues [3]. The ideal technique must be fast, reliable, and cost efficient, imposing minimal morbidity on the patient [4]. Considerable debate involving immediate versus delayed reconstruction continues. The reconstructive process may involve multiple staged surgical procedures, for which the patient will require extensive preoperative counseling.

Advocates of delayed treatment wait months to years after the original surgical resection [5]. Factors that disfavor an immediate approach include the covering of the primary site and therefore the inability to detect a recurrence, a longer surgical time, the possibility of seeding cancer cells in newly dissected tissue planes, and an increased risk of graft infection from the contaminated salivary environment [6]. In contrast, Markowitz and colleagues [7] were not able to demonstrate any advantage for delayed reconstruction. In fact, secondary surgery, or two-stage reconstruction, is associated with higher overall complication rate, longer hospital stay, and greater cost [8]. Heller and associates [9] studied the long-term benefits in 47 patients who underwent immediate reconstruction of the mandible and found acceptable functional and long-term survival results. Leaving the patient unreconstructed was advocated by those who felt that an adequate follow-up period to detect recurrence was required before complete reconstruction. Since the advent of extensive noninvasive imaging systems such as computed tomography (CT), magnetic resonance imaging (MRI), and single photon emission CT (SPECT) technology, physicians are better able to identify an early recurrence. Over the past decade, one-stage reconstructive efforts using musculocutaneous flaps and microvascular free tissue transfers have significantly improved the quality of life of such patients. When such a reconstruction is performed during the primary surgery, it allows postoperative radiation treatment to be administered in a timely fashion. Delaying postoperative radiation can result in increased morbidity and increase the risk of recurrence [10]. Furthermore, delayed reconstruction is preceded by considerable fibrosis and soft tissue contraction, increasing the difficulty of subsequent reconstruction and compromising functional and cosmetic restoration.

The advantages of immediate or early reconstruction in summary are as follows: reduction in the total number of surgical procedures, less time that the patient must endure deformity and morbidity, protection and preservation of vital structures, reduced economic cost of treatment, and rapid oral rehabilitation and return to normal social lifestyle [4]. The surgical result after cancer resection of the oral cavity and oropharynx is a significant functional and cosmetic defect. For example, a partial glossectomy leaves a patient with varying degrees of articulation and swallowing difficulties, depending on the amount of tongue tissue removed. Bony resection of the involved mandible produces masticatory problems, as well as alteration of facial contour.

A multidisciplinary team is often involved in the assessment and treatment of cancer patients. This team consists of head and neck surgeons, plastic surgeons, oral and maxillofacial surgeons, maxillofacial prosthodontists, radiation oncologists, medical oncologists, radiologists, pathologists, speech and occupational therapists, internists, and psychologists. Preoperative evaluation of the patient must include a full assessment of the patient's overall health, ability to tolerate prolonged general anesthesia and blood loss, emotional and intellectual abilities, motivation, and expectations. In addition, the status of the patient's airway and nutritional needs must be addressed. Preoperative physical examinations, endoscopies or panendoscopy, and radiologic evaluation (CT scans, MRI) must outline the tumor size, location, and tissue type (biopsy) and rule out other concomitant lesions. The choice of which reconstructive modality is used depends on the extent of the defect preoperatively. The stage of the disease, the type of node dissection, and the availability of neck vessels are determined by the surgeon. Transverse CT scan and a lateral cephalogram provide the model of the mandible in two dimensions. Enhanced three-dimensional reconstructive CT scans further outline the preoperative mandibular contours and provide a more complete model. Before surgery, it is equally important that the patient be evaluated by a prosthodontist to aid in the achievement of proper bimaxillary arch alignment for postsurgical dental rehabilitation. Angiograms or noninvasive Doppler studies of the recipient and donor vessels are obtained if their adequacy is in doubt, providing information regarding their vascular status. Successful outcome can be ensured when the overall medical condition of the patient, the extent of the disease and prognosis, and the potential donor sites are thoroughly evaluated in the preoperative setting. [11]

Reconstruction in head and neck cancer patients requires a thorough understanding of function and tissue defects needs to be restored. Anatomically, a classification system for maxillofacial rehabilitation has been described.

Maxillary defects encompass minor defects of the hard and soft palate to extensive hard and soft tissue losses from resections of the maxilla, soft palate, sinuses, and adjacent structures (i.e., orbit and cheek).

Mandibular defects include alveolar segments with associated soft tissues, as well as portions of the tongue and floor of the mouth.

Facial defects include structures of the orbit, nose, ear, and/ or cheek. Defects of the oral cavity and oropharynx of small to moderate size can be successfully closed primarily, as long as tongue mobility and the gingival sulcus are not compromised. The goal of reconstructive surgery is to achieve coverage of the soft tissue defect, providing a definitive separation between the oral cavity and the neck. This can be accomplished by use of either split-thickness or full-thickness skin grafts or local, regional flaps. Functional and aesthetic outcomes become less favorable as the extent of resection increases. Large defects, depending on the location, require vascularized skin, soft tissue, and muscle. The advantages of myocutaneous flaps are abundant blood supply, greater reliability, better effectiveness and predictability. These pedicled osteomyocutaneous flaps facilitate resistance to infection and resorption, which is directly related to the osseous vascular supply. Flap geometry, bone availability, and muscle bulk restrict the degree to which the pedicled flap will adapt to the defect [12]. The use of free microvascular flaps is another option for reconstruction in this region. The free microflaps provide vascularized skin and bone to regions formerly considered impossible to reconstruct owing to limitations of the donor site tissue. The most widely used free microvascular flaps are radial forearm flaps for the floor of the mouth defects involving segments of the mandible. Flap selection is based on the quantity and contour of bone required, as well as the volume of soft tissue necessary to accommodate the patient's needs. Whenever possible, it is best to use adjacent soft tissue. If this is not feasible, then a regional flap (e.g., pectoralis major myocutaneous flap or deltopectoral flap) may be required. Reconstruction of mandibular defects requires the use of myocutaneous and microvascular free flaps, in conjunction with osseointegrated dental implants, to provide satisfactory masticatory function. The goal of reconstructing a tooth-bearing mandible with adequate strength, with appropriate vestibular sulci, and without excessive soft tissue bulk continues to invite surgeons to develop new treatment options. Once the mandibular segments are properly aligned to restore a normal relationship with the maxilla, oral rehabilitation is easily accomplished by a maxillofacial prosthodontist. One area of oromandibular reconstruction that has challenged reconstructive surgeons is the restoration of preoperative sensory and motor functions. Both pedicled and free tissue flaps are large, insensitive tissue blocks that are used to replace oral tissues, thus compromising swallowing and speech mechanisms. It has been difficult to reproduce the complex neurosensory and muscular activities of the oral and pharyngeal viscera. There is a need for thin, pliable, sensate tissue to facilitate oral rehabilitation. Radial forearm, dorsalis pedis, lateral thigh, lateral arm, and fibular osteocutaneous flaps all possess thin, pliable tissue and identifiable sensory nerves that may be integrated into the reconstructive plan. [4] Urken and Moscoso [13] reported 80% sensory recovery in 40 cases of mandibular reconstruction with radial forearm flaps. Reconstruction of other bony defects typically requires bone grafting (cortical versus cancellous), bone containing vascularized pedicled or free flaps, and free nonvascularized bone grafts. With the advent of rigid fixation, bone grafting techniques have been enhanced, allowing broader applications. Alloplastic materials such as silicone and hydroxyapatite have been used to "fill in" bony defects and not to replace functional and structural tissue loss. The success of bone grafting is completely dependent on adequate stabilization, immobilization, and healthy soft tissue coverage. Once tissue has been irradiated, its repair capacity is compromised. In bone, hypovascularity, damage to osteoprogenitor cells and hypoxic tissue are responsible.

When a patient has received doses greater than 5000 rads (50 Gy) after ablative tumor surgery, significant reconstructive difficulties are encountered. Grafts placed into irradiated tissue beds have high rates of complications.

Hyperbaric oxygen (HBO) has been reported to help poorly perfused tissues by allowing hyperoxygenation [14], providing antimicrobial activity (cidal to anaerobes and static to microaerophilic organisms) [15], increasing fibroblastic proliferative activity [16], improving neovascularization and angiogenesis [17], increasing bone matrix formation [18], increasing mineralization [19], promoting osteoclastic activity to remove necrotic bone[20]; and enhancing the transport capacity of erythrocytes by increasing their deformability [21]. Ganstrom [22] suggested a protocol for HBO delivery: The patient is seated in a pressurized closed chamber that is above one atmospheric pressure. The patient breathes 100% oxygen, with oxygen toxicity avoided by regulating time and dose limits. Routinely, a single treatment (dive) varies from 90 to 120 minutes once or twice a day. Another protocol developed by Marx''' is as follows:

http://dx.doi.org/10.5772/59746

20 sessions of HBO at 2.4 atmospheres (ATA) for 90 minutes of oxygen breathing, once daily for 5 or 6 days per week. This is followed by the surgical procedure. Postoperatively, the patient undergoes 10 sessions of HBO, following the same preoperative regimen. The disadvantage of HBO is time consumption without improvement in the quantity of tissue; only the quality is enhanced. Also, HBO is expensive, ranging up to $50,000 for a treatment sequence. There are some contraindications to receiving hyperbaric oxygen, including optic neuritis, immune deficiency states, and end-stage chronic obstructive pulmonary disease. It is therefore very important to make a thorough assessment of the patient's medical history, pulmonary status, and chest radiograph. Occasionally, pulmonary function testing and ophthalmologic evaluation are required.

2. Grafts

2.1. Free skin grafting

Healthy skin grafts usually retain the same color as the donor area and retain the texture and appearance of normal skin (Figure. 1). Skin grafting to the oral cavity has been indicated for the correction of periodontal defects, minor and major preprosthetic defects, and implant surgery, as well as for the reconstruction of traumatic, congenital cleft, and tumor ablative surgery.

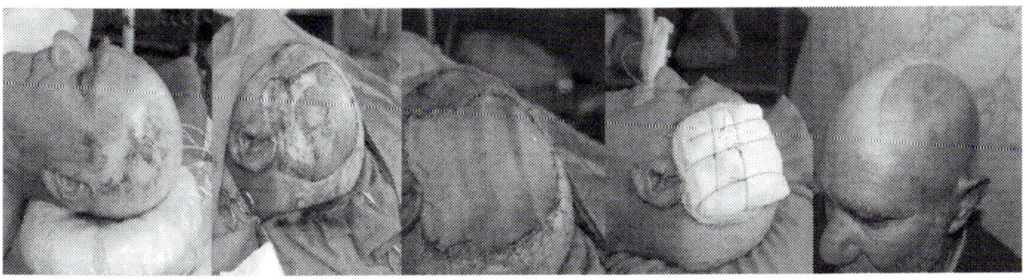

Figure 1. Free skin graft of the scalp.

Free grafting of the oral mucosa was first described by Propper [23] and was later refined by using mucotome and expanded mesh graft techniques. Skin grafts may be taken from a variety of donor sites. The anterior and lateral aspects of the thigh are frequently used because they can provide a sufficient quantity of graft material using a relatively simple procedure. The buttocks are also used as a donor site when cosmesis is a concern. Full-thickness skin grafts from a retroauricular location are chosen when a good color match is desired for facial reconstruction. For mucosal grafting, the cheek and palate are the two sites most widely used for oral transplantation. Theoretically, the tissue that is intended for reconstruction must closely match the nature of that which was removed. For example, lost periodontal tissues would best be replaced by palatal mucosa, as its thick keratinized nature allows it to withstand the mechanical insults of brushing. Split-thickness skin grafts may be harvested by adjusting the dermatome to control the thickness of the graft and to confine the amount of donor tissue being removed. The desired thickness of the graft is generally dependent on the correct adjustment on the dermatome, manual dexterity, pressure, advancement of the dermatome, and experience. A similar harvest can be obtained using a scalpel and sharp dissection of the epidermis and dermis from the underlying connective tissues. Oral mucosal grafts from the palate are taken free handed with a scalpel. A Mormann mucotome with a 6-mm blade is also suited for instrumentation. Skin grafts are preferably outlined before injection with a local anesthetic solution. In this way, the tissues are not distorted with the infused solution. If using a dermatome, a donor site with evident capillary bleeding from the dermal layer can be dressed with a Telfa cover sponge impregnated with 1:100,000 epinephrine solution and placed over the site for approximately 10 minutes for hemostatic control. A dressing is then placed to prevent infection and to promote rapid healing. Traditionally, a dressing with petroleum jelly gauze over the donor site works well. There is no need for antibiotics unless there is clinical evidence of infection. When using the free-hand technique for skin graft acquisition, the donor site must be closed primarily, which is relatively easy in the lateral thigh, buttocks, and inguinal regions. The subcutaneous tissues are undermined widely to allow for a tension-free closure. Sutures are placed in the subcutaneous layer, as well as in the skin. There is no need for a drain, provided that dead space has been eliminated using the layered closure. The graft is then placed on a wet gauze towel, which helps prevent folding of the graft edges. A "mesher" can be used to cut multiple slits in the graft to transform it into a lattice, which increases its area two to three times its original size. A meshed graft also has greater pliability to follow irregular contours. The use of slits also creates sites where blood and wound exudate can escape, providing optimal healing conditions. In order for skin grafting to be successful, graft immobility is of primary importance, especially during the early healing phase of revascularization. There have been various methods to achieve this goal: sutures, splints, wires, bone screws, and fibrin adhesive. Stents can be produced in advance using conventional dental impression materials and techniques. Ideally, graft immobility should be maintained for 5 to 7 days. Essentially, a graft that is not protected has a greater likelihood of failure. The use of freeze-dried allergenic grafts has been shown in studies to be comparable to skin grafts for maintaining vestibular depth. Lyophilized dura as a wound dressing after periodontal surgery was reported to delay healing time, with subsequent hematoma formation. There have been many similar studies comparing the effectiveness of allografts and xenografts with that of traditional fresh autogenous skin grafts. At present, there are no benefits in using such materials for oral and maxillofacial reconstruction.

2.2. Bone grafting

When faced with a patient who requires reconstruction of significant hard tissue losses of the mandible, bone grafting is the most viable treatment option. The continuity defect must be prepared with a graft that provides several functions. The principles of bone induction and conduction have been studied extensively over the years. The graft must be able to provide a source of viable osteogenic cells, such that it maintains sufficient osseous bulk and resists resorption for subsequent prosthetic rehabilitation. It must also act as a precursor for bone production and maturation by the bone induction principle. The graft must physically correct any facial form deficiencies resulting from underlying hard tissue losses.

2.2.1. *Autogenous bone grafts*

Autogenous bone is a viable treatment option. It can be particulate cancellous bone marrow, cortical blocks, or a combination of corticocancellous blocks. Particulate bone and cancellous marrow grafts contain numerous osteoprogenitor cells and allow a rapid revascularization. However, owing to their particulate nature, they require some form of containment via either soft tissue envelope-type pockets or rigid mandibular trays. The nonvascular corticocancellous blocks provide structure and bulk. The most common sites for acquisition are the anterior and posterior ilium, rib, and cranial bone. These types of grafts transplant more mineral content rather than osteocompetent cells. When grafting autogenous bone for reconstruction, one must pay close attention to the anatomic detail of the donor site as well as the amount, quality, and contour of bone to be used.

The iliac crest is widely accepted because it provides the greatest absolute amount of cancellous bone volume, as well as providing a cortical plate with significant structure and contour. When approaching the anterior ilium, the position and course of sensory cutaneous innervation must be considered. The nerve most often affected in this dissection is the iliohypogastric nerve, which courses over the area of the tubercle. The subcostal nerve traverses over the tip of the anterior superior iliac spine. The lateral femoral cutaneous nerve provides cutaneous sensory innervation to the lateral thigh region. It is located medially between the iliacus and psoas major muscles and then dives deep to the inguinal ligament, piercing the tensor fascia lata muscle. The incisions are therefore made lateral to the crest, avoiding the lateral femoral cutaneous nerve, extending from 2 cm posterior to the iliac tubercle, away from the subcostal nerve, to 1 cm posterior to the anterior superior spine. This places the incision away from the belt and waistband area, preventing excessive impingement. The blood supply to the anterior ilium is from terminal branches of the deep circumflex iliac artery. This lies medially and is avoided in the dissection. A roll is placed under the supinepositioned patient to elevate the iliac crest by lateral rotation at the hip. The patient is then prepped with povidone-iodine (Betadine) soap and paint and draped in a standard sterile fashion. Before sharp dissection, local infiltration of 1 % lidocaine with 1:100,000 epinephrine is used at the planned incision site for its local anesthetic and vasoconstrictive properties. A No. 15 blade is used to make the skin incision, extending to the subcutaneous tissues. Electrocautery is used to gain hemostatic control. The incision can then be manipulated to be centered over the crest. A sharp dissection is completed through the external and internal oblique musculature and periosteal layers to gain access to the bony crest. A subperiosteal reflection of the iliac crest in the medial direction is preferred, to avoid dissection of the tensor fascia lata muscles laterally, creating gait disturbances. Elevation of the iliacus muscle on the medial aspect of the ilium allows adequate access and visualization of the crest for retrieval of the desired bone graft. One must take care in this medial dissection to avoid accidental perforation of the peritoneum and/or bowel. Several osteotomy approaches, with either conventional mallet and osteotomes or air or electrical-driven saw blades, have been described to gain access to the cancellous bone. For small quantities of particulate cancellous bone marrow (PCBM), the "clamshell" approach requires an osteotomy in the midcrestal position to a depth just through the cortical plates. The medial and lateral cortices can be "split" and greensticked apart to allow a route of entry to the cancellous graft. The "trap-door" technique allows access by creating a midline osteotomy and reflecting either medial or lateral cortices, pedicled on adjacent muscles. The "hollowed crest" approach osteotomizes the crest in a horizontal fashion by "de-capping" the crest and reflecting the crest cap laterally to gain access to the central marrow (e.g., Tschapp approach). Finally, Tessier's approach attempts to maintain the contour of the crest by performing oblique osteotomies off the lateral and medial aspects and retrieving the bone deep to the crest itself. If a corticocancellous block is desired, full-thickness osteotomies are completed on the medial aspect, detaching the block at the most medial aspect. Once cancellous marrow has been found, bone can be harvested using a 3/8- or 1/2 inch bone gouge and series of curettes. Upon maximal retrieval, closure of the donor sites begins. Any sharp edges are smoothed with bone files. Hemostasis can be achieved with electrocautery of small perforating vessels, placement of bone wax, or microfibrillar bovine collagen (Avitene) to tamponade bleeding. A drain is usually required, exiting at a site away from the incision and suctioned at a low intermittent strength to avoid continuous aspiration of marrow blood. Closure is achieved primarily, first reapproximating periosteal layers with 2-0 Vicryl suture, muscular layers with 4-0 Vicryl suture, subcutaneous tissues with 3-0 chromic gut suture, subcuticular with running, pull-out, and skin with 4-0 nylon/praline suture. A pressure dressing is helpful in the immediate postoperative setting and can be accomplished with cover sponges and foam tape [24].

Rib harvesting provides an alternative source of autogenous bone (Figure 2).

At the present time, its primary indication is to reconstruct the mandibular articulation with good adaptation to the temporal fossa and reestablishment of ramus height, and also to augment an atrophic mandible. Depending on size and contour, fourth, fifth, and sixth ribs are best. The sixth rib is most widely used because it can be accessed through an inframammary crease incision. At this level, minimal muscle is transected, as the dissection is between the pectoralis major and rectus abdominis muscles, thus preserving these for future muscle flaps. With the patient in the supine position, an inframammary incision is made through the skin and subcutaneous tissues until fibers from the pectoralis major muscle (from above) and rectus abdominis muscle (from below) are seen attaching on the sixth rib. A periosteal incision is placed at the greatest convexity on the lateral aspect of the rib, and with the use of periosteal elevators, the rib is exposed from its costochondral junction anteriorly to a posterior length as much as 18 cm. The length is limited posterolaterally by the latissimus dorsi muscle.Careful elevation of the periosteum with Molt and Freer elevators is most effective in preventing small tears in the pleura, as small projections of the pleural cortex may tear with the use of large elevators. Once reflection is completed, the resection is begun at the cartilage site, taking only 3 mm of cartilage medially in both adults and children. Including more than 3 mm increases the chance for cartilage separation from bone, especially in children. Once the anterior end is separated from the sternum, the rib can be elevated by placing an instrument on the undersurface of the rib, protecting the parietal pleura as the posterior extent is reached. The posterior end is then cut, and the host end is smoothed with files. At this time, it is prudent to evaluate the pleura for tears. This can be done either visually or with the use of saline irrigation; the latter produces air bubbles if an air leak is present. Closure begins with periosteal approximation, followed by a muscle layer, subcutaneous tissue layer, and skin. Drains are usually not indicated. In children, a full morphologically normal rib will regenerate within 1 year, whereas in adults, an incomplete bone ossicle resembling a rib slowly forms over 1 to 3 years. [25]

Calvarial bone grafting for oral and maxillofacial surgery has progressed since its described use by Harsha and colleagues [26]. It has been widely used for vertical augmentation of maxilla and reconstruction of orbital wall and floor defects. It has a unique characteristic of early revascularization, which is directly related to the numerous vascular systems. As a result, the graft survives with little dimensional change. The paramedian portion of the parietal bone is the most likely area for harvest because it is the thickest, it is away from any vital structures (e.g., the superior sagittal sinus), and there is less chance that the scar will be visible in patients with male pattern baldness. The approach to this area requires a hemicoronal or bicoronal incision, posterior to the ear, and is carried through the five scalp layers (skin, subcutaneous tissues, galea-aponeurotic layer, loose connective tissue, and periosteum). Bleeding skin vessels are hemostatically controlled with Raney clips. The use of electrocoagulation may destroy hair follicles and result in patchy alopecia. A bur is used to create the shape of the desired graft in the outer cortex to the level of the cancellous marrow. Then, with the use of curved osteotomes, the outer table can be cleaved from the inner table in the plane of the interposed cancellous marrow. The incision is closed primarily in layers. Pressure dressings with "crani-caps" are placed to allow adaptation of the elevated tissues to bony scalp.

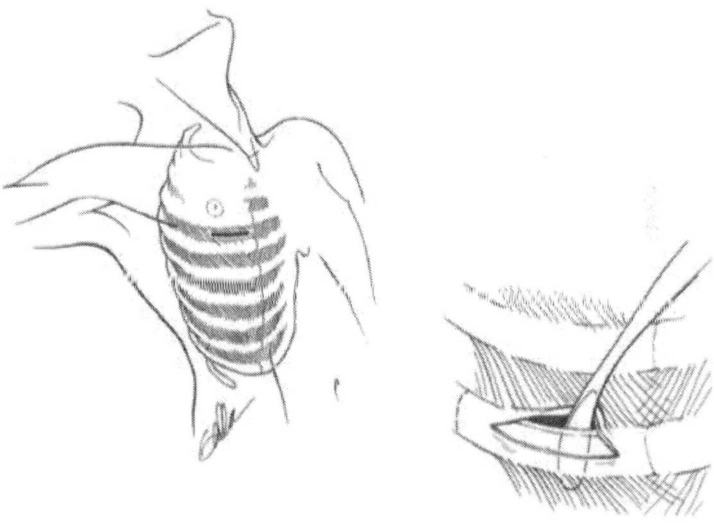

Figure 2. Rib harvesting

Rigid plate fixation [27] has resolved the problems with nonunion, but resorption continues to occur due to the stress shielding. Branemark and colleagues [28] in 1975 first reported the successful use of a block bone graft stabilized by a titanium plate in traumatic cases. Rigid plates have been well adapted to the preselected mandible to achieve the functional contours necessary for reconstruction. Li and associates [29] established a technique to maintain mandibular position with respect to the temporomandibular joint. Before resection, the mandible is placed in maximal intercuspation, with condyles seated firmly in the fossa.

Miniplates and screws are spanned bilaterally from the maxillary zygomatic processes to the mandibular ascending ramus. The plate is then adapted to the contour of the existing mandible, and the resection takes place. In this technique, the posterior facial height is maintained, as well as accurate adaptation of the condyle to the fossa. Ardary [30] also commented on the importance of adequately stabilizing the free bone graft with the use of a mandibular reconstruction plate in a report of nine consecutive cases with successful results. Absolute stability promotes neovascularization of the graft by permitting vascular ingrowth while simultaneously allowing for immediate postsurgical jaw function. Boyne [31] compared segmental defects in dogs that were bridged together with block bone or stabilized with a plate or with particulate bone and marrow within a Vitallium tray. He found significant resorption with the block bone, whereas complete bony regeneration and union were evident when the PCBM and tray were used. Dacron urethane mandibular trays were used with autogenous iliac crest bone in one study that showed retention of 80% of bony height over a 3-year period, with little alteration in the complication rate compared with standard reconstructive techniques [32]. The Dacron tray is a lightweight, biologically inert structure that is easy to adapt to the mandible, requiring a more limited access. Its radiolucency allows one to appreciate the radiographic monitoring of the bone graft. And, finally, reconstruction of the bone graft with fixation plates and metallic trays requires a second surgical procedure before endosseous dental implant placement, whereas the Dacron tray does not require removal. Mandibular reconstruction with reimplantation of resected mandibles that are hollowed out and function like a tray has been studied by Jisander and coworkers [33]. The prepared segments act as a matrix for new bone formation and as a carrier for transplanted cancellous bone. [34].

2.2.2. *Allogenic bone grafts*

Allogenic grafts are those taken from the same species but transplanted into a different individual. [35]. The major disadvantage of FFB is the small risk of disease transmission. [36] Bone substitutes, or alloplastic materials, have been used to recontour alveolar defects and as extenders in bone graft systems for reconstruction of major continuity defects. One such substitute is hydroxyapatite. It does not have the mechanical properties necessary for reconstructing major defects but provides a temporary matrix for future bone growth because of its osteoconductive nature.

Xenografts of bone and cartilage such as bovine bone mineral have been used as fillers or spacers in orthognathic and preprosthetic surgeries, as well as sinus grafting procedures (Figure 3) and alloplastic trays are commonly used to bridge the gap and to carry PCBM to fill mandibular defects. Its drawback is the risk of disease transmission. The Dacron-coated polyurethane crib is flexible, lightweight, biologically inert, easy to trim and adapt to the mandible, and radiolucent, which allows assessment of postoperative bone graft healing. Its disadvantages include its reliability in long-span mandibular defects, where intermaxillary fixation or internal reinforced metal rods are used for added rigidity.

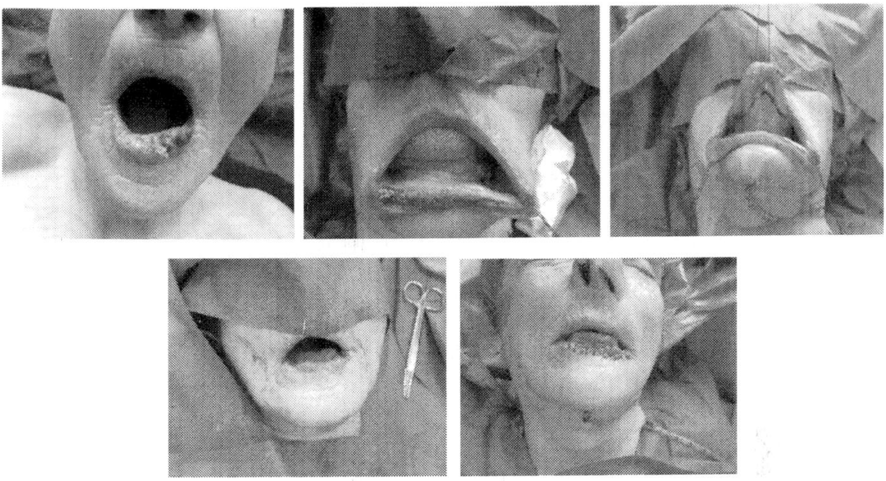

Figure 3. Polyurethane crib (left), alveolar bone grafting (right)

Metallic alloplastic trays have the ability to maintain the normal relationship of the residual mandibular segment without additional fixation, so the patient resumes normal functions earlier. The titanium tray is harder than the Dacron tray but softer than cobalt-chromium and stainless steel trays. The disadvantages of metallic cribs are that they have very high flanges in order to carry an adequate volume of bone, thus interfering with preprosthetic procedures and dental prostheses. This leads to tray removal. A simple technique was recently reported by Tayapongsak and coworkers [37] in designing a custom-made inferior border titanium crib (IBTC). The disadvantages of the custom-made IBTC are the use of intermaxillary fixation and its nonresorptive ability.

3. Flaps

Soft tissue flaps can be classified according to the method of movement (i.e., local or distant); according to blood supply, such as axial or random pattern; and according to the composition of the flap, such as cutaneous, myocutaneous, osteomyocutaneous, or fasciocutaneous. Random flaps consist of skin with the underlying subcutaneous tissues and frequently muscle. Their blood supply is provided by the plexuses from the dermal and subdermal regions. Axial patterned flaps have their perfusion from dominant vessels present with the flap. They may also contain secondary vessels to increase the flap's viability.

3.1. Local flaps

3.1.1. Lingual tongue flap

The use of tongue flaps was described as early as 1909 by Lexer, for the repair of cheek defects. Since then, tongue flaps have been described for facial and labial reconstruction [38]. Flaps from the dorsum of the tongue are designed lengthwise, usually paramedian, with a posterior or anterior base. Transverse flaps do not cross the midline of the body of the tongue, because its blood flow would be compromised. The posteriorly based dorsal tongue flap relies on the dorsal lingual artery for its survival. It usually runs the entire length of the tongue, from the circumvallate line to its anterior tip. The thickness of the flap is approximately 8 mm and is uniform, to avoid a wedge-shaped cross section. The flap includes mucosa and the adherent stratum of the superior lingual musculature. The flap, once elevated, can be rotated laterally and backward to repair the defect in the retromolar trigone or tonsillar region on the ipsilateral side, or to repair a cheek defect. This donor region is closed by direct suture, with meticulous attention to hemostasis. Dead space is eliminated by interrupted buried sutures, thus preventing hematoma formation and airway compromise. This closure does not affect the tongue's lingual function.

The anteriorly based dorsal tongue flap offers greater mobility, because the pedicle is on the free end of the tongue, and is thus more versatile. The tip of the tongue is supplied by the anastomotic ranine arch, which is the terminal branch from the forward continuation of the lingual artery. This vessel gives off numerous branches as it ascends to the tip. Thus the flap, which appears delicate and friable, is more robust than imagined. This type of flap is indicated mainly to repair anterior cheek and commissural defects. With outward rotation, it can be used to replace the lining and vermilion of the lips. With downward rotation, it is able to repair floor of the mouth defects in the anterior region, as well as anterior lateral defects when rotated through a window in the median raphe of the tongue. And by forward reflection, it can cover oronasal defects in cleft patients and excisional defects of the hard palate. As opposed to the posterior-based flap, the anterior one requires second-stage surgery to divide the tongue at its pedicle in order to maintain speech and swallow function.

The transverse dorsal tongue flap is usually created in bipedicle form, such that the flap is transferred anteriorly from the tongue to the floor of the mouth or to the lip, and the donor defect is closed primarily by approximation. The disadvantage is that tongue length is diminished and blunting of the free end occurs. This type of flap is recommended in cases in which length is not a factor.

The perimeter flap is developed by a vertical incision just inside and parallel to the border of the tongue. These flaps are narrow and may be uni- or bipedicle in design. Their use is indicated mainly for repair of lip vermilion defects, and variations in flap design are possible. Because of the anastomotic ranine arch, there is no compromise of vascular supply.

Dorsoventral flaps are derived from the lingual tip by a horizontal incision, inside and parallel to the edge, and are wider than they are long. They can be reflected dorsally on a posterior base to reconstruct the lining of the upper lip. The flap can also be reflected ventrally on an anterior base for lower lip reconstruction. A combination of both types of flaps can be incorporated to reconstruct vermilion and lining. The only drawback in creating these flaps is the resultant shortening of the tongue, which may affect speech and swallow mechanisms.

Ventral-based flaps have been described for repairs of anterior floor of the mouth defects, where two parallel lengthwise posterior-based flaps are reflected and rotated to the anterior defect. The resultant donor site cannot be closed primarily because of obvious contraction of the tongue. In this case, a skin graft can be placed to cover the donor site and is in fact well tolerated, with minimal effect on tongue mobility. This flap also has good results for vermilion reconstruction [38] (Figure 4)

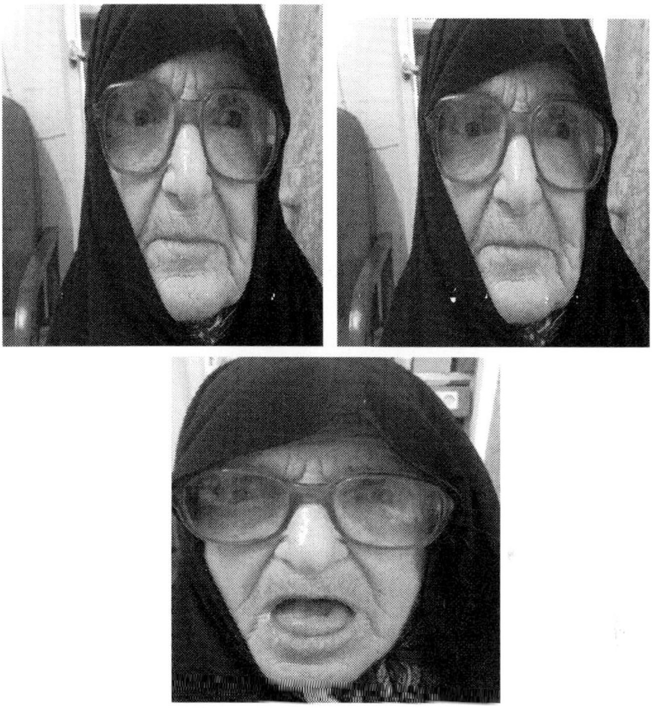

Figure 4. Reconstruction of the lower lip with a pedicled tongue flap.

3.1.2. Nasolabial flap

Nasolabial flaps are more useful for intraoral reconstruction when they are based inferiorly. With this design, floor of the mouth, tongue, and anterior mandibular defects can be reconstructed (Figure 5). In the dissection, it is important to include a thick portion of the underlying subcutaneous tissues to provide adequate blood supply to the flap. Its primary supply is from the branches of the facial artery. The flap can be based superiorly for upper alveolar or palatal resurfacing. A long, tapered flap is designed on the hairless skin edge along the nasolabial fold. The epithelium is removed at the base and tunneled through the cheek. It is then sutured in the oral cavity at the desired site and to its contralateral counterpart as the flaps lie side by side to provide wide coverage of the deficiencies.

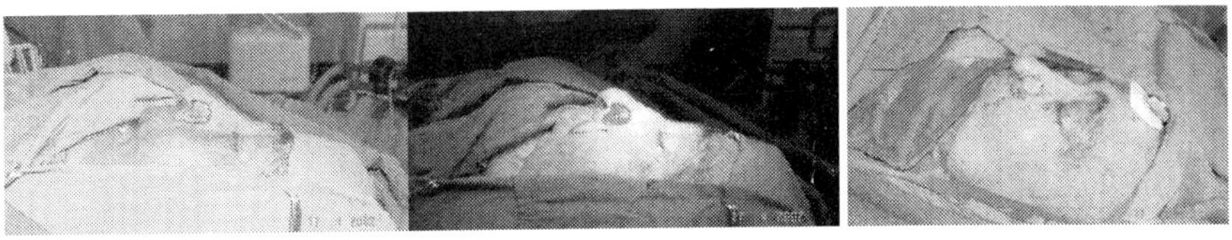

Figure 5. Nasolabial flap.

3.1.3. *Cervical island skin flap*

For defects that include the oral mucosa, gingiva, and part of the mandible after excision of gingival carcinomas, a cervical island skin flap has been described for reconstruction, alongside a bone graft for the hard tissue mandibular bony defect [39]. The cervical island flap was first described by Farr and colleagues [40]. The size of the skin island depends on the extent of the resected oral mucosa and gingiva, which in most cases is 2 to 2.5 cm in width and 4 to 5 cm in length. A skin margin of 3 mm is elevated to suture the skin of the flap to the oral mucosa (Figure 6).

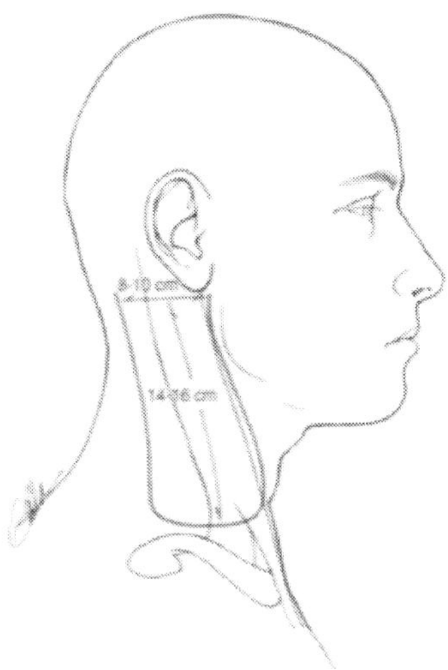

Figure 6. Cervical Island Skin Flap

The flap is passed under the mandible and introduced medial to the mucosal defect. The margin of the denuded distal part of the flap is sutured to the lingual edge of the cut surface of the remaining mandible. The border of the skin island is sutured to the mucosa of the floor of the mouth and the anteroposterior adjoining gingiva, thus forming a partition. The lateral margin of the skin island is sutured to the buccal mucosa. This creates a pocket from the cervical flap. The pocket can then be filled with autologous PCBM or hydroxyapatite granules. The study by Tashiro and associate [39] showed successful reconstruction using this technique. Reconstructed mandibles lost approximately 8% to 22% of their bone height, with patients wearing their prostheses comfortably. Minimal necrosis of the flaps was noted.

3.1.4. Bilobe skin flap

Bilobe flaps are double transposition flaps that share a single base (Figure 7). Similar to single transposition flaps, bilobe flaps move around pivotal points located at their base and develop standing cutaneous deformities as they pivot. Since each flap or lobe moves around an independent pivotal point, each lobe develops and individual standing cutaneous deformity. The greater is the arc of movement about their pivotal points, the larger are the standing cutaneous deformities.

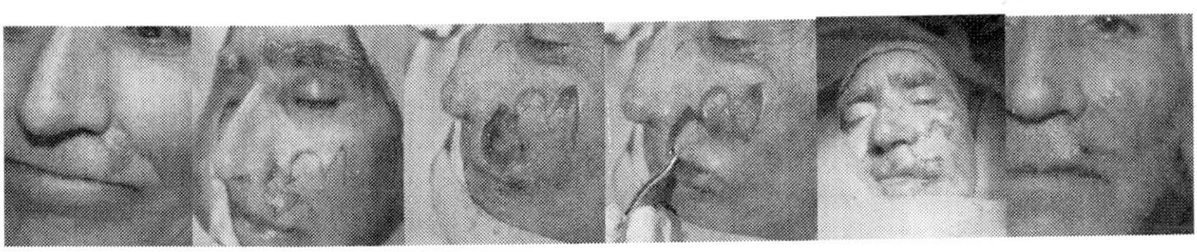

Figure 7. Bilobed skin flap

3.2. Regional flaps

3.2.1. Pedicled fasciocutaneous/myocutaneous/muscle flaps

The pectoralis major myocutaneous flap was first introduced by Ariyan [41] in 1979, and along with the forehead flap, it was the most commonly used flap for head and neck reconstruction in the early 1980s. However, these flaps consisted of only epithelium and some subcutaneous tissue and therefore were not appropriate for defects in which bulk had to be restored. The total scheme of soft tissue reconstructive management is dependent on the type of pathology being treated. For example, the management of oral cancer requires immediate soft tissue reconstruction. Also, in areas where reconstructive bone plates are used, it is usually paramount to have the plate covered with a muscle flap when postoperative adjuvant radiotherapy will be used, which helps prevent skin dehiscence overlying the bone plate.

3.2.2. *Sternocleidomastoid myocutaneous/ muscle flap*

The sternocleidomastoid (SCM) myocutaneous flap was first described by Owen [42] in 1955. This type of flap has been reported in the literature for a variety of indications[43]. These include aiding in mucosal reconstruction by providing an epithelial lining; creating a facial cover to close orocutaneous fistula; releasing scar contractures, especially around the angle and submandibular regions; providing additional tissue to allow for a passive, tension free closure; and, when used as a muscle flap, obliterating dead space around a bone graft. It is also a very vascular flap that, when used in an irradiated tissue bed, provides additional perfusion to the bone graft material. This strap muscle originates at the medial third of the clavicle (muscular) and near the manubrium (tendon). The SCM is innervated by a branch of the spinal accessory nerve, which is found between the internal carotid artery and the internal jugular vein, outside the carotid sheath, and enters the deep surface of the muscle. The dominant blood supply is from branches of the occipital artery and corresponding vein. The muscle also receives blood supply from the superior thyroid artery and vein, and the entire muscle and overlying skin remain viable (Figure 8). The inferior third aspect of the muscle is supplied by a branch of the inferior thyroid artery and a branch of the thyrocervical trunk, which may be sacrificed if not contained in the desired flap design. The dissection begins by outlining the skin paddle at the anterior and posterior borders with a scalpel and dissecting through skin, subcutaneous tissues, and platysmal muscle until the SCM is reached. The myocutaneous flap is then separated from the clavicular and sternal origins and deeply dissected to the level of the carotid sheath. This dissection is carried superiorly, always taking care to avoid trauma to the contents of the carotid sheath. At the level of the carotid bifurcation and anterior to the muscle, the branches of the superior thyroid artery are found. Just below the level of the bifurcation, the spinal accessory nerve enters the posterior dorsal surface of the muscle. It is important that this nerve be preserved, to maintain the function of the trapezius muscle. Thus, neuromuscular blocking agents are not recommended. The flap is developed until adequate length to reach the recipient site without tension is achieved. One of the drawbacks of this flap is the limited size and arc of rotation. For this reason, these flaps are not used for defects involving the anterior floor of the mouth. Functionally, use of the SCM muscle for reconstructive purposes does not lead to the inability to rotate the head to the contralateral side, as this function is maintained by other muscles (splenius capitis, trapezius, and suprahyoid muscles of the contralateral neck).

3.2.3. *Temporalis muscle flap*

Temporalis flap can provide abundant tissue for soft tissue reconstruction of the upper two thirds of the face, as well as reconstruction of the oropharynx (Figure 9). Use of this flap has been studied extensively. It was first described by Golovine, who used the flap for the obliteration of dead space after orbital exenteration as cited by Huttenbrink [44]. It is used to reconstruct composite defects of the maxilla, as well as areas of scar contracture and soft tissue deficiencies. Cheung [45] described the use of the temporalis flap for intraoral defects after maxillectomies in cats and the healing mechanisms of the flap in the oral cavity. He found a biologic response similar to that of humans, with regeneration of smooth palatal mucosa,

http://dx.doi.org/10.5772/59746

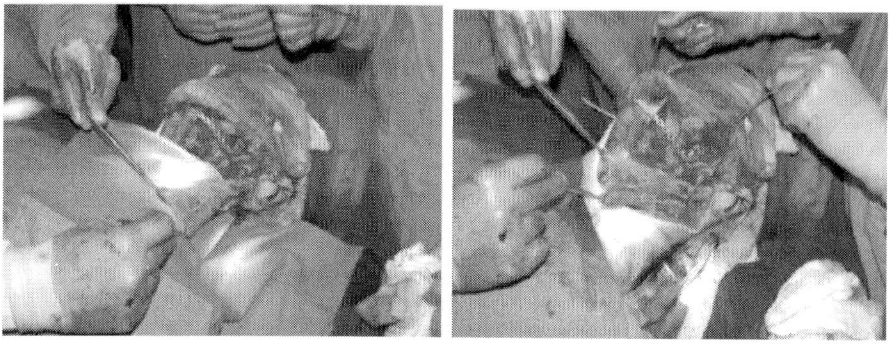

Figure 8. Sternocleidomastoid Myocutaneous/ Muscle Flap

without ruga formation. Anatomically, the fan-shaped, bipennate temporalis muscle is based on the main vascular supply from the anterior and posterior deep temporal arteries, which arise from the second division of the maxillary artery. The anterior deep temporal artery enters the muscle approximately 1 cm anterior to the coronoid process, whereas the posterior branch is 1.7 cm posterior to the bony landmark. Thus, the mobilized flap, consisting of the fascia, muscle, and pericranium, can be split into anterior and posterior flaps.

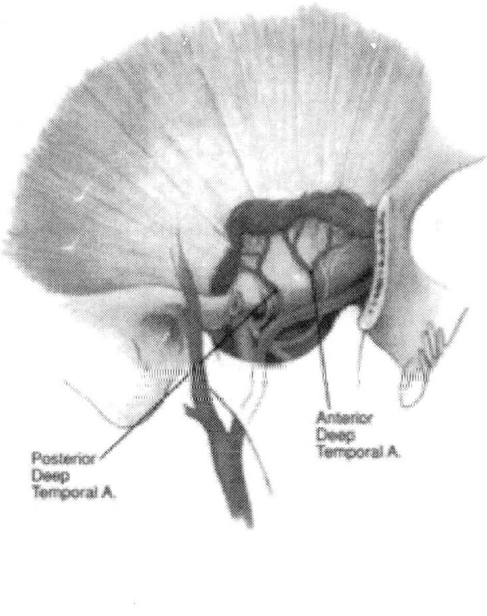

Figure 9. Temporalis muscle

An additional flap can be pedicled from the middle temporal artery, which arises from the superficial temporal artery immediately superior to the zygomatic arch. Located immediately deep to the subdermal layer is the superficial temporal fascia, which is a thin, highly vascular layer of moderately dense connective tissue. On its deep aspect, a very loose areolar tissue separates it from the deep temporal fascia. A temporoparietal fasciocutaneous flap described by Upton and colleagues [46] can be raised, as it is based on the superficial temporal artery. It is a prefabricated flap, in that a full-thickness skin graft is placed on the temporoparietal fascia 2 weeks before reconstruction. Access to the temporal flap is via a bicoronal incision and flap. It has the advantage of being very thin and quite sturdy and is suitable for the maxillofacial region. The dissection extends to the deep temporal fascia until the entire muscle is exposed. In this way, the temporal branch of the facial nerve (cranial nerve VII) is protected. In a subperiosteal plane, the muscle is then stripped of the temporal bone. When used for reconstructing the oral cavity, passage to enter the mouth requires fracturing the zygomatic arch as far posteriorly and anteriorly as possible and displacing it laterally, providing a tunnel into the mouth. The flap can then be rotated by dividing the coronoid process carefully, so as not to sever the vascular pedicle. Its ability to provide a large amount of tissue for reconstructing facial defects results in a mild cosmetic deformity at the donor site (i.e., hollowing of the temporalis fossa). However, with time, the depression may be hidden either by scar tissue or by hairstyle. If only an anterior flap is being used, the posterior flap can be rotated to fill in the prominent depression. Alloplastic materials, such as acrylic, have been used to fill in the defect.

3.2.4. Forehead myocutaneous flap

The forehead flap is a powerful tool in nasal and surrounding area reconstruction and is currently the method of choice for resurfacing large nasal defects [47]. It has evolved from its ancient roots as a broad-based flap with significant donor site morbidity and excessive bulk to an elegant procedure using a narrow pedicle with adequate length and appropriate thickness to achieve an esthetically pleasing result for both the patient and surgeon [48] (Figure 10).

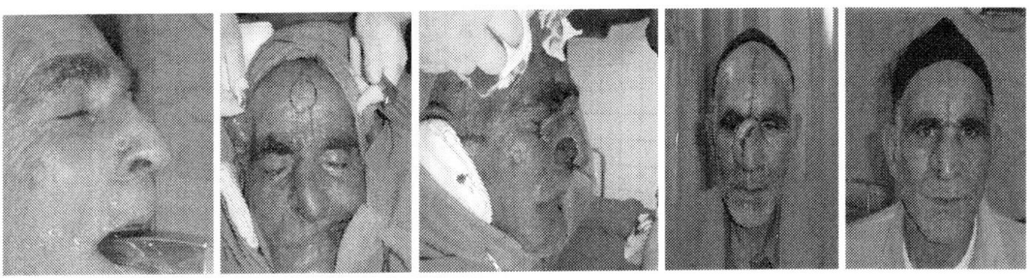

Figure 10. Forehead Myocutaneous Flap

Advances in understanding of the anatomic basis for forehead flaps have allowed surgeons to expand the versatility of the pedicle without compromising viability. The midline skin paddle has advantages, which include a favorable donor site scar [49]. The forehead flap is multilamellar, consisting of skin, subcutaneous tissue, frontalis muscle, and a thin, areolar layer. Elevated as a full thickness flap based on a paramedian pedicle, its supratrochlear vessels pass deeply over the periosteum at the supraorbital rim and travel vertically upward through the muscle to lie at an almost subdermal position under the skin at the hairline. It is both a myofascial and axial flap, and highly vascular [50] (Figure 11).

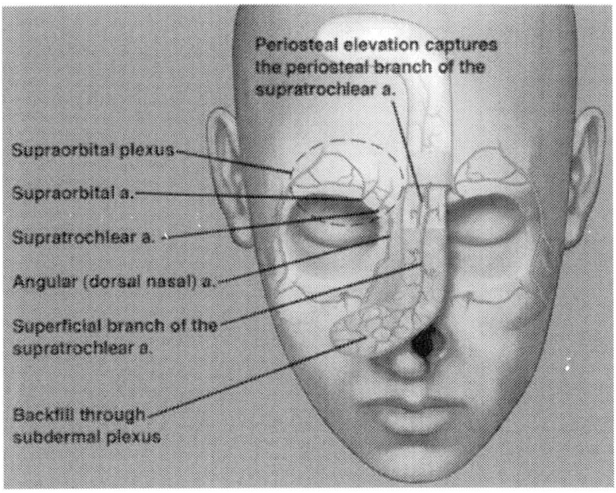

Figure 11. Forehead Myocutaneous Flap

The use of tissue expansion in conjunction with this flap has been an important, managing factor for these problems (Figure 12). [51]

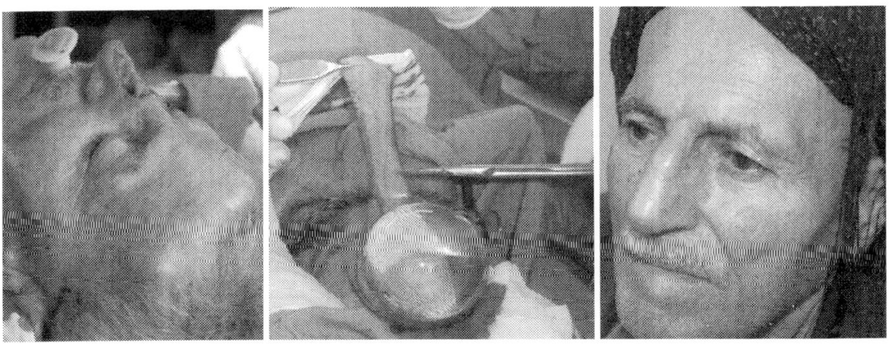

Figure 12. Forehead Myocutaneous Flap

3.2.5. Temporoparietal fasciocutaneous flap

Over the years, many uses have been found for the well-vascularized and long-reaching pedicled temporoparietal fascial (TPF) flap (Figure 13).

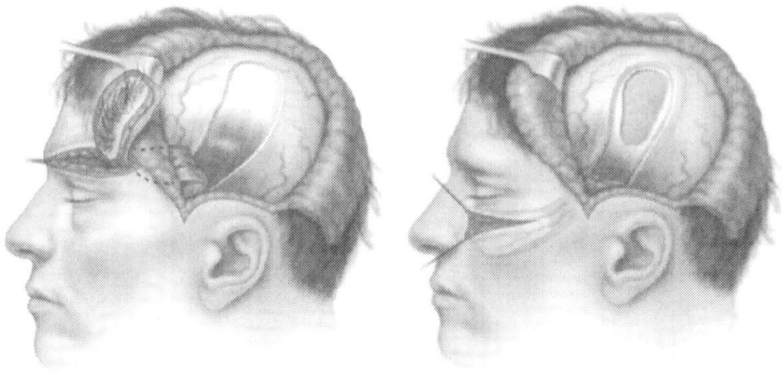

Figure 13. Temporoparietal Fasciocutaneous Flap

It has been used for several reconstructive situations, including functional and esthetic restoration of the extended maxillectomy; mandibulectomy; anterior skull base; oral cavity; base of tongue; and pharyngeal, orbital, auricular, mastoid, scalp, dura, cheek, lip, eyelid, and brow deficits. It also provides excellent vascular inflow for cases of infection such as with osteoradionecrosis of the facial or mandibular bones, or coverage for carotid protection [51]. When confronted with a head and neck defect following tumor resection or trauma, especially in a chemoradiated field, one must call upon a hardy, reliable and flexible flap for reconstruction, such as the TPF flap. Additionally, the TPF flap avoids the relatively awkward positioning of free flaps and musculocutaneous flaps and still is richly vascular. There are several variations of the TPF flap, including the superficial temporal vessels-pedicled pericranial-galea flap, which can be used in combination with an iliac bone graft to reconstruct the orbital floor, and palate in total maxillectomy defects with globe preservation [51]. The TPF flap can be used in composite with outer-table or full-thickness calvarial for maxillectomy/ orbital floor or mandibular deficits. This modification was originally described by Conley [51] but with the entire temporalis muscle. This tissue also has been used as a free microvascular flap.

3.2.6. Scalp myocutaneous flap

The scalp consists of five layers: skin, subcutaneous tissue, galea aponeurotica, subaponeurotic areolar tissue and pericranium. The three outer layers are closely joined, and function as a single entity. Skin thickness in this region ranges from 3 to 8 mm, making it the thickest in the body. The adnexal tissues, nerves, lymphatics, and principal scalp vessels are located in a dense layer of subcutaneous tissue underlying the skin. The paired occipitalis and frontalis muscles are connected at the vertex by the galea aponeurotica which is an elastic musculofascial layer supported by the areolar tissue in the sub- aponeurotic space. This is by far the strongest and most important layer. The primary function of the subaponeurotic layer is to enable scalp mobility. It is comprised of loose, thin, connective tissue facilitating this movement. The pericranium is the innermost layer of the scalp. Generally, scalp flaps are elevated superficial to this layer. There are many different types

http://dx.doi.org/10.5772/59746

of rotation flap techniques that may be used for reconstruction of scalp defects. The reconstructive surgeon has used rotation, sliding, and direct advancement bipedicled flaps since the mid-twentieth century. Rotation flaps are used primarily for small defects. Transposition flaps are used for larger defects (Figure 14).

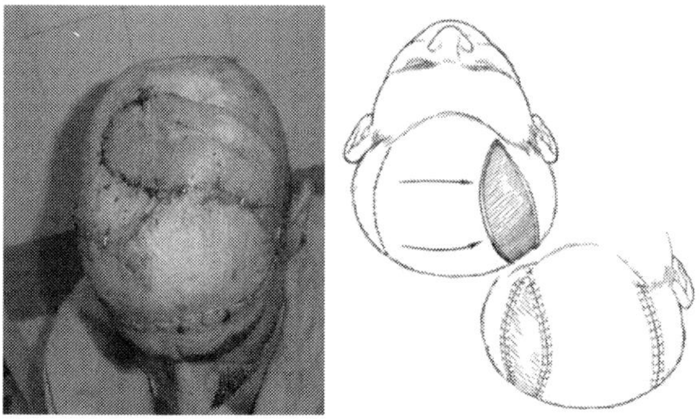

Figure 14. Scalp Myocutaneous Flap

The use of tissue expansion in scalp reconstruction has been an important in managing these problems (Figure 15).

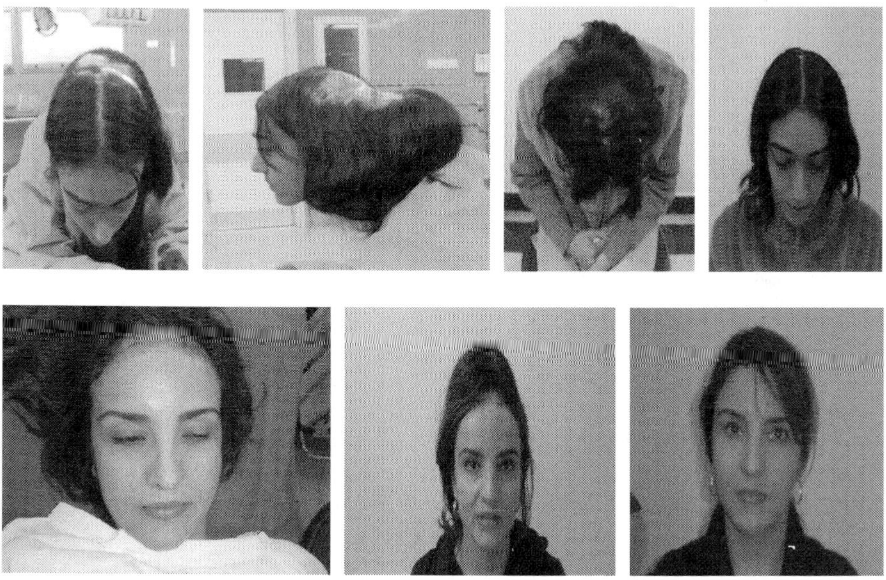

Figure 15. Scalp Myocutaneous Flap

3.2.7. Platysmal myocutaneous flap

The platysmal flap has been described as an axial flap used for soft tissue reconstruction in oral and maxillofacial surgery. It has significant advantages in reconstruction of the buccal mucosa after excision of lesions such as squamous cell carcinoma; the flap is close to the site of reconstruction, as well as being a thin and generally hairless tissue surface that is adequate to line the buccal mucosa. Also, carcinomas of the buccal mucosa rarely require neck dissections. In situations in which neck dissection is performed, the major vascular branch to this flap, the submental branch of the facial artery, is likely to be sacrificed, therefore obviating the use of this type of flap. The flap is not indicated in patients with previous irradiation, because the small perforators supplying blood to the subdermal plexus may provide inadequate perfusion to the flap. This type of flap is indicated for stage I and II gingival squamous cell carcinomas that require oral lining. It can cover an exposed area of mandible where other types of coverage, such as skin grafts, would not survive. It can be used as a bipedicle neck flap for closure of a tight neck during bone graft reconstruction and as a random pattern flap for closure of bone graft dehiscence. This muscle of facial expression originates from the skin just inferior to the clavicle and inserts into the skin of the face superior to the body of the mandible. Its motor function is supplied by cranial nerve VII (the facial nerve), and sensory innervation of the overlying skin is by the cutaneous nerves of the cervical plexus (C2 and C3). Again, the major artery for the pedicle is the submental branch of the facial artery. It also has a minor pedicle that is supplied by the superficial branch of the transverse cervical artery. The overlying skin is supplied by small perforators from these two main vessels. This is a technically easy flap that can be harvested in the same operative field, providing a thin and pliable flap for resurfacing deficiencies. The skin paddle is outlined by determining the size of the recipient defect. The skin paddle is placed in the supraclavicular fossa when the site to be reconstructed is located in the upper neck or oral cavity. Skin incisions are made over the anterior and posterior aspects of the muscle or parallel to the midline and are carried down to the midline, taking care to avoid cutting through the muscle. The deep aspect of the muscle is dissected down to the investing layer of the deep cervical fascia. The flap is then undermined superficially to the investing fascia and mobilized superiorly, where the submental branch of the facial artery is coursing in a horizontal fashion over the submandibular gland. The dissection is continued until adequate mobility of the flap is achieved to cover the defect [43]. Esclamado and coworkers [52] described 12 consecutive patients undergoing reconstruction for T2 and small T3 lesions of the oral cavity and oropharynx. They reported a flap survival rate of 92%, whereas earlier studies had reported 80% to 85%. Their complications were related to skin paddle loss, pharyngocutaneous fistula, and intraoral wound dehiscence, related to excessive tension on the muscle pedicle as it was rotated to the recipient site. The apron flap is a musculocutaneous flap incorporating the platysmal muscle. It can provide an adequate amount of thin tissue to resurface defects involving the floor of the mouth. It is usually outlined in the lower part of the neck. The base is frequently de-epithelialized in order to turn the flap under the mandible and into the floor of the mouth in a one-step procedure. The donor site can be closed primarily by undermining skin edges to achieve advancement of the adjacent tissues of the cervical skin. This reconstruction provides a thin lining to the remaining mandible and reconstructed floor of the mouth.

http://dx.doi.org/10.5772/59746

3.3. Pedicled osteomyocutaneous flaps

In the development of mandibular reconstruction techniques, it was evident that nonvascular bone grafting was a less reliable technique, because there was a high rate of infection secondary to salivary contamination, and vascularity to the graft was limited by the vascularity of the recipient bed in cases of previous irradiation. As a result, a poor success rate was obtained. [53-60] Using vascularized bone implies the maintenance of an intact blood supply to the bone during transplantation. This enables the donor bone to retain its original volume when incorporated for mandibular defects. The additional blood supply also aids in resisting infection and extrusion of the graft. The bone remains viable and does not need to be replaced by "creeping substitution." The healing time is therefore shortened, and function is regained earlier. An early study compared vascularized bone grafts with nonvascularized types and concluded that free grafts undergo resorption but pedicled bone grafts have greater survival [61-63]. Pedicled osteomyocutaneous flaps have the advantages of ease of flap harvest, relatively short operative time, decreased resorption, improved healing, and decreased infection rate. Their disadvantages include limited amount of bone for grafting, a variable vascular supply, and limited maneuverability of the bone. These factors contribute to an overall lower success rate compared with that of composite free tissue transfers, which is about 95%. However, the latter flap designs require increased sophistication and expertise and prolonged operative time. The following pedicled osteomyocutaneous flaps are clinically useful techniques for head and neck skeletal reconstruction.

3.3.1. Sternocleidomastoid osteomyocutaneous flap

Conley and Gullane [64] first described the SCM flap with a bone component for head and neck repairs. It was further described by Siemssen and colleagues [65] in 1978 for reconstruction of traumatic mandibular fractures, osteoradionecrosis, and mandibular defects following cancer resection. Barnes and associates [66] in 1981 made further technical modifications and cited a 3- year follow-up with no bone resorption. The SCM osteomyocutaneous flap was recently used by Friedman and Mayer [67] for tracheal reconstruction using clavicular periosteum with an SCM pedicle in cases of long-standing subglottic or tracheal stenosis. They were able to conform the clavicular periosteum to that of the trachea, with resulting bone formation to provide stability to the airway. The technique for raising an SCM osteomyocutaneous flap is to use the contralateral muscle and bone for reconstruction. After tumor resection, the clavicle is measured to obtain the desired segment to fill the mandibular defect. The clavicle that is harvested must include its medial portion and at least two thirds of the lateral clavicular body. Once the SCM muscle is dissected, preserving the clavicular attachments, the thyrocervical trunk, its blood supply, is identified and transected. The superior thyroid trunk is preserved superiorly, as is the spinal accessory nerve. Once the clavicle is released from all its attachments except for the SCM, it is rotated on the muscular pedicle across the midline into the defect and fixated with conventional bone fixation systems. The intraoral defect is closed primarily, the external skin flap is repositioned, and the neck is closed in a standard layered closure. The primary problem with this type of flap is the tripartite blood supply to the SCM muscle. The flap as described is a superior based one, which has the occipital artery as the major supply to the superior aspect of the muscle only. Thus the skin component of the flap is unreliable. Other disadvantages include the exposure of the great vessels of the neck after mobilization and a resulting contour deformity of the neck. However, the flap is a rapid, technically easy flap to elevate for one-stage immediate reconstruction of oromandibular defects.

3.3.2. Pectoralis major-rib osteomyocutaneous flap

In 1979, the pectoralis myocutaneous flap was first introduced, and it has been modified over the years. Cuono and Ariyan [68] first reported a case in which they used a rib graft for mandibular reconstruction and proved its viability 3 months postoperatively. Multiple studies have reported on the inconsistencies of this flap, with the primary limitations involving the tenuous blood supply, which hinders manipulation and contouring of the transferred bone. The size of the skin island is also limited, and it cannot be manipulated on the pedicle to achieve the desired closure. Additional graft resorption occurs, as well as pectoralis muscle atrophy, loss of cartilage, and separation of the graft from the mandible. Therefore, several other modifications have been designed to overcome these limitations. The pectoralis osteomyocutaneous flap has its dominant vascular pedicle based on the pectoral branch of the thoracoacromial artery, which is located beneath the clavicle at the midsuperior edge of the muscle. Other vascular pedicles include that which contains the lateral thoracic artery and other perforating arterial branches at the first through sixth intercostal spaces off the internal mammary artery. The skin island is chosen to lie in a transverse axis over the fifth rib between the nipple and sternum. Placement in the inframammary crease is an alternative site, especially in female patients. The elliptic skin island is incised through skin and subcutaneous tissues to the level of the pectoralis major muscle. The muscle is dissected from the inferior sixth, seventh, and eighth ribs, and the dissection proceeds in a cephalad direction toward the fifth and sixth intercostal spaces. Laterally, the pectoralis muscle is bluntly dissected off pectoralis minor muscle to expose the vascular pedicle while maintaining the attachments to the fifth rib. The intercostal muscles between the fifth and sixth ribs are divided, with reflection of the pleura from the undersurface of the rib performed carefully. The rib is then sectioned at its lateral and medial desired extent with rib cutters. This rib segment, along with its muscle attachments, is released from the anterior chest wall, with increased mobilization of the flap gained by dividing the humeral, sternal, and clavicular attachments. A segment of the clavicle may also be excised to increase mobility. The flap is then transferred under the deltopectoral skin bridge. The rib segment harvested with the skin pedicle is secured to the remaining mandibular segment. The skin island can then be secured to the intraoral mucosa. The donor site is closed primarily by undermining the adjacent wound margins. Advantages of this reconstructive design include the technical ease of harvest and a versatile and durable flap that contains a long pedicle. However, the rib segment does not provide adequate bone stock for reconstruction, there is an increased risk of pneumothorax, and the limited vascular supply to the bone segment may lead to long-term bone resorption and muscular atrophy.

3.3.3. Temporalis osteomuscular/ osteomusculofascial Flap

The temporalis osteomuscular flap is an option for reconstruction of maxillary and mandibular deficiencies. Its advantageous location permits the arc of rotation of the flap to facilitate

http://dx.doi.org/10.5772/59746

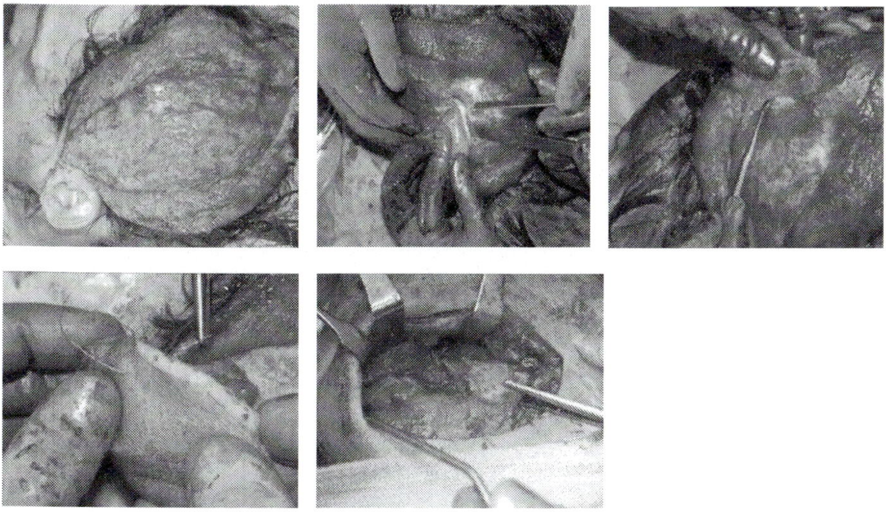

Figure 16. Temporalis Osteomuscular/ Osteomusculofascial Flap

reconstruction of the facial skeleton at all anatomic levels. [69] Conleys [70] designed an osteomuscular flap incorporating the temporalis muscle and the underlying bone, using the deep temporal artery and its perforators for flap viability. In 1984, McCarthy and Zide [71] designed a composite flap for orbital and frontal reconstructions but encountered limited mobility due to an anatomic obstruction by the intact zygoma and lateral orbital rim. The dissection was modified to include division of the arch and removal of the coronoid process, which allowed maximal mobility of the muscle flap by basing the pedicle on the deep temporal artery. The involvement of the membranous calvarial bone provides further advantages, including superior viability of bone (as compared with endochondral bone), greater bone availability, single operative field with minimal associated morbidity, and a cosmetic result. Weaknesses include the previously mentioned poor anterior mobilization, increased bulk of the flap, and a donor site volume defect that may affect jaw function and range of motion. Choung and colleagues [72] recently developed a bone-facial-periosteal flap, not using muscle, to overcome the aforementioned limitations. They successfully reconstructed zygomaticoorbital complexes and maxillary and mandibular defects, including hemifacial microsomia. This new design provides a long, thin pedicle that is easily rotated into the defect, allowing simultaneous use of cranial bone. They found a low incidence of temporal volume loss and adverse effects on jaw movements. The side that is ipsilateral to the defect is often chosen, and the dissection begins in the supragaleal plane to expose the superficial temporal artery and vein. The pedicle may be designed with the use of a template, such that the center of the pedicle is overlying the vessels with sufficient length to the pedicle. The desired facial island is incised to the pericranium, and the parietotemporal fascia is elevated to the limits of the designed bone and folded over the bone. The bone is then harvested, avoiding the sinuses with burs and osteotomies, producing full- or partial-thickness bone grafts. The muscle is anchored to the zygomatic arch by the deep temporal fascia. Dividing these attachments allows anterior mobilization of the flap. Again, the zygomatic arch may be divided, and the coronoid process may be transected to provide maximal transposition of the flap. The muscle's arc of rotation is thus increased, as it is isolated on its neurovascular pedicle. The flap can be used for external reconstruction of maxillary and mandibular defects but can also be tunneled intraorally to reach the ipsilateral canine region. The bone segment is fixed to the surrounding bone by standard fixation materials, such as wires or plates. The wound is then closed in a two-layered fashion with the appropriate use of drains (Figure 16).

4. Free flaps

4.1. Free fasciocutaneous flaps

4.1.1. Radial forearm flap

Originally developed in China [73], the radial forearm flap has developed into one of the most utilized techniques for reconstruction. Initially, it was used for the correction of cervical skin contracture in burn patients. It was then applied for reconstruction of total thumb defects using a portion of the radial bone. In 1983, Soutar [74] introduced this technique to oromandibular reconstruction. Urken [75] followed in 1989 by re-innervating the oral cavity with modifications of the flap design, using medial and lateral antebrachial cutaneous nerves of the forearm anastomosed with the transected branches of the greater auricular nerve. This was a major breakthrough in the restoration of sensory function in the oral cavity. The radial forearm flap with or without incorporation of radial bone stock has many attributes that make it ideal for the reconstruction of intraoral defects. It is composed of a hairless surface that is relatively thin and pliable and allows easy three-dimensional restoration of the oral cavity. There is flexibility in skin paddle design, allowing for the creation of independent skin islands to resurface intraoral defects. The vascular pedicle that can be obtained has a generous length and caliber, which facilitates revascularization, especially if recipient vessels are at a distance. The rich vascularity of the flap promotes rapid healing and minimizes wound-healing complications, and there is a potential for sensory reinnervation. Finally, the flap can be harvested at the same time as tumor ablation is performed. Anatomically, the major blood supply to the flap is from the branches of the radial artery that course along the lateral intramuscular septum of the forearm, between the brachioradialis and flexor carpi radialis muscles. There are 9 to 17 septal perforators that supply the deep forearm fascia superficial to muscle and the overlying skin. The septal perforators and the direct branches of the radial artery supply the tendons of the brachioradialis, flexor carpi radialis, and palmaris longus muscles. Vascularized segments of the lateral cortex of the distal radius can be included in the flap, based on a periosteal circulation supplied by direct fascioperiosteal branches of the radial artery and musculoperiosteal vessels. The maximal length that can be harvested is 12 cm, based on the pronator teres muscle insertion proximally and the brachioradialis insertion distally. The sensory nerves, the medial and lateral antebrachial cutaneous nerves, run in close proximity to the superficial veins of the

http://dx.doi.org/10.5772/59746

forearm and can be incorporated by dissecting proximally to obtain adequate length to anastomose to recipient vessels (Figure 17).

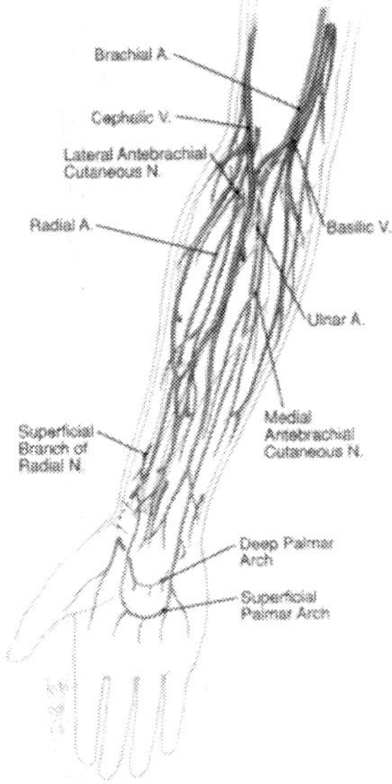

Figure 17. Forearm anatomy

The nondominant arm is usually selected for flap harvest, after documentation of adequate palmar circulation by Allen's test. Under sterile conditions, the extremity is exsanguinated, followed by application of a tourniquet. The skin paddle is then outlined, with its configuration dependent on the size and shape of the defect. It is usually projected over the course of the radial artery and one of the subcutaneous veins. The paddle is frequently outlined over the distal radius to obtain a vascular pedicle of greatest length. A flap may also be designed to provide a second, proximal skin island that is exteriorized in the lower neck to serve as an external monitor of flap viability. Intervening tissue is often used to provide coverage to the carotid vessels and augment soft tissue defects in radical neck cases. Once the distal incision is made, the radial vessels are identified and ligated just lateral to the flexor carpi radialis tendon. The incisions are carried through the deep muscular fascia, and flap elevation proceeds deep to this plane and extends proximally toward the intramuscular septum of the forearm. As the septum is approached, the septal perforators are encountered. The flap is then elevated for the flexor muscles of the wrist, where care is taken to preserve the paratendon, as this provides the vascularized bed for the healing of skin grafts. Once the intramuscular septum is widely exposed, the radial vessels are elevated sharply from the groove between the flexor carpi radialis and the brachioradialis muscles. The dissection continues proximally until the bifurcation of the brachial artery, which requires careful separation of the muscle bellies. At this proximal aspect, the antebrachial cutaneous nerves are identified next to the cephalic vein. The tourniquet is then released while the flap is still attached to its vascular pedicle, so the flap is reperfused until ready for transfer to the donor site. If radial bone is to be used, a cuff of muscle and periosteum is preserved along the anterior radial border in continuity with the lateral intramuscular septum. The periosteum and muscle are carefully incised along the ulnar border of the radius. Holes are drilled into the bone, which are subsequently joined by a fissure bur, and the osteotomy is completed with a reciprocating saw. Only 40% of the anterior radius can be harvested in full thickness. The bone is then lifted and segmentalized by greenstick fractures in order to be adapted to the bony defect. Each segment is attached by a screw to a precontoured titanium reconstruction plate [76]. The harvested fascia is then adapted to the bony contours and sutured to provide a watertight seal. Following tissue transfer, the wound is closed and bolstered with split-thickness skin grafts. Full-thickness skin grafts that are defatted and taken from the abdomen provide an excellent alternative to the traditional split thickness grafts, which are associated with complications [77]. An ulnar transposition flap may be used to close a small residual donor defect. An ulnar immobilizing splint is then applied for approximately 1 week. The wrist is in slight extension to eliminate dead space between the brachioradialis and flexor carpi radialis muscles, where a hematoma may form. Radial forearm flaps have been applied mostly to reconstruction of the oral cavity and pharyngeal defects. They provide tissue with an independent blood supply capable of healing in a contaminated and irradiated wound. It has been shown in many studies that an improved level of oral cavity function occurs after skin graft reconstruction as opposed to using tongue or myocutaneous flaps alone [78]. The radial forearm flap, without its bony counterpart, is well suited for the reconstruction of tongue and floor of the mouth defects. A bilobed design has been used by Urken and Biller [79] to restore shape and volume of the tongue with one lobe and to resurface the floor of the mouth and gingiva with the second lobe. They reported that mobility, oral alimentation, articulation, and sensory reinnervation occurred in the majority of their patients (Figure 18).

In those cases in which tumor ablation involves segmental mandibulectomy, the radial forearm flap with its radial bone, or in conjunction with bone stock from other sites such as iliac crest free flap or scapular bone, achieves functional mandibular reconstruction with a sensate soft tissue component. Nakatsuka and colleagues [80] described their experience using dual free flap transfers combining the radial forearm flap with an osteocutaneous free bone flap. Despite a high complication rate of 41 %, the technique is useful for obtaining good alveolar ridge height. Circumferential defects of the hypopharynx or cervical esophagus can be restored with the use of tubed radial forearm free flaps, allowing rehabilitation of the swallowing mechanism. Soft palatal defects can be reconstructed by using this flap design, folded over on itself to provide lining for the oro- and nasopharynx. Utilizing the tendons, as incorporated in flap design, allows total lip and chin reconstruction, with the palmaris longus tendon acting as a sling to assist in maintaining the vertical height and support of the lip [81] Complications of using the radial forearm flap include those encountered with other designs, such as flap necrosis, delayed wound healing due to failure of the skin graft to take over the exposed flexor tendons of the wrist, radial bone fracture, lack of sensation over the grafted donor site, vascular

http://dx.doi.org/10.5772/59746

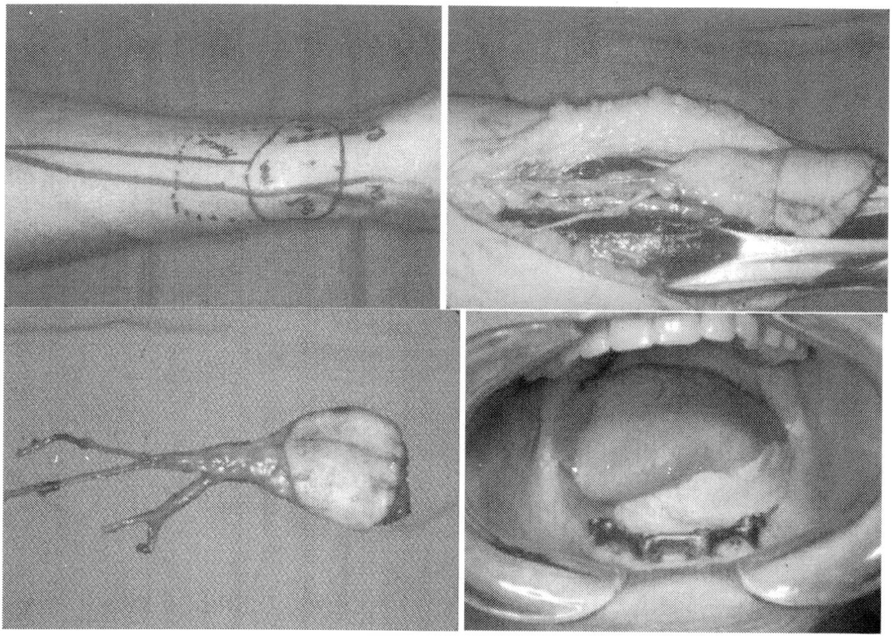

Figure 18. Radial Forearm Flap

insufficiency of the hand, stiffness or swelling of the wrist, reduced hand or wrist length, and sympathetic dystrophy. Disfigurement of the forearm was noted to be acceptable in men but was not as well tolerated in women [82].

4.1.2. Lateral thigh flap

This type of flap was first described by Baek [83] in 1983, when it was used for reconstruction of pharyngoesophageal defects, as well as for regions of skin contraction secondary to burn contractures in the anterior neck. It has been described as a fasciocutaneous flap from the lower limb used primarily for pharyngoesophageal defects [84]. This flap provides a more abundant surface area than any other skin flap. The overlying skin in women is frequently thin, pliable, and hairless. The more proximal aspect of the flap is used to provide bulk, whereas the thinner distal aspect can be used to reconstruct the thin oral and pharyngeal mucous membranes. This is useful when there is a subtotal loss of the tongue base and loss of the lateral pharyngeal wall and soft palate. The thicker portions of the flap can fill the tongue defect with bulk, and the thinner aspects can be used to reconstruct the pharyngeal wall and soft palate. In regions of subtotal and total glossectomies, the flap can serve as a sensate fasciocutaneous flap, with the lateral femoral cutaneous nerve anastomosed with the glossopharyngeal or lingual nerves. This flap also has a long vascular pedicle, which may lend itself to the repair of cranial base defects by incorporating fascia lata with the flap. The flap has also been used without its skin for a vascularized facial graft for facial augmentation, as it has sufficient fat deposits and can be harvested while the patient remains in the supine position. The lateral thigh flap offers large vessel diameters, which make microvascular anastomosis easier (Figure 19).

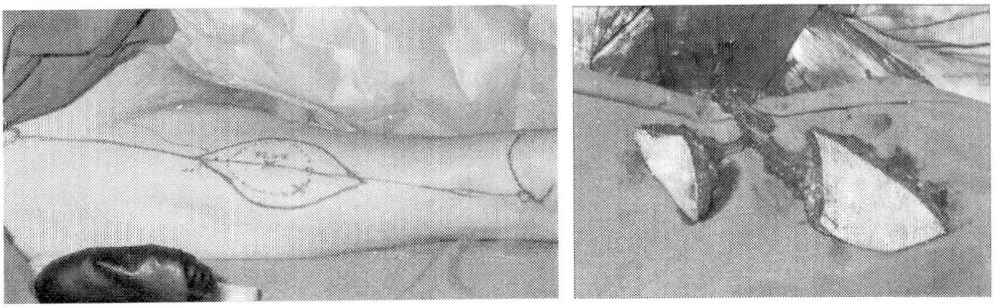

Figure 19. The lateral thigh flap

This flap has not gained popularity largely owing to technical difficulties. However, for large laryngopharyngectomies, it should be a first-line reconstructive choice.

4.2. Free osteomyocutaneous flaps

Primary mandibular reconstruction in patients treated with preoperative radiation therapy is often unsuccessful, failing be- cause of ineffective healing, lack of neovascularization, or infection from salivary contamination. The use of vascularized free flaps has decreased the morbidity and mortality, as well as the length of hospital stay, for patients who have undergone oral cavity reconstruction. The use of myocutaneous vascularized flaps has been criticized, because they result in bulky tissues in the oral cavity, which has a major adverse affect on deglutition and articulation, and dental appliances often fail in these settings. Free vascularized bone flap transfers from distant sites have revolutionized mandibular reconstruction. [85-89] The postoncologic mandibulectomy defect is unique, in that oral contamination, radiation changes, and decreased blood supply hinder the use of nonvascularized tissues. Furthermore, rehabilitation of the dental arch is possible with the simultaneous use of vascularized osteocutaneous flaps and osseointegrated implants, which results in improved postoperative masticatory function. A variety of donor sites exist for oromandibular reconstruction, including the iliac crest, fibula, scapula, radius, metatarsus, and rib [90]

4.2.1. Iliac crest osteocutaneous free flap

Free microvascular flaps in oromandibular reconstruction have proved to be reliable in the face of adverse environmental conditions [91]. Of the sites that have been described, the iliac crest composite free flap has distinguished itself as being the most efficacious and has become the principal reconstructive option (Figure 20).

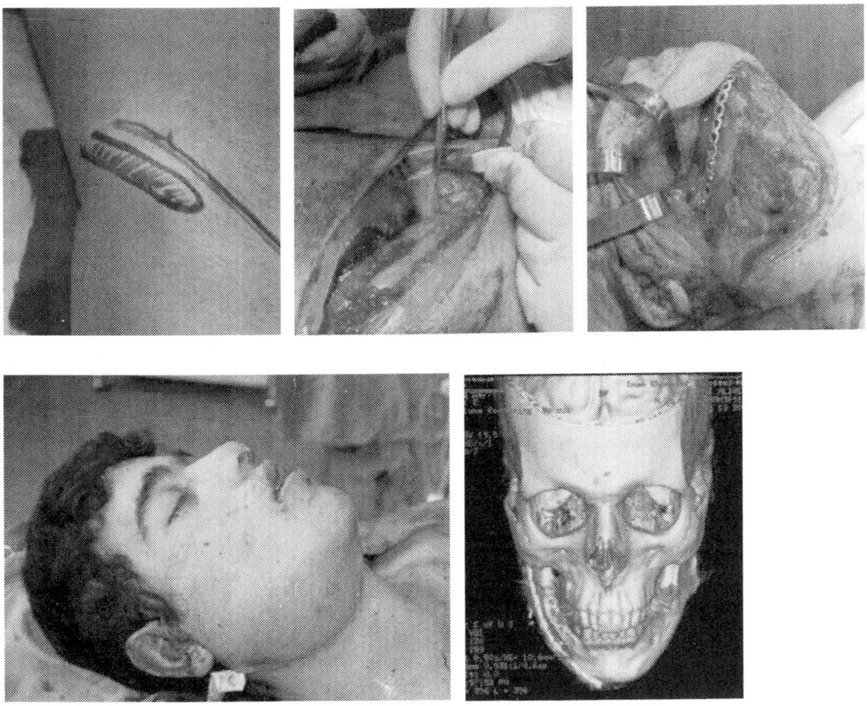

Figure 20. Iliac Crest Osteocutaneous Free Flap

The corticocancellous iliac crest yields sufficient bone for reconstruction, as well as providing the appropriate contour to parallel the mandible. The cancellous portion promotes rapid healing, while the dense cortex maintains strength and contour and allows the use of rigid fixation and restoration with osseointegrated implants. The soft tissue free flap provides extensive soft tissue coverage. With the incorporation of the internal oblique muscle, the oral cavity can be lined, and articulation can be improved following glossectomy. Use of the iliac crest free flap allows for immediate reconstruction, thus preventing distortions in contour. This is accomplished by the use of fixation stabilization achieved before initial resection. This approach is also amenable to use of a dual surgical team, improving the efficiency of harvest. The flap can be raised as an osteocutaneous, myo-osseous, or osteomyocutaneous flap. Review of Urken's report suggests a success rate of 96%. [29] This type of reconstructive option also has limitations; for example, it is technically difficult in obese patients. Removal of a bicortical block produces significant donor site deformity and asymmetry. Encroachment on the abdomen may occur, producing weakness or hernia development. The associated skin paddle may be difficult to mobilize and thus difficult to orient and position. The bulky bony mass often requires secondary revision to improve or create ideal contours. Postoperative sequelae include injury to the lateral femoral cutaneous and ilioinguinal nerves, which can produce unpleasant dysesthesia and/or anesthesia. A number of refinements have taken place over the years to prevent some of these adverse postoperative sequelae. The split inner cortex iliac crest microsurgical free flap preserves the outer cortex to anchor the abdominal wall musculature and fascia and produces a firm, dependable closure, preventing abdominal wall weakness and subsequent hernia formation. The advantages of liberating a single cortex are that it is technically easier, takes less time to harvest, reduces blood loss, and decreases the incidence of hematoma or seroma formation. Of course, the amount of harvested bone is limited and less reliable for contouring osteotomies, internal fixation, and osseointegration. However, the breadth of the single cortex is comparable to that of the intact mandible. The iliac bone is perfused by a number of vessels, including the deep, lateral, and superficial circumflex iliac arteries; the superficial inferior epigastric artery; and the superior deep branch of the superior gluteal artery. The osteomyocutaneous flap is based on the deep iliac artery as the principal blood supply, with accompanying perforators to augment perfusion to the overlying skin.

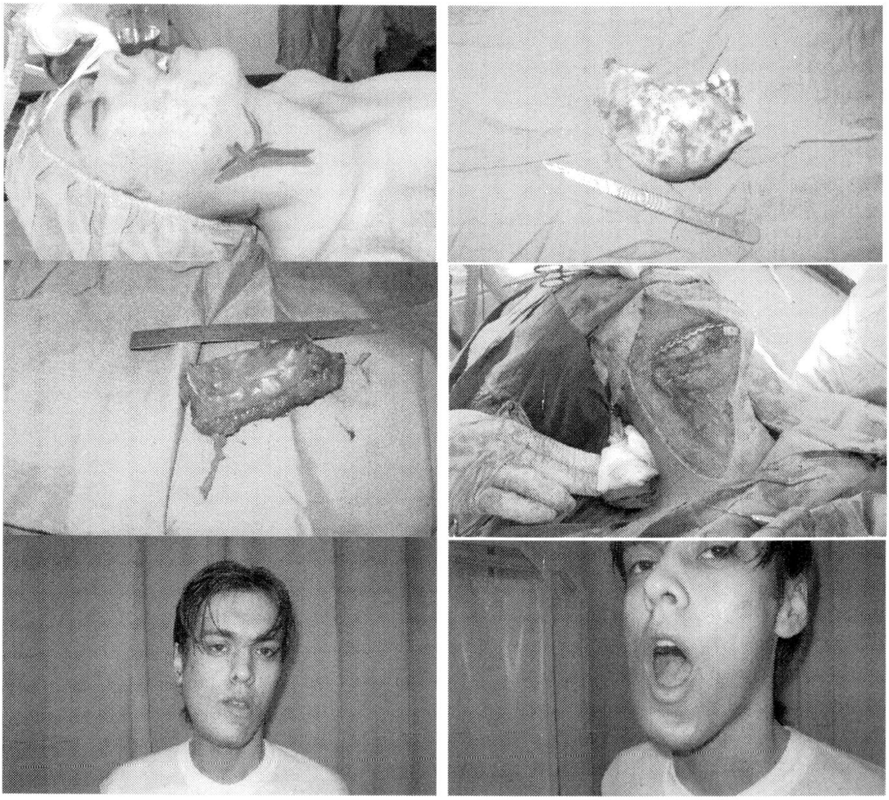

Figure 21. Iliac Crest Osteocutaneous Free Flap

http://dx.doi.org/10.5772/59746

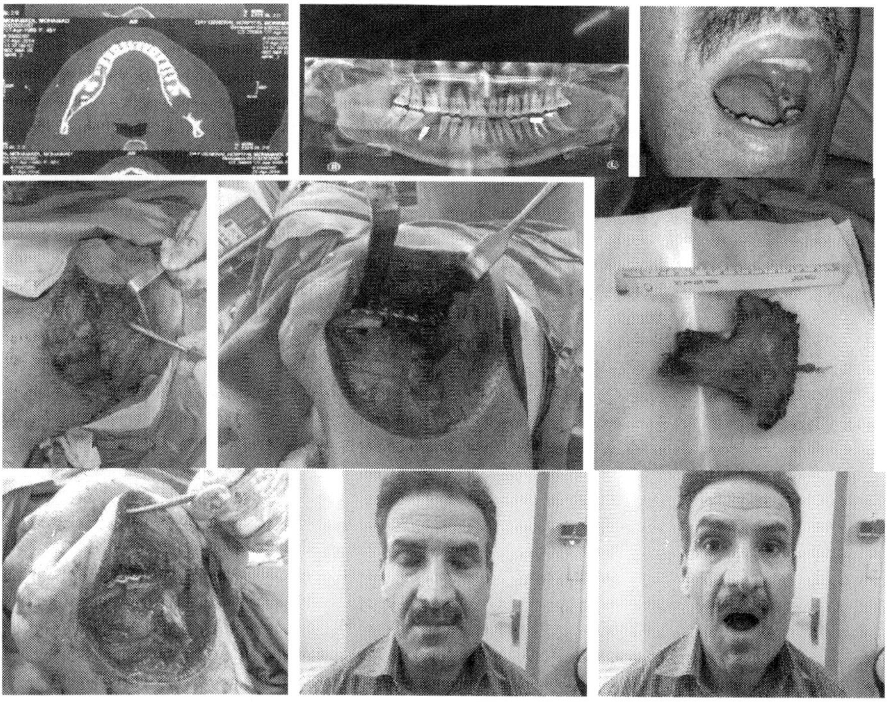

Figure 22. Iliac Crest Osteocutaneous Free Flap

The deep circumflex iliac artery originates from the external iliac just proximal to the inguinal ligament and courses toward the iliac spine in a plane deep to the transverse fascia and parallel to the inguinal ligament. In this path, it is crossed by the ilioinguinal and lateral femoral cutaneous nerves. The dissection begins with a skin incision parallel to the inguinal ligament in the direction of the anterior superior iliac spine. A vertical incision over the major femoral vessels is made approximately 5 cm in length, forming a final inverted-L--shaped incision. The deep circumflex vessels are identified and dissected to their origin. Care is taken to identify the ascending branch of the deep circumflex artery, which takes off from the parent artery 1 cm before the anterior iliac spine. It is important to preserve this vasculature, as it is the major supplier to the internal oblique muscle. If required, a skin paddle can be excised over the crest. The skin, subcutaneous tissues, and fascia are elevated as one unit, with an adjoining 2.5- cm protective cuff of muscle. The skin flap is then undermined to the superior border of the crest, where the periosteum is divided in the midline of the crest. With adequate elevation of the periosteum in the medial and lateral dimensions, the two cortices can be osteotomized with a sagittal saw. The internal oblique muscle flap can then be fashioned, with the iliacus muscle divided and dissected to a level below the deep circumflex artery. The medial cortical plate can then be accessed for the osteotomy. The shape of the reconstructed mandible is dependent on the sites of the osteotomy. The vascular pedicle follows behind the newly designed mandibular angle with a length sufficient to reach the external carotid system, where anastomoses of the donor vessels will take place. The donor site is closed in layers, where the residual internal oblique muscle is reapproximated with the residual periosteum, and the external oblique muscle is anchored to the outer cortex of the iliac crest. Drains are frequently used in the wound site and covered with fascia and skin. This donor site provides a long vascular pedicle that can be fashioned to fit the defect precisely (Figure 21).

Incorporation of the internal oblique muscle flap provides a source of oral lining to aid in the reconstruction of compound deficiencies. Durable internal fixation of free vascularized bone grafts is accomplished with reconstructive plating systems (e.g., THORP, AO). Placement of the plates before initial resection maintains contour and eliminates the need for intermaxillary or external fixation (Figure 22).

4.2.2. Fibula free flap

Among the free flap donor sites used for mandibular reconstruction, the fibula is becoming a popular choice (Figures 23). [92]

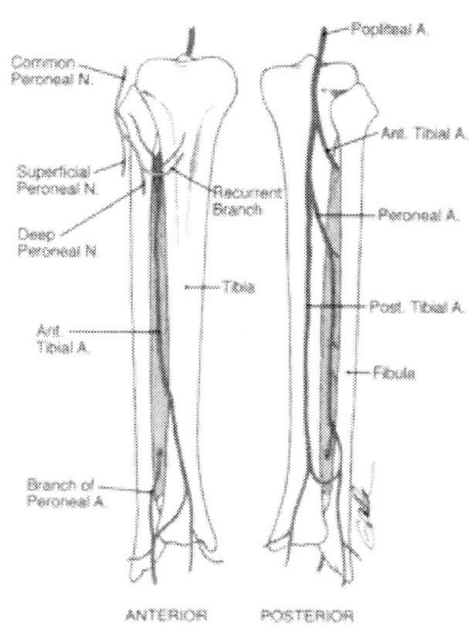

Figure 23. Fibula anatomy

It provides enough bone stock, with up to 25 cm of bone, and can maintain a consistent shape throughout its length for shaping a mandibular defect. Its blood supply courses along with it, in parallel, guaranteeing adequate vascularity to the osteotomized segments. The muscle segment also parallels the bony segment, enabling the soft tissue defect to be filled in adequately. It provides a rigid, strong, tubular-shaped cortical bone similar to the anatomic structure of the mandible, and it is easily contoured without compromising vascularity [93]. Simultaneous reconstruction, both internally and externally, can be reliably performed with an associated skin island based on the septocutaneous blood supply. Finally, the graft site is located distally enough so that two teams can work simultaneously. Most anterior mandibular reconstructions, where defects can exceed 12 cm and where external skin or floor of the mouth defects mandate replacement, are accomplished primarily with fibula free flaps. Other indications include hemimandibular defects with adjacent lateral floor of the mouth or buccal mucosa loss. Carroll and Esclamado recently suggested the use of preoperative angiography in all patients undergoing reconstructions using fibular osteocutaneous flaps [94]. They found that subclinical and marked atherosclerotic disease may be detected in patients with clinically benign lower extremity examinations, and that aberrant arterial anatomy exists in 5% to 7% of the population. However, a dominant peroneal artery occurs in a very small number of patients in a population, and an angiogram is not justified. Moreover, a diseased peroneal artery can be safely used for microvascular anastomoses. But if the peroneal artery must be used in the free flap transfer, adequate foot runoffs must be present. Primary reconstruction provides the optimal setting for obtaining the best surgical result. Graft shaping is easily accomplished when the resected segment is directly visualized. In secondary reconstruction, distortion of the anatomy, secondary to soft tissue contracture, makes the reconstruction a "mystery." Before tumor ablation, miniplates are easily contoured to the existing mandible. They provide a high degree of precision, without the bulk of AO reconstruction plates. When planning on which donor leg to use, the ipsilateral fibula is generally used [95]. When the same side is used, the flexor hallucis longus muscle lies under the fibula to aid in filling in the soft tissue defect. The skin island can then be easily rotated up and over the fibula to reach the oral cavity and reconstruct a mucosal defect. The skin island is designed to run along the length of the fibula to preserve all its septal blood supply. The long axis is centered over the fibula's posterior border, such that the septal blood supply is captured. The width of the island is approximately 4 cm on average, which usually allows primary closure of the donor site (Figure 24).

A larger skin island requires some type of skin graft closure. Dissection begins from a lateral approach, with the skin incised anteriorly. The lateral compartment, separated from the anterior by the intramuscular septum, is divided, and muscles from both groups are divided, with the use of electrocautery to gain hemostasis. A cleft posteriorly between the soleus and flexor hallucis muscles is created by blunt dissection, and the soleus is separated with electrocautery from the fibula (Figure 25).

Osteotomies are performed at the proximal neck of the fibula and at a distal site 4 to 6 cm proximal to the lateral malleolus. The peroneal vessels and the flexor hallucis longus muscle are divided distally. At the distal site, traction on the bone outward exposes the posterior tibialis muscle and its median raphae; the former is then divided along the latter in a distal to proximal direction. The peroneal and tibial vessels are usually safe as long as the muscle is divided along the raphae. The recipient vessels are dissected in preparation for a microvascular transfer. The facial artery and external carotid artery are used most frequently, and the superior thyroid artery is used as an alternative. However, the external jugular vein is generally

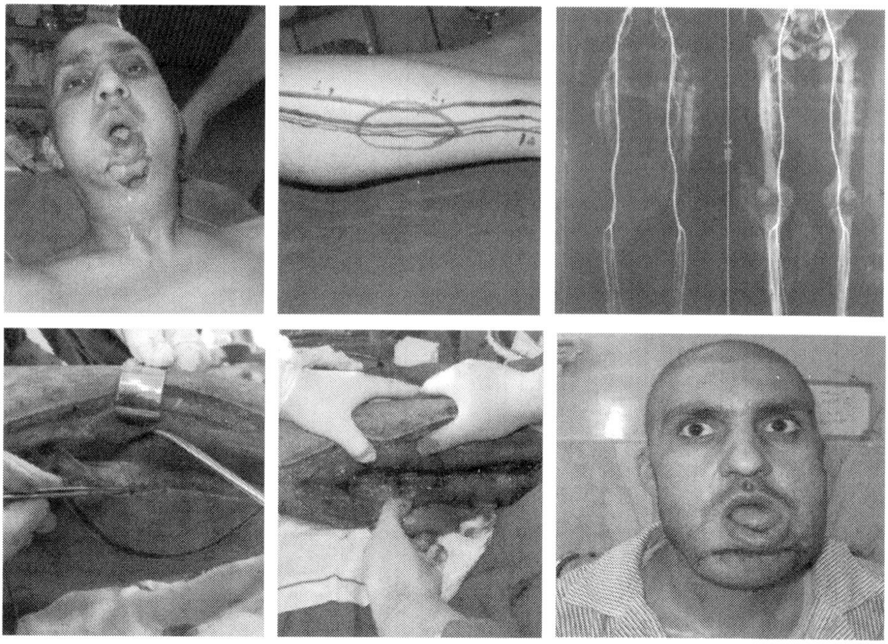

Figure 24. Free fibula flap

preferred, because it is more superficial and has an ideal diameter for anastomosis. In general, to prevent lengthy ischemia times, the fibula is shaped as much as possible before the pedicle is divided. The graft is completely shaped, and then the final osteotomies that determine the overall length are performed before the insetting process. The process of shaping is facilitated by prefabricated templates. Osteotomies in the desired positions are created and stabilized with miniplates. Once microvascular anastomosis is complete, the skin island is rotated up and over the mandible into the oral cavity. The flexus hallucis longus muscle can be used to fill in the submental soft tissue loss. Postoperatively, graft monitoring can be difficult unless intraoral reconstruction was done. The intraoral skin island can be followed for any color or capillary refill change. The peroneal artery patency can be followed with Doppler examination. The successful grafts can then be recipients for osseointegrated implants to complete the functional reconstruction. Wells [96] stated that the fibula flap is more technically difficult to elevate but is an excellent reconstructive modality, because it provides superior bone stock for mandibular reconstruction. Another disadvantage is insufficient height to restore the mandible, but this has been corrected with the use of a double fibula graft (i.e., the double barreled flap). Sensibility can be restored using this neurocutaneous fibular free flap by repairing the lateral cutaneous nerve of the calf to the lingual nerve. A vascularized jump graft can be accomplished by using the sural communicating nerve to bridge the inferior alveolar nerve defect [97]. There has been ongoing controversy regarding the reliability of the skin island associated with the fibular osteocutaneous flap in mandibular reconstruction. Jones and

http://dx.doi.org/10.5772/59746

coworkers [98] recently addressed this topic by studying a new flap design in 60 cadavers. They found that a major perforator through the soleus muscle or flexor hallucis muscle can provide perfusion to the skin flap, without the need to incorporate portions of the muscle. The reliability of the skin island is based on the design's more distal location (that is, it is placed more distally over the distal third of the lower leg); preoperative identification of the perforators with Doppler mapping so as not to sacrifice them during dissection; and protection of the septocutaneous perforators that traverse the posterior periosteum when performing wedge osteotomies of the fibula. Violations of this design may be responsible for the poor outcomes previously reported regarding the reliability of the fibular osteocutaneous flap for mandibular reconstruction (Figure 26).

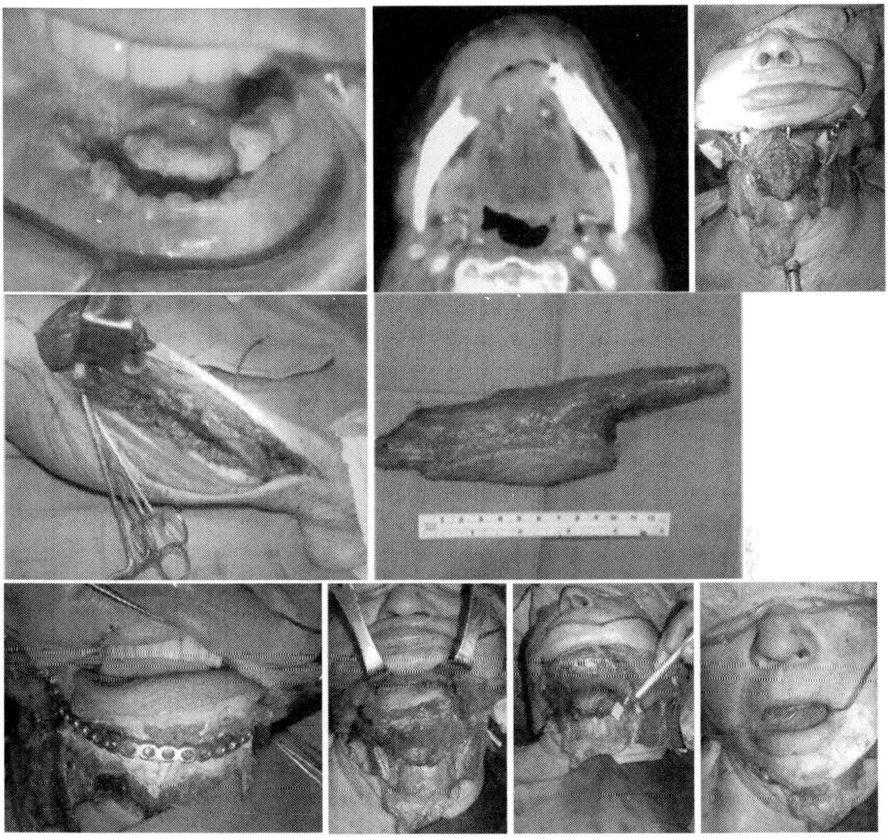

Figure 25. Free fibula flap

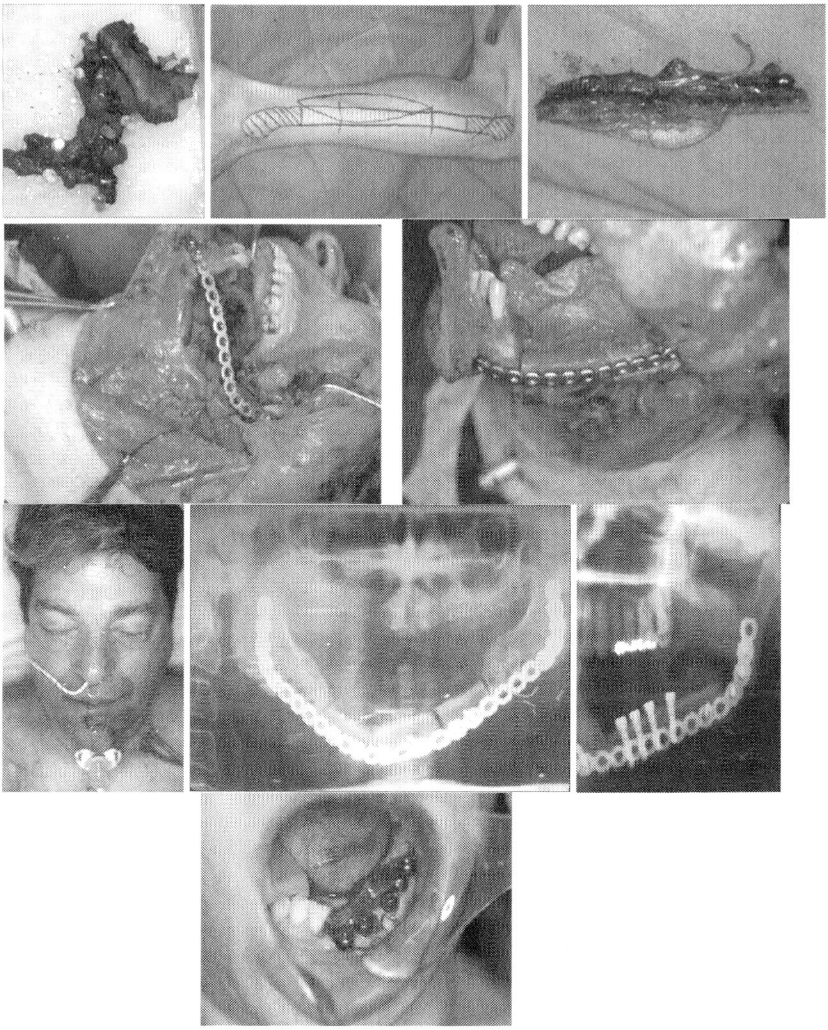

Figure 26. Free fibula flap reconstruction

4.3. Other free flaps in head and neck reconstruction

4.3.1. Linked free flaps

The goal of reconstructive surgery is to replace bone and soft tissue in a manner such that functional and aesthetic problems are minimized. For this reason, a large number of pedicled myo-osteocutaneous flaps and free tissue transfers have been developed. Patients who have

http://dx.doi.org/10.5772/59746

undergone previous surgery and radiation develop poor recipient beds. In these cases, vascularized bone has become a viable treatment option. In cases in which complex soft tissue and bony defects have resulted from tumor extirpation, multiple head and neck surgical operations, and past irradiation, limited recipient vascularity requires reconstructive modalities other than a single osteocutaneous flap. Because of their limitations, linking of free flaps has become a preferred method of reconstruction for complex composite head and neck defects. The use of sequentially linked free flaps is best suited to cases of composite defects that cannot be adequately restored by a single flap, large through-and-through head and neck defects, limited native vasculature from either previous surgical excisions or preoperative radiation, lack of availability of local or regional flaps, and defects that require both adequate bony stock and a thin mucosal lining for intraoral coverage. [99-117]

Wells and coworkers [118] described their technique for using the radial forearm flap in conjunction with a free fibular transfer. Similar experiences were shared by Camilleri and associates [119] reporting survival rates of 98%. Elevation of the flaps occurred simultaneously and independently of each other, as described earlier. The peroneal vessels and vein from the contoured fibular flap and the radial artery vessels and cephalic vein were anastomosed in an end-to-end fashion, respectively. The long pedicle of the forearm flap allowed for primary anastomosis of the linked flaps without the use of intervening vein grafts. The radial artery was then anastomosed end to end to a branch of the external carotid artery, and the cephalic vein was anastomosed to the external or internal jugular vein in an end-to-end configuration. This technique is advantageous because there is no ideal osteocutaneous free flap that provides both an unlimited amount of bone and a reliable cutaneous component. The fibula provides ample bone stock to reconstruct the entire mandible, and the forearm furnishes a thin, reliable, hairless sensate flap for intraoral lining. The potential disadvantage is the risk of proximal thrombosis, which results in the loss of two free tissue transfers. Also, extra operative time is involved in the microvascular reconstruction. However, if the two donor sites are appropriately spaced, the use of two surgical teams may reduce operative time. Penfold and colleagues [120] described the combination serratus anterior-rib flap with the latissimus dorsi myocutaneous flap for mandibular reconstruction. Their technique accesses both flaps through a single skin incision placed along the anterior border of the latissimus muscle. After elevating this muscle, the lower part of the serratus anterior muscle is exposed. A segment of rib (either sixth or seventh in this location) with its associated periosteum and a cuff of muscle above and below is elevated on the serratus muscle pedicle. The superior part of the latissimus dorsi muscle is then divided, and the combined flap is transferred on a common pedicle of the thoracodorsal vessels. The donor site is closed primarily. The vascular anastomosis can then be performed in an end-to-side fashion to the external carotid artery and vein, or to the facial artery and vein. The amount of tissue provided by the latissimus dorsi muscle flap for transfer is ideal for reconstructing large mandibular defects, which are often associated with extensive soft tissue losses involving the floor of the mouth. The disadvantages of using such a combined flap include those associated with serratus-rib composite flaps, such as insufficient bony stock to allow for placement of osseointegrated implants. Even though bulky tissue is required for reconstructing extensive soft tissue defects, the combined flap may provide excessive tissue bulk in the neck, resulting in poor cosmesis. Another variation in flap design is the combined

V-shaped scapular osteocutaneous and latissimus dorsi myocutaneous flap, used for primary or secondary reconstruction of the mandible, intraoral mucosa, and external skin. The design, reported by Yamamoto and coworkers [121], is based on the vascular network including the angular branch from the thoracodorsal artery, the dorsal scapular artery, the circumflex scapular artery arising from the subscapular artery, and the suprascapular artery. They reported seven cases in which this reconstructive option was employed, citing six successful cases. The fact that this combined flap is nourished by the angular branch allows the graft to have an independent long arc of rotation. The V shape of the grafted bone has a reliable blood supply from the vascular network. Combining this bone graft with a myocutaneous component, the latissimus dorsi flap, allows the reconstruction of large soft tissue losses in the oral floor or submandibular region. The latissimus dorsi muscle may also restore tongue volume when large tongue defects coexist. As already mentioned, the main disadvantage of using the latissimus dorsi flap in conjunction with a scapular bone flap is the necessity of patient repositioning for flap harvest. Thus, the operation is usually prolonged. Also, the quality of bone retrieved from the scapula is not adequate to accept dental reconstructive implants, unless the lateral border or inferior angle of the scapula is obtained.

5. Site specific reconstruction problems

5.1. Mandibular reconstruction

Mandibular reconstructive procedures have conventionally consisted of bone graft replacing the resected defect. Historically, Macewen [122] discussed the reconstruction of defects using a tibia harvested graft. Blocker and Stout [123] described the use of iliac crest in the mandible. Development of other donor sites was sought, with disappointing results. Metallic cribs and mesh trays to contain the grafts were designed but were suboptimal for primary reconstruction. Furthermore, in patients who had been irradiated or who presented with extensive soft tissue defects, successful reconstruction was difficult to achieve, as there was a greater chance of postoperative infection due to diminished blood circulation, ingress of oral flora, and an absent blood supply to the grafted bone. One technique that would provide increased resistance to infection was to use pedicled grafts. Conley [124] and Snyder [125] published the first case reports using osteomyocutaneous flaps in the immediate reconstructive setting. Numerous other flaps followed, with minimal reliability and poor success rates. They were subsequently considered unacceptable for primary mandibular reconstruction. Because the defect site is plagued with soft tissue loss, oral contamination, and compromised irradiated tissues, free vascularized grafts were thought to be the ideal choice. McKee [126] and Daniel [127] were the first to report the outcomes of free vascularized composite rib flaps in a large series of patients. Success rates have increased for microvascular free tissue transfers using iliac crest and scapular free flaps, reaching 96% [128]. With the recent development of rigid fixation systems, reconstruction of the mandible with a combination of metallic plate and pedicled osteomyocutaneous flap or microvascular free tissue transfer has been advocated. Essentially, reconstruction of the mandible with bone grafting must be dimensionally and

http://dx.doi.org/10.5772/59746

structurally stable, capable of withstanding the functional demands of prosthesis. The graft must be able to maintain a correct arch form and continuity, with significant bone height and osseous bulk for full prosthetic rehabilitation and an acceptable facial form. The primary goals of mandibular reconstruction are to achieve primary wound closure and to achieve adequate range of motion with a stabilized, repetitive occlusion, dependent on the maintenance of physiologic condylar position. Bony reconstruction is of importance when acceptable facial aesthetics are required. If a defect in the anterior symphysis or chin region were not addressed, an "Andy Gump" deformity would result, with posterior and inferior collapse. Lateral defects stabilize jaw symmetry and contour. Functionally, masticatory difficulties result from poor bony reconstructive efforts. Inadequately repaired regions result in jaw deviation and inability to fabricate an acceptable prosthesis. Soft tissue attachments to the mandible are also affected (i.e., lip, floor of the mouth, tongue, hyoid musculature). Thus, poor restoration of a mandibular defect results in oral incompetence and difficulties with speech, mastication, and swallowing functions. Bony mandibular defects are classified by the amount of hard tissue loss specific to an anatomic region. For example, class I mandibular defects involve the alveolus, but with preservation of mandibular continuity; class II defects involve loss of continuity distal to the canine; class III involves loss up to the mandibular midline region; class IV deficiencies involve the lateral aspect of the mandible but are augmented to maintain pseudoarticulation of bone and soft tissue in the region of the ascending ramus; class V involves the symphysis and parasymphyseal regions only, augmented to preserve bilateral temporomandibular articulations; class VI is similar to class V, except that mandibular continuity is not restored. Similar functional deficits can occur with inadequate soft tissue reconstruction. For example, inadequate mucosal replacement can create restricted tongue mobility and insufficient space for dental reconstruction.

5.2. Reconstruction of symphysis, condyle, and ramus

Symphyseal mandibular defects resulting from cancer ablation continue to be a surgical problem. Many techniques using autologous bone grafts, osteomyocutaneous regional and free flaps, and alloplastic and allogeneic materials have been described in the literature, with variable results. As in all reconstructive surgical cases, the primary goals are restoration of function and cosmesis. Recently, distraction osteogenesis has been used in mandibular reconstruction. In essence, a vascularized bony segment is stretched, or distracted, across a defect, inducing new bone formation from the native bone. This process has been well described in the orthopedic surgical literature for the reconstruction of long bones in lower extremities. Bony defects of the symphysis create a great cosmetic and functional problem. Annino and associates [129] created iatrogenic mandibular symphyseal defects in the canine model and reported great success with the use of a trifocal distraction osteogenetic appliance. Mandibular body segmental defects were also reconstructed by distraction osteogenesis, and biomechanical testing revealed the newly generated bone to have approximately 77% the strength of the native bone. Owing to the complexity of applying this device, it is not recommended for the reconstruction of mandibular condylar or ramus regions.

5.3. Reconstruction plates

The AO stainless steel plate has been available for many years as an effective means of mandibular replacement. Mignogna and colleagues [130] commented on their experiences using the AO reconstruction plate with a sternal osteomyocutaneous flap in primary mandibular reconstruction. They replicated the mandible with a malleable pattern before excision and transferred its shape to an AO reconstruction plate, which was then positioned to the unresected portions of the mandible with drilled pilot holes. Once resection takes place, the pectoralis myocutaneous flap is harvested, and the sternum is split to the size of the defect. The osteocutaneous flap is placed at the defect site, and the AO plate is rigidly fixed into position using noncompression screws. Closure of the myocutaneous portion of the flap is carried out meticulously to prevent oral contamination. Mignogna and colleagues believe that the increased operative time, high failure rate, frequent need for operative rescue, and need for specialized training, care, and facilities make reconstruction with vascularized free flaps an impractical option for reconstructive surgeons. In the titanium hollow screw system (THORP), hollow screws integrate at the surface level and permit ingrowth of bone that locks each screw in place. Before resection, the plate is bent and shaped to the existing contours of the mandible [131]. The resected mandible may also serve as a template for plate bending and hole drilling. The plate is generally contoured to the inferior border of the mandible to avoid tooth roots, maintain facial contour, leave space for osseointegration, and keep it well away from the oral mucosa to lessen the chance of intraoral exposure. Metallic fatigue and plate exposure are some of the complications that require removal and replacement. Intraoral exposures are frequently associated with granulation tissue that heals in the immediate postoperative period. Nonetheless, it remains an excellent method of fixing a vascularized bone graft.[132] The plates, in general, provided better cosmetic results than autogenous bone grafting, because there is greater flexibility in contouring a metal plate as opposed to a linear bone strut. Alloplastic metallic plates provided a more rapid postoperative oral rehabilitation and have become a viable reconstructive option. Cordeiro and Hidalgo [133] studied the effects of soft tissue coverage for titanium reconstructive plating systems. They compared patients who received pectoralis major flaps with those who received soft tissue-free flaps. Forty-four percent of the patients with pectoralis flaps had extrusion of the hardware, requiring its subsequent removal. They commented that the excessive tension placed on the flap, from the shoulder-based pedicle; create this high risk of failure. Moreover, despite the increased operative time to acquire free tissue for transfer, as well as the complexity of its harvest; free flap patients had shorter hospital stays, higher overall success rates, and fewer additional procedures. Their data suggest that a free flap provides more reliable soft tissue coverage of reconstruction plates than does a pectoralis flap.

Recently, Blackwell and colleagues [134] looked at the outcomes of using various soft tissue free flaps in conjunction with mandibular reconstruction plates. Even though the added morbidity associated with harvesting free vascularized bone grafts is higher than that for harvesting soft tissue alone, they found a high rate of delayed failure (40%) using metallic reconstruction plates and soft tissue. Thus, they advocate the practice of using vascularized bone-containing free flaps or a combination of free flaps for patients who are undergoing primary reconstruction of lateral mandibulectomy defects. Kudo and associates [135] evaluated the use of various mandibular reconstructive techniques. They commented on the excellent long-term results when using AO-type reconstruction plates, citing successful reconstruction lasting over 10 years, provided sufficient soft tissues exist. When there is a lack of soft tissue, avoidance of plate exposure is best handled by using a myocutaneous flap. Immediate reconstruction of the posterior region of the mandible was most appropriately treated with a metallic plate or a myocutaneous flap and bone graft. Anterior mandibular regions that were immediately reconstructed with autogenous bone grafts resulted in postoperative infection. The authors recommended delayed bone grafting after immediate fixation using a metallic plate to bridge the mandibular defect. An extensive defect of the anterior region requires immediate reconstruction with a myocutaneous flap and bone graft.

5.4. Reconstruction of maxillary and midfacial defects

Tumors of the midface account for a small subset of head and neck cancers. Malignancies of the paranasal sinuses make up 0.2% of the total number of malignancies and 3% of all cancers in the aerodigestive tract. Tumors of the palate are uncommon, representing 8% of all oral cancers and 5% of all aerodigestive carcinomas. The goal in treatment and reconstruction of these cancers is extirpation in toto and cure of the patient with restoration of aesthetic form and function [136]. In many situations, the surgical resection results in a significant functional loss, causing feeding and speech developmental problems with oral-antral communication and velopharyngeal incompetence. Loss of the orbital floor and Lockwood's ligament may result in the loss of orbital support, with ensuing exophthalmoses and orbital dystopia. Reconstructive options are determined primarily by the extent of the midfacial skin deficit, the extent of maxillary buttress resection, the size of the palatal defect, and the loss of orbital support (Figure 27).

Type I defects are those with loss of midfacial skin of the cheeks and lips only. The underlying bony skeleton is not affected. These cutaneous defects can be restored with standard soft tissue reconstructive techniques, from simple primary closure in areas of lax surrounding soft tissue to skin grafts and use of cervicofacial flaps. Larger tissue deficits require regional or distant flaps, such as, latissimus dorsi, temporalis, or forehead flaps. Larger aesthetic units may require resurfacing with free tissue transfers.

Type II and III defects result from partial maxillectomy procedures in which the palate is complete or a portion of the palate is lost, respectively. Traditionally, these midfacial defects are satisfactorily restored by fabrication of a maxillofacial prosthesis in which the denture and palatal obturator close the oral antral fistula and provide projection of the midface. The only requirement for success is that there is an adequate residual palatal arch with enough surrounding soft tissues to support the prosthesis. The impression is taken of the defect well after swelling has subsided, approximately 3 to 4 weeks. The silicone prosthesis constructed from the impression is custom made and attached by previously inserted integrated fixtures and abutments. Other patients may benefit from reconstruction with autogenous tissues, with the use of ipsilateral or bilateral temporal muscle flaps or facial artery musculomucosal flaps, which are often used to reconstruct small oroantral fistulae and palatal defects.

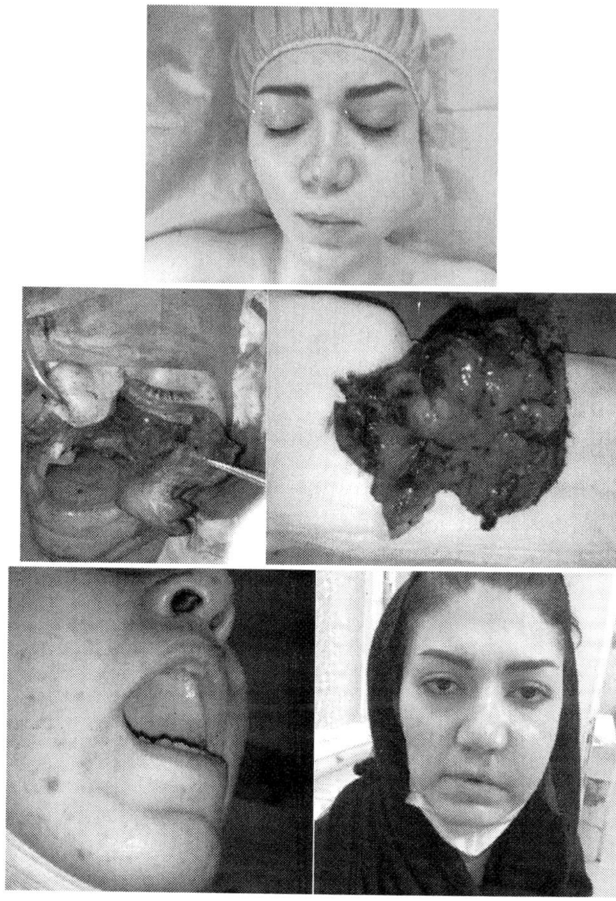

Figure 27. Maxillary tumor reconstruction

Type IV defects that result after total maxillectomy with a concomitant palatectomy are best served by reconstruction with autogenous tissue via regional or distant flaps. The aforementioned pedicled flaps and free tissue transfers are all indicated to redrape defects in the middle third of the face. The bony component is addressed with vascularized bone with its cutaneous counterparts, or bone combined with separate free soft tissue flaps used as linked flaps. For example, by combining the bony reconstruction with scapular and parascapular paddles, massive defects of the midface can be reconstructed with primary closure of the donor site. In this case, the muscular portion of the transfer can be used to obliterate the dead space of the maxillary sinus defect, and the cutaneous aspect can be used to resurface the face and palate.

Type V defects are type IV defects that extend into the orbital floor. Tumors that require exenteration of the orbit should be followed by reconstructive procedures that obliterate the

http://dx.doi.org/10.5772/59746

orbital cavity and restore facial contour. Orbital support procedures, described by Ilankovan and Jackson [137], include split-thickness vascularized calvarial bone pedicled on either the temporalis or the superficial temporalis muscle to reconstruct the orbital floor. A temporoparietal facial flap has been used for orbital and eyelid reconstruction. Free transfer flaps are advocated for this reconstructive challenge, as there are no limitations with

rotation and the goals of maintaining facial structural stability and contour are upheld. Sadove and Powell [138] described a one-stage reconstruction of the subtotal maxillectomy and hemimandibulectomy with a free fibular osteocutaneous flap. After harvesting a vascularized fibular bone flap, multiple osteotomies allow the surgeon to shape the bone and simultaneously apply the segments to the maxilla and mandible. The technique applied was taken from Jones and colleagues [139]. In their "double-barreled" bone graft, transverse osteotomies produce two vascularized bone struts that can be folded parallel to each other and connected by the periosteum and muscle cuff pedicle. Here, three bone struts were employed; the distal end of the fibula was rigidly fixed to the small remaining portion of the maxilla, and a transverse osteotomy allowed a 90-degree turn of the segment. A second osteotomy was then performed to allow fixation to the remaining zygomatic fragment, and all osteotomies were rigidly fixated with miniplates and screws. A third osteotomy in the remaining third portion of the harvested fibula allowed removal of a 3- cm segment, which would account for the distance between the maxilla and mandible. The remaining vascularized bony segment was then rotated and used to bridge the mandibular bony defect, and rigid fixation was similarly applied. The accompanying peroneal vessels were anastomosed end to side with a radial artery, from a radial artery forearm flap. The combination of radial forearm and fibular fasciocutaneous flaps offers excellent versatility to meet the extreme three-dimensional demands of reconstruction of massive injuries to the face.

5.5. Lip reconstruction

The overall survival rate for carcinomas involving the lip has increased over the past 30 years to 85% to 90%. Because regional spread is uncommon in the behavior of lip cancers, reconstruction after tumor ablation becomes paramount in these patients. Most neoplastic processes occur in the lower lip, and almost all lesions are epidermoid or squamous cell carcinomas. Upper lip malignancies are almost exclusively basal cell cancers. The primary function of the lip is oral competence, along with its role in speech, deglutition, and beauty. The competence is provided by the sphincter muscles, the orbicularis oris muscle, and a number of elevator and depressor muscles. Its primary blood supply is from the superior and inferior labial arteries, which are direct branches of the facial artery. When performing lip reconstruction, one must attempt to retain the sphincter muscle function, obtain a watertight oral seal, and allow sufficient opening for daily dietary habits. In defects of 30% to 65%, upper lip tissue may be transferred by a pedicle flap based on the labial artery [140]. The oral commissure is preserved when using this in conjunction with the Abbe technique or when the flap is rotated around the commissure using the Eastlander method. The flap on the upper lip is designed with the medial incision on the philtrum ridge to allow closure of the donor site on this natural landmark. The largest flap that can be designed is approximately 2 cm, and one fourth of the upper lip can be excised and closed primarily. The Karapandzic technique also uses lip tissue by advancing and rotating segments of skin, orbicularis muscle, and mucosa. However, the principal disadvantage is the creation of microsomia. Local flaps are preferable to regional flaps for closing defects of less than two thirds of the lip width because of their skin color and texture match and the availability of mucous membrane for internal lining. Defects greater than two thirds of the entire lip are best reconstructed using adjacent cheek flaps. Large defects of the upper lip may be reconstructed by excising crescent-shaped peri-alar cheek tissue and advancing the flaps medially. For larger defects, between 65% and 80%, the cheek tissue can be advanced as in the Webster-Bernard approach. This technique, however, has led to the development of chronic tension, resulting in a poorly functioning lower lip. Karapandzic lip rotation has been used, without inevitable microstomia. This approach requires dissection of the remaining lower lip segment, the modiolus bilaterally, and the lateral upper lip tissue, and then advancement of these components to reconstruct the lower lip deficiency. Defects greater than 80% to 85% have been reconstructed with inferiorly based nasolabial flaps. Massive defects of the lip, chin, and mandible are reconstructed with the use of distant flaps, transferring composite flaps of skin and bone revascularized by microvascular techniques. The radial forearm flap, incorporating the plantaris tendon, provides excellent support to the circumoral structures (Figure 28).

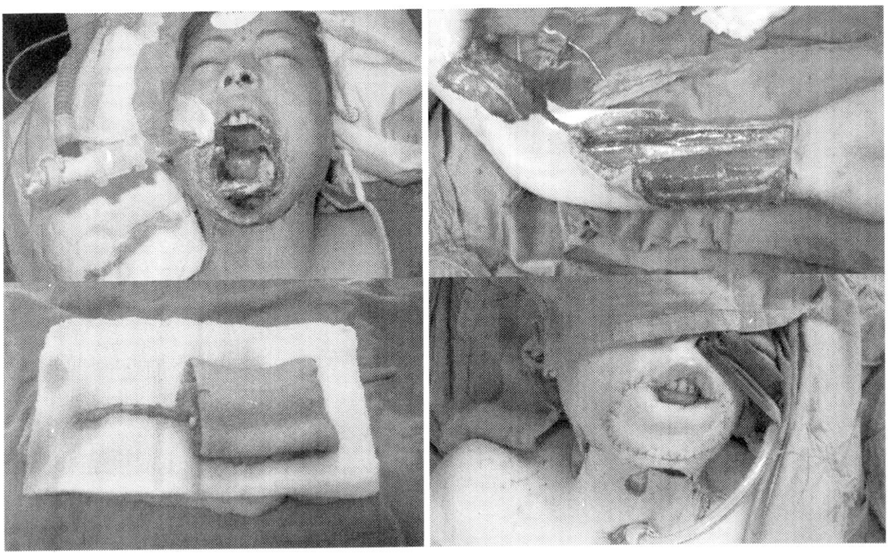

Figure 28. Total reconstruction of the lower lip

Sensation can be restored by suturing the antebrachial cutaneous nerve of the flap to the stump of mental neural tissue. To effectively reconstruct the lower lip, the skin, mucosa, and functioning muscle must be replaced. Dissection of the platysma myocutaneous flap with an extended muscle pedicle including the cervical branch of the facial nerve would greatly improve its motor function. This has yet to be demonstrated clinically. The temporal forehead flap can be used for total upper lip reconstruction, but a secondary cosmetic deformity precludes its common use. More recently, the pectoralis major myocutaneous flap has been used for lip reconstruction; it has the advantage of being an axial myocutaneous flap that may be elevated as a strip of muscle, and a portion of the flap may be turned on itself to provide tissue for the inner aspect of the lips or anterior floor of the mouth [141]. The development of microvascular techniques has allowed reconstruction of concomitant defects of the lip, chin, and anterior mandible by transferring free composite osteomyocutaneous flaps, providing vascularized bone grafts for mandibular reconstruction.

5.6. Tongue reconstruction

Reconstruction of hemiglossectomy requires a thin-tissue flap. Many flaps have been advocated for this purpose. The forearm flap is easily retrieved, but the donor site must receive skin grafting coverage. Because this is an area of daily exposure, its appearance may not be well tolerated by patients. The forehead flap is also easy to harvest, but one of the complications is facial nerve palsy from damage to the temporal branch of the facial nerve. In order to restore the tongue's sensation, a neurovascular radial forearm flap and lateral arm flap could potentially fulfill a sensory function if anastomosed to the lingual or inferior alveolar nerve (Figure 29).

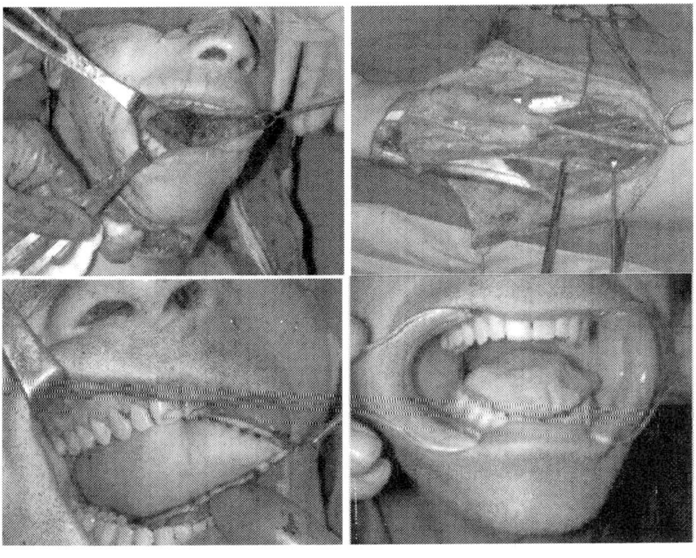

Figure 29. Tongue reconstruction

The dorsalis pedis flap has recently received attention, as it is thinner than the lateral forearm flap. The donor site is well covered, and its distal location allows simultaneous harvest and ablation. The only functional disturbances are related to slight sensory alterations, which have been shown to improve over time. No motor deficits or impairments have been reported. Initially, preoperative angiography was recommended, but a Doppler flowmeter is able to detect dorsalis pedis artery patency. The largest skin island that can be obtained is approximately 9 by 8 cm. The flap is designed to include the dorsalis pedis artery and the first metatarsal dorsal artery. Distally, the flap is elevated and the dorsalis pedis artery is located laterally to medially. The extensor hallucis brevis tendon should be cut because it crosses the first metatarsal artery. If a long pedicle is desired, the inferior extensor retinaculum is incised to elevate the tibialis anterior artery and dorsalis pedis artery. The donor site is then covered by a split-thickness skin graft [142].

5.7. Nasal reconstruction

The most common causes of nasal defects are wide surgical excisions of nasal tumors, followed by trauma and infection. Most nasal skin tumors are basal cell carcinomas, with squamous cell carcinomas accounting for up to 50% of all aggressive tumors. Frequently, treatment of these neoplastic processes requires hemirhinectomy or total rhinectomy to achieve cure. Historically, the use of a nasal prosthesis attached to spectacles was cosmetically acceptable but could be troublesome and lead to patient noncompliance. In fact, more patients have opted for immediate reconstruction [143]. The principles of nasal reconstruction are to replace the lost mucosal lining, reconstruct the skeletal framework, and achieve adequate external skin coverage. The mucosal lining is best replaced by folding full thickness adjacent nasal skin or by using nasolabial flaps or a fold-down median forehead flap (the Kazanjian flap) (Figure 30). [144]

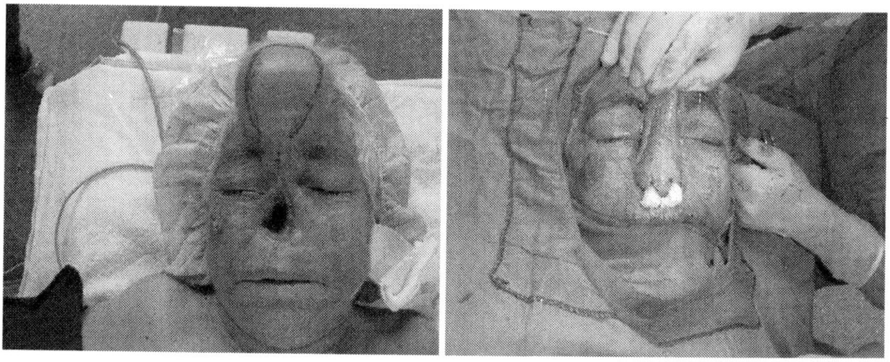

Figure 30. Nasal reconstruction using tissue expansion

The skeletal framework provides support to prevent sagging of overlying tissues, which can lead to nasal stenosis and a poor cosmetic result. The framework can be made by advancing the remaining septal cartilage or using a composite conchal graft, cartilage xenograft, Silastic prosthesis, or cantilever bone graft, which is usually a strut of rib bone graft fixed at its base to the nasal or frontal bones by osteosynthesis wires or plates. The problem arises when trying to match color and texture to replace the external skin covering. This has led to the development of many types of flap designs, including median forehead flaps, based on the supraorbital and supratrochlear vessels, and the scalping forehead flap, which resembles the nasal skin in color and texture and is based on the superficial temporal artery. Primary closure of these forehead flaps can be accomplished with the use of tissue expanders. This, however, requires multiple staged procedures, which may affect patient willingness. The retroauriculotemporal flap, or Washio flap [145], is based on the anastomosis between the posterior branches of the superficial temporal and retroauricular vessels. Its advantage is that the donor site is hidden and composite skin and conchal cartilage are available. Distant pedicled flaps from the arm or neck have been used but require prolonged periods of immobilization and often have poor cosmetic results. Free microvascular tissue transfer can also provide tissue coverage, as well as bony support (Figure 31).

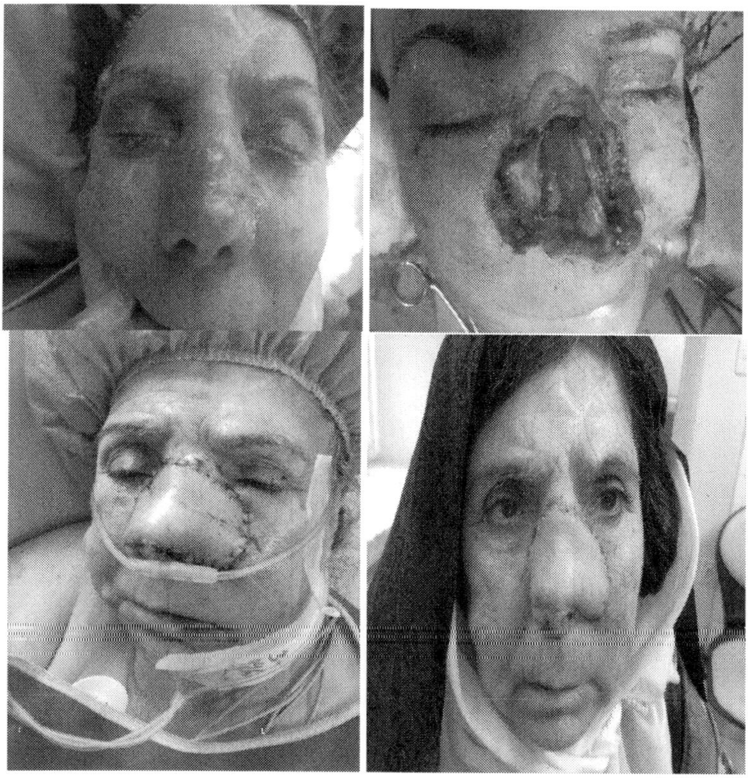

Figure 31. Free flap nasal reconstruction

For example, in the dorsalis pedis osteocutaneous flap, skin is taken from the dorsum of the foot, associated with a vascularized bone graft from the second metatarsal bone.

5.8. Reconstruction of the buccal mucosa

Cancers occurring in the buccal mucosa account for only 10% of all oral cavity carcinomas. There is a higher distribution in the southeastern United States, where "snuff dipping" is a common practice. These lesions tend to occur along the occlusal plane or just below it, and affect the mandible more than the maxilla. These types of lesions are readily treated with surgical ablative surgery, followed by reconstructive efforts to restore the defect. Smaller lesions can be successfully treated with local and buccal flaps. When larger defects are left from surgical excision of larger tumors, more substantial flap designs are required. The buccal cavity allows for expansion of the oral cavity during opening and chewing. Limitation in this region affects jaw function and vestibular loss. Because the buccal mucosa requires a thin, soft, pliable flap for its reconstruction [146], a deltopectoral flap is an ideal choice. It is, however, a two-stage procedure that gives a significantly better result than simple myocutaneous flaps. A thin flap reconstruction can also be achieved with a microvascular free tissue transfer of jejunum used as a patch graft, or with a radial forearm flap. Large full-thickness defects have historically been reconstructed using forehead flaps, temporalis muscle flaps, or pectoralis, latissimus, or trapezius muscle flaps [147]. The operative combination of lower lip splitting incisions and composite anterior oromandibular reconstruction creates a pre- disposition to increased lip and labial sulcus deformities related to abnormal wound healing, which is commonly caused by extensive anterior floor of the mouth and oral lining defects combined with partial skin paddle necrosis, inadequate intraoral lining replacement, closure under excess tension, over projection of mandible reconstruction, and improper draping of the soft tissues of the chin to the reconstructed mandible. The lower lip deformity is called a reverse whistling deformity [148]. It is a vertically short lip with central notching associated with oral incontinence and an inadequate lower labial sulcus. To repair this cosmetically displeasing complication, the scar contractures are released with excisions, and vertical musculomucosal turnover flaps are combined with bilateral lip advancement to improve the deficient lip height and labial sulcus. The blood supply to these flaps is based on inferior labial artery and submental artery distributions, which are branches of the facial artery.

5.9. Craniofacial reconstruction

Large resections during cranial surgery produce severe disfigurement and emotional anguish, with significant functional impairment for the patient. After surgical management of skull-based malignancies, the reconstructive surgeon is faced with the extensive task of not only restoring the anatomic defects but also preventing potentially life-threatening complications, such as ascending meningitis from the close proximity of the paranasal sinuses and nasopharynx to the dura. Reconstructions may be immediate or delayed. Although immediate reconstruction after extensive resection of aggressive or recurrent tumors has been recommended, it is not routinely practiced, because extensive immediate reconstruction may lead to delayed detection of early recurrence. Also, the ideal reconstructive option, which is usually the first major reconstruction, would be sacrificed. The two indications for immediate reconstruction are to prevent ascending infection from an open nasopharynx or to close the frontal sinus, and to prevent exposure of brain and/or bone. Historically, many cranial base defects were treated with the use of local flaps through a "patch" design. Myocutaneous flaps were then developed, with the pectoralis major and latissimus dorsi flaps becoming the most widely employed. Finally came the advent of free tissue transfer for larger defects requiring well-vascularized tissue with bulk, not restricted by pedicles. As experience with free flap harvest has been gained, complication rates have dropped. The correct selection and application of these reconstructive methods require that the surgeon appreciate the capabilities of each technique. Often a combination of techniques is required for optimal reconstruction. The most common combination is an internal fixation device and a bone graft. In the reconstruction of cranio-orbital defects, the following goals are addressed: achieve a tight dural seal to isolate the intracranial contents from the aerodigestive tract, obliterate dead spaces in the sinuses to remove potential sources of infection, suspend and support neural structures, provide bone and soft tissue coverage, maintain function, and achieve optimal cosmetic result [149]. The likelihood of recurrence of the disease and its concealment by the reconstruction has been a major deterrent to midface reconstruction. Calvarial grafts, having a membranous bony quality with delayed resorption, are excellent replacements for the orbital floor and nasal dorsum. Stability is maintained with rigid fixation. When combined with the temporoparietal fascia, a calvarial graft provides an excellent source of vascularized tissue for enhancing soft tissue reconstruction to the orbit and maxilla. However, because it is based on a pedicle, its arc of rotation limits its flexibility. Free tissue transfer using microvascular anastomosis has alleviated this problem. The scapula, radial forearm, and dorsalis pedis osteocutaneous flaps all have fairly long pedicles and can carry both skin and bone reliably. The deep circumflex iliac artery flap has a short pedicle, thick skin, and little mobility, making it more difficult to maneuver. A modification of the scapular flap using the angular artery, which supplies the entire lateral border of the scapula, can increase the pedicle from 4 to 9 cm to 13 to 18 cm; this allows the skin and bone to have much longer, independent arcs of rotation, so that they can be used in different parts of the reconstruction, such as skin for the palate and lateral nasal wall and bone for the infraorbital rim, with the two segments supplied by the same subscapular pedicle [150]. Preoperative planning for osseous reconstruction begins with a careful and thorough history and physical examination. Radiographic imaging with standard cephalometric radiographs and CT with three dimensional reconstructive images are very useful. Reconstructions of the cranial base are divided by their anatomic designs. Classifications by Jones and Jacksons have been widely used to integrate the anatomic boundaries with tumor growth patterns in different regions. Region I corresponds to defects extending from the anterior midline to the posterior wall of the orbital cavity, but including an extension down the clivus to the foramen magnum. This region houses tumors from the maxilla, maxillary antrum, parotid gland, and midfacial skin. Initially, reconstruction was aimed at covering the exposed dura with the use of nonvascularized split-thickness skin grafts, such as tensor fascia lata grafts. Failures would occur in 50% of the cases in which dural leaks of cerebrospinal fluid occurred [151]. Thus, covering the defect with a vascularized tissue seemed appropriate. Forehead flaps, glabella flaps, pericranial flaps, and galea flaps have all been advocated. Defects of the anterior cranial fossa can be covered by using a laterally positioned temporalis muscle flap. Myocutaneous flaps have also been used and provide a number of distinct advantages. They are well vascularized, provide additional bulk that aids in eliminating dead space, and provide acceptable soft tissue contouring and aesthetic results. The pectoralis major flap is used to reach the orbital region, but it must be exteriorized to reach this site, thus adding a second operation. The latissimus dorsi muscle flap can access the orbit without a subsequent exteriorization procedure, but the patient must be repositioned for its harvest. A trapezius flap is also available, but its use must be carefully assessed in a previously irradiated patient or one in whom a radical neck dissection was performed. Again, this technique requires repositioning of the patient. In larger defects, free tissue transfer provides a well-vascularized, bulky tissue, without the restrictions of a pedicle. The most frequently used is the rectus abdominis free flap; simultaneous ablation of the tumor and flap harvest by two surgical teams reduces operative time and patient mortality. Region II defects essentially include the boundaries of the middle cranial fossa. It comprises the infratemporal and pterygomaxillary fossae and the overlying segment of the skull base. Tumors of this area include basal and squamous cell carcinoma of the external ear and scalp, invasive parotid tumors, and tumors of the middle ear. Access to the middle cranial vault is primarily through an infratemporal approach but may also be combined with a mandibulotomy, lateral mandibulotomy, anterior mandibulotomy with swing, or anterior displacement of the mandible. Also, via a hemicoronal incision, a transtemporal approach can provide access to the tumor. The location and the size of the defect dictate which reconstructive option is used. Historically, large scalp rotation flaps [152] and deltopectoral flaps have provided adequate restoration. Smaller defects can be repaired with temporalis muscle flaps. However, when larger defects may be inadequately treated with these local flaps-that is, when communications between the nasopharynx and dura persists-free flaps become the procedure of choice, specifically, the rectus abdominis free flap.

Region III includes the posterior segment of the middle cranial fossa, as well as the entire posterior section. The most common tumors encountered here are glomus tumors and schwannomas. Through a transtemporal approach, tumors are readily excised, and small defects can be closed with local flaps such as temporalis, deltoid, and sternocleidomastoid. Larger defects are more definitively reconstructed with latissimus dorsi flaps or the rectus abdominis free flap. Eye socket reconstruction requires not only a mucosal lining but also supportive tissue to mimic the tarsus. Traditionally, full- or split-thickness skin grafts without any supportive tissue failed owing to severe contracture formation. Millard [153] in 1962 used a composite nasal cartilage-mucosa graft. In 1985, Siegel [154] discussed the use of the palatal mucosa for reconstruction of the eyelid. The palatal mucosa is thick and rigid tissue that has been used for the reconstruction of the lip, gingiva, nasal vestibular lining, and tracheal wall defects. The "socket plasty" described by Yoshimura and coworkers [155] uses a palatal mucosa graft to maintain the dimensions of the socket to accept an orbital prosthesis. The palatal mucosa is sutured to deepen the fornix and keep the maximal dimensions of the graft for at least 10 to 14 days. An artificial eye or Silastic rubber ball is inserted to maintain the newly formed socket during the initial healing period. The donor site usually heals unremarkably, with little patient discomfort. Orbital floor defects have been treated with many materials, including autografts, allografts, xenografts, and alloplasts. The ideal material is fresh autogenous bone, but this requires a second surgical procedure. Harvested auricular cartilage provides an excellent source of autogenous tissue for repairing orbital floor defects. This fresh cartilage maintains adequate structure and volume many years after transplantation [156] In fact, less resorption occurs if the perichondrium is left intact. Two approaches to auricular harvesting have been described: patients susceptible to keloid formation benefit from a posterior approach, and others undergo the anterior approach. The anterior approach involves a semicircular incision made through skin and perichondrium within the edge of the concha bowl to hide the scar. The skin-perichondrial flap is elevated anteriorly with blunt dissection to expose the graft conchal cartilage. Once the desired amount is excised with its associated perichondrium, the donor site can be closed with single-layer closure. The graft can then be sculpted to its desired shape, thus allowing it to be custom fitted. The posterior approach uses a posterior auricular incision to expose the posteromedial aspect of the concha. Using blunt dissection with a Freer elevator, the cartilage is accessed and excised from its native site. The auricular wound is closed in a similar fashion as that described for the anterior approach. Both techniques require a pressure dressing to prevent hematoma formation. This procedure is quick, is in the same location as the recipient site, and has minimal associated morbidity [157]. Shestak [158] described the reconstruction of combined midfacial and palatal defects with the use of a latissimus dorsi musculocutaneous free flap with separate skin paddles to reconstruct multiple tissue surfaces. After tumor excision, the recipient vessels of free flap are selected in the ipsilateral neck. The latissimus dorsi flap is harvested in a standard fashion, with the proximal end of the inscribed skin paddle designed at least 5 cm below the tip of the scapula to allow an ample length of the thoracodorsal artery and vein. The palatal inset is performed first using everting horizontal mattress sutures to obtain a watertight seal. An area of the skin is then de-epithelialized to accept remnants of facial skin and lip segments. The vascular pedicle is passed through a tunnel to the recipient vessels in the neck. Revascularization occurs by microvascular anastomosis. Because of the latissimus dorsi's accessibility, pedicle length, reliability of skin paddles, and ample available tissue, this flap is a viable treatment option for soft tissue reconstruction of complex craniofacial defects. Shestak reported 12 reconstructions using the same technique with satisfactory functional and aesthetic outcomes.

6. Implants in reconstruction

After extensive ablation of maxillofacial tumors, reconstruction of the head and neck region is attempted to restore the external cosmetic and functional deficits. However, masticatory function continues to be a problem in the rehabilitation of these patients. Without dental implants, the area of reconstruction does not allow placement of a dental prosthesis. Implants eliminate the requirement for adjacent natural soft tissue support for the prosthesis. Endosseous implants placed in bone grafts have been shown to stimulate bone growth and minimize its resorption. Therefore, when one reconstructive option is chosen over another, not only the quantity but also the quality of the bone that will ultimately receive endosseous implants should be a consideration [20]. Implants can be placed after a reconstruction has been performed or at the time of immediate reconstruction [159] Stoler and Hill [160] were the first to report a case in which oromandibular reconstruction was performed for a patient who had undergone ablative surgery for fibrous dysplasia using a combination of both free cranial and microvascular iliac crest grafts, as well as osseointegrated implants placed in vitro and then grafted onto the reconstructed mandible. The advantages of immediate placement are the ease of access and ability to avoid any adjacent alloplastic materials, such as bone plates and screws. One possible problem associated with immediate placement is improper position of the implant. A delayed placement has the advantage of providing better control for placement in the correct position. However, disadvantages of the delayed technique are the necessity for a secondary surgical procedure, the need to deal with abnormal intraoral soft tissues, and the need to be aware of the position of the vascular pedicle as it relates to the reconstructed mandible [161]. Moscoso and associates [162] analyzed the effect of osseointegration in various donor sites for vascularized bone used for oromandibular reconstruction. The results of the study confirmed that the iliac crest is the most uniform implantable source of vascularized bone for the reception of osseointegrated implants. This was followed by scapula, fibula, and radius. They also pointed out some gender differences. Male fibulas were statistically equivalent to the iliac crest in terms of implantability. In females, however, only one third of proximal scapulas and 50% of proximal to midfibulas would allow implant placement. The long-term stability of a successfully osseointegrated implant is dependent on implant dimension, the structural integrity of the bone to withstand functional loading, and allowances for loss of marginal bone height [163] In cases in which the iliac crest is not accessible owing to previous bone grafting attempts or disruption of vascular anatomy from previous groin vascular surgery, or when the excessive tissue bulk associated with the osteomyocutaneous iliac flap is not desired, an alternative is to use osseointegrated implants in free vascularized radial bone grafts. The radial bone graft provides the ideal mucosal replacement tissue from the associated forearm skin paddle. Radial bone was previously reported as being too thin to accept implants. Mounsey and Boyd [164] reported their experiences using implants placed in vascularized radial bone flaps.

They showed that for small, straight, bony defects, the radius is a good alternative. In larger defects, the contoured iliac crest is a better option. However, the radial bone may be osteotomized to attempt to create the desired mandibular contour. They reported excellent results following implant placement in small- to moderate-size lateral defects, as well as small anterior or anterolateral defects. Further reports using radial bone and dental implants were made by Martin and colleagues [165], with similar success. They do not advocate one-stage reconstruction and primary implant placement because of the possibility of jeopardizing its periosteal blood supply. The microvascular free fibular transfer is an excellent option for reconstruction of large mandibular defects. Its bicortical nature mimics that of the native mandible and seems to be ideal for inserting implants as primary stabilization is achieved [166]. However, dental restoration with traditional removable oral appliances has failed owing to diminished denture-bearing regions as tongue dysfunction. Zlotolow and associates [167] studied the use of the fibular free flap with osseointegrated implants. They reported seven successful cases and concluded that with microvascular bony reconstruction with osseointegrated implants, the quality of life is greatly enhanced by bringing the patient closer to the predisease state.

In 1994, Donovan and coworkers [168] described a new technique combining calvarial onlay bone grafts with osseointegrated implants-more specifically, the Branemark system. The use of such membranous grafts stemmed from previous reports stating that less resorption is seen with membranous bone grafts, compared with endochondral onlay grafts [169]. After harvesting the outer cortical table of calvarial-parietal bone in strips, two grafting techniques are used. The vertical technique is used primarily in the atrophic maxilla, and the graft is secured to the lateral aspect of the remaining maxillary bone or alveolar processes with a rigid screw system. This is followed by a period of healing, approximately 6 to 8 months, before definitive placement of dental implants. They reported an 86% success rate with this onlay procedure, attributing possible failures to varying degrees of soft tissue ingrowth, as well as the cortical strip of bone being further away from its source of blood supply. The horizontal technique, which enjoyed a 98% success rate, places the calvarial bony strips in a horizontal fashion in the anterior maxillary region, where the nasal spine is separated from its most inferior bony attachment. The cortical struts are then placed in a horizontal fashion superiorly at the level of the nasal floor as well as inferiorly, augmenting the height of the maxillary ridge. The "sandwiched" maxilla is then stabilized with its grafts with the placement of osseointegrated implants from one canine eminence to the other. These implants, in contrast to those used in the vertical technique, have bicortical stabilization and are placed close together to aid in stress load distribution. These success rates are comparable to those seen when reconstructing the anterior mandible. All patients were restored with implant-supported prostheses, resulting in good function, a stable prosthesis, lack of donor site morbidity, early ambulation, and a short hospital stay.

6.1. Maxillofacial prosthodontics

The demand for maxillofacial prosthodontic devices for the rehabilitation of patients with postsurgical defects has intensified in recent years. The extensive surgical procedures necessary to eradicate cancer of the head and neck often leave extremely large physical defects that may not be amenable to surgical reconstruction. The prosthodontist can provide surgical stents, radiation carriers and shields, intraoral cone stents, palatal augmentation prostheses for glossectomy patients, and immediate transitional and definitive prostheses, as well as extraoral prostheses to replace ears, nose, and facial defects. Thus, the maxillofacial prosthodontist must have knowledge of the disease, etiology, diagnosis, treatment, and rehabilitation in order to be a member of the team that is responsible for enhancing the patient's quality of life [170]. Prosthetic and prosthodontic appliances are required for realignment and fixation of mandibular fragments in adequate dental occlusal relationships with the teeth of the opposing jaw; as obturators for the occlusion of defects of the palatal region; for the maintenance of facial form and contour so as to prevent contracture of the tissues during the healing period; as a temporary or transitional modality before or during surgical treatment; and for the restoration of facial features, such as the nose, auricle, or orbital region [171]. The maxillary defects that result from ablative cancer surgery vary in complexity, but prosthetic rehabilitation may provide a functional and aesthetic result. The purpose of the obturator prosthesis is to re-establish the normal contour of the oral cavity to allow normal speech and swallowing. The size of the defect determines the size of the obturator, or bulb portion that closes the surgical defect. The loss of this supporting tissue can be offset by gaining retention from the peripheral tissues. The maturity of the defect also determines how the obturator is tolerated. The more mature the defect, the more readily it is tolerated. A skin graft can provide a firm tissue base that resists abrasion and reduces mucus secretion, minimizing poor hygienic environments. The opposing mandibular ridge is important to the stability of the obturator. Prosthetic rehabilitation of the maxillectomy patient is performed in three phases. Stage one starts with the placement of the surgical packing and surgical obturator, which is retained for 5 to 7 days by screw or wire fixation. This helps re-establish oral contours and allows the patient to start a liquid diet almost immediately postoperatively, bypassing the need for nasogastric feeding. In the second stage, the surgical obturator is removed and modified with a tissue conditioner. As the obturator is modified, the patient learns how to swallow less forcefully, and leakage around the prosthesis decreases. The third stage can be anywhere from 3 months to over a year after maxillectomy, when the definitive obturator prosthesis is fabricated [172]. In maxillectomy patients, osseointegrated implants may be placed in the residual alveolar ridge or horizontal palate. An edentulous maxillectomy defect has the poorest prognosis for accepting an obturator. It is impossible to achieve retention of a complete maxillary denture. Thus, endosseous implants may aid in retention, stability, and support of the obturator prosthesis; a bar and clip, magnet, and ball-0-ring gasket-type keeper are widely used in these situations. The bar and clip assembly provides the obturator prosthesis with improved stability and retention. For patients with significant extraoral tissue loss, the facial prosthesis also has limitations related to retention and stability. The extraoral application of implants has been a significant advance in maxillofacial prosthetics (Figure 32).

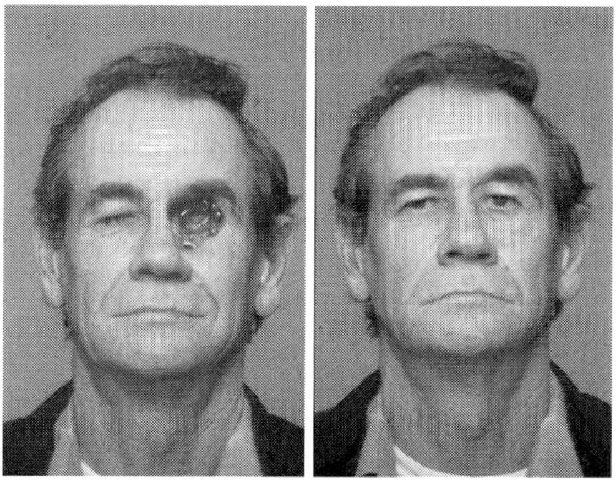

Figure 32. Orbit prosthesis

For example, implants placed in the mastoid bone or the temporal bones allow an auricular implant to be fixated via bar splinting. A nasal prosthesis can use a similar retention technique and have its fixtures placed in the floor of the nose. And in situations in which tumor ablation included the orbit, implants can be placed in the supraorbital rim region [173]. As with intraoral dental implants, extraoral sites require proper hygiene practices to ensure tissue health.

http://dx.doi.org/10.5772/59746

7. Pediatric reconstruction

Mandibular reconstruction and rehabilitation in a 7-year-old with osteosarcoma were recently reported by Richardson and Cawood [174]. They made every effort to maintain the functional matrix so as not to disturb the normal growth processes of the face. After tumor ablation with a partial mandibulectomy, immediate reconstruction with a titanium mesh tray was performed without bone graft. This technique allowed the tray to function as a space maintainer. When the patient approached the onset of puberty, the tray was removed and a composite circumflex iliac crest free flap was used to restore the continuity and soft tissue deficiencies. Microvascular anastomosis of the donor and recipient sites was used. Two years later, osseointegrated implants were placed, with a subsequent vestibuloplasty with a split-thickness skin graft. They concluded that the multidisciplinary approach to the care of this patient, along with the introduction of revascularized free tissue transfer with osseointegrated implants, revolutionized the reconstruction of pediatric orofacial defects following extensive tissue losses.

8. Postoperative evaluation

The postoperative care and management of complications require an understanding of osseous wound healing and the potential causes of failure. Loss of skeletal stability as a result of loss of fixation allows for motion at the wound interface, with secondary impairment of vascularization. Early recognition of flap compromise is associated with improved chances of flap salvage. The ideal flap monitoring technique should be reliable, reproducible, easily interpretable, inexpensive, noninvasive, rapidly responsive to changes in microcirculation, and able to provide continuous monitoring in the immediate postreconstructive period. The clinical examination should focus on capillary refill time (>3 seconds is the cutoff), which provides information on the adequacy of the arterial supply. Early venous outflow obstruction results in capillary refill that is too brisk. The color of a flap can also provide information about arterial insufficiency. A pale flap signifies poor flap perfusion, whereas one with outflow obstruction is congested and hyperemic. Skin temperature can assess the adequacy of circulation in digits but is of little use when applied to flaps for reconstruction, as changes in ambient temperature affect the measured surface temperature readings. The most invasive monitoring method is blood flow from the flap. Flow of oxygenated blood, from a needle puncture, indicates good perfusion, whereas dark red blood or sluggish flow is a prognostic indicator.

Buried flaps, or flaps used for pharyngoesophageal reconstruction, require some other form of monitoring technique, because direct visualization is not possible. Flexible fiberoptic telescopes have been used, but this method cannot be performed on a continual basis. To visualize a segment of jejunum used for pharyngeal reconstruction, a sheet of silicone rubber (Silastic) is placed over the segment of jejunum and the skin is left open to provide a "window" to allow a direct view of the jejunum. A flap can be designed with a segment externalized so that the surgeon can readily visualize it. The cutaneous part can often be partially externalized and incorporated in the wound closure to serve as an indicator of graft survival; this also decreases wound tension. Tissue that is unnecessary for reconstruction and is supplied by the vascular pedicle can be externalized and observed for impairment of blood supply.

There are a number of adjunctive monitoring devices that can be used to assess the adequacy of tissue perfusion. An electromagnetic flowmeter determines the absolute blood flow in a vessel by electromagnetic induction and allows immediate and continuous readings to see slow or rapid changes. The ultrasonic Doppler flowmeter has been in clinical use for more than 30 years and is useful if one is certain that the flow signal heard is from the vascular pedicle. Arterial thermometry is a system that measures temperature difference across a vascular anastomosis with implanted thermocouple probes. Fluorescein has been used to identify flaps with inadequate perfusion; when injected intravenously, it diffuses out to the capillaries into the interstitial fluid. The staining can then be visualized under ultraviolet illumination. The more intense the staining, the better the perfusion, and vice versa. The dermofluorometer enables the clinician to quantify minute degrees of fluorescence and uses smaller doses of the drug to prevent allergic reactions. Radioisotope washout of xenon 133, sodium pertechnetate Tc99m, iodine 131, and sodium 24 has been used to indicate the adequacy of perfusion; after administration of an isotope, clearance from the flap is monitored and correlated with flap perfusion (i.e., greater clearance equals greater flap perfusion). Pulse oximetery can detect pulsatile blood flow until the artery is 95% occluded. Laser-Doppler velocimetry is currently the best tool for objective monitoring of flaps. It must be in place when the flap is known to have good perfusion, because changes in this initial value are the important parameter. The laser-Doppler velocimeter can provide an accurate, easily interpretable readout of tissue perfusion that is rapidly responsive to changes in perfusion. Duplex Doppler ultrasonography is capable of identifying and characterizing blood flow from small, superficially located vessels, similar to those involved with microvascular surgery. Different shades of gray are assigned to stationary areas, whereas color is assigned to areas of motion such as blood flowing within a vessel. Vessels as small as 1 mm in diameter can be identified. Transcutaneous oxygen monitoring is also an option, where Po2 is measured directly to assess the state of microcirculation. Finally, changes in interstitial fluid hydrostatic pressures can reflect changes in blood flow [175]. Radiologic literature on bone graft evaluation is sparse. Follow-up assessment of skeletal reconstruction with plain radiographs and cephalometric studies in the immediate postoperative period is needed to document the position of bone segments and the location of hardware. However, data on the evaluation of primary bone tumors and bone allografts stress the role of plain film radiography. In 1992, Soderholm and colleague [176] studied the effectiveness of using plain film radiography in the follow-up and prognosis of non-vascular bone grafting used in mandibular reconstruction. They concluded that narrow-beam radiography and spiral tomography are excellent tools for the evaluation of bone resorption and bony healing of mandibular grafts. Panoramic radiographs are able to visualize the whole mandibular bone and are used for a general assessment; tomography is used for specified, selected diagnostic tasks, such as to visualize bone resorption within the graft and under the plate. After reconstruction of large defects in the oral cavity or the oropharynx with myocutaneous or free microvascular flaps, physical rehabilitation by a therapist trained in speech and swallowing is of paramount importance, as these reconstructive procedures cannot fully restore the patient's ability to masticate, swallow, or speak. The major aims of physical therapy are to decrease the amount of facial deformity and to limit the loss of oral opening. Oral opening exercises are initiated as soon as the patient can tolerate them. Stretching exercises three to four times a day are adequate home regimens. A specialized therapist may use the Therabite mouth opener (Therabite Co., Bryn Mawr, PA) to improve maximal opening. Also, those patients who have had neck dissections require physical therapy for shoulder pain and trapezius weakness. Range-of-motion exercises are necessary to prevent frozen shoulder and worsening pain.

Author details

Ata Garajei[1,2,3*], Ali Arabkheradmand[2], Mohammad Hosein Kalantar Motamedi[4,5], Alex E. Pazoki[6] and Ashkan Rashad[7]

*Address all correspondence to: atagarajei@tums.ac.ir

1 Department of Oral and Maxillofacial Surgery, School of Dentistry, The Cancer Institute, Tehran

2 Department of Head and Neck Surgical Oncology and Reconstructive Surgery, The Cancer Institute, Tehran, Iran

3 Craniomaxillofacial Research Center, Tehran University of Medical Sciences, Tehran, Iran

4 Trauma Research Center, Baqiyatallah University of Medical Sciences, Tehran, Iran

5 Department of Oral and Maxillofacial Surgery, Azad University of Medical Sciences, Dental College, Tehran, Iran

6 Department of Oral and Maxillofacial Surgery, Johns Hopkins University, Baltimore, USA

7 Department of Oral and Maxillofacial Surgery, Bremerhaven Hospital (Reinkenheide); Bremerhaven, Germany

References

[1] Marx RE, Schiff WM, and Saunders TR: Reconstruction and rehabilitation of cancer patients. In Fonseca RJ, Davis WH (eds): Reconstructive Preprosthetic Oral and Maxillofacial Surgery, ed 2. Philadelphia, WB Saunders, 1995, p 1057.

[2] Ferraro NF, August M: Reconstruction following resection for maxillofacial tumors. Oral Maxillo fac Surg Clin North Am 1993;5:355.

[3] Markowitz BL, Calcaterra TC: Preoperative assessment and surgical planning for patients undergoing immediate composite reconstruction of oromandibular defects. Clin Plast Surg 1994; 21:9.

[4] Martin PJ, O'Leary MJ, Hayden RE: Free tissue transfer in oromandibular reconstruction: Necessity or extravagance? Otolaryngol Clin North Am 1994; 27:1141.

[5] Lowlicht RA, Delacure MD, and Sasaki CT: Allogeneic (homograft) reconstruction of the mandible. Laryngoscope 1990; 100:837.

[6] Lawson W, Biller H: Reconstruction of the Mandible. In McCarthy JG (ed): Plastic Surgery, Ed 2. Philadelphia, WB Saunders, 1990, p 2069.

[7] Markowitz B, Taleisnik A, and Calcaterra T, et al: Achieving mandibular continuity with vascular bone flaps. J Oral Maxillofac Surg 1994; 52:114.

[8] Kroll SS, Schusterman MA, and Reece GP: Costs and complications in mandibular reconstruction. Ann Plast Surg 1992; 29:341.

[9] Heller KS, Dubner S, Keller A: Long-term evaluation of patients undergoing immediate mandibu lar reconstruction. Am J Surg 1995; 170:517.

[10] Shockley WW, Weissler MC: Reconstructive alternatives following segmental mandibulectomy. Am J Otolaryngol 1992; 13:156.

[11] Cordeiro PG, Hidalgo DA: Conceptual considerations in mandibular reconstruction. Clin Plast Surg 1995; 22:61.

[12] Kuriloff DB, Sullivan MJ: Mandibular reconstruction using vascularized bone grafts. Otolaryngol Clin North Am 1991; 24:1391.

[13] Urken ML, Moscoso JF: Sensate cutaneous flaps in oral cavity and pharyngeal reconstruction. Oper Tech Otolaryngol Head N eek Surg 1993; 4:141-144.

[14] Strauss MB: Chronic refractory osteomyelitis: Review the role of hyperbaric oxygen. Hyperbaric Oxygen Review 1980; 1:231.

[15] Hyperbaric Oxygen Therapy: A Committee Report: Mechanisms of Action. Bethesda, MD, Undersea Medical Society, 1986, pp 5-9.

[16] Hunt K, Pai MP: The effect of varying ambient oxygen tensions on wound metabolism. and collagen synthesis. Surg Gynecol Obstet 1972; 12:77.

[17] Nemiroff PM, Lungu AP: The influence ofhyperbaric oxygen and irradiation on vascularity in skin flaps: A controlled study. Surg Forum 1987; 37:565.

[18] Nilsson LP, Albrektsson T, Granstrom G, et al: The effect of hyperbaric oxygen treatment on bone regeneration: An experimental study in the rabbit using the bone harvest chamber (BHC). J Oral Maxillofac Implants 1988; 3:43.

[19] Granstrom G, Nilsson LP, Magnusson BC, et al: Experimental mandibular practice: Effect on bone healing after treatment with hyperbaric oxygen. Proceedings of the 25th EUBS Scientific Meeting, Eilat, Israel, 1989, pp 290-297.

[20] Marx RE, Johnson RP, Kline SN: Prevention of osteoradionecrosis: A randomi'zed prospective clinical trial of hyperbaric oxygen versus penicillin. J Am Dent Assoc 1985; 14:49.

[21] Mathiew D, Coget J, Vinckier F, et al: Red blood cell deformability and hyperbaric oxygen therapy. Med Subaquat Hyperbar 1984; 3:100.

[22] Ganstrom G: The use of hyperbaric oxygen to prevent implant loss in the irradiated patient. In Worthington P,.Branemark PI (eds): Advanced Osseointegration Surgery. Chicago, Quintessence, 1989, p 336.

[23] Propper RH: Simplified ridge extension using free mucosal grafts. J Oral Surg 1964;22:469-474.

[24] Marx RE: Philosophy and particulars of autogenous bone grafting. Oral Maxillofac Clin North Am 1993;5:599.

[25] Shirota T, Ohno K, Motohashi M, et al: Histologic and microradiologic comparison of block and particulate cancellous bone and marrow grafts in reconstructed mandibles being considered for dental implant placement. J Oral Maxillofac Surg 1996; 54:15.

[26] Harsha BC, Turvey TA, Powers SK: Use of autogenous cranial bone grafts in the maxillofacial surgery: A preliminary report. J Oral Maxillofac Surg 1986; 44:11.

[27] Kudo K, Shoji M, Yokota M, et al: Evaluation of mandibular reconstruction techniques following resection of malignant tumors in the oral region. J Oral Maxillofac Surg 1992; 50:14.

[28] Branemark PI, Lindstrom J, Hallen 0, et al: Reconstruction of the defective mandible. Scand J Plast Surg 1975; 9:116.

[29] Li KK, Cheney ML, and Teknos TN: The importance of mandibular position in microvascular mandibular reconstruction. Laryngoscope 1996; 106:903.

[30] Ardary WC: Reconstruction of mandibular discontinuity defects using autogenous grafting and a mandibular reconstruction plate: A prospective evaluation of nine consecutive cases. J Oral Maxillofac Surg 1993; 51:125.

[31] Boyne PJ: Autogenous cancellous bone and marrow transplants. Clin Orthop 1992; 73:253.

[32] Gheung LK, Samman N, Tong ACK, et al: Mandibular reconstruction with the Dacron urethane tray: A radiologic assessment of bone remodeling. J Oral Maxillofac Surg 1994; 52:373.

[33] Jisander S, Aspenberg P, Salemark L, et al: Mandibular reconstruction by secondary reimplanta tion of resected segments: A preliminary report. Int J Oral Maxillofac Surg 1995; 24:288.

[34] Tayapongsak P, O'Brien DA, Monteiro CB, et al: Autologous fibrin adhesive in mandibular reconstruction with particulate cancellous bone and marrow. J Oral Maxillofac Surg 1994; 52:161.

[35] Perrott DH, Smith RA, and Kahan LB: The use of fresh frozen allogeneic bone for maxillary and mandibular reconstruction. Int J Oral Maxillofac Surg 1992; 21:260.

[36] Dong Y, Zhang G, Wandg S, et al: The use of immediate frozen autogenous mandible, for benign tumor mandibular reconstruction. Br J Oral Maxillofac Surg 1996;34:58.

[37] Tayapongsak P, Pijut J, and Scheffer RB: Inferior border titanium cribs in mandibular reconstruction. Oral Surg Oral Med Oral Pathol 1995; 79:30.

[38] Bakamjian VY, Calame PM: Oropharyngeoesophageal reconstructive surgery. In Converse JM (ed): Reconstructive Plastic Surgery, vol 5, Ed 2. Philadelphia, WB Saunders, 1977, p 2700.

[39] Kheradmand AA, Garajei A: Ventral tongue myomucosal flap: a suitable choice for shaved lower vermilion border reconstruction. Journal of Craniofacial Surgery 2013; 24 (2), e114-e116.

[40] Tashiro H, Sasaguri M, Ozeki S, et al: Mandibular reconstruction using hydroxyapatite granules, autogenous bone, and a cervical island skin flap. J Oral Maxillofac Surg 1993; 51:1327.

[41] Farr HW, Jean-Gilles B, Die A: Cervical island skin flap repair of oral and pharyngeal defects in the composite operation for cancer. Am J Surg 1969; 118:759.

[42] Ariyan S: The pectoralis major myocutaneous flap: A versatile flap for reconstruction in the head and neck. Plast Reconstr Surg 1979; 63:73.

[43] Owen N: Compound neck pedicle designed for repair of massive facial defects. Plast Reconstr Surg1955; 15:369.

[44] Carlson ER: Regional flaps in maxillofacial reconstruction. Oral Maxillofac Clin North Am 1993; 5:667.

[45] Huttenbrink K: Temporalis muscle flap: An alter- native in oropharyngeal reconstruction. Laryngoscope 1986; 96:1034.

[46] Cheung LK: An animal model of maxillary reconstruction using a temporalis muscle flap. J Oral Maxillofac Surg 1996; 54:1439.

[47] Upton J, Ferraro N, Healy G, et al: The use of prefabricated facial flaps for lining the oral and nasal cavities. Plast Reconstr Surg 1994; 94(5): 573.

[48] Roopenian A. Kazanjian V: Median forehead flaps in the repair of defects of the nose and surrounding areas. Tr Am Acad Oahth and Oto 1956; 60:557.

[49] Shumrick KA, Smith TL: The anatomic basis for the design of forehead flaps. Arch Otolaryngol Head Neck Surg 1992; 118:373.

[50] Burget GC, Menick FJ: Aesthetic Reconstruction of the Nose. St. Louis, Mosby, 1994, p 123

[51] Millard, DR: Reconstructive rhinoplasty for the lower half of a nose. Plast. Recontr. Surg 1974; 53:133.

[52] Kheradmand AA, Garajei A, Motamedi MH: Nasal reconstruction: Experience using tissue expansion and forehead flap. J Oral Maxillofac Surg 69:1478-1484, 2011

[53] Panje WR, Morris MR: The temporoparietal fascia flap in head and neck reconstruction. Ear Nose Throat J 70:311-317,1991

[54] Ladrach K, Raveh J, Lizuka T: Reconstruction of the midface and fronto-orbital region following tumor resection and trauma, in Maniglia AJ, Stucker FJ, Stepnick DW (eds): Surgical Reconstruction of the Face and Anterior Skull Base. Philadelphia, PA, Saunders, 1999, pp 113-140

[55] Conley J: Use of composite flaps containing bone for major repairs on the head and neck. Plast Reconstr Surg 49:522-527, 1972

[56] Esclamado RM, Burkey BB, Carroll WR, et al: The platysma myocutaneous flap: Indications and caveats. Arch Otolaryngol Head Neck Surg 1994; 120:32.

[57] Bakamjian VY: A two-stage method for pharyngoesophageal reconstruction with a primary pec toral skin flap. Plast Reconstr Surg 1965; 36:173.

[58] Murphy JB, Weisman RA, and Kent K: The use of stabilization plates in the immediate repair of defects following mandibular resection. Oral Surg Oral Med Oral Pathol 1989; 68:380.

[59] Marx RE, Smith BR: An improved technique for development of the pectoralis major myocutaneous flap. J Oral Maxillofac Surg 1990; 48:1168.

[60] Kingdom TT, Singer MI: Enhanced reliability and renewed applications of the deltopectoral flap in head and neck reconstruction. Laryngoscope 1996; 106:1230.

[61] Ijsselstein CB, Hovius SER, ten Have BLEF, et al: Is the pectoralis myocutaneous flap in intraoral and oropharyngeal reconstruction outdated? Am J Surg 1996; 172:259.

[62] Lehtimaki K, Pukander J: Primary mandibular reconstruction after ablative cancer surgery. Acta Otolaryngol Suppl 1992; 492:160.

[63] Ord RA: The pectoralis major myocutaneous flap in oral and maxillofacial reconstruction: A retrospective analysis of 50 cases. J Oral Maxillofac Surg 1996; 54:1292.

[64] Haers PE, Gratz KW, Sailer HF: The bilobed myocutaneous pectoralis major flap in closure of combined intra- and extraoral defects. Int J Oral Maxillofac Surg 1994; 23:214.

[65] Baadsgaard K, Medgysi S: Muscle pedicle bone grafts. Acta Orthop Scand 1965; 35:279.

[66] Panje W: Mandible reconstruction with the trapezius osteomusculocutaneous flap. Arch Otolaryngol 1985; 111:223-229.

[67] Kimura Y, Nakamura T, Tojima H, et al: Trapezius osteomyocutaneous flap in reconstructive surgery for mandibular and oral defects. Acta Otolaryngol Suppl 1994; 511:179.

[68] Conley J, Gullane PJ: The sternocleidomastoid muscle flap. Head Neck Surg 1980; 2:30F.

[69] Siemsen SO, Kirkby B, and O'Connor TP: Immediate reconstruction of a resected segment of the lower jaw, using a compound flap of clavicle and sternocleidomastoid muscles. Plast Reconstr Surg 1978; 61:724.

[70] Barnes DR, Ossof RH, Pecano B, et al: Immediate reconstruction of mandibular defects with composite sternocleidomastoid musculoclavicular graft. Arch Otolaryngol 1981;107:711.

[71] Friedman M, Mayer AD: Laryngotracheal reconstruction in adults with the sternocleidomastoid myoperiosteal flap. Ann Otol Rhinol Laryngol 1992; 101:897.

[72] Cuono CB, Aryan S: Immediate reconstruction of a composite mandibular defect with a regional osteomusculocutaneous flap. Plast Reconstr Surg 1980; 65(4): 4 77.

[73] Gratz KW, Siler HF, Haers PE, et al: Mandibular reconstruction with full thickness calvarial bone and temporal muscle flap. Br J Oral Maxillofac Surg 1996; 34:379.

[74] Conley JE: Cancer of the head and neck. New York, Appleton-Century-Crofts, 1967, p 274.

[75] McCarthy JG: Side bar. The spectrum for calvarial bone grafting: Introduction of the vascularized calva.rial flap. Plast Reconstr Surg 1984;74(1):10.

[76] Choung PH, Nam IW, Kim KS: Vascularized cranial bone grafts for mandibular and maxillary reconstruction: The parietal osteofascial flap. J Craniomaxillofac Surg 1991;19(6):325.

[77] Moscoso JF, Urken ML: Radial forearm flaps. Otolaryngol Clin North Am 1994; 27:1119-1140.

[78] Soutar DS, Scheker LR, Tanner NS, et al: The radial forearm flap: A versatile method for in traoral reconstruction. Br J Plast Surg 1983; 36(1): 1.

[79] Urken ML, Weinberg H, Vickery C, et al: The neurofasciocutaneous radial forearm flap in head and neck reconstruction: A preliminary report. Laryngoscope 1990; 100(2): 161.

[80] Vaughan ED: The radial forearm free flap in orofacial reconstruction. J Craniomaxillofac Surg 1990; 18:2.

[81] Gaukroger MC, Langdon JD, Whear NM, et al: Repair of the radial forearm flap donor site with a full-thickness graft. Int J Oral Maxillofac Surg 1994; 23:205-208.

[82] Teichgraeber J, Bowman J, and Geopfert H: New test series for the functional evaluation of oral cavity cancer. Head Neck Surg 1985; 8:9.

[83] Urken ML, Biller HF: A new bilobed design for the sensate radial forearm flap to preserve tongue mobility following significant glossectomy. Arch Otolaryngol Head Neck Surg 1994; 120:26.

[84] Nakatsuka T, Harii K, Yamada A, et al: Dual free flap transfer using forearm flap for mandibular reconstruction. Head Neck 1992; 14:452.

[85] Sadove RC, Luce EA, and McGrath PC: Reconstruction of the lower lip and chin with composite radial forearm-palmaris longus free flap. Plast Reconstr Surg 1991; 88:209.

[86] Fenton OM, Roberts JO: Improving the donor site of the radial forearm lap. Br J Plast Surg 1985; 38:504.

[87] Baek SM: Two new cutaneous free flaps: The medial and lateral thigh flaps. Plast Reconstr Surg 1983; 71:354.

[88] Hayden RE: Lateral thigh flap. Otolaryngol Clin North Am 1994; 27:1171.

[89] Schliephake H, Schmelzeisen R, Neukam FW: The free revascularized rectus abdominis myocutaneous flap for the repair of tumor related defects in the head and neck area. Br J Oral Maxillofac Surg 1996; 34:18.

[90] Schusterman MA, Kroll SS: Reconstruction strategy for temporal bone and lateral facial defects. Ann Plast Surg 1991; 26:233.

[91] Kroll SS, Baldwin BJ: Head and neck reconstruction with the rectus abdominis free flap. Clin Plast Surg 1994; 1:97.

[92] Kroll SS, Reece GP: Reconstruction of the face for cancer therapy. Adv Plast Surg 1993; 9:127.

[93] Arons JA, Guyuron B: Use of rectus abdominis osteomyocutaneous double island flap based on internal mammary vessels. Br J Oral Maxillofac Surg 1995; 48:145.

[94] Moscoso JF, Urken ML: The iliac crest composite flap for oromandibular reconstruction. Otolaryngol Clin North Am 1994; 27:1097.

[95] Shenaq SM, Klebuc MJA: The iliac crest microsurgical free flap in mandibular reconstruction. Clin Plast Surg 1994; 21:37.

[96] Reychler H, Ortabe JI: Mandibular reconstruction with the free fibula osteocutaneous flap. Int J Oral Maxillofac Surg 1994; 23:209.

[97] Lee JH, Kim MJ, Kim JW: Mandibular reconstruction with free vascularized fibular flap. J Craniomaxillofac Surg 1995; 23:20.

[98] Carroll WR, Esclamado R: Preoperative vascular imaging for fibular osteocutaneous flap. Arch Otolaryngol Head Neck Surg 1996; 122:708.

[99] Hidalgo DA: Fibula free flap mandibular reconstruction. Clin Plast Surg 1994; 21:25.

[100] Wells MD: Part I. Mandibular reconstruction using vascularized bone grafts. J Oral Maxillofac Surg 1996;54(7):883.

[101] O'Leary MJ, Martin PJ, Hayden RE: The neurocutaneous free fibula flap in mandibular reconstruction. Otolaryngol Clin North Am 1994; 27:1081.

[102] Jones NF, Monstrey S, Gambier BA: Reliability of the fibular osteocutaneous flap for mandibular reconstruction. Anatomical and surgical confirmation. Plast Reconstr Surg 1996;97:707.

[103] Saijo M: The vascular territories of the dorsal trunk: A reappraisal for potential flap donor sites. Br J Plast Surg 1978;31(3):200.

[104] Ostrup LT, Fredrichson JM: Distant transfer of a free, living bone graft by microvascular anastomoses. An experimental study. Plast Reconstr Surg 1974;54(3):274.

[105] McKee D: Microvascular bone transplantation. Clin Plast Surg North Am 1978;5:283.

[106] Genden E, Haughey BH: Mandibular reconstruction by vascularized free tissue transfer. Am J Otolaryngol 1996;17:219.

[107] Turk JB, Vuillemin T: Revascularized bone grafts for craniofacial reconstruction. Otolaryngol Clin North Am 1994;27:955.

[108] Carrel A: The surgery of blood vessels. Johns Hopkins Hosp Bull 1907;19:15.

[109] Jacobson JH II, Suarez EL: Microsurgery in anastomosis of small vessels. Surg Forum 1960; 11:247.

[110] Haughey BH: The jejuna! free flap in oral cavity and pharyngeal reconstruction. Otolaryngol Clin North Am 1994;27:1159.

[111] Yamamoto Y, Kunihiko N, Yoshihisa S, et al: Mes Enteric flap in free jejuna! transfers: A versatile technique for head and neck reconstruction. Head Neck 1995;17:213.

[112] Hayden RE: Free flap transfer for restoration of sensation and lubrication to the reconstructed oral cavity and pharynx. Otolaryngol Clin North Am 1994; 27:1185.

http://dx.doi.org/10.5772/59746

[113] David D: Use of an innervated deltopectoral flap for intraoral reconstruction. Plast Reconstr Surg 1977; 60:377.

[114] Franklin J, Withers E, Madden J, et al: Use of the free dorsalis pedis flap in head and neck repairs. Plast Reconstr Surg 1979; 63:195.

[115] Hermanson A, Dalsgaard C, Arnander D, et al: Sensibility and cutaneous reinnervation in free flaps. Plast Reconstr Surg 1987; 79:422.

[116] Hayden RE: Sensate flaps for oral and pharyngeal reconstruction: The next frontier. COSM, Triologic Society, Palm Beach, FL, 1990.

[117] Urken ML, Weinberg H, Vickery C, et al: The combined sensate radical forearm and iliac crest flaps for reconstruction of significant glossectomymandibulectomy defects. Laryngoscope 1992; 102(5): 543.

[118] Urken ML, Weinberg H, Vickery C, et al: Oromandibular reconstruction using microvascular composite free flaps: Report of 71 cases and a new classification scheme for bony, soft tissue and neurologic defects. Arch Otolaryngol Head N eek Surg 1991; 117:733.

[119] Hayden RE, O'Leary M: Osseointegrated neuroasciocutaneous fibula flap for complete oromandibular reconstruction. COSM, American Academy of Facial Plastic and Reconstructive Surgery, Waikoloa, HI, 1991.

[120] Papachristou DN, Trichilis E, Fortner JG: Experimental use of free gastric flaps for repair of pharyngoesophageal defects. Plast Reconstr Surg 1979; 64:336.

[121] Mah SM, Durham JS, Anderson DW, et al: Functional results in oral cavity reconstruction using reinnervated versus nonreinnervated free fasciocutaneous grafts. J Otolaryngol 1996; 25:75.

[122] Wells MD, Luce EA, Edwards AL, et al: Sequentially linked free flaps in head and neck reconstruction. Clin Plast Surg 1994; 21:59.

[123] Camilleri I, Wilson GR, McLean NR: Mandibular reconstruction using a "parasitic" flap. Br J Oral Maxillofac Surg 1994; 32:373.

[124] Penfold CN, Davies HT, Cole RP, et al: Combined latissimus dorsi-serratus anterior/rib composite free flap in mandibular reconstruction. Int J Oral Maxillofac Surg 1992; 21:92.

[125] Yamamoto Y, Nohira K, Yamashita T, et al: Combined V figure-shaped scapular osteocutaneous and latissimus dorsi myocutaneous flap for composite mandibular reconstruction. Head Neck 1995; 17:219.

[126] Macewen W: The Growth of Bone. Glasgow, J Mackhose, 1912.

[127] Blocker TG, Stout RA: Mandibular reconstruction in World War II. Plast Reconstr Surg 1949;4:153.

[128] Conley J: Use of composite flaps containing bone for major repairs in the head and neck. Plast Reconstr Surg 1972;49:522.

[129] Snyder C: Mandibulofacial restoration with live osteocutaneous flaps. Plast Reconstr Surg 1979;64:14.

[130] McKee K: Microvascular bone transplantation. Clin Plast Surg 1978;5:283.

[131] Daniel R: Mandibular reconstruction with free tissue transfers. Ann Plast Surg 1978;2:346.

[132] Urken ML: Composite free flaps in oromandibular reconstruction: Review of the literature. Arch Otolaryngol Head Neck Surg 1991;117:724.

[133] Annino DJ, Goguen LA, Karmody CS: Distraction osteogenesis for reconstruction of mandibular symphyseal defects. Arch Otolaryngol Head Neck Surg 1994;120:911.

[134] Mignogna FV, Rankow R, Garay KF: A-0 reconstruction plate and sternal osteomyocutaneous flap in primary mandibular reconstruction. Am J Surg 1993;166:416.

[135] Boyd JB: Use of reconstruction plates in conjunction with soft-tissue free flaps for oromandibular reconstruction. Clin Plast Surg 1994;21:69.

[136] Irish JC, Gullane PJ, Gilber RW, et al: Primary mandibular reconstruction with the titanium hollow screw reconstruction plate: Evaluation of 51 cases. Plast Reconstr Surg 1995;96:93.

[137] Cordeiro PG, Hidalgo DA: Soft tissue coverage of mandibular reconstruction plates. Head N eek Surg 1994; 16:112.

[138] Blackwell KE, Buchbinder D, Urken ML: Lateral mandibular reconstruction using soft-tissue free flaps and plates. Arch Otolaryngol Head Neck Surg 1996;122:672.

[139] Kudo K, Shoji M, Yokota, et al: Evaluation of mandibular reconstruction techniques following resection of malignant tumors of the oral region. J Oral Maxillofac Surg 1992;50:14.

[140] Wells MD, Luce EA: Reconstruction of midfacial defects after surgical resection of malignancies. Clin Plast Surg 1995;22:79.

[141] Ilankovan V, Jackson IT: Experience in the use of calvarial bone grafts in orbital reconstruction. J Oral Maxillofac Surg 1992;30:92.

[142] Sadove RC, Powell LA: Simultaneous maxillary and mandibular reconstruction with one free osteocutaneous flap. Plast Reconstr Surg 1993; 92:141.

[143] Jones NF, Swartz WM, Mears DC, et al: The "double-barrel" free vascularized fibular bone graft. Plast Reconstr Surg 1988;81:378.

[144] Luce EA: Reconstruction of the lower lip. Clin Plast Surg 1995;22:109.

[145] Baker SR, Krause CJ: Pedicle flaps in reconstruction of the lip. Fae Plast Surg 1983;1:61.

[146] Takeichi Y, Kamei S, Oyama S, et al: Mobile tongue reconstruction with the free dorsalis pedis flap. Acta Otolaryngol Suppl 1996;525:30.

[147] Stanley RJ, Olsen KD: Rhinectomy for malignant disease: A 20-year experience. Arch Otolaryngol Head Neck Surg 1988;114:1307.

[148] Kazanjian VH: The repair of nasal defects with median forehead flap lining. Surg Gynecol Obstet 1946;83:37.

[149] Washio H: Further experiences with the retroauricular-temporal flap. Plast Reconstr Surg 1972;50:160.

[150] Yousif NJ, Matloub HS, Sanger JR, et al: Softtissue reconstruction of the oral cavity. Clin Plast Surg 1994;21:15.

[151] Wells MD, Edwards AL, Luce EA: Intraoral reconstructive techniques. Clin Plast Surg 1995;22:91.

[152] Wagner JD, Ress A, Coleman JJ: Repair of midline vertical lower lip deficiency after mandible reconstruction. Am J Surg 1996;172:625.

[153] Neligan PC, Boyd JB: Reconstruction of the cranial base defect. Clin Plast Surg 1995;22:71.

[154] Coleman JJ: Osseous reconstruction of the midface and orbits. Clin Plast Surg 1994;21:113.

[155] Ketcham AS, Hoye RC, Van Buren JM, et al: Complications of intracranial facial resections for tumors of the paranasal sinuses. Am J Surg 1966;112:591.

[156] Westbury G, Wilson JSP, Richardson A: Combined craniofacial resection for malignant disease. Am J Surg 1975;130:463.

[157] Millard DR Jr: Congenital nasal tip retrusion and three little composite ear grafts. Case report. Plast Reconstr Surg 1971;40(5):501.

[158] Siegel RF: Palatal grafts for eyelid reconstruction. Plast Reconstr Surg 1985;26(3):411.

[159] Yoshimura Y, Nakajima T, Yoneda K: Use of palatal mucosal graft for reconstruction of the eye socket. J Craniomaxillofac Surg 1995;23:27.

[160] Motoki DS, Mulliken JB: The healing of bone and cartilage. Clin Plast Surg 1990;17:527.

[161] Hendler BH, Gateno J, Smith BM: Use of auricular cartilage in the repair of orbital floor defects. Oral Surg Oral Med Oral Pathol 1992;74:719.11.

[162] Shestak KC: Soft-tissue reconstruction of craniofacial defects. Clin Plast Surg 1994;21:107.

[163] Sclaroff A, Haughey B, Gay WD, et al: Immediate mandibular reconstruction and placement of dental implants: At the time of ablative surgery. Oral Surg Oral Med Oral Pathol 1994;78:711.

[164] Stoler A, Hill T: Parts I, II. Mandibular reconstruction: Combined intra-oral and in vitro placement of osseointegrated implants into a free and vascularized bone graft. J Oral Implantol 1992;18(1):38.

[165] Taylor TD, Rieger WP: Alloplastic implants: Their role in reconstruction of the mandible. Clin Plast Surg 1994;21:79.

[166] Moscoso JF, Keller J, Genden E, et al: Vascularized bone flaps in oromandibular reconstruction. Arch Otolaryngol Head Neck Surg 1994; 120:36.

[167] Albrektsson T: A multicenter report on osseointegreated oral implants. J Prosthet Dent 1988; 60:76.

[168] Mounsey RA, Boyd JB: Mandibular reconstruction with osseointegrated implants into free vascularized radius. Plast Reconstr Surg 1994; 94:457.

[169] Martin IC, Cawood JI, Vaughan ED, et al: Endosseous implants in the irradiated composite radial forearm free flap. Int J Oral Maxillofac Surg 1992;21:266.

[170] Reychler R, Ortabe JI, Pecheur A, et al: Mandibular reconstruction with a free vascularized fibula flap and osseointegrated implants: A report of four cases. J Oral Maxillofac Surg 1996;54:1464.

[171] Zlotolow IM, Huryn JM, Piro JD, et al: Osseointegrated implants and functional prosthetic reha bilitation in microvascular fibula free flap reconstructed mandibles. Am J Surg 1992;165:677.

[172] Donovan MG, Dickerson NG, Hanson LJ, et al: Maxillary and mandibular reconstruction using calvarial bone grafts and Branemark implants: A preliminary report. J Oral Maxillofac Surg 1994;52:588.

[173] Peer L: Transplantation of Tissues, vol 1. Baltimore, Williams & Wilkins, 1955.

[174] Skinner FA: Maxillofacial prosthodontics: An aid to the oncology patient. J Med Assoc Ga 1992;81:331.

[175] Valauri AJ: Maxillofacial Prosthetics. In McCarthy JG (ed): McCarthy's Plastic Surgery, ed 2. Philadelphia, WB Saunders, 1990.

[176] King GE, Martin JW: Complete dentures for the obturator patient. Dent Clin North Am 1996; 40:217.

[177] Sharma AB: Case studies in maxillofacial reconstruction using osseointegrated implants. Oral Maxillofac Surg Clin North Am 1993;5:395.

[178] Richarson D, Cawood JI: Mandibular reconstruction and rehabilitation in childhood. Br Dent J 1995;179:141.

http://dx.doi.org/10.5772/59746

[179] Stepnick DW, Hayden RE: Postoperative monitoring and salvage ofmicrovascular free flaps. Otolaryngol Clin North Am 1994;27:1201-1217.

[180] Soderholm AL, Hallikainen D, Lindqvist C: Radiologic follow-up of bone transplants to bridge mandibular continuity defects. Oral Surg Oral Med Oral Pathol 1992;73:253

Chapter 29

Virtual Surgical Planning in Craniomaxillofacial Reconstruction

Eric Zielinski, Ryan J. Jacobs, Eric Barker,
Kate Rodby and Anuja K. Antony

Additional information is available at the end of the chapter

http://dx.doi.org/10.5772/59965

1. Introduction

Craniomaxillofacial reconstruction poses inherent and unique challenges due to the three-dimensional configuration of the proposed construct and the critical importance to restore speech, swallowing, mastication and symmetrical facial contour. Additionally, reconstruction results are often inconsistent and learning curve dependent.[1-43] Until recently, the overall success in bony reconstruction of the craniomaxillofacial skeleton has relied mainly on the use of surgical trial-and-error and 2D imaging modalities. Virtual surgical planning (VSP) and computer aided design (CAD) / computer aided modeling (CAM) is an exciting new technology that presents advantages in complex craniomaxillofacial reconstruction, with potential to transform the approach and execution of challenging head and neck reconstructions.[30] Among the reported benefits of VSP- CAD/CAM are increased reconstructive accuracy, reduced OR and graft ischemia time, improved patient satisfaction and ease of use.[1, 9, 19] VSP- CAD/CAM is gaining traction in craniomaxillofacial reconstruction applications and offers opportunity for increased accuracy, improved efficiency, enhanced outcomes and ease of use.[34, 43] To illustrate this point, the usage of this technology in different applications is presented in subsequent sections with an emphasis and case study example for an oncologic indication.

2. Applications

VSP- CAD/CAM is a novel technology which has been described for a range of surgical applications ranging from trauma to oncologic reconstruction. Widening utilization in craniomaxillofacial reconstruction is largely due to its unique capability that allows the surgical team to visualize and manipulate patient-derived virtual and stereolithographic models in three dimensions during the virtual pre-operative planning phase. Due to refinements in pre-operative planning, many studies, though limited, have reported improved outcomes through CT evaluation of actual verses planned height and width dimensions, volumes, osseous graft overlap, and aesthetic outcomes.[24] For these reasons, VSP-CAD/CAM has been of benefit for the following applications:

Craniomaxillofacial / Orthognathic procedures–VSP-CAD/CAM is a useful technology to address craniofacial anomalies or maxillofacial deficiencies. Until recently, traditional imaging methods only allowed for 2D images in a single plane to visualize the irregular and uniquely shaped donor-graft and recipient sites.[3] While multiple imaging studies may aid in forming a pre-surgical plan, the outcomes of movements outside the plane of imaging cannot be reliably predicted. Therefore, complex reconstructions requiring correction for craniofacial and maxillofacial applications can induce asymmetry since the traditional radiological studies cannot plan movements in three dimensions; a capability that VSP-CAD/CAM offers.[23] In addition, pre-made guides for harvesting and transplanting autografts as well as customized allograft materials (e.g. pre-bent plates) facilitate achieving a result consistent with the craniofacial reconstructive plan.[23, 43] In maxillofacial procedures, VSP-CAD/CAM eliminates several other sources of error when planning midline correction by allowing the surgeon to account for the natural yaw, pitch, roll of a head position, and assessing heights and widths; virtual manipulations of the patient model to millimeter precision can be performed to achieve accurate maxillofacial balance and appropriate orthognathic relationships. Pre-bent fixation plates further promote accurate translational movements intraoperatively that are pre-planned in the virtual environment. When compared to the 'classic' method of building acrylic intermaxillary occlusal splints using plaster models, VSP-CAD/CAM was shown to be superior when evaluating post-operative maxillary position and centrality of the condyles in the temporomandibular joint.[43]

Trauma–VSP-CAD/CAM has been utilized for reconstruction of traumatic facial injuries, including comminuted mandible and panfacial fracture reduction and repair. Three-dimensional modeling of craniomaxillofacial injuries facilitates precise intraoperative reduction of displaced bone fragments, while CAD/CAM produces occlusal splints that allow superior restoration of facial symmetry, appearance, and function to those fitted intraopertively.[35] Avulsed or necrotic areas can be replaced with grafts or covered with custom implants. Additionally, implementation of VSP-CAD/CAM offers use of pre-manufactured cutting guides for improved accuracy and reduced trial-and-error when harvesting and shaping autologous implants, thus helping to ensure optimal bone-to-bone contact and aesthetic outcome. Pre-bent fixation plates decrease intraoperative time and limit the extent of subperiosteal dissection, thus minimizing avascularization of bony fragments.[35] Utilization of VSP-CAD/CAM starting at initial presentation of traumatic facial injury does not result in increased time to reconstruction and has been shown to better preserve facial height and width.[6, 35]

TMJ reconstruction – Traditional temporomandibular joint (TMJ) reconstruction is a two-stage approach beginning with gap arthroplasty followed by postoperative CT to plan implant design and fabrication. A subsequent procedure is then required to inset the pre-designed TMJ implant. VSP-CAD/CAM however, enables single-stage reconstruction of the TMJ as gap arthroplasty simulation and TMJ implant pre-fabrication can be performed on a virtual 3D

http://dx.doi.org/10.5772/59965

model.[23] Planning and simulation of TMJ movements and jaw occlusion can also be assessed on stereolithographic models prior to implant in-setting resulting in improved functional outcomes and reduced postoperative complications.[23]

Mandibular Atrophy –In a case series of seven patients, VSP-CAD/CAM was utilized to repair atrophic mandibular alveolar crest defects in patients after all other treatment modalities had failed.[28] A free iliac crest transplant was harvested and anastamosed to the thoracodorsal artery and vein in the axilla. Grafts were harvested three months later, after having developed a whitish tissue layer on the bone, which was used as a mucous membrane following fixation to the mandible. All grafts fit the mandible as predicted in the initial pre-reconstructive planning phase and no implants were lost after 7 years of follow up.[28]

Oncologic resection and reconstruction–Craniomaxillofacial reconstruction using free fibula flaps, as first described by Hidalgo, has traditionally relied on surgical skill, judgment, and intra-operative trial and error to create the neomandible.[2, 3] Reconstruction of the mandible and maxilla has therefore been considered to be learning curve dependent, often with inconsistent results during the skill acquisition phase.[1] Furthermore, preoperative planning and communication between the oncologic and reconstructive teams has been limited by the lack of data regarding the anatomy of the lesion, precise margins of resection, and anatomy of the graft recipient site, which prior to use of VSP-CAD/CAM, are only revealed in the operating room.[6] Thus,for a procedure requiring a high degree of precision for optimal orthognathic and aesthetic outcomes, craniomaxillofacial reconstructive success has historically been hindered by prolonged intraoperative time and suboptimal reconstructions.[12] VSP-CAD/CAM offers significant benefits for use in complex oncologic osseous head and neck reconstruction by providing enhanced cooperation between surgical teams, pre-operative planning, and the ability to customize models to patient's individual characteristics, which offers potential for considerable intraoperative time saving.[1]

VSP-CAD/CAM allows for a cooperative team approach to plan the resection and reconstruction by synergistically facilitating pre-operative collaboration between the extirpative and reconstructive teams, maximizing chances for tumor-free resection margins.[1, 3, 20] Additionally, as the extirpative surgeon is provided with pre-operative 3D CT visualization of the lesion borders and a comprehensive plan from the reconstructive team, he may be more inclined to plan liberal resection margins initially; thus potentiating decreased local recurrence rates and intraoperative time.[1] Similarly and in reciprocal fashion, reconstructive planning may be better realized for the reconstructive surgeon with advance knowledge of the resection plan. As refinements in the VSP-CAD/CAM interface have become progressively more user-friendly for both the extirpative and reconstructive surgeon, adoption of this technology and coordinated pre-operative planning has continued to increase.[30]

3. Process

Computer-assisted craniomaxillofacial surgery is based on four specific, well-described phases, which are all necessary in order to achieve predictable outcomes: planning, modeling, surgery, and evaluation.[3, 19] these steps are detailed as follows[24]:

The first phase, planning, begins with a high-resolution computed tomographic (CT) scan of the craniofacial skeleton and the possible donor sites, (e.g. lower extremities) if considered necessary. A 3D reconstruction of the CT images is performed and then forwarded to the desired modeling company. A web-based teleconference is then held between the surgical teams and a biomedical engineer to allow participation from remote locations. During this phase, the resection and reconstruction is virtually planned, with key parameters including resection margins, osteotomies, placement of the vascularized bone graft in oncologic reconstruction, accurate reduction of the fractured bony segments for traumatic injuries, and the staged virtual movement of the jaws in orthognathic procedures.

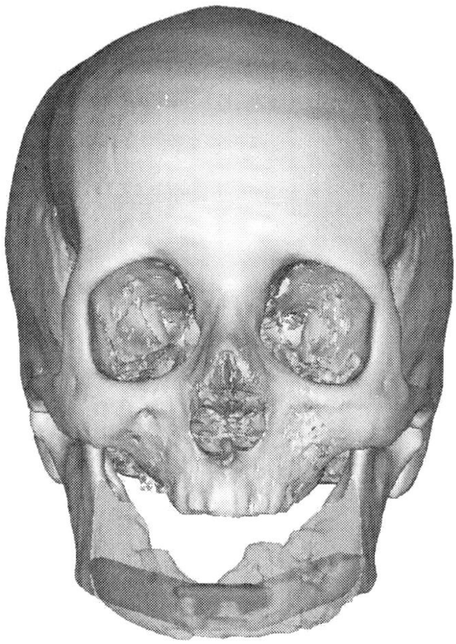

Figure 1. Overlay of the planned reconstruction with the native diseased mandible after virtual planning of the osteotomies.

The modeling phase begins Based on the virtual surgical plan. Stereolithographic models are manufactured of the area of the craniomaxillofacial skeleton of interest, along with specific cutting guides for both the resection and the vascularized bone graft that will be used for oncologic bony reconstruction (e.g. fibula), if indicated. In orthognathic procedures, pre-bending of plates allows for accurate translation of the osteotomized segments for advancement/ setback and precise execution of the pre-operative plan (e.g. LeFort I, Bilateral Sagittal Split Osteotomy). In oncologic reconstruction, this also allows for manufacturing of a reconstruction plate or plate-bending template; the specific guides and templates can be tailored to

http://dx.doi.org/10.5772/59965

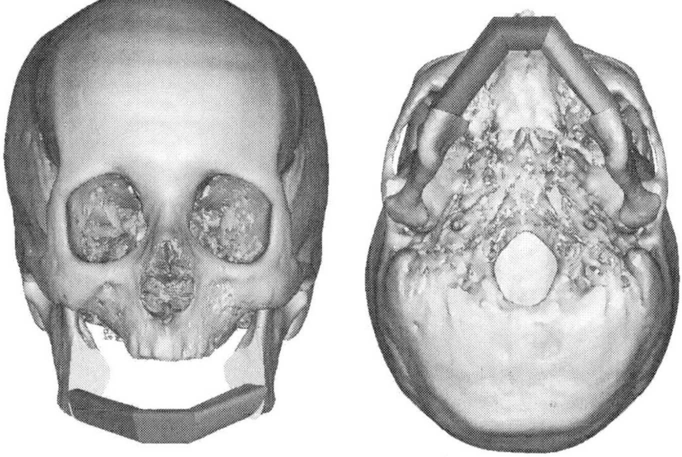

Figure 2. Positioning of the designed neomandible adjusted to optimize bony contact and restore the anticipated mandibular defect. Note the osseous segments to be produced via guided cuts of the free fibula graft.

the surgeon's preference and the stereolithographic models can help to create pre-bent plates prior to reconstruction[17, 19]

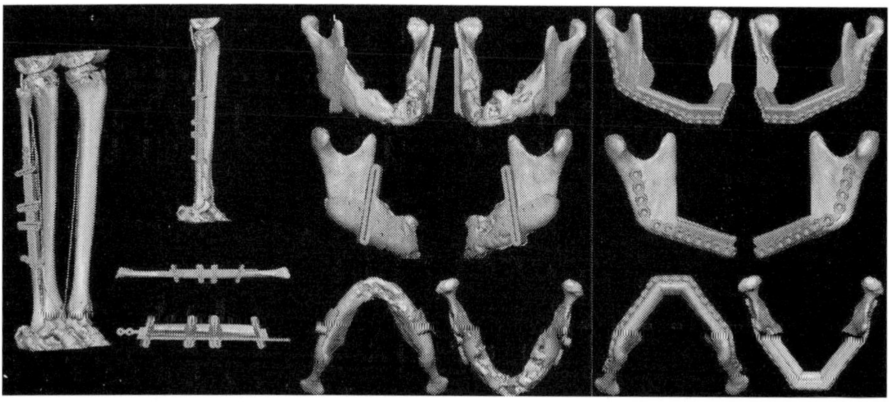

Figure 3. Virtual positioning of the pre-manufactured graft osteotomy guides on the fibula (A), extirpative osteotomy guides on the diseased mandible (B), and fibula grafts secured to the pre-bent reconstruction plate aligned to the native mandible.

During the surgery phase plate-bending templates and pre-bending of plates also expedites the fixation step. Osteotomies are made in the mandible or maxilla based on the cutting guides, typically after maxillomandibular fixation is achieved. In the case of oncologic reconstruction, the harvested osseous flap is also cut and osteotomized in-situ based on the cutting guides and typically fixed to the reconstruction plate before the composite unit is secured into the maxillofacial/mandibular defect. With the bony foundation restored, the soft tissue reconstruction can be carried out synergistically.

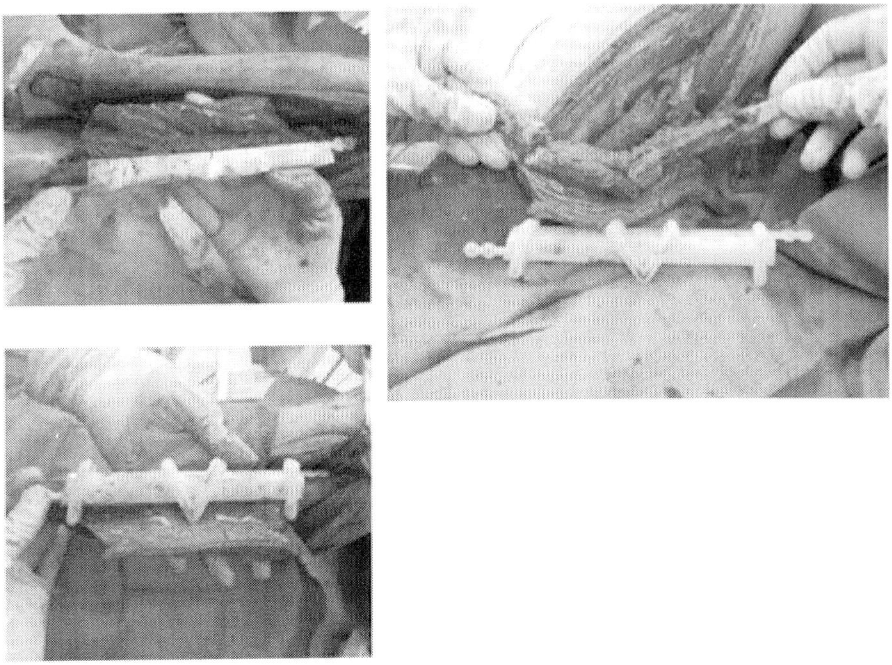

Figure 4. Intraoperative placement of osteotomy guide to fibula facilitating guided cuts for the neomandible.

The evaluation phase begins in the post-operative period, with a repeat high-resolution CT scan performed, based on the same preoperative protocol.[17] While the method of evaluation varies between institutions, a postoperative CT scan allows for a quantitative evaluation of the surgical outcomes and can complement subjective assessments by the surgeon and patient of restored oral and maxillofacial function. 3D models of the post-operative results are overlaid with the pre-operative plan to determine accuracy and success of reconstruction including actual mandibular angle and margins of bony contact in addition to accuracy of the VSP- CAD/CAM plan including: bony segment overlap (repeatability) and mean service deviation, overall positioning, osteotomy site differences, and reconstructive plate overlap.[3, 9, 25, 20] Clinical parameters can then be correlated in the evaluation phase with functional parameters including occlusion, mastication, and speech, in addition to overall aesthetic outcome, and patient satisfaction.

http://dx.doi.org/10.5772/59965

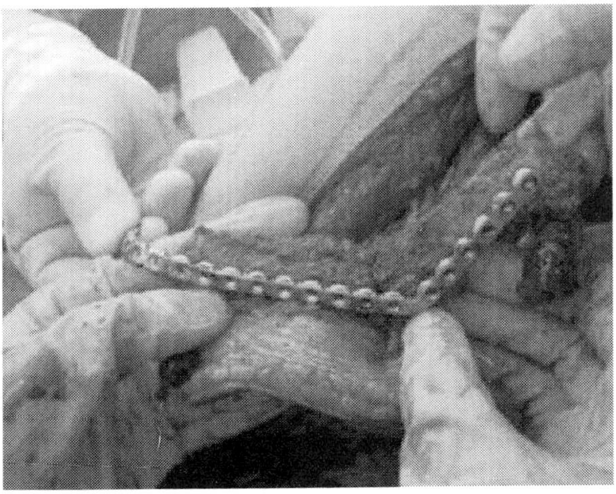

Figure 5. Intraoperatively, the fibular grafts are secured to the reconstruction plate.

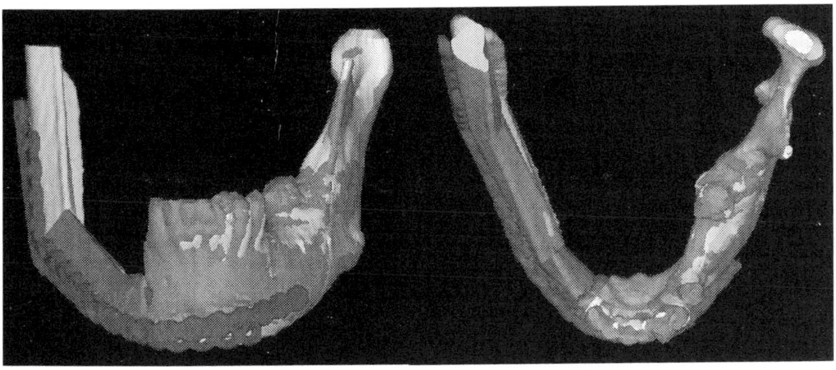

Figure 6. Overlay of the designed neomandible (blue segments) with the actual postoperative mandibular reconstruction (green segments) evaluated by 3D CT.

Oncologic Case – A 61-year-old male patient presented to an oral surgeon for evaluation of the right posterior mandible for potential chronic osteomyelitis. He stated that he had felt a "dull pain" since nine months prior. Teeth #31 and #32 were extracted 16 and 9 months ago, respectively. Since extraction, the patient had completed multiple courses of antibiotics, most recently Augmentin 500mg.

On exam the patient displayed normal facial symmetry with a non-tender movable lymph node <1cm right Level 1b without erythema, discharge or skin changes. The right mandible was slightly tender to palpation with only minimal expansion, with slight "crepitus" appreciated upon opening, concerning for osteolysis. Radiographic appearance on panorex was notable for significant bone distraction appreciated on the right mandible involving the body to the inferior border. Initial workup of the patient included an incisional biopsy and curettage of the area under local anesthesia in order to rule out osteomyelitis. The pathology report described a well-differentiated squamous cell carcinoma of right posterior mandible. The patient was referred to oral-maxillofacial surgery for extirpation of the affected region of the mandible with adequate margins and concomitant right free fibular osteocutaneous flap reconstruction of the mandible by plastic and reconstructive surgery. High-resolution CT scans were performed and sent to an outside company for modeling via CAD/CAM software.

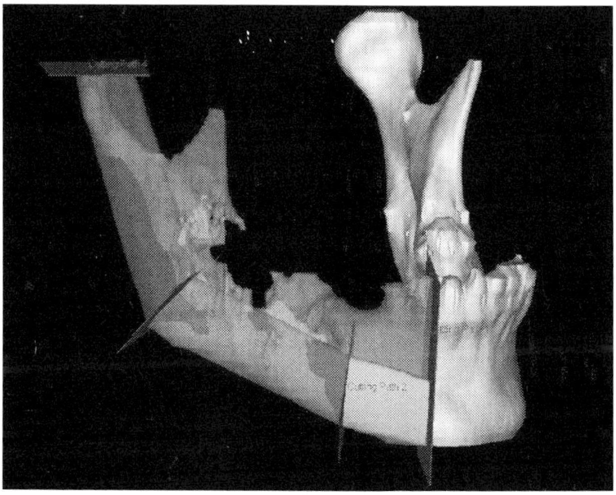

Figure 7. Overlay of the virtual planned multiple fibular graft segments to reconstruct the mandible (blue segments), over the diseased mandible (green).

After rendering the virtual models, the extirpative and reconstructive teams formulated a surgical approach and consulted the modeling company for manufacturing of the desired guides.

The virtual three-dimensional model of the craniofacial skeleton was first used to plan the resection of the lesion and then the subsequent reconstruction of the defect by the extirpative and reconstructive teams respectively in a joint teleconference facilitated by the biomedical engineer from the modeling company. During the surgical phase, the oral-maxillofacial team first excised the diseased mandible as planned using the prefabricated cutting guides. The fibular osteocutaneous flap was then harvested by the reconstructive team; prefabricated templates and guides were used by both the extirpative and reconstructive teams to ensure the precise location and angle of osteotomies. The harvested, osteotomized flap was fixed to the pre-bent plate in-situ and subsequently inset to the mandibular defect. The free condylar end of the graft was contoured to fit the articular disk of the temporomandibular joint and the

http://dx.doi.org/10.5772/59965

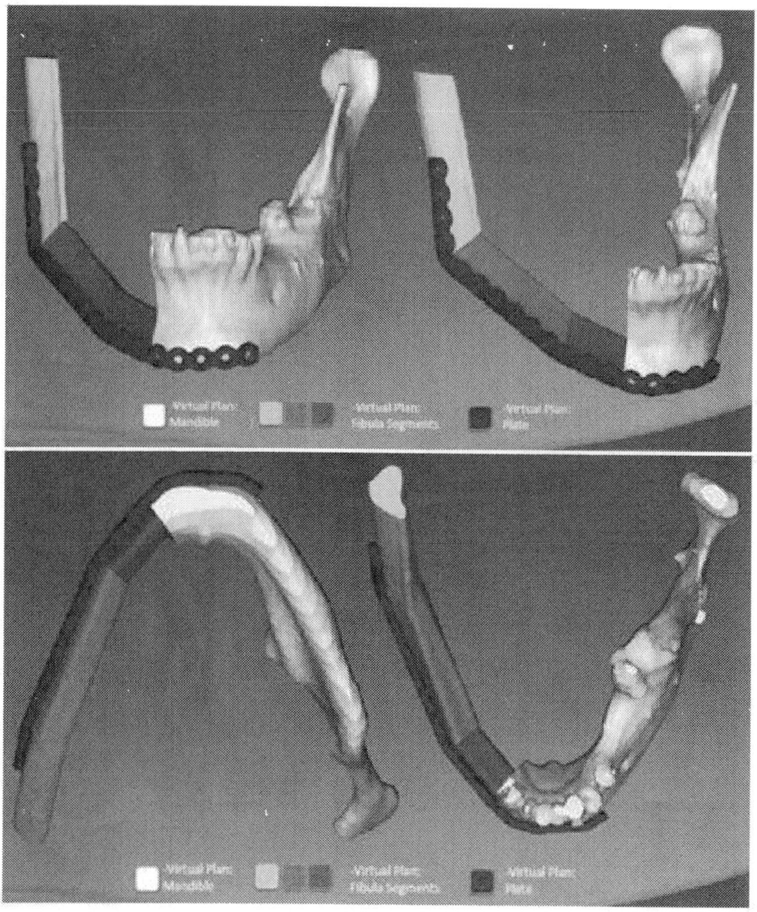

Figure 8. Positioning of the designed neomandible in the expected right hemimandible defect after virtual planning of the osteotomies with positioning of the planned reconstructive plate.

graft placed into position. After successful fixation of the plate and graft to native bone, the donor cutaneous flap was tailored for use in reconstruction of the oral mucosa. The flap vasculature was then anastamosed, adequate circulation ensured, and both sites were closed in a layered fashion.

After surgical completion, a high-resolution CT scan was obtained and sent to the original modeling company for evaluation of reconstructive success. Comparisons were made between the anatomical dimensions of the pre-operative and post-operative skull and mandible. Reconstructive plate overlap was considered to be acceptable and the patient achieved excellent functional and aesthetic results. The evaluation phase allowed for review of surgical outcomes in a multidisciplinary fashion to further refine the technique.

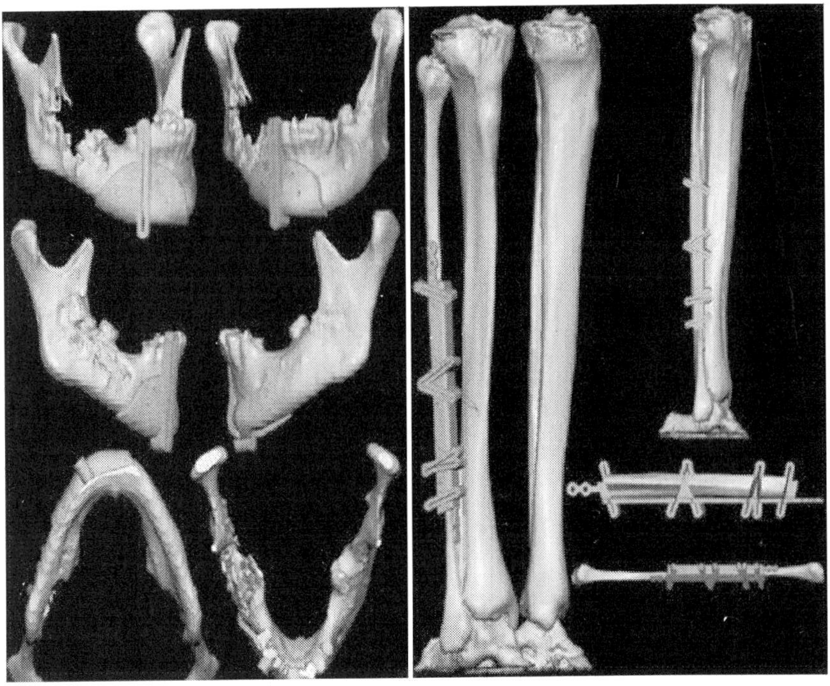

Figure 9. Virtual placement of the pre-manufactured extirpative osteotomy guide on the patient's native mandible and resection /osteotomy guide on the patient's fibula for creation of the neomandible.

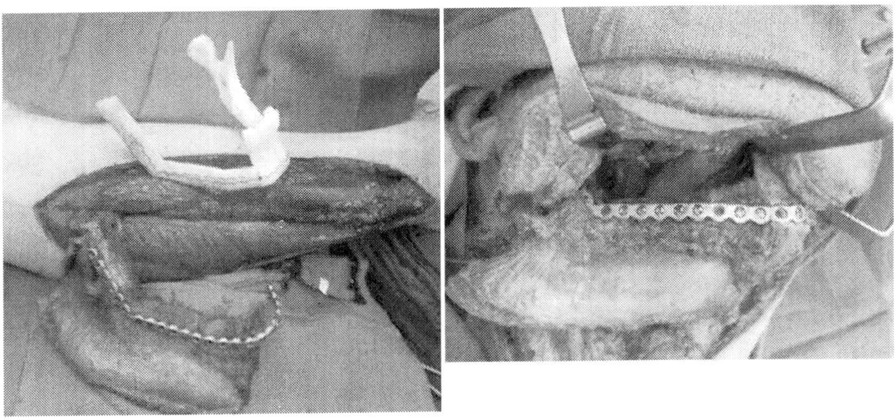

Figure 10. Intraoperative comparison of the virtual surgical planned reconstruction model with the fibular osteomyocutaneous flap segments secured to the pre-bent reconstruction plate (left). Placement of the plate secured fibula graft to the native mandible (right).

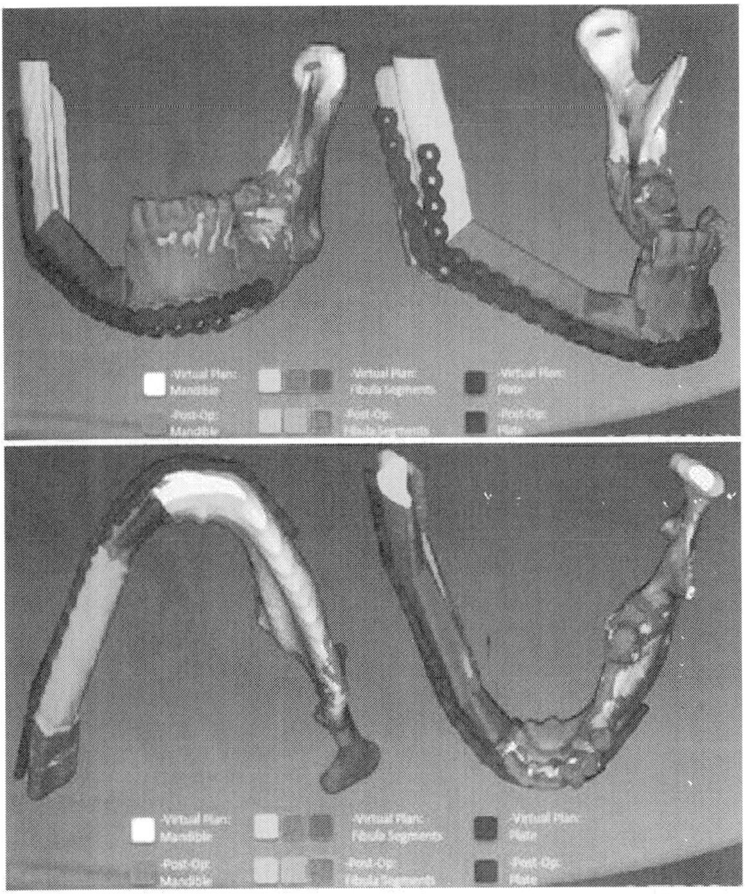

Figure 11. Post-operative evaluation by 3D CT of the virtually planned neomandible (blue segments) with the actual mandibular reconstruction (green segments)

4. Advantages

Heightened aesthetic outcomes and reconstructive accuracy are realized with the multi-stage implementation of virtual surgical planning throughout the four phases of computer-assisted craniomaxillofacial surgery and the use of cutting guides, stereolithographic models and pre-fabricated plates. In particular, the surgical course with VSP-CAD/CAM implementation, specifically in the oncologic reconstruction of the mandible and maxilla, has been favorably altered when compared to intraoperative planning and in-situ plate bending.[2, 23] More pervasive use of the technology throughout the reconstructive process reduces translational error due to human error.[24] The virtual model data allows manufacturing of cutting guides, plate bending templates, prefabricated reconstruction plates, and also stereolithographic models to facilitate an accurate execution of the virtual plan in the operating room.[11, 13] Pre-operative simulation of the maxillo-mandibular relationship facilitates proper alignment of the graft for proper dental occlusion and proper orthognathic relationships.[4, 10] As the majority of the planning of this process has occurred pre-operatively, total operating time is also reduced concordantly.

While achieving reconstructive success was previously reliant on the surgeon's experience and intra-operative trial-and-error using 2-D imaging, VSP-CAD/CAM offers cited benefits over traditional methods which include increased bone-to-bone contact, better dental alignment, improved aesthetic contour, reduced complication rates and decreased intraoperative time.[10, 13] In our review of surgeon-reported benefits, increased reconstruction accuracy in 92% of cases proved to be a major perceived advantage demonstrated by this technology.[24] Furthermore, a future direction of the VSP-CAD/CAM technology includes planning of osseointegrated implants for mandibular reconstruction at the initial virtual planning session to greater improve functional outcomes.[31, 34]

Quantifiable patient satisfaction surveys, subjective outcome evaluations, and clinical assessment can help to measure functional and aesthetic outcomes.[1, 11, 20, 21, 32, 33, 36] Likely Results from more true-to-plan reconstructions attained by use of this technology, VSP-CAD/CAM has been purported to translate to increased patient satisfaction. In a 2012 study comparing VSP-CAD/CAM with conventional surgery, patients were asked to report satisfaction on a scale of 0-100. Patients who underwent virtually planned surgery reported an average score of 88 compared to an average score of 68 by those patients undergoing traditional reconstruction.[21]

The technical accuracy achieved as a consequence of VSP-CAD/CAM utilization can be enumerated with evaluation of the final reconstruction with the virtual plan via comparison of pre-operative and post-operative three-dimensional CT scans. Performing osteotomy with use of cutting guides has been shown to assist in more accurately designed free flaps, while use of pre-manufactured reconstruction plates versus hand-bent reconstruction plates has been shown to promote true-to-plan reconstructive results.[4],`[9, 2] `Additionally, a noted decreased difference in the overall positioning between the native and reconstructed mandibles was found in VSP-CAD/CAM aided reconstructions when comparing standard technique reconstructions.[9] Thus, improved reconstructive accuracy via the reduction of human error can be achieved with pre-manufacturing of the reconstructive plates and implementation of VSP-CAD/CAM more pervasively throughout the reconstructive process.[24] It follows that application of VSP-CAD/CAM to refine preoperative planning, intraoperative contouring, and postoperative orthodontic relationships in each surgical step can improve functional and aesthetic outcomes.[22] With completion of the VSP process to the final evaluation phase, 3D comparison imaging not only permits assessment of the reliability of the technology, it allows the collaborative discussion between surgical teams to assess technique and identify areas for improved performance.[25]

http://dx.doi.org/10.5772/59965

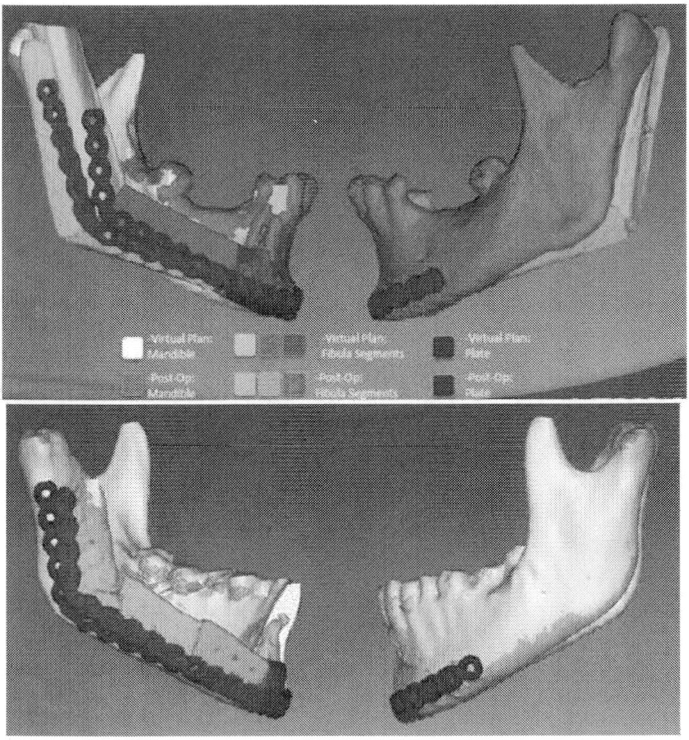

Figure 12. Overlay of the virtually planned reconstruction (blue segments) with the native mandible demonstrating translational error using a hand-bent plate (top). Post-operative overlay demonstrating improved match between actual and virtual segments using a pre-bent reconstructive plate (bottom).

Pre-operative planning of the resection and reconstructive segmental osteotomies results in enhanced operative time efficiency so that the extent of surgical time required is optimized to precisely execute the previously developed plan.[1]Intraoperative surgical planning is thereby converted to a preoperative event so that substantial savings in intraoperative time and reductions in the surgical learning curve may be realized.[1] Such savings may be further realized in reduced surgeon fatigue and concomitant reduced surgical error. Decreased operative time and increased accuracy have been noted in multiple reconstructive series, further illustrating the utility of VSP-CAD/CAM in dealing with complex head and neck reconstruction for various surgical indications.[6, 28, 35] in mandibular reconstructions using fibula free flaps, Hanasono reported a significant decreased mean intraoperative time when utilizing VSP- CAM/CAD.[8] While Seruya et. al did not find a significant decrease in operative time; they described a decrease in mean ischemic time in CAD assisted mandibular reconstructions.[29] Reduced ischemia time has been shown to result in decreased flap loss and overall post-operative complications.[27, 29] Enhancing overall intra-operative efficiency is facilitated by the use of pre-manufactured cutting guides and models which enables faster and more accurate osteotomies and graft placement. [7, 31] Use of manufactured pre-bent reconstructive plates can also significantly decrease the total operative time; total reconstructive operative time was reported in one case to be less than 90 minutes.[3, 19, 31]

5. Disadvantages

With regard to the current economic climate in healthcare, potential limitation of widespread incorporation of VSP-CAD/CAM technology is its added cost and the resultant financial burdens that may be placed on the patient and medical system.[8, 17, 28, 34] Given the economic healthcare constraints, the improved patient outcomes seen with VSP-CAD/CAM have to be balanced against the cost of the technology.[24, 39] Potential costs are further increased with the use of the manufactured pre-bent reconstruction plates. Given the qualitative nature of many benefits of VSP-CAD/CAM and the paucity of data currently available, the total value added and cost efficiency of VSP-CAD/CAM utilization has not been formally evaluated and still remains the subject of future studies.[24] As previously discussed, reductions in ischemia and/or overall operative time is a potential source of cost reduction. Additionally, the decreased complications and patient morbidity, and generalized improved outcomes seen signify cost savings that may offset the technological costs.[24] However, the clinical implications and economic benefits have yet to be formally analyzed with the added cost of VSP-CAD/CAM in the context of various expanding clinical applications including trauma, temporomandibular joint reconstruction, cancer, and skull base surgery.[6, 28, 35, 38] In head and neck cancer reconstruction, patient lifespan, risk for tumor recurrence and disease progression, and quality of life are additional factors that add complexity to the cost-benefit evaluation of the technology in an oncologic setting.

6. Summary

VSP-CAD/CAM is a novel technology that holds potential to consistently and predictably advance reconstructive outcomes, both aesthetically and functionally. This technology is suited for use in spatially complex reconstructive cases due to its ability to visualize and virtually manipulate 3D configurations of the craniomaxillofacial skeleton in a collaborative, synergistic fashion. Its applications are expanding for cases of varying levels of complexity that require precise millimeter precision particularly in trauma, orthognathic procedures and oncology to obtain optimized function and aesthetic outcomes. Implementation of VSP-CAD/CAM into each stage of the reconstruction affords the opportunity to reduce human translational error and facilitates intra-operative decision-making with expedition of the surgical phase.[1, 10, 11, 13, 21, 24] VSP- CAD/CAM technology is attaining acceptance across the multiple surgical disciplines as efforts towards validating its use are increasing, thereby holding promise as an mainstay, innovative solution in the management of challenging head and neck reconstruction cases.

http://dx.doi.org/10.5772/59965

Author details

Eric Zielinski[1], Ryan J. Jacobs[1], Eric Barker[3], Kate Rodby[2] and Anuja K. Antony[3*]

*Address all correspondence to: akantony@uic.edu

1 University of Illinois at Chicago, USA

2 Mount Sinai Medical Center, USA

3 Rush University Medical Center, USA

References

[1] Antony A, Chen W, Kolokythas A, Weimer K, Cohen M. Use of virtual surgery and stereolithography-guided osteotomy for mandibular reconstruction with the free fibula. Plast Reconstr Surg 2011;128(5);1080-4.

[2] Bell RB, Weimer KA, Dierks EJ, Buehler M, Lubek JE. Computer Planning and Intraoperative Navigation for Palatomaxillary and Mandibular Reconstruction With Fibular Free Flaps. Journal of Oral and Maxillofacial Surgery 2011;69;724-32.

[3] Ciocca L, Mazzoni S, Fantini M et al. A CAD/CAM-prototyped anatomical condylar prosthesis connected to a custom-made bone plate to support a fibula free flap. Med Biol Eng Comput 2012;50(7);743-9.

[4] Ciocca L, Mazzoni S, Fantini M, Marchetti C, Scotti R. The design and rapid prototyping of surgical guides and bone plates to support iliac free flaps for mandible reconstruction. Plast Reconstr Surg 2012;129(5);859-61.

[5] Cohen A, Laviv A, Berman P, Nashef R, Abu-Tair J. Mandibular reconstruction using stereolithographic 3-dimensional printing modeling technology. Oral Surgery, Oral Medicine, Oral Pathology, Oral Radiology, and Endodontology 2009;108;661-6.

[6] Foley BD, Thayer WP, Honeybrook A, McKenna S, Press S. Mandibular Reconstruction Using Computer-Aided Design and Computer-Aided Manufacturing: An Analysis of Surgical Results. Journal of Oral and Maxillofacial Surgery 2013;71;e111-9.

[7] Haddock N, Monaco C, Weimer K, Hirsch D, Levine J, Saadeh P. Increasing bony contact and overlap with computer-designed offset cuts in free fibula mandible reconstruction.. J Craniofac Surg 2012;23(6);1592-5.

[8] Hanasono MM, Skoracki RJ. Computer-assisted design and rapid prototype modeling in microvascular mandible reconstruction. Laryngoscope 2013;123;597-604.

[9] Hanasono M, Skoracki J. Improving the speed and accuracy of mandibular reconstruction using preoperative virtual planning and rapid prototype modeling. 2011.

[10] Hayden R, Mullin D, Patel A. Reconstruction of the segmental mandibular defect: current state of the art. Curr Opin Otolaryngol Head Neck Surg 2012;20(4);231-6.

[11] He Y, Zhu Hg, Zhang Zy, He J, Sader R. Three-dimensional model simulation and reconstruction of composite total maxillectomy defects with fibula osteomyocutaneous flap flow-through from radial forearm flap. Oral Surgery, Oral Medicine, Oral Pathology, Oral Radiology, and Endodontology 2009;108;e6-e12.

[12] Hirsch DL, Garfein ES, Christensen AM, Weimer KA, Saddeh PB, Levine JP. Use of Computer-Aided Design and Computer-Aided Manufacturing to Produce Orthognathically Ideal Surgical Outcomes: A Paradigm Shift in Head and Neck Reconstruction. Journal of Oral and Maxillofacial Surgery 2009;67;2115-22.

[13] Hou J, Chen M, Pan C et al. Immediate Reconstruction of Bilateral Mandible Defects: Management Based on Computer-Aided Design/Computer-Aided Manufacturing Rapid Prototyping Technology in Combination With Vascularized Fibular Osteomyocutaneous Flap. Journal of Oral and Maxillofacial Surgery 2011;69;1792-7.

[14] Hu YJ, Hardianto A, Li SY, Zhang ZY, Zhang CP. Reconstruction of a palatomaxillary defect with vascularized iliac bone combined with a superficial inferior epigastric artery flap and zygomatic implants as anchorage. Int J Oral Maxillofac Surg 2007;36;854-7.

[15] Jedrzejewski P, Maciejewski A, Szymczyk C, Wierzgon J. Maxillary Reconstruction Using A Multi-Element Free Fibula Flap Based on a Three-Dimensional Polyacrylic Resin Model. Pol Przegl Chir 2012;84(1);49-55.

[16] Juergens P, Krol Z, Zeilhofer H et al. Computer Simulation and Rapid Prototyping for the Reconstruction of the Mandible. Journal of Oral and Maxillofacial Surgery 2009;67;2167-70.

[17] Lee J, Fang J, Chang L, Yu C. Mandibular Defect Reconstruction with the Help of Mirror Imaging Coupled with Laser Stereolithographic Modeling Technique. J Formosan Med Assoc 2007;106;244-50.

[18] Leiggener C, Messo E, Thor A, Zeilhofer H-, Hirsch J-. A selective laser sintering guide for transferring a virtual plan to real time surgery in composite mandibular reconstruction with free fibula osseous flaps. Int J Oral Maxillofac Surg 2009;38;187-92.

[19] Lethaus B, Poort L, Böckmann R, Smeets R, Tolba R, Kessler P. Additive manufacturing for microvascular reconstruction of the mandible in 20 patients. Journal of Cranio-Maxillofacial Surgery 2012;40;43-6.

[20] Liu X, Gui L, Mao C, Peng X, Yu G. Applying computer techniques in maxillofacial reconstruction using a fibula flap: a messenger and an evaluation method. J Craniofac Surg 2009;20(2);372-7.

[21] Modabber A, Legros C, Rana M, Gerressen M, Riediger D, Ghassemi A. Evaluation of computer-assisted jaw reconstruction with free vascularized fibular flap compared to conventional surgery: a clinical pilot study. The International Journal of Medical Robotics and Computer Assisted Surgery 2012;8;215-20.

[22] Moore E, Hinni M, Arce K, Salinas T. Mandibular alveolar reconstruction using three-dimensional planning. Curr Opin Otolaryngol Head Neck Surg 2013;21.

[23] Patel A, Otterburn D, Saadeh P, Levine J, Hirsch DL. 3D Volume Assessment Techniques and Computer-Aided Design and Manufacturing for Preoperative Fabrication of Implants in Head and Neck Reconstruction. Facial Plastic Surgery Clinics of North America 2011;19;683-709.

[24] Rodby K, Turin S et al. Advances in Oncologic Head and Neck Reconstruction: Systemic Review and Future Considerations of Virtual Surgical Planning and Computer Aided Design / Computer Aided Modeling. J Plast Reconstr Aesthet Surg. 2014 Sep; 67(9):1171-1185.

[25] Roser SM, Ramachandra S, Blair H et al. The Accuracy of Virtual Surgical Planning in Free Fibula Mandibular Reconstruction: Comparison of Planned and Final Results. Journal of Oral and Maxillofacial Surgery 2010;68;2824-32.

[26] Saad A, Winters R, Wise M, Dupin C, St.Hilaire H. Virtual Surgical Planning in Complex Composite Maxillofacial Reconstruction. Plast Reconstr Surg 2013;132(3);626-9.

[27] Schepers R, Raghoebar G, Lahoda L et al. Full 3D digital planning of implant supported bridges in secondarily mandibular reconstruction with prefabricated fibula free flaps. Head Neck Oncol 2012;4(2);44.

[28] Schultes G, Kärcher H, Gerzanic L. Prefabricated Iliac Crest Transplant. Journal of Oral and Maxillofacial Surgery 2013;71;428-32.

[29] Seruya M, Fisher M, Rodriguez E. Computer-Assisted versus Conventional Free Fibula Flap Technique for Craniofacial Reconstruction: An Outcomes Comparison. Plast Reconstr Surg 2013;132(5);1219-28.

[30] Sharaf B, Levine J, Hirsch D, Bastidas J, Schiff B, Garfein E. Importance of computer-aided design and manufacturing technology in the multidisciplinary approach to head and neck reconstruction. J Craniofac Surg 2010;21(4);1277-80.

[31] Shen Y, Sun J, Li J, Li M, Huang W, Ow A. Special considerations in virtual surgical planning for secondary accurate maxillary reconstruction with vascularised fibula osteomyocutaneous flap. Journal of Plastic, Reconstructive & Aesthetic Surgery 2012;65;893-902.

[32] Shen Y, Sun J, Li J et al. Using computer simulation and stereomodel for accurate mandibular reconstruction with vascularized iliac crest flap. Oral Surgery, Oral Medicine, Oral Pathology and Oral Radiology 2012;114;175-82.

[33] Sink J, Hamlar D, Kademani D, Khariwala S. Computer-Aided Stereolithography for Presurgical Planning in Fibula Free Tissue Reconstruction of the Mandible. J R 2012;28(6);395-404.

[34] Tepper O, Hirsch D, Levine J, Garfein E. The New Age of Three-Dimensional Virtual Surgical Planning in Reconstructive Plastic Surgery. Plast Reconstr Surg 2012;130(1); 192-4.

[35] Tepper OM, Sorice S, Hershman GN, Saadeh P, Levine JP, Hirsch D. Use of Virtual 3-Dimensional Surgery in Post-Traumatic Craniomaxillofacial Reconstruction. Journal of Oral and Maxillofacial Surgery 2011;69;733-41.

[36] Ueda K, Tajima S, Oba S, Omiya Y, Byun S, Okada M. Mandibular contour reconstruction with three-dimensional computer-assisted models. Ann Plast Surg 2001;46(4);387-3893.

[37] Wang WH, Zhu J, Deng JY, Xia B, Xu B. Three-dimensional virtual technology in reconstruction of mandibular defect including condyle using double-barrel vascularized fibula flap. Journal of Cranio-Maxillofacial Surgery 2013;41;417-22.

[38] Wang T, Tseng C, Hsieh C et al. Using Computer-Aided Design Paper Model for Mandibular Reconstruction: A Preliminary Report. Journal of Oral and Maxillofacial Surgery 2009;67;2534-40.

[39] Xia J, Phillips C, Gateno J, Teighgraeber J, Christensen A, Gliddon M, Lemoine J, Liebschner M. Cost-Effectiveness Analysis for Computer-Aided Surgical Simulation in Complex Cranio-Maxillofacial Surgery. j.joms.2005.12.072

[40] Yeung RWK, Samman N, Cheung LK, Zhang C, Chow RLK. Stereomodel-Assisted Fibula Flap Harvest and Mandibular Reconstruction. Journal of Oral and Maxillofacial Surgery 2007;65;1128-34.

[41] Zheng G, Su Y, Liao G et al. Mandible reconstruction assisted by preoperative virtual surgical simulation. Oral Surgery, Oral Medicine, Oral Pathology and Oral Radiology 2012;113;604-11.

[42] Zhou L, Shang H, He L et al. Accurate Reconstruction of Discontinuous Mandible Using a Reverse Engineering/Computer-Aided Design/Rapid Prototyping Technique: A Preliminary Clinical Study. Journal of Oral and Maxillofacial Surgery 2010;68;2115-21.

[43] Zinser M, Sailer H, Ritter L, Braumann B, Maegele M, Zoller J. A Paradigm Shift in Orthognathic Surgery? A Comparison of Navigation, Computer-Aided Designed/ Computer-Aided Manufactured Splints, and "Classic" Intermaxillary Splints to Surgical Transfer of Virtual Orthognathic Planning. Journal of Oral and Maxillofacial Surgery; 2014;72(10);A1-A26

Chapter 30

Reconstruction of Maxillofacial Osseous Defects with Computer-Aided Designed/Computer-Aided Manufactured Devices

Jan Rustemeyer

Additional information is available at the end of the chapter

http://dx.doi.org/10.5772/58955

1. Introduction

Over the past years, virtually planned surgery has been increasingly utilised in maxillofacial reconstructive surgery. The concept of computer-aided surgery uses surgical simulation and three-dimensional (3-D) computer-aided designed/computer-aided manufactured (CAD/CAM) tools such as cutting guides and jigs rather than relying exclusively on intraoperative manual approximation for facial reconstruction [1].

The advantage of virtually planned surgery over conventional surgery has indisputably less deviation between reconstructed and natural bony landmarks [2]. Nevertheless, the amount of time saved by using the CAD/CAM approach is subject to controversy. On the one hand, microsurgical craniofacial reconstruction using computer-assisted techniques, such as for fibula-flap harvesting, has yielded significantly shorter ischemia times even with a larger number of osteotomies compared with conventional techniques [3]. On the other hand, the time savings should be considered in light of the additional time needed to complete the preoperative virtual modeling session, which can take up to an hour. So if saving time were a means of recouping the added cost of the CAD/CAM technique, the overall operative time should not be different from that of the conventional technique [4]. However, no differences between the techniques exist with respect to perioperative and long-term outcomes, length of hospital stay, recipient-site infection, partial and total flap loss, or rate of soft-tissue and bony-tissue revisions [3].

We report herein our experiences using CAD/CAM techniques in five separate cases and discuss them on the basis of recent criteria for the usage of CAD/CAM techniques given in the literature.

2. Materials and methods

2.1. Classification systems of osseous maxillofacial defects

Osseous defects of the maxillofacial region are described using international classification systems. The applied classification of mandibular defects refers to the HLC classification described by Boyd et al. [5]. The *H* represents a defect compromising a lateral segment of any length containing a condyle and not substantially crossing the midline, *L* stands for the same defect but without a condyle, and *C* represents the anterior segment between the incisor foramina. The classification of maxillopalatine defects refers to the classification given by Okay et al. [6]. Class Ia summarizes defects with no involvement of the tooth-bearing alveolus; Class Ib, preservation of both canines; Class II, resection of one canine or less than 50% of the hard palate; Class III, resection of both canines or greater than 50% of the hard palate.

2.2. CAD/CAM technique

The CAD/CAM technique was applied for the reconstruction procedures. An exemplary operational sequence of virtual osseous reconstruction with CAD/CAM technique is given in Figure 1. Planning was performed on 3-D images generated from high-resolution, helical computed tomography (CT) scans of the maxillomandibular region and the chosen donor site, respectively. The patient's natural anatomy was restored virtually by mirroring the unaffected side (case 1 to 4). The mirroring protocol is not possible in defects involving both sides of the mandible or maxilla. Therefore the solution is having a database from other patients which can be imported as a reference (case 5). The selected osseous donor site was virtually harvested, trimmed, and inset using the tools contained in the appropriate planning software of the CAD/CAM tools-providing company (case 1 to 4: MedX, Xilloc Medical B.V., Maastricht, The Netherlands; case 5: ProPlan CMF, Synthes/Materilise, Leuven, Belgium). Patient-specific cutting guides for the donor site, as well as for the recipient site (if applicable), were created using a 3-D printer. The prepared cutting guides should ensure the accurate segmentation and implementation of the harvested bone.

2.3. Subjects

All patients were recruited and treated at the Department of Oral and Maxillofacial Surgery and Plastic Operations. In all cases of applying the CAD/CAM technique, the bony reconstruction was intended to provide a basis for implant loading and prosthetic rehabilitation of the patient. Subjects gave written informed consent to publish their medical records and accompanying images. An overview of the presented cases with applied CAD/CAM technique for maxillofacial reconstruction including their histories, chief complaints, affected sites and types of reconstruction is given in table 1.

http://dx.doi.org/10.5772/58955

Case	Age	Gender	History	Chief complains	Affected site	Class	Reconstruction
1	72	M	SCC of the lateral floor of the mouth and alveolar ridge, partial mandibular resection	Missing bony width and height	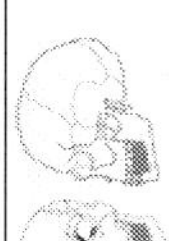	L	Free iliac crest
2	54	F	Chronic osteomyelitis, mandibular continuity resection	Recurrent facial pain and swelling	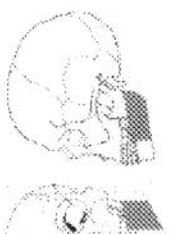	L	Vascularised iliac crest and ASIS
3	72	F	SCC of the lateral floor of the mouth, ORN of mandible, mandibular continuity resection	Deviation and severe scaring of lower face	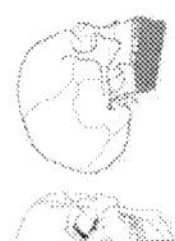	LC	Vascularised two-segment osteomyocutaneous fibula flap
4	43	F	Maxillary ACC, hemimaxillectomy	Wide opening of maxillary sinus and nasal cavity	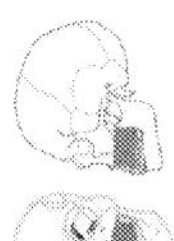	III	Double Flap technique: vascularised osteomyocutaneous double-barrelled fibula flap and RFF
5	45	M	Toxic induced subtotal maxillary osteonecrosis	Wide opening of maxillary sinus and nasal cavities	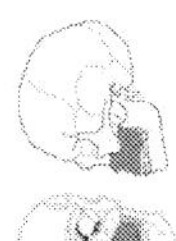	III	Vascularised three-segment osteomyocutaneous fibula flap

SCC = Squamous Cell Carcinoma, ASIS = Anterior Superior Iliac Spine, ORN = Osteoradionecrosis, ACC = Adenoidcystic Carcinoma; RFF = Radial Forearm Flap

Table 1. Overview of cases with applied CAD/CAM technique for maxillofacial reconstruction.

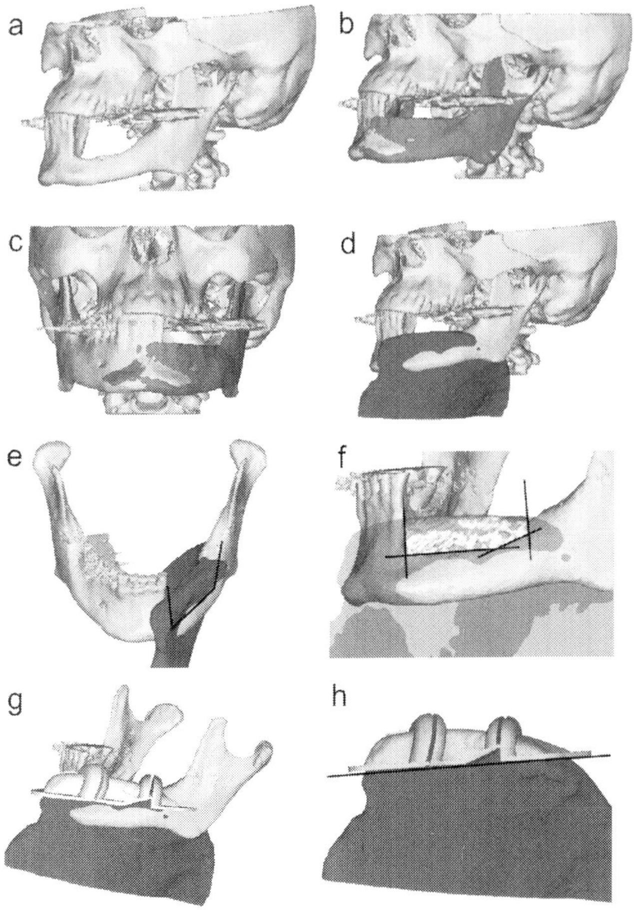

Figure 1. Exemplary operational sequence of virtual osseous reconstruction with CAD/CAM technique. (a) Initial findings in 3-D CT, (b) and (c) Mirroring the unaffected side for virtual reconstruction, (d) Selecting a proper harvesting site by precisely superimposing the virtually reconstructed side, (e) and (f) Virtually harvesting, trimming and insetting of the osseous transplant, (g) and (h) Designing patient-specific cutting guides for 3-D printing.

3. Clinical case studies

3.1. Case 1

A 72-year-old male was admitted to our centre with squamous cell carcinoma (SCC) of the left lateral floor of the mouth and the adjacent alveolar ridge. He underwent tumour resection including partial resection of the left mandible with scarifying of the ipsilateral canine, premolars, and molars, leaving a Class L defect. No mandibular resection in continuity was necessary. Hence, it was possible to preserve the inferior alveolar nerve (IAN) and the base of the mandible to ensure stability without osteosynthesis.

One year after primary surgery, reconstruction of the mandible was virtually planned to augment the missing bony width and height (Figure 2). An additional soft tissue transfer was not necessary since the residual soft tissue would provide a sure and tensionless wound closure. Within the intraoperative use of a CAD/CAM cutting guide for harvesting a left iliac crest bone part, the anterior superior iliac spine (ASIS) could be preserved. Using an intraoral approach, we inset the harvested free iliac crest bone and rigidly anchored it with two osteosynthesis platelets (2.0 mm system, Stryker Corp, Freiburg, Germany). On the anterolateral aspect, a space of 1.5 mm was left between the transplant and the preserved alveolar ridge of the mandible. Therefore, it was necessary to bridge this gap with cancellous bone. Both, postsurgical wound healing and further recovery were uneventful.

3.2. Case 2

In a 54-year-old female, chronic osteomyelitis of the left mandible from the premolar region up to the ascending ramus was detected with bone scans consisting of scintigraphy using single-photon-emission computed tomography (SPECT) and CT scans (Figure 3). A recurrent intravenous antibiotic regime with piperacillin 3 × 2 g and sulbactam 3 × 1 g and local decortication did not lead to an enduring remission.

We consequently decided to resect the involved mandibular segments, achieving a Class L defect, and to perform an immediate osseous reconstruction in one operative session. The IAN was already compromised, leaving an anaesthetic area of corresponding ipsilateral skin, mucosa, and lower lip. Virtual planning revealed that the best reconstruction could be obtained using the ipsilateral ASIS and accompanying parts of the iliac crest.

At surgery, CAD/CAM cutting guides were used for mandibular resection, and iliac bone harvesting ensured an exact fit of the osseous reconstruction. Vascular, pedicled iliac bone was harvested, inset, and fixed with osteosynthesis platelets before microvascular anastomoses were done. Following resection of the mandible, the condyle-bearing portion of the mandible immediately rotated clockwise and was repositioned upon inset of the iliac bone flap. No further augmentative features were necessary because the intraoperative findings were in strict accordance with the planned situation. No complications occurred during the postoperative course and no further episodes of inflammatory osteomyelitis were realised during a follow-up of 6 months.

3.3. Case 3

A 72-year-old female suffering from SCC had tumour resection of the anterior and right lateral floor of the mouth. Soft tissue reconstruction was performed with a radial forearm flap (RFF). Postsurgically, necessary radiotherapy led to severe osteoradionecrosis (ORN) of the mandible, compromising the area of the contralateral canine region up to the ipsilateral mandibular

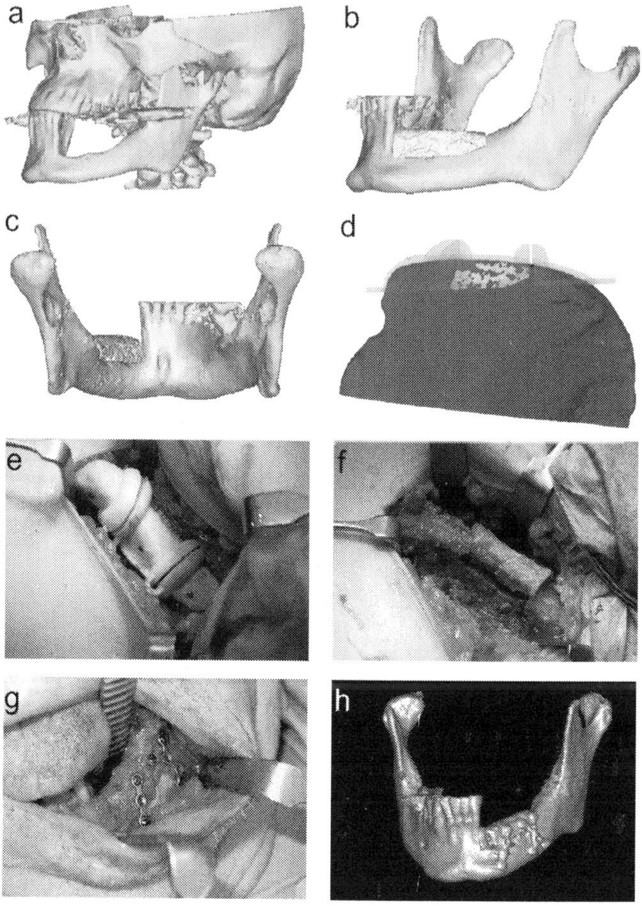

Figure 2. Case 1. (a) 3-D CT shows the left mandibular defect. (b) and (c) Virtual reconstruction of osseous defect. (d) Virtual iliac crest with planned cutting guide and transplant. (e) Intraoperative positioning of the cutting guide. (f) Harvesting of the iliac crest bone. (g) The transplant inset and fixed. (h) Postoperative 3-D CT findings with iliac crest for mandibular augmentation.

angle. The affected parts of the mandible were completely resected without further reconstruction, leaving a class LC defect.

During follow-ups, the patient complained about ipsilateral deviation of the lower face after muscle contraction and scar formation. No applicable prosthetic solution could be devised. After 1 year and without any further evidence of ORN, mandibular reconstruction was planned using CAD/CAM tools for harvesting a vascularised osteomyocutaneous fibula flap (Figure 4). Intraoperative cutting guides for the mandibular stumps were used to assure straight osteotomy lines. Another cutting guide was needed to produce a two-segment fibula

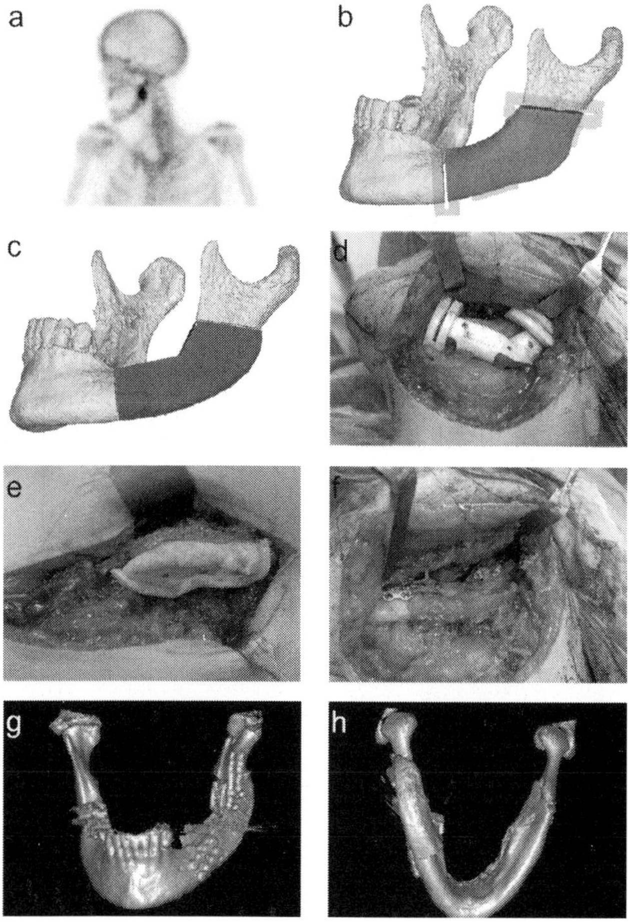

Figure 3. Case 2. (a) SPECT shows osteomyelitis of the left mandible. (b) and (c) Virtual resection and reconstruction of mandible. (d) and (e) Intraoperative positioning of the cutting guides on the mandible and the iliac crest and ASIS. (f) Vascularised iliac bone flap inset and fixed. (g) and (h) Postoperative 3-D CT showing incorporated iliac bone flap.

to reconstruct the mandibular angle, corpus, and the anterior part. A skin paddle containing two septocutaneous perforators was placed extraorally over the chin area to provide volume for the resulting skin defect after dissolving the scars and repositioning the soft tissue chin in the facial midline. Intraorally, the former RFF provided stable soft tissue coverage. The segmented fibula was stabilised and fixed to the prepared mandibular stumps with osteosynthesis platelets before microvascular anastomosis was carried out. The fitting was in accordance with the planned situation, including repositioning both condyles. No trimming or application of cancellous bone was necessary. The wounds healed primarily and the further postsurgical course was uneventful.

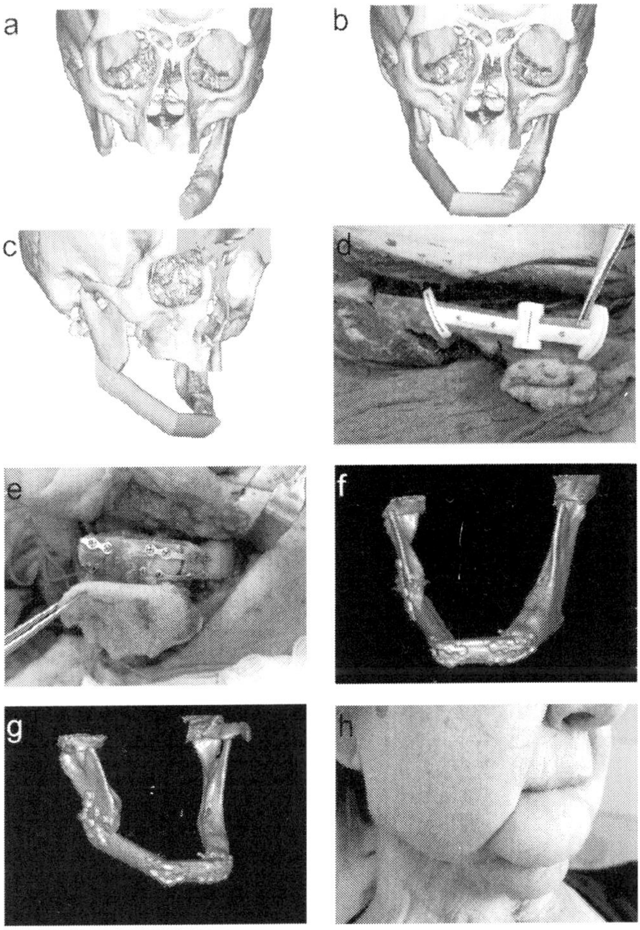

Figure 4. Case 3. (a) Initial mandibular defect in the 3-D CT. (b) and (c) Virtual reconstruction with a two-segment fibula flap. (d) Intraoperative positioning of the fibular cutting guide. (e) Inset of the prepared and osseous segmented osteomyocutaneous fibula flap. (f) and (g) Postoperative 3-D CT of reconstructed mandible. (h) Complete wound healing after 4 weeks.

3.4. Case 4

In a 43-year-old female, an adenoidcystic carcinoma of the left maxilla and hard palate was histologically confirmed. Tumour surgery consisted of a hemimaxillectomy up to the zygomatic arch and resection of the left and part of the right hard palate to achieve clear margins. The maxillary sinus, nasal cavity, and septum were widely exposed, comprising a Class III defect. No primary reconstruction was carried out. Radiotherapy was applied postsurgically, as suggested by the tumour board.

http://dx.doi.org/10.5772/58955

One year after initial therapy and with no evidence of recurrence, reconstruction was virtually planned and realised by performing a double-flap technique for covering the soft and hard tissue defects (Figure 5). During one operation, a fibula flap, with a wide muscular cuff to provide bulkiness, was harvested. The fibular bone was then segmented using a CAD/CAM cutting guide and prepared as a double-barrelled fibula by folding upward a precisely determined distal portion of the fibula. This technique was chosen to apply the necessary bony height to fill the osseous maxillary resection defect. After osteosynthesis between both fibular parts and between the fibula and the preserved maxilla, microvascular anastomosis was carried out. In the next step, an RFF was harvested to cover the muscle cuff of the fibular flap and to provide adequate soft tissue coverage for the palatal defect. The postoperative course was uncomplicated and both flaps were successfully incorporated.

3.5. Case 5

At first presentation, a 44-year-old male complained of chronic facial pain and nasal outflow of fluid and food for at least two years. Clinical inspection revealed a desolate intraoral situation with osteonecrosis of the nearly edentulous upper jaw and palate with oroantral and oronasal fistulas. After careful inquiry, the patient admitted chronic abuse of alcohol, nicotine and of the illicit drug methamphetamine (MA) for at least 25 years. For the past 20 years, he had synthesized MA for his own consumption and for illegal disposal in his home country. Furthermore, he confessed to extracting teeth himself since he became addicted to MA. After further investigation, a history of bisphosphonate intake for any reason or radiation of the head and face was definitely ruled out. In the last year the patient had successfully completed a drug intervention and rehabilitation program and he was successfully cured of his addiction to toxic substances and illegal drugs.

Upon hospitalization, an intravenous antibiotic regime with piperacillin 3 × 2 g and sulbactam 3 × 1 g was initiated. Bone scans consisting of SPECT and 3-D CT of the head and neck showed extensive bony destruction of the maxilla and an accompanying osteomyelitis up to the zygomatic arches. The surgical treatment comprised a step-by-step approach. In the first step, the affected necrotic parts of the maxilla were resected to achieve clear margins. During surgery, the infraorbital and zygomatic region showed bleeding spots and vital solid bone. The diagnosis of osteonecrosis was confirmed by histopathology. In a second step two weeks later, reconstruction of the maxilla was performed using a vascularized osteomyocutaneous fibula flap from the left side (Figure 6).

To imitate the natural maxillary arch in the planning sessions, the fibula was divided into three segments and folded in the transverse plane. After inset of the osteomyocutaneous fibular flap and subcutaneous tunneling of the preauricular region, microvascular anastomoses were carried out using the left superficial temporal artery and vein as recipient vessels for the peroneal artery and the accompanying dominant vein. Surgery and postsurgical course were uneventful and a remarkably good accordance between the virtually-planned and the real outcome was recognized on postoperative CT scans. Immediately after surgery, nasal outflow ceased and facial pain was remarkably minimized.

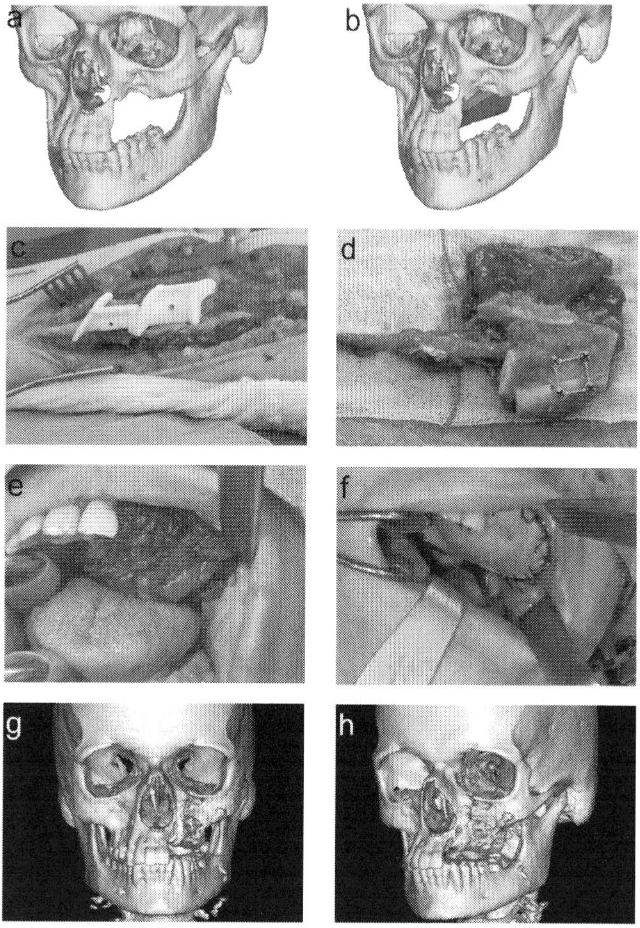

Figure 5. Case 4. (a) Initial finding of the maxillopalatine defect in the 3-D CT. (b) Virtual reconstruction with a double-barrelled fibula flap. (c) Positioning of the fibular cutting guide. (d) and (e) Prepared double-barrelled fibula flap inset into the defect area. (f) Inset of radial forearm flap for intraoral cutaneous covering. (g) and (h) Postoperative 3-D CT findings with incorporated fibula flap for osseous reconstruction.

4. Discussion

In this clinical study, we presented five different cases bearing for us some indications for the application of CAD/CAM techniques. Our report included a regional mandibular defect after tumour ablation (Case 1), extensive loss of mandibular continuity as a result of chronic osteomyelitis and ORN (Cases 2 and 3), and maxillopalatine defects (Case 4 and 5). Recent literature provides somewhat different criteria compared with ours for the application of CAD/CAM technique for osseous reconstruction [7-9]. The former comprise the requirement of

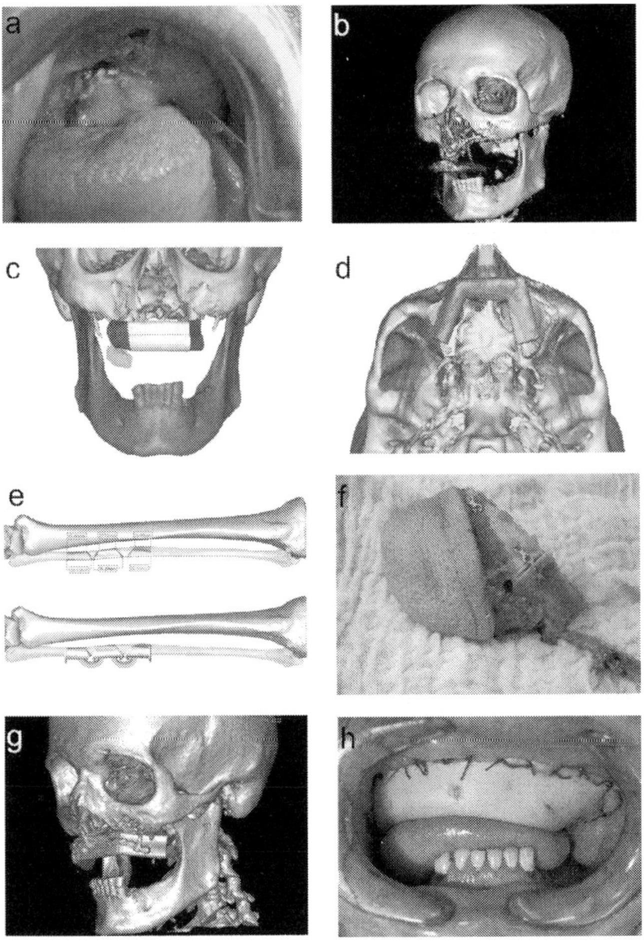

Figure 6. Case 5. (a) and (b) Extensive osteonecrosis and extensive bony destruction of the upper jaw. (c) and (d) Virtually restored native anatomy and virtually inset of fibula bone to imitate the natural maxillary arch. (e) Cutting guide for the three-segment fibula. (f) Prepared osteomyocutaneous fibula flap before inset. (g) and (h) Postoperative 3-D CT and total soft tissue covering of the former subtotal maxillary defect.

multiple osteotomies for an osseous flap, the need for multiple simultaneous free flaps, history of ORN or radiation therapy to the head and neck, and high-velocity ballistic injury with significant tissue loss. However, it is remarkable that no evidence-based studies covering these criteria are available and mostly refer to anecdotal case studies.

Keeping this in mind and following the criteria given above, only three of our presented cases should be appropriate for the CAD/CAM technique. These cases comprise osseous reconstructions obviously more complex because of having to produce segmented bone flaps (Cases

3 to 5) and employ a two-flap technique (Case 4). The two cases not meeting the criteria include the harvesting of a free iliac bone flap (Case 1) and a vascularised iliac bone flap (Case 2). Indeed, the latter cases were simpler with respect to the literature criteria and compared with Cases 3, 4 and 5. However, our experience was that the CAD/CAM technique facilitated finding and harvesting bone segments that closely duplicated the shape of the natural mandible in even less complex cases of osseous reconstruction. Without the CAD/CAM technique and cutting guides, surgery might have required further trimming and blurring of the osseous transplant without improving accuracy. At worst, it might have resulted in unnecessary scarifying of the ASIS in Case1 with further comorbidity.

However, the latter case was the only one in which compromises were necessary with respect to the accuracy of the anterolateral junction of the osseous transplant and the residual mandibular bone. Besides, the discrepancy between virtual planning and the actual finding was within the scope of a reported distance between the real and virtual osteotomies of 1.30 ± 0.59 mm [1]. Retrospectively, the source of this error is difficult to detect. Possible reasons for this inaccuracy are purely hypothetical, including movement artefacts during CT scans, metallic artefacts from filled teeth, too much play of the oscillating saw in the slots of the cutting guides, calculation errors, or simply being unfamiliar with a new method. Further studies are warranted to clarify these hypotheses.

While performing surgery with CAD/CAM devices, we experienced in Cases 2 and 3 an additional helpful aspect. After we resected the aforementioned mandibular part in Case 2, including parts of the ascending ramus, the condyle-bearing stump rotated clockwise as a result of contraction of the temporal muscle tendon. Hand-setting alone would have resulted in considerable bias when repositioning the condlye. However, by seamlessly insetting the osseous transplant, we were able to replace the condyle exactly in its initial position without further effort. Accordingly in Case 3, initial findings showed that the ascending rami were pathologically rotated medially and the condyles laterally. During virtual planning, the rotated parts were derotated and the segmented fibula flap was planned for the new position. Within the inset of the prepared fibula we achieved the planned derotation of the condyles by setting the residual mandibular stumps and fibula in a strictly axial and seamless bone-to-bone contact. Hence, the outcomes of these cases suggest that the CAD/CAM technique presents both the opportunity to accurately reconstruct osseous parts of the maxillofacial region and to solve arising or existing pathological conditions.

5. Conclusion

Our case report has fulfilled the challenge in the literature to improve upon traditional shaping methods, especially to justify the added costs [4, 10]. Furthermore, our report suggests that the possible applications of CAD/CAM techniques have not yet to be exhausted. At the current state of the art, we believe that the application of CAD/CAM techniques for osseous reconstruction in the field of maxillofacial surgery should not be restricted to obviously complex reconstructions.

http://dx.doi.org/10.5772/58955

Author details

Jan Rustemeyer

Department of Oral and Maxillofacial Surgery, Plastic Operations, Klinikum Bremen-Mitte, School of Medicine of the University of Göttingen, Bremen, Germany

References

[1] Roser SM, Ramachandra S, Blair H, Grist W, Carlson GW, Christensen AM, Weimer KA, Steed MB. The accuracy of virtual surgical planning in free fibula mandibular reconstruction: comparison of planned and final results. J Oral Maxillofac Surg 2010;68(11) 2824-2832.

[2] Hanasono MM, Skoracki RJ. Computer-assisted design and rapid prototype modeling in microvascular mandible reconstruction. Laryngoscope 2012; 123(3) 597–604.

[3] Seruya M, Fisher M, Rodriguez ED. Computer-assisted versus conventional free fibula flap technique for craniofacial reconstruction: an outcomes comparison. Plast Reconstr Surg 2013;132(5) 1219-1228.

[4] Matros E, Disa JJ. Discussion: Computer-Assisted versus Conventional Free Fibula Flap Technique for Craniofacial Reconstruction: An Outcomes Comparison. Plast Reconstr Surg 2013;132(5) 1229-1230.

[5] Boyd JB, Gullane PJ, Brown DH. Classification of Mandibular Defects. Plast Reconstr Surg 1993;92(7) 1266-1275.

[6] Okay DJ, Genden E, Buchbinder D, Urken M. Prosthodontic guidelines for surgical reconstruction of the maxilla: a classification system of defects. J Prosthet Dent 2001;86(4) 352-363.

[7] Saad A, Winters R, Wise MW, Dupin CL, St Hilaire H. Virtual surgical planning in complex composite maxillofacial reconstruction. Plast Reconstr Surg 2013; 132(3) 626-633.

[8] Ghazali N, Collyer JC, Tighe JV. Hemimandibulectomy and vascularized fibula flap in bisphosphonate-induced mandibular osteonecrosis with polycythaemia rubra vera. Int J Oral Maxillofac Surg 2013; 42(1) 120-123.

[9] Tepper OM, Sorice S, Hershman GN, Saadeh P, Levine JP, Hirsch D. Use of virtual 3-dimensional surgery in post-traumatic craniomaxillofacial reconstruction. J Oral Maxillofac Surg 2011;69(3) 733–741.

[10] Hanasono MM, Jacob RF, Bidaut L, Robb GL, Skoracki RJ. Midfacial reconstruction sing virtual planning, rapid prototype modeling,and stereotactic navigation. Plast Reconstr Surg 2010; 126(6) 2002–2006.

Section 12

Basic and Advanced Rhinoplasty

Chapter 31

Contemporary Rhinoplasty Techniques

Payam Varedi and Behnam Bohluli

Additional information is available at the end of the chapter

http://dx.doi.org/10.5772/59811

1. Introduction

Rhinoplasty has evolved during the past two decades. The popular trend to have a smaller nose is gradually changing to having a normal looking nose. Nowadays, functional considerations are an integral part of any treatment plan. A major effort is usually made to detect any deficits in the nasal airway before aesthetic surgery to be solved or improved by a proper treatment plan. Grafting and suturing techniques have replaced some older destructive techniques. This chapter gives an overview of current concepts in rhinoplasty; we also present logical approaches in case selection and evaluation.

2. Preoperative evaluations

Like any other aesthetic procedure, a comprehensive preoperative evaluation, may directly affect the final outcome of the operation. The first step is usually started by a thorough psychological assessment, and then functional assessment of the nose is performed. Structural and aesthetic evaluations are usually the last stages followed by the treatment plan and finally operation [1].

2.1. Psychological evaluation

Psychological assessment of the rhinoplasty candidates is the first step to build up a proper treatment plan. Unrealistic demands and personality disorders are best detected at this stage. An open discussion with the patient may clarify many potential problems. Any previous psychological medications or therapies should be clarified. Patient may be asked to bring up their ideal nose models; computerized simulation is another modality that may help the surgeon communicate with the patient and seek their real demands and expectations. It is clear that an ideal surgery with perfect results in an unsatisfied patient is a big failure and is best prevented in this preoperative phase [2-3].

2.2. Functional evaluation

The human nose bears a complex physiologic and functional role in breathing and smelling. For this reason it is logically expected that this delicate organ be preserved and even improved during aesthetic surgery. This evaluation usually starts with verbal interview with the patient. Any breathing problems may be easily detected. Exacerbating factors or problems are usually best described by the patient, and then the evaluation continues with direct inspection of the nose. Any deviation or deformity should be observed and documented. To assess the septum and turbinates sufficient light and a nasal speculum are necessary. A few drops of a vasoconstrictor such as phenylephrine in each nostril may be applied for better visualization [4-7].The final step is to check the valve. The Cottle test is a known method to assess the internal nasal valve. The patient is asked to take a deep breath through the nose, and then inhalation is repeated while the patient is retracting his/her nasal side wall. If a considerable improvement occurs (positive Cottle test), this means a serious weakness exists in the internal nasal valve (Figure1). [8].It is clear that a reinforcement or total reconstruction of the internal valve should be considered in treatment planning. This test should be done on both sides and documented properly.

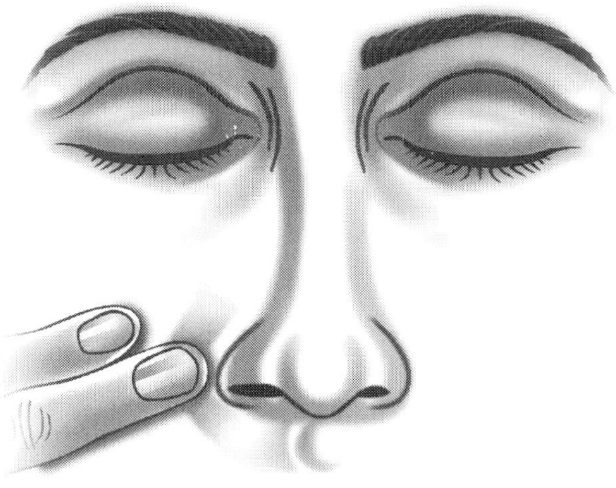

Figure 1. Cottle test.

To assess the external valves the patient is asked to tilt the head backward and take a deep. The nose is closely observed by the surgeon. This test may be documented by simple standard photography. Excessive medial movements of the nostrils and/or collapse means that some kind of reinforcement technique needs to be considered in the rhinoplasty procedure [9-10].

3. Additional diagnostic techniques

Water's view radiograph is commonly used to evaluate the maxillary sinuses and nasal septum. In case a complex deformity or deviation is found, CT scan may help the surgeon better analyze the problem.

Lateral nasal view may help the surgeon measure the length and height of the bony vault though measurement, palpation and tactile sensation may easily provide the same data for the surgery.

CT scans are commonly used to assess internal compartments of the nose. Septal deformities and spicules are easily detected and documented. Nasal turbinates and paranasal sinuses are also clearly observed on CT scans. Nasal valve diameters are sometimes measured and documented as well.

4. Structural assessment

Structurally the nose is formed from cartilage, bone, muscle, connective tissue and skin. It is clear that the quantity and quality of these components play a determining role in the outcome of aesthetic nasal surgery. For structural evaluation, the nose is gently palpated by the surgeon. The quality and thickness of the overlying skin is size and length of the bony vault is grossly measured and then subtle finger pressure is applied over the tip to determine the strength and support of the cartilage framework. Then, the patient is asked to smile. Excessive drooping of the nose or unpleasant widening may be an indicator of muscular hyperactivity or structural weakness that both may be easily corrected with a thorough treatment plan.

5. Basic techniques in rhinoplasty

5.1. Incisions

Open approach rhinoplasty needs two basic incisions namely, skin incision and rim incisions. These two incisions are connected to each other and skeletonization is started.

5.2. Skin incisions

The skin incision is placed in the mid-columellar skin. An inverted-V (Figure 2) or stair-step (Figure 3) design will provide a longer incision line and logically better healing and less visible scar. On the other hand, the geometric incision may help the surgeon return the flap to its exact position thus, distortion or deformities are prevented.

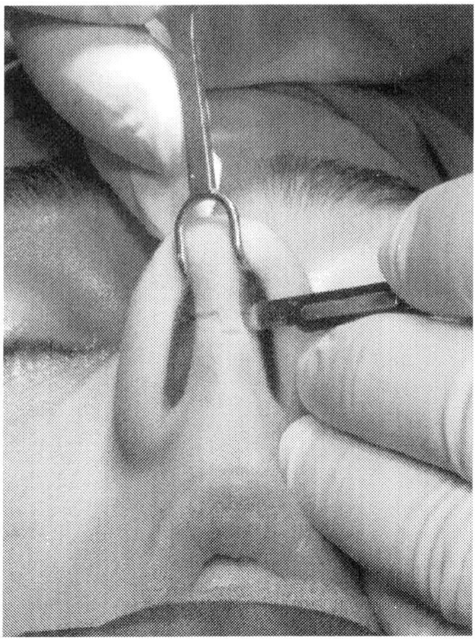

Figure 2. Inverted-V incision

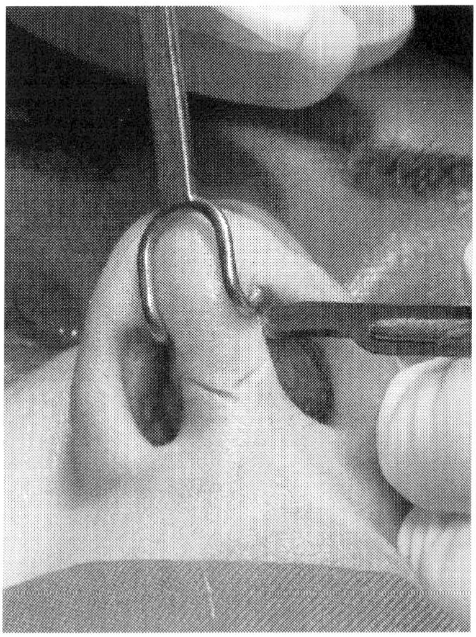

Figure 3. Stair-step incision

5.3. Rim incision

The rim incision is an intranasal incision along the caudal edge of the lower lateral cartilages (Figure 4).Care should be taken to remain close to the cartilage edge. In this way a proper incision will follow the normal anatomy of the lower lateral cartilages. For this reason, the incision line will be close to the nostril margins in the dome area and will move caudally as it is continued along the border of the lateral crural cartilage.

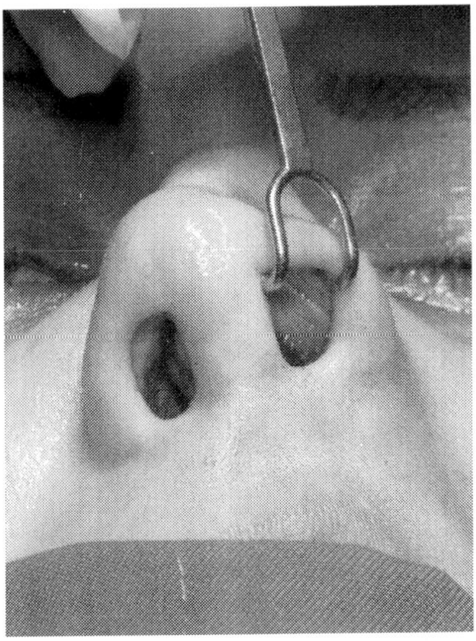

Figure 4. Rim incision

5.4. Skeletonization

Skeletonization is usually done to gain access to cartilaginous and bony framework of the nose. To do so, columellar and marginal incisions are connected to each other and with delicate scissors the skin flap is reflected gradually. Care is usually taken to move close to the cartilage and bone during dissection (Figure 5). A deeper plane will provide a skin coverage that will conceal subtle irregularities while intradermal dissections may lead to color changes or surface irregularities.

5.5. Tip-plasty

Tip-plasty is a combination of many reductive, suturing and grafting techniques that are done to refine or shape a malformed asymmetric tip. Basic techniques are usually enough in most cases. Though in some complicated noses such as revision or cleft noses some advanced methods may be applied that require skill and training.

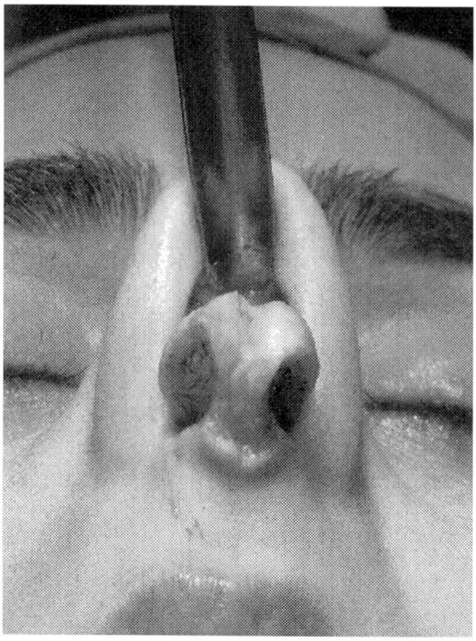

Figure 5. Skeletonization is completed.

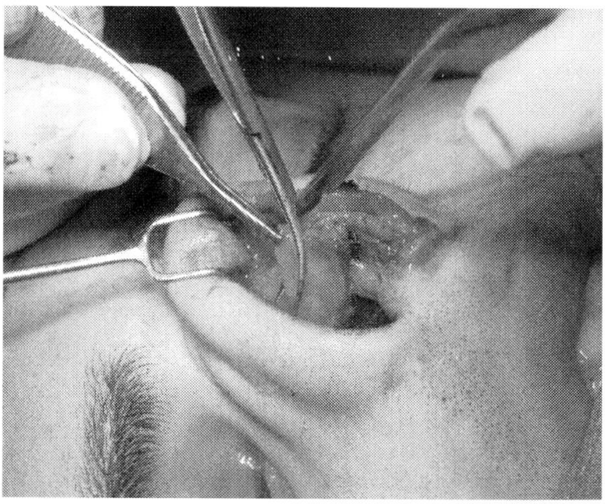

Figure 6. Cephalic trimming.

5.6. Cephalic trimming

In this technique, a narrow strip of lateral crural cartilage is marked, incised and separated from underlying skin. The main purpose of cephalic trimming is to refine the tip and make enough space for tip rotation (Figure 6). [11].

http://dx.doi.org/10.5772/59811

5.7. Salient points

This technique is potentially destructive and may weaken the tip. Vigorous cartilage resection may result in severe pinch deformities and external nasal valve incompetency. As a rule all respective techniques must be done conservatively and is best avoided in narrow or weak lower lateral cartilages.

5.8. Tip spanning suture

Tip spanning suture is a mattress suture that is done on each dome. This suture will make a sharper dome on each side and as result more definition of the tip will be apparent (Figure 7).

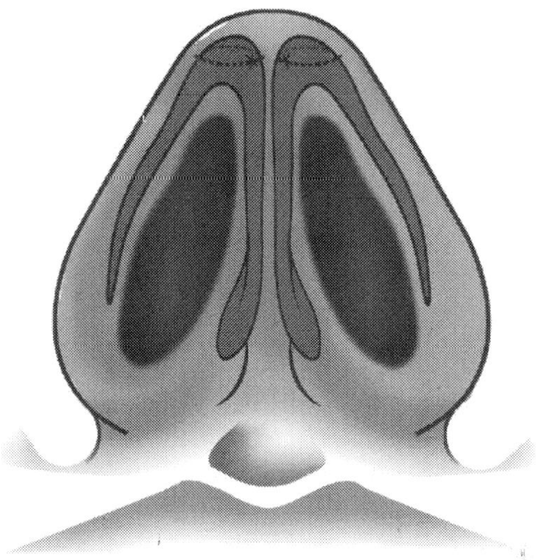

Figure 7. Tip spanning suture

5.9. Common mistakes

Big suture bites over the dome area or over-tightening of the tip spanning suture may lead to a pinch deformity or tip destruction. Gentle tightening of sutures and use of delicate suture material (PDS 6-0) is enough to shape the structure of the lower lateral cartilages.

6. Interdomal suture

Interdomal suture is a simple suture that approximates the two lateral crura. This simple suture is the most effective approach to correct a boxy and/or bifid tip (Figure 8.(

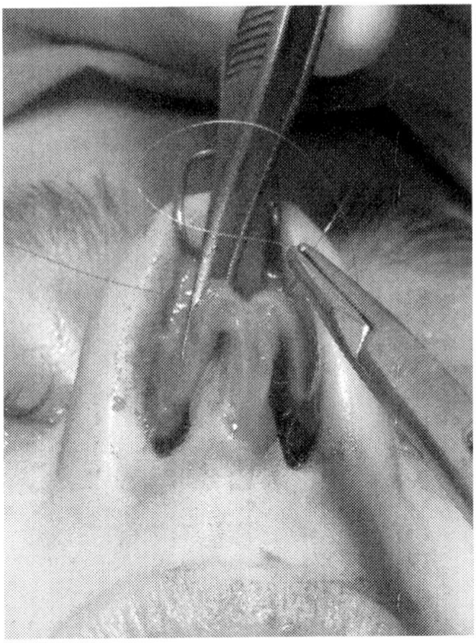

Figure 8. Interdomal suture

6.1. Common mistakes

The interdomal suture should be done in a way that two domes form a 45 degree angle to each other. Careless non-anatomic interdomal suturing will provide a pointed tip that has no definition and is not aesthetically pleasing. [12-15].

7. Basic grafts in tip plasty

7.1. Collumellar strut

The columellar strut is a quadrangular piece of cartilage that is inserted and fixed, in a pocket between the two medial crura. The columellar strut is aimed to reinforce tip support; the strut may indirectly have positive effects on tip rotation and increasing tip projection (Figure 9). [16].

7.2. Cap graft

The cap graft is a small ovoid cartilage that is prepared from septal cartilage, remnants of excised cephalic trimming or choncal cartilage. This graft is placed and fixed over the domes (Figure10). Cap grafts may have several aesthetic results namely:

1. Slightly increases tip projection

2. Shapes the tip

http://dx.doi.org/10.5772/59811

3. Covers the irregularities of the tip cartilages

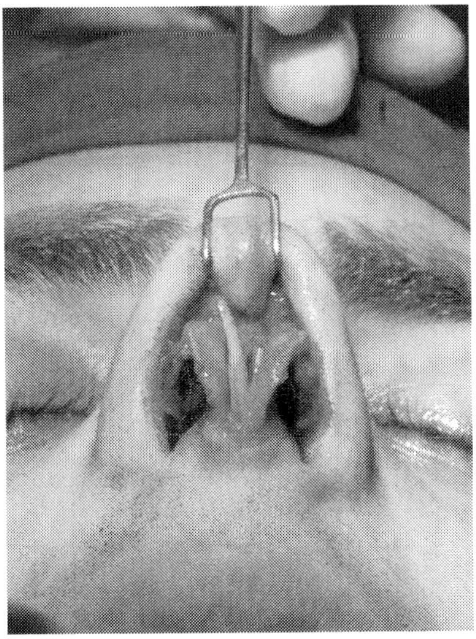

Figure 9. Collumellar strut

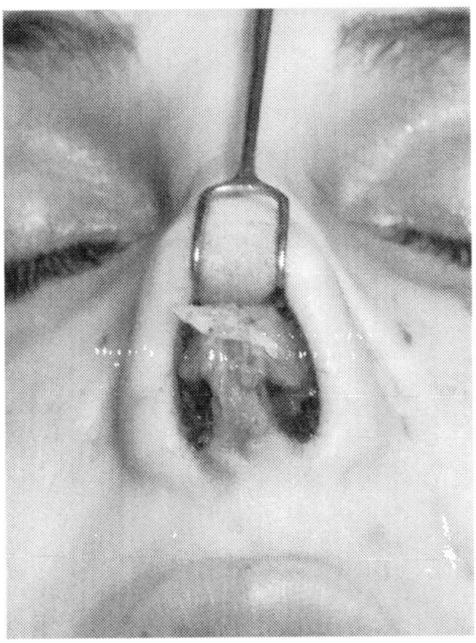

Figure 10. Cap graft

7.3. Shield graft

Shield graft is a quadrangular piece of a cartilage that is formed and trimmed according to the aesthetic needs of the deformity. A shield graft is generally placed and fixed caudal to the medial crural cartilages (Figure 11).This graft has nearly the same role as a cap graft though its heavier and stronger; there are two specific uses for it:

1. To form the bulky tip
2. To increase tip projection [17-21]

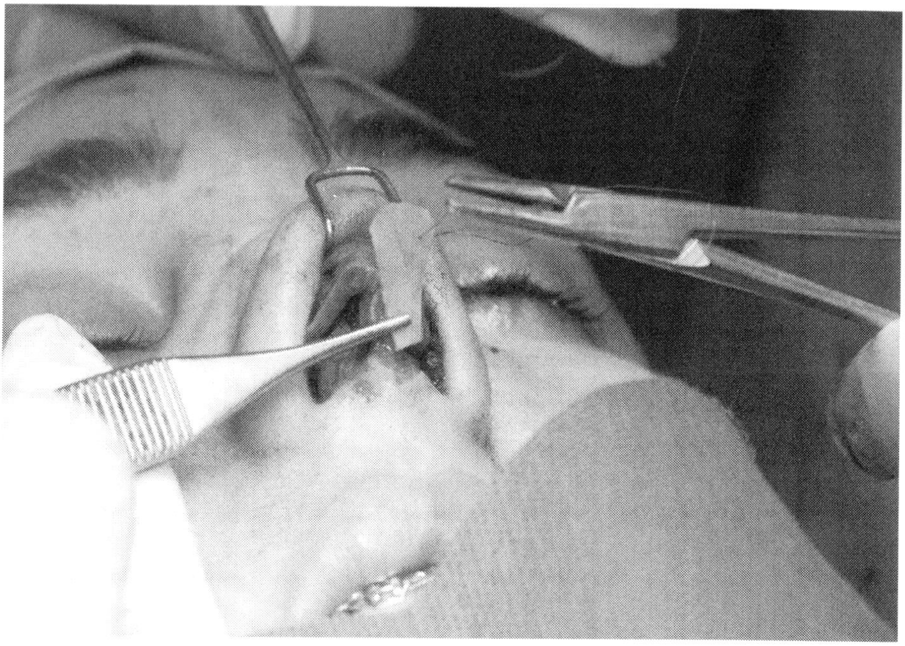

Figure 11. Shield graft

8. Crushed cartilage

A small piece of cartilage is placed in a crusher and with few strokes of a mallet, a smooth soft texture is provided that may be used to cover the irregularities or fill subtle deformities(Figure 12).Tip grafts are best fixed by delicate 6-0 PDS sutures to prevent any future dislodgment or displacement. The skin may be re-draped several times to seek any spicules. Sharp edges or shadows of tip grafts are corrected intra-operatively to avoid later revisions. [22]

http://dx.doi.org/10.5772/59811

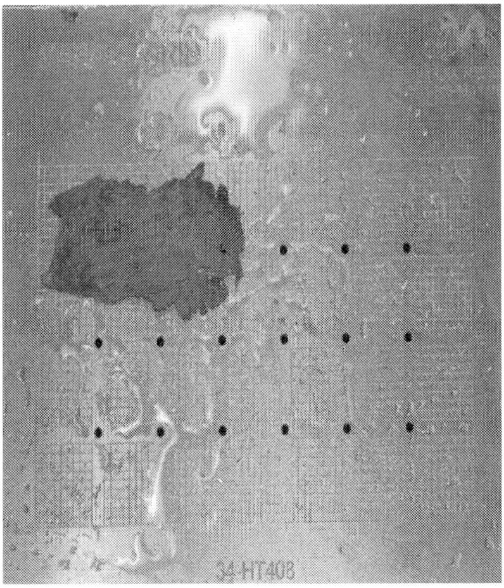

Figure 12. Crushed cartilage

9. Hump modification

The dorsal hump is a complex anatomic component of the nose. The nasal hump is formed by two upper lateral cartilages, the septal cartilage and two nasal bones. Dorsal modification is usually started with resection of excessive parts and in some cases augmentation of shallow and defective parts. Hump resection may be done in a way that all excessive parts are resected in one piece (composite resection) or in a way that each component is trimmed and resected separately in an incremental manner (component resection).

9.1. Composite hump surgery

When it is planned to remove a maximum of 2 or 3mm of dorsal hump, composite resection may be done. In this technique, cartilaginous part is cut by surgical knife and a hump osteotome is inserted beneath the cut cartilage and hump resection is continued with mallet strokes to cut the excessive bone; then the resected hump is simply removed (Figure 13).

9.2. Salient points

1. Integrity of the underlying mucous is crucial in internal nasal valve function so this technique is best preserved for minor resections and in case further resection is necessary component resection should be performed.

2. The resected hump is a potential graft material that may be used as a strut, tip graft or as an ideal material for dorsal augmentation.

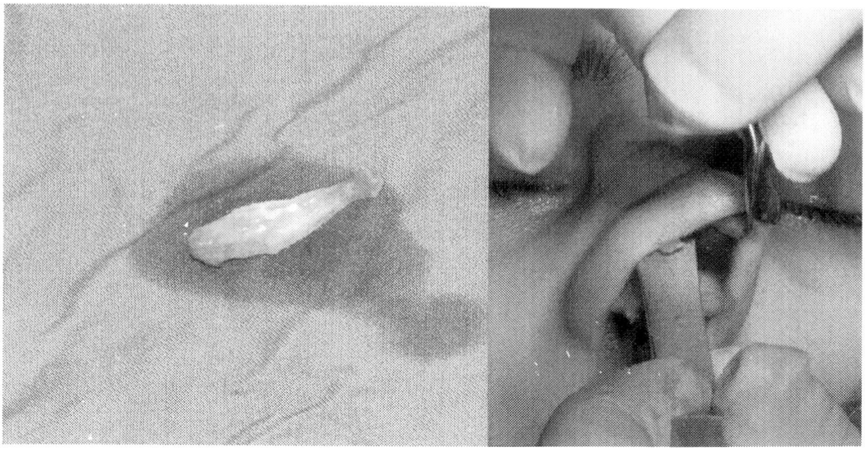

Figure 13. Composite hump surgery

9.3. Component hump resection

In this technique the upper lateral cartilages are precisely separated from the nasal septum and underlying mucosa, then excessive septal cartilage is trimmed until the ideal position is achieved. To adjust the bony part, a bone rasp or osteotome is used. In final steps excessive upper laterals may be trimmed very conservatively.

9.4. Important points

1-In major hump resections (more than 3mm), the dorsal hump may be reconstructed to avoid breathing problems and to provide a pleasant aesthetic brow line. A spreader graft is the gold standard with which to reconstruct the internal nasal valve; additionally, autospreader grafts and splay grafts are also effective methods in indicated cases [23-24].

10. Basic grafting techniques in dorsal surgery

10.1. Spreader grafts

Spreader grafts are two quadrangular pieces of cartilage (3mm in width and 20mm in length) that may be modified according to the patients' specific needs. These cartilages are placed on both sides of nasal septum and fixed with 5-0 PDS sutures. This grafting technique will change the geometry of internal nasal valve and prevent internal nasal valve incompetency (Figure 14). [25-27].

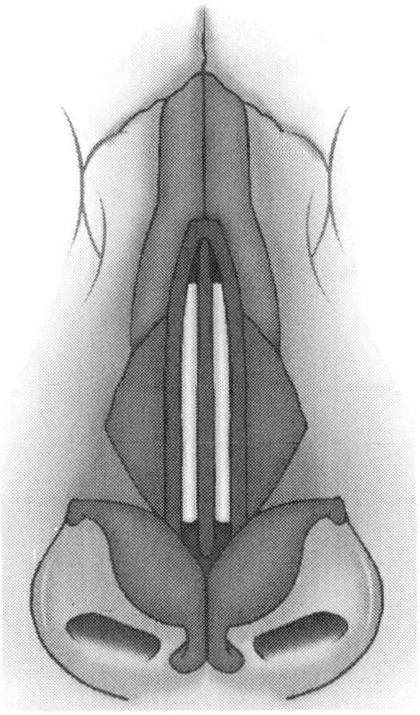

Figure 14. Spreader grafts.

10.2. Crushed cartilage

Crushed cartilage is an ideal augmentation material that may be precisely added to defective dorsal segments and cover irregularities.

10.3. Temporalis fascia

Temporalis fascia is a soft smooth graft material that is frequently reported to be used in augmentation rhinoplasty. This graft easily blends-in with normal nasal tissues and does not make shadows or visible borders. To harvest temporalis fascia a 5cm curvilinear incision is made on the posterior hairline. With upward and anterior subcutaneous dissection, ideal access to temporalis fascia is obtained then adequate fascia is harvested and placed in the recipient site in the nose. This approach provides ideal access to the area. A direct incision in hair-bearing areas of the temporalis area is also frequently used.

10.4. Lateral osteotomy

Lateral osteotomy is generally done to narrow a wide bony vault and/or to close an open roof deformity. This is beneficial to reshape a malformed bony vault (like traumatic noses).Lateral osteotomy may be done by two main options; external perforating osteotomy or internal continuous osteotomy. Both techniques have their own advantages and disadvantages; the literature has shown that both work well in the hands of skilled and trained surgeons.

10.5. External perforating osteotomy

The osteotomy line is planned and marked over the skin. A small stab incision is made on the nasal skin, midway of the bony vault; then a 2mm osteotome is inserted through the incision line. Using sweeping movements of the osteotome it finds its proper place at the beginning of marked osteotomy line under the periosteum of the bony vault. Then, with mallet strokes the osteotomy is started. After performing one osteotomy site, the osteotome is gently pulled out of the bone in a way that it stays inside the skin incision and is guided in the planned osteotomy line and the next osteotomy site is done adjacent to first one. In this way several osteotomy holes are made along the planned line. Then a gentle finger pressure is applied over the bony vault and the osteotomized bony segment is moved medially. Gauze soaked in cold serum is pressed over the osteotomy region and held for a few minutes to control bleeding and edema (Figure 15).

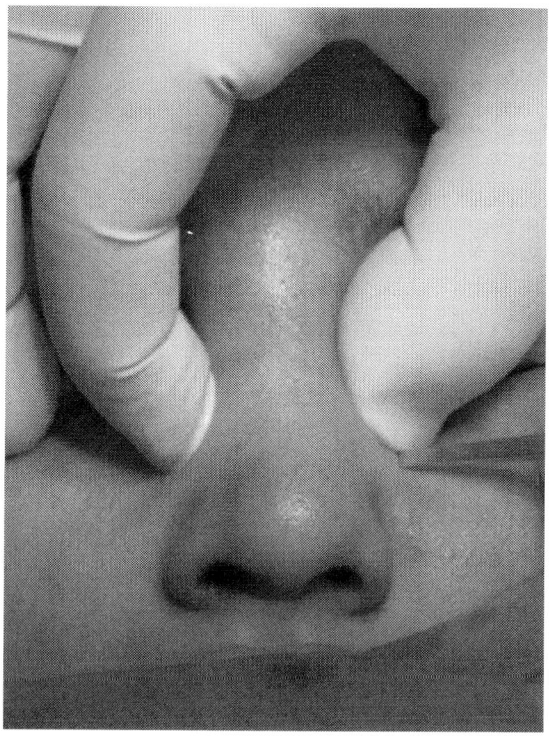

Figure 15. External perforating osteotomy

http://dx.doi.org/10.5772/59811

10.6. Internal continuous osteotomy

A 3 to 4mm guided osteotomy is usually used in this method of osteotomy. First a nasal speculum is used to find the best place in pyriform aperture. A small 5 mm incision is done. Then the osteotome is inserted inside the incision in a way that the guide stays laterally and blade medially toward the nostrils. With mallet strokes, the osteotomy is started and continues toward the medial canthus in the planned line. Then gentle finger pressure is applied to medialize the bony segment. The same procedure is done on the other side and gauze is pressed over the bony nasal vault and held for few minutes to control the bleeding and edema.

10.7. Salient points

1. Medial movements of the bony pyramid can be done by gentle finger pressure after lateral osteotomy. Failing to do so means that inadequate osteotomy is performed and osteotomy should be repeated properly. Aggressive use of force to in-fracture the bony segments by the surgeon or osteotome handle may dislodge the segments or lead to severe bony collapse.

2. It is generally suggested to limit the osteotomy line up to the medial canthus; further extension does not lead to acceptable results and will add the possibility of complications [28-32].

11. Nasal base surgery

The nasal base is a triangular view of the nose that is formed by two nostrils, nasal columella that separates these two nostrils and nasal lobule or the area above the nostrils. Nasal base surgery is usually based on thorough preoperative evaluations. It should be kept in mind that this stage of rhinoplasty is quite irreversible and any mistake in design or incision line will result in valve incompetency, nasal base deformity and visible scars (Figure 16).

11.1. Suturing and taping

After finishing the operation the skin flap is turned back to its proper place and all the details are checked several times. When the surgeon is sure that the desired result is achieved, suturing is done. As a rule, all the incisions must be closed by sutures to avoid unfavorable scars or dead spaces. It is suggested to irrigate the wound during suturing to avoid clot formation over incision lines. The incisions are immediately covered by antibiotic ointment. Taping helps to control dead spaces and edema; after suturing, a one centimeter tape is applied to re-drape the skin flap over newly formed cartilaginous and bony structure. This taping is applied immediately after suturing and is continued for one month or longer after operation.

11.2. Intranasal splint fixation

Internal splints usually have small tubes that help the patient breathe through the nose in the first post-operative days. It's believed that internal splints prevent intranasal edema and

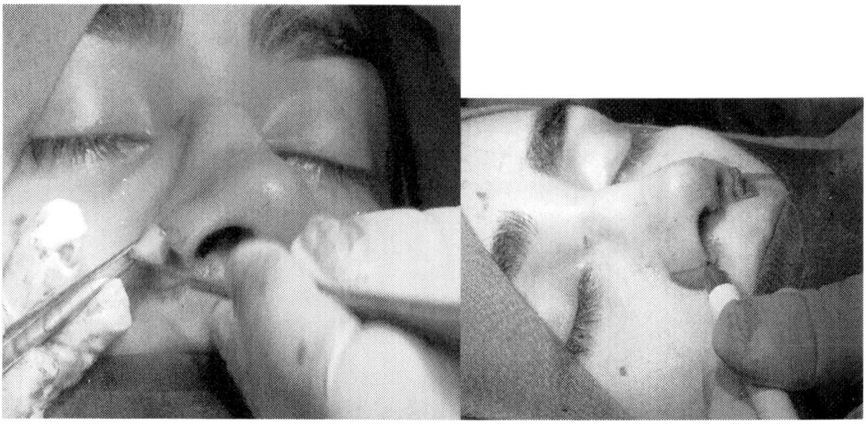

Figure 16. Nasal base surgery

synechia. Internal splints may be removed after 24 hours; however, it is possible to preserve it for one week or longer according to septal or turbinate manipulations done during surgery.

11.3. External splint application

External splints are usually thermoplastic stents softened in warm water and trimmed to provide suitable protection. The splint is gently placed over the taped nose. Irrigation with cold water will fix the splint in place. The splint is held for 5 days to one week. It is believed that external splints will hold the bony segments in their new position and will help the skin envelope re-drape over its new structure [33-35].

11.4. Post-operative care

Careful post-operative care will help the operated nose achieve its ideal shape in a predictable period of time. Sutures are usually removed in 5-7 post-operative days. Internal and external splints are usually removed on the same day though in some cases due to some specific indications such as extensive septoplasty splints may be preserved for a longer period of time. Clot and debris are gently cleaned in periodic postoperative visits. Frequent normal saline rinse by the patient and phenylephrine drops (only for three days after operation) may help the patient breathe better in the immediate post-op period. Taping is continued for one month. Patients are asked to avoid moderate sport activities for one month though vigorous activities such as contact sports or professional exercises are best postponed for three months.

11.5. Important points

1. Diluted corticosteroids (triamcinolone) may be beneficial to control the edema and granulation tissues post-operatively.

2. Selective taping is an effective method to shape subtle deformities. In this method prominent edematous points such as supratip area may be pressed under tight taping while other points that are susceptible to slight depression are left without taping or covered with light taping

3. Any major revision is best postponed for 6 months to one year after the first operation while smaller revisions such as alar base surgeries may be done sooner according to specific conditions of patient after the first operation.

Author details

Payam Varedi[1,2*] and Behnam Bohluli[2,3]

*Address all correspondence to: payam.varedi@yahoo.com

1 Department of Oral and Maxillofacial Surgery, Qazvin University of Medical Sciences, Qazvin, Iran

2 Department of Oral and Maxillofacial Surgery, Craniomaxillofacial Research Center, Shariati Hospital, Tehran University of Medical Sciences, Tehran, Iran

3 Department of Oral and Maxillofacial Surgery, Buali Hospital, Islamic Azad University of Medical Sciences, Tehran, Iran

References

[1] Swamy RS, Sykes JM, Most SP. Principles of photography in rhinoplasty for the digital photographer Clin Plast Surg. 2010 Apr;37(2):213-21.

[2] Ziglinas P, Menger DJ, Georgalas C. The body dysmorphic disorder patient: to perform rhinoplasty or not? Eur Arch Otorhinolaryngol. 2014 Sep;271(9):2355-8.

[3] Belli H, Belli S, Ural C. Psychopathological evaluation of patients requesting cosmetic rhinoplasty: a review. West Indian Med J. 2012 Mar;61(2):149-53.

[4] Chauhan N, Warner J, Adamson PA. Aesthetic outcomes Plast Surg. 2010 Aug;34(4): 510-6

[5] Tan S, Rotenberg B. Functional outcomes after lateral crural J-flap repair of external nasal valve collapse. Ann Otol Rhinol Laryngol. 2012 Jan;121(1):16-20.

[6] Saleh AM, Younes A, Friedman O. Cosmetics and function: quality-of-life changes after rhinoplasty surgery. Laryngoscope. 2012 Feb;122(2):254-9.

[7] Zoumalan RA, Larrabee WF Jr, Murakami CS. Intraoperative suction-assisted evaluation of the nasal valve in rhinoplasty. Arch Facial Plast Surg. 2012 Jan-Feb;14(1):34-8.

[8] Fung E, Hong P, Moore C, Taylor SM. The effectiveness of modified cottle maneuver in predicting outcomes in functional rhinoplasty.

[9] Duron JB, Nguyen PS, Jallut Y, Bardot J, Aiach G. Middle third of the nose and internal valve. Alar wall and external valve. Ann Chir Plast Esthet. 2014 Jul 30. pii: S0294-1260(14)00105-8.

[10] Riechelmann H, Karow E, DiDio D, Kral F. External nasal valve collapse - a case-control and interventional study employing a novel internal nasal dilator (Nasanita).Rhinology. 2010 Jun; 48(2):183-8.

[11] Bohluli B, Varedi P, Nazari S, Bagheri SC. Lateral crural suspension flap: a novel technique to modify and stabilize the nasolabial angle.J Oral Maxillofac Surg. 2013 Sep;71(9):1572-6.

[12] Xavier R.Nasal tip plasty: the delivery approach revisited. Aesthetic Plast Surg. 2013 Feb; 37(1):16-21.

[13] Gruber RP, Chang E, Buchanan E. Suture techniques in rhinoplasty. Clin Plast Surg. 2010 Apr; 37(2):231-43.

[14] Gruber RP, Weintraub J, Pomerantz J. Suture techniques for the nasal tip. Aesthet Surg J. 2008 Jan-Feb; 28(1):92-100.

[15] Lee KC, Kwon YS, Park JM, Kim SK, Park SH, Kim JH. Nasal tip plasty using various techniques in rhinoplasty. Aesthetic Plast Surg. 2004 Nov-Dec; 28(6):445-55.

[16] Atighechi S, Sajadinejad BS, Baradaranfar MH, Dadgarnia MH, Shahbazian H. Caudal extension graft versus columellar strut with plumping graft for acute nasolabial angle correction in rhinoplasty surgery.Eur Arch Otorhinolaryngol. 2014 Aug 18.

[17] McCollough EG, Mangat D. Systematic approach to correction of the nasal tip in rhinoplasty. Arch Otolaryngol 07:12, 1981.

[18] Daniel RK. Rhinoplasty: creating an aesthetic tip. Plast Reconstr Surg 80:775, 1987.

[19] Xavier R. Nasal tip plasty: the delivery approach revisited. Aesthetic Plast Surg. 2013 Feb;37(1):16-21.

[20] Lee KC, Kwon YS, Park JM, Kim SK, Park SH, Kim JH. Nasal tip plasty using various techniques in rhinoplasty. Aesthetic Plast Surg. 2004 Nov-Dec;28(6):445-55. Epub 2004 Dec 2.

[21] Hwang K, Hwang JH, Park JH, Kim DJ, Shin YH. J Experimental study of autologous cartilage, acellular cadaveric dermis, lyophilized bovine pericardium, and irradiated bovine tendon: applicability to nasal tip plasty. Craniofac Surg. 2007 May;18(3):551-8.

[22] Antohi N, Isac C, Stan V, Ionescu R.Dorsal nasal augmentation with "open sandwich" graft consisting of conchal cartilage and retroauricular fascia. AesthetSurg J. 2012 Sep;32(7):833-45.

[23] Temiz G, Yeşiloğlu N, Sarici M, Filinte GT. Congenital isolated aplasia of lower lateral cartilage and reconstruction using dorsal hump material. J Craniofac Surg. 2014 Sep;25(5):e411-3.

[24] Rohrich RJ, Muzaffar AR, Janis JE. Component dorsal hump reduction: the importance of maintaining dorsal aesthetic lines in rhinoplasty. PlastReconstr Surg. 2004 Oct;114(5):1298-308; discussion 1309-12.

[25] Varedi P, Bohluli B, Bayat M, Mohammadi F. Spreader graft placement: A simplified technique for young surgeons. Int J Oral Maxillofac Surg. 2014 Oct;43(10):1216-7.

[26] Kucuker I, Ozmen S. Extended spreader graft placement before lateral nasal osteotomy. Aesthetic Plast Surg. 2013 Aug;37(4):684-91.

[27] Grigoryants V, Baroni A.The use of short spreader grafts in rhinoplasty for patients with thick nasal skin. Aesthetic Plast Surg. 2013 Jun;37(3):516-20.

[28] Varedi P, Shirani G, Bohluli B, Besharati R, Keyhan SO. A simplified approach to the external lateral nasal osteotomy: a technical note. J Oral Maxillofac Surg. 2013 Aug; 71(8):1435-8.

[29] Rootman D, DeAngelis D, Tucker N, Wu A, Hurwitz J. Cadaveric anatomical comparison of the lateral nasal wall after external and endonasal dacryocystorhinostomy Ophthal Plast Reconstr Surg. 2012 Mar-Apr;28(2):149-53.

[30] Bohluli B, Moharamnejad N, Bayat M.Dorsal hump surgery and lateral osteotomy. Oral Maxillofac Surg Clin North Am. 2012 Feb;24(1):75-86.

[31] Levie P, Horoi M, Claes J, Monnoye JP, Verheyden PJ, Monnoye V, Lefebvre J, Millet B, Dartevelle D, Lemaire FX, Hatert AS, de Burbure C. External or internal lateral osteotomy: why I choose the external percutaneous approach. B-ENT. 2010;6Suppl 15:49-50.

[32] Helal MZ, El-Tarabishi M, MagdySabry S, Yassin A, Rabie A, Lin SJ. Effects of rhinoplasty on the internal nasal valve: a comparison between internal continuous and external perforating osteotomy. Ann Plast Surg. 2010 May;64(5):649-57.

[33] Yi CR, Kim YJ, Kim H, Nam SH, Choi YW. Comparison study of the use of absorbable and nonabsorbable materials as internal splints after closed reduction for nasal bone fracture. Arch Plast Surg. 2014 Jul;41(4):350-4.

[34] Cayonu M, Acar A, Horasanlı E, Altundag A, Salihoglu M. Comparison of totally occlusive nasal pack, internal nasal splint, and transseptal suture technique after septoplasty in terms of immediate respiratory distress related to anesthesia and surgical complications. Acta Otolaryngol. 2014 Apr;134(4):390-4.

[35] Drezner DA. Thermoplastic splint for use after nasal fracture. Otolaryngol Head Neck Surg. 1994 Jul;111(1):146-7

Chapter 32

Advanced Techniques in Rhinoplasty

Behnam Bohluli and Payam Varedi

Additional information is available at the end of the chapter

http://dx.doi.org/10.5772/59745

1. Introduction

Basic techniques of rhinoplasty are known to experienced aesthetic surgeons; however, post-traumatic nasal deformities, secondary cases and ethnic demands require advanced techniques. These modern techniques are generally aimed to provide a more normal looking nose while a great attempt is made to preserve or return the normal function of the nose while improving some existing functional shortcomings during the surgery. This chapter presents a problem-based approach to some complex nasal deformities. Current solutions to each deformity are presented and advantages and limitations of each technique are discussed.

2. Nasal tip deformities

2.1. Under-projected tip

Many techniques are known to increase tip projection all of which may be effectively used according to patient's special needs and indications:

1. **Tip sutures**: A tip spanning suture is a mattress suture that is used on each dome area to refine the angle between lateral crura and medial crura cartilages (Figure 1).This suture has been shown to increase tip projection.

2. **Cap graft**: Cap graft is a small piece of cartilage that is precisely formed and trimmed and fixed over the cartilaginous tip (Figure 2). The main indication of this graft is necessity to form and refine the tip; though this graft slightly increases tip projection in this technique.

3. **Shield graft** (Sheen graft): The shield graft is the only technique that may arbitrarily add to tip projection. A usual approach is to prepare and fix a bigger piece of cartilage. This

oversized graft is incrementally trimmed and tailored until the ideal tip projection and contour is achieved (Figure 3).[1,8]

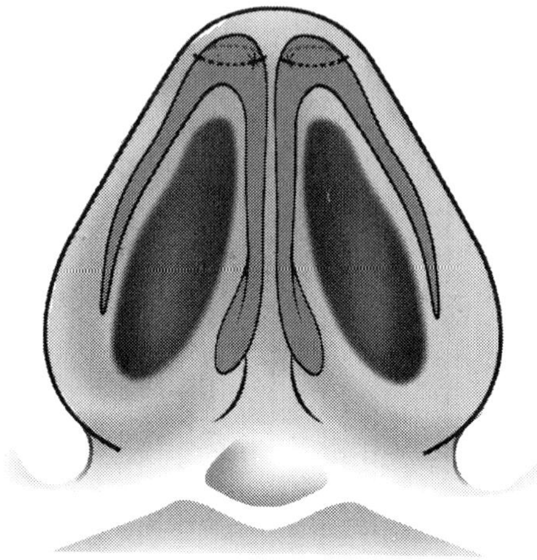

Figure 1. Tip spanning suture

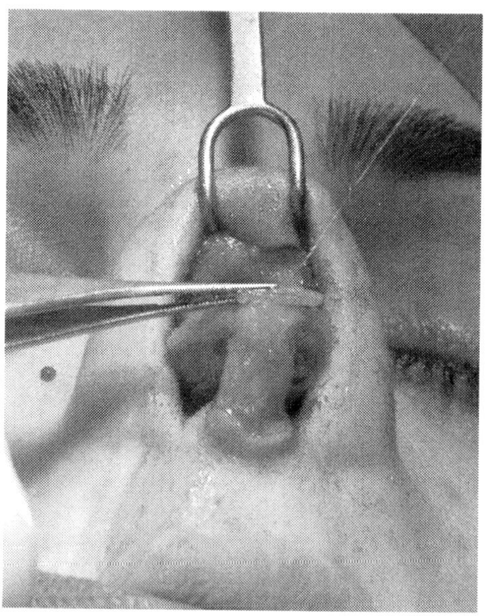

Figure 2. Cap graft

http://dx.doi.org/10.5772/59745

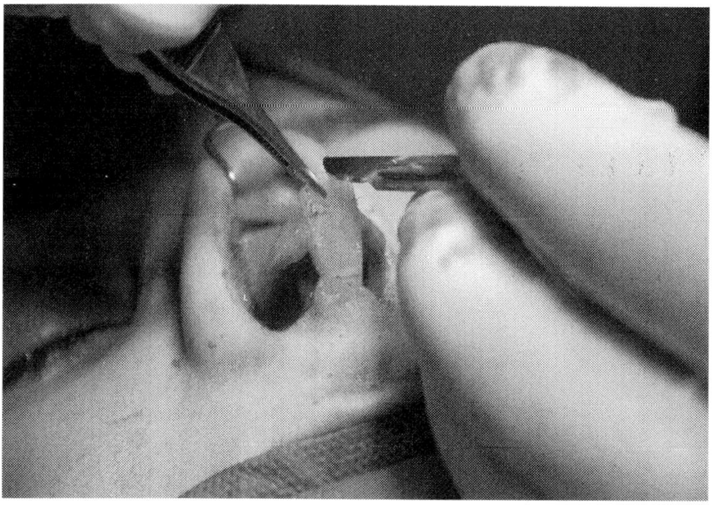

Figure 3. Shield graft (Sheen graft)

2.2. Over-projected tip

An over-projected nasal tip is a common finding that must be detected in preoperative assessments. Two general groups of techniques are applied to decrease the projection for all over-projected noses. In the first group it is tried to sever normal tip support mechanisms that will result in small decrease in tip projection. In the second group lower lateral cartilages are interrupted in some parts. A few millimeters of cartilage are resected and a new tripod with smaller limbs is formed.

1. Transfixion incision: All the resective techniques that are done on lower lateral cartilages may decrease the projection; although, the transfixion incision is the only one that is specifically done to decrease projection of the nose. This incision may decrease projection up to 3 mm (Figure 4).

2. Dome splitting: In this technique lower lateral cartilages are divided in dome area, then a few millimeter of excessive cartilage is resected and a new dome is formed by precise suturing. A small piece of crushed or morselized cartilage may be placed over dome area to cover the sutures and sharp edges of cartilages [9,13]

2.3. Drooping tip

There are many modalities to correct the drooping tip or acute nasolabial angle.

1. **A wedge is sometimes resected** from the caudal part of the septum to provide enough space for tip rotation (Figure 5).

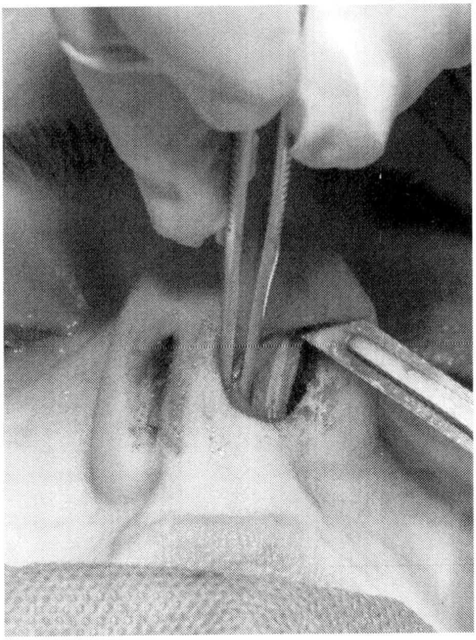

Figure 4. Transfixion incision

2. **Cephalic trimming of lower lateral cartilages and**

3. **Collumellar strut insertion**

These are other modalities that are basically done to increase nasolabial angle. In case basic techniques fail to provide the ideal result, the following techniques may be effectively applied [14,16]

4. **Tip rotating suture**

This is an effective method to increase and hold the nasolabial angle. In this technique a mattress suture is used to anchor lower lateral cartilages to the nasal septum, by incremental tightening of the suture, ideal nasolabial angle is achieved, then with several subsequent ties this nasolabial angle is fixed and stabilized.

2.4. Important points

Tip rotating suture easily changes the tip position, though it is clear that a single suture suspension may lose its effect gradually and will not lead to permanent results; to achieve stable results, tip support mechanisms should be improved (i.e. application of collumellar strut) and appropriate space be provided for new tip position (i.e. conservative cephalic trimming and caudal resection of septum) [17,18]

http://dx.doi.org/10.5772/59745

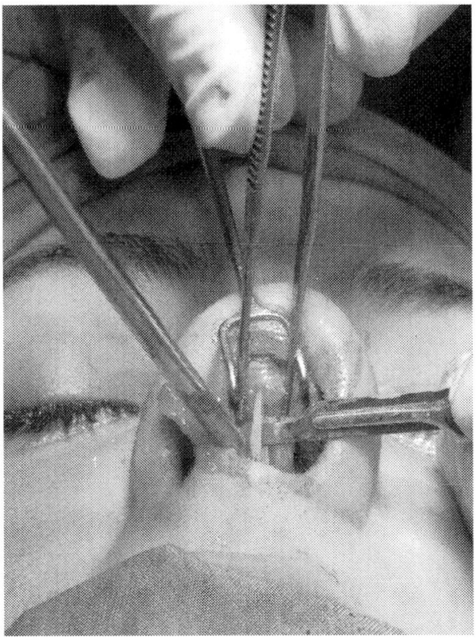

Figure 5. A wedge is resected from caudal part of the septum to provide enough space for tip rotation.

3. Tongue in groove

In this technique two medial crura cartilages are completely separated from each other. Then upper lateral cartilages are stripped off the nasal septum. Medial crural cartilages are pushed back in a way that each medial cru covers the nasal septum on one side. A delicate needle is used to temporarily fix the medial crura cartilages to the septum. Skin flap is turned back to its original position for several times. When the ideal nasolabial angle is achieved, medial crura are fixed to the septum with several PDS sutures. In this method the lower lateral cartilages (nasal tip) are permanently fixed to the nasal septum. [19]

4. Lateral crural anchorage flap

In this technique, excessive parts of the lateral crural cartilages that are routinely excised and resected in tip plasty are marked on both sides. Cartilage incisions are made and excessive cartilage is separated from its underlying skin in a way that its medial attachments remain intact. Excessive cartilages are easily omitted while two cartilage flaps with a strong attachment to medial crural cartilage are available. These two flaps are used to rotate the nasal tip. Cartilage flaps are fixed with a needle to the nasal septum. The maneuver may be done for several times to find the ideal tip position. Then the flaps are precisely fixed with sutures to the nasal septum. [17]

4.1. Important points

This technique is based on two cartilage flaps that are in fact excessive parts of the lower lateral cartilages. These cartilages are supposed to be trimmed and resected in normal rhinoplasty. It is clear that in weak cartilage, or in case a small strip of cartilage is to be trimmed this approach will not be possible.

4.2. Weak lower lateral cartilages and pinch deformity

Strength and consistency of lower lateral cartilages play an important role in shape and function of the lower one third of the nose. Many techniques have been proposed to reinforce and reshape the lower lateral cartilages; all may be used in specific indications:

1. **Batten grafts**: a batten graft is a thin oval piece of cartilage that is used over deficient or weak cartilaginous part of the nose to reshape and reinforce the nose. This graft is frequently fabricated from septal cartilage or chonchal cartilage. It may be used on one side or bilaterally according to specific needs and indications. [20,22]

2. **Lateral crural strut graft**: Unlike batten grafts the lateral crural strut graft is placed beneath the lower lateral cartilages, so after adequate injection of local anesthetic under the lower lateral cartilages, the lateral crura is precisely stripped off from its underlying skin and a quadrangular piece of cartilage is fixed under the lateral crura.

This technique:

a. Restores pinch deformities

b. Reinforces external nasal valve

c. Corrects moderate to severe cephalic positioning of lower lateral cartilages [23,24]

d. **Alar contouring grafts**: Alar contour or alar rim grafts are quite simple and effective techniques frequently used for several aesthetic and functional indications. These grafts are narrow strips of cartilage placed in a pocket anterior to the lower lateral cartilages. This graft is made from septal or chonchal cartilage.

Indications:

a. To reinforce external nasal valve

b. To correct minor cephalic positioning of lower lateral cartilages

c. To provide a pleasant nostril borders [25]

d. **Lateral crural transposition flap**: In this technique excessive parts of lower lateral cartilages that are usually trimmed and discarded in rhinoplasty, are folded inside, in this way, wide lateral crural cartilages are reshaped while excessive cartilage is used to reinforce the lateral crural cartilage. [26]

5. Dorsal problems

5.1. Shallow radix

In some patients pre-operative evaluations show that radix augmentation will help gain a pleasant aesthetic appearance. A complete familiarity with common autografts, their potentials and limitations will help the surgeon to select a predictable and stable graft with acceptable results in each specific indication. [27,28]

5.2. Low dorsum

Augmentation of a low dorsum is an important task in current concepts of rhinoplasty. Many modalities and techniques are proposed, though all of them have their own advantages and disadvantages and no one technique seems to cover all the indications for dorsal augmentation. Proper case selection and familiarity with characteristics of each technique are prerequisites for a successful dorsal augmentation.

5.3. 1-rib graft

Rib grafts are extensively used in reconstructive nasal surgery. Considerable amounts of cartilage and bone, acceptable mechanical properties such as strength and load bearing as well as its resistance to resorption has made it the gold standard for massive cartilaginous augmentations and reconstructions. Availability of other autografts, potential drawbacks of rib cartilage and patient compliance has limited its use to severe deformities and the need for excessive amount of graft material.

5.4. Important points

Graft distortion (warping) is a common complication in rib cartilage grafting. Many modalities have been proposed to control this unwanted effect. Some authors drill the core of the graft with a long delicate orthopedic bur and insert a strong Krishner wire to control any possible distortion. Sometimes it is thought that core of the graft has the least potential for warping so it is suggested to trim the periphery of the graft and to use the core of rib cartilage as the graft material.[29,31]

6. Temporalis fascia

Temporalis fascia is a well-established augmentation material in rhinoplasty. To harvest temporalis fascia, after proper application of local anesthesia, a 5 cm incision is done in posterior neck hair line with anterior and upward dissections adequate access is gained to the superficial layer of the deep temporalis fascia. Adequate amount of fascial tissue is harvested and the donor site is precisely sutured after complete control of bleeding. Temporalis fascia provides a soft and smooth layer that may cover dorsal irregularities. It may be used for minimal dorsal augmentations and for greater amounts of augmentation it should be combined with other grafting techniques otherwise alternatives may be selected. [32,33]

6.1. Postauricular fascia

Postauricular and mastoid fascia provide a thick fascial tissue that is easily harvested with a 4cm curvilinear incision exactly behind the ears; incision lines are completely concealed behind the ears in normal skin creases and the risk of complications comparing to donor sites in the temporalis fascia is quiet low. This fascial tissue may be used in moderate dorsal augmentations (Figure 6). [34]

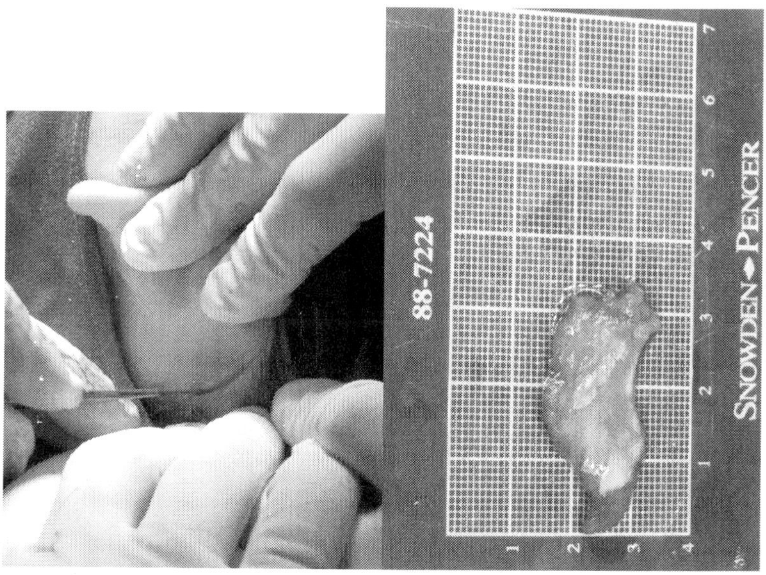

Figure 6. Post-auricular fascia harvesting

6.2. Turkish delight

Turkish delight is an efficient technique that was originally designed by Erol in 2000. This technique was aimed to solve essential problems that were frequently encountered in the use of cartilage blocks from the nasal septum or ribs. In Erol's original report rib cartilage was delicately diced into small particles, then soaked in blood and wrapped in Surgicel. Daniel wrapped the diced cartilages in temporalis fascia to omit the unpredictable behavior of Surgicel (oxidized cellulose) coverage. Diced cartilage wrapped in fascia is now commonly utilized in augmentation rhinoplasty and is reported to have acceptable results (Figure 7). [35,36]

http://dx.doi.org/10.5772/59745

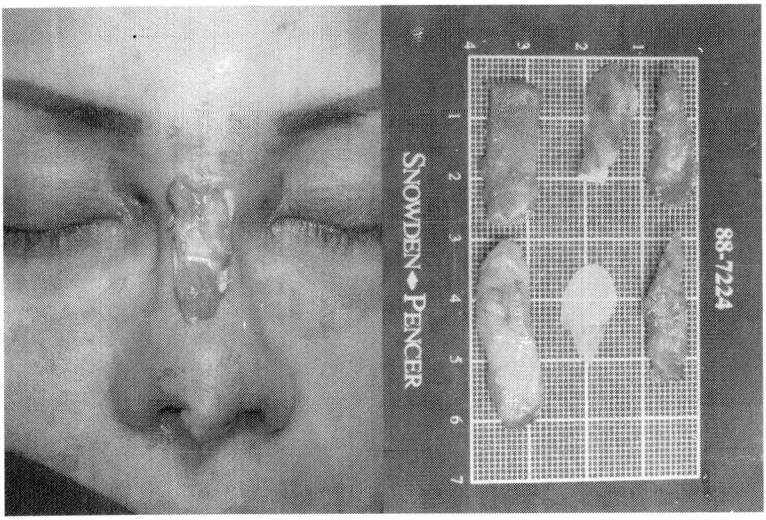

Figure 7. Turkish delight

6.3. Fascia-cartilage sandwich technique

Fascia-cartilage sandwich is reasonable alternative to rib grafts. In this technique temporalis or mastoid tissue is harvested, cartilage block from nasal septum or chonchal tissue is trimmed and formed in its ideal contour, and then it is covered with fascia. In fact cartilage provides the bulk of augmentation material and fascia covers the possible irregularities and shadows of a cartilage block graft [37]

6.4. Internal nasal valve incompetency

Sometimes pre-operative evaluations show that one or both internal nasal valves are incompetent and do not work well. On the other hand in major hump resections (more than 3mm); nasal valve reconstruction will be necessary. For this reason, internal nasal valve reinforcement is commonly indicated and may be indicated in most cases. The followings are some of effective valve reinforcement techniques:

1. **Spreader graft**: Spreader grafts were first introduced in 1981 by Jack Sheen and are now considered the gold standard in internal nasal valve reinforcements. A spreader graft is a piece of quadrangular cartilage that is placed between upper lateral cartilage and septum. Spreader grafts are usually used on both sides though due to some specific needs such as asymmetries unilateral spreaders may be utilized. [39]

2. **Autospreader**: In this technique, after incremental trimming of the nasal septum, the upper lateral cartilages are folded inside. It is thought that this technique prevents unnecessary graft harvesting and will provide the same effects as spreader grafts though

the main advantage of this technique is its reversibility and when an ideal result is not obtained intra-operatively, the sutures can be removed. Upper lateral cartilages are conservatively trimmed and other standard valve reconstruction techniques such as spreader grafts may be applied (Figure 8).[40-42]

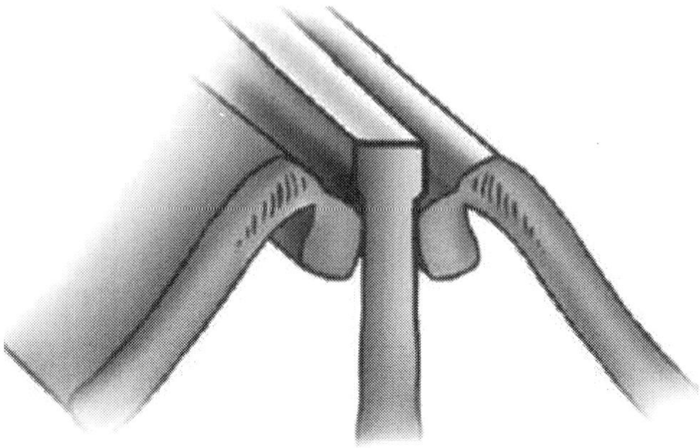

Figure 8. Autospreader

3. **Docile splay graft**: The docile splay graft is a piece of septal cartilage that is gently crushed and is placed over the nasal septum in a way that it covers the nasal septum and the two upper lateral cartilages are located laterally to the graft. It is believed that this simple graft will prevent upper lateral cartilages from functional movements and collapse [43]

6.5. Important points

1. Spreader grafts may be indicated to straighten a curved nasal dorsum that is not corrected in normal septoplasty techniques [39]

2. Internal nasal valve reconstruction prevents and corrects inverted V deformities and plays a substantial role in providing aesthetic brow lines.

7. Septal deformities

In most cases basic techniques will result in a straight functional nasal airway though in complicated cases more aggressive approaches may be necessary.

7.1. Complicated septal deformities

Sometimes the nasal septum is deviated in several different planes, and insisting on basic septoplasty techniques does not solve the problem and may lead to septal perforation and many other complications. Extracorporeal septoplasty is a known modality that may be applied by experienced surgeons. In this technique, after an open approach skeletonization, the upper lateral cartilages are completely stripped off from nasal septum and then septal cartilage is precisely detached from all its anatomic connections and is taken out completely. The deformed nasal septum, which is now on the surgical table, is completely re-evaluated. Broken and deformed parts are excised and omitted in a way that a heavy strong L strut remains or is reconstructed. This newly formed septum is placed back inside the nose and tightly fixed to the bony vault and upper lateral cartilages [44-47]

7.2. Inadequate osteotomy

Sometimes intraoperative evaluations show that in spite of clear lateral osteotomy lines, medialization of bony segments is not achieved; in these cases medial osteotomy (in internal continuous osteotomy) and lateral oblique osteotomy (in external perforating osteotomy) may be indicated.

7.3. Medial osteotomy

In most rhinoplasty cases, lateral osteotomy will fulfill all the aims of osteotomy and there are limited indications for medial osteotomy; in indicated cases medial osteotomy may resolve some potential complications and will complete the bony vault surgery such as:

1. **Exteremely wide noses**: Sometimes in wide noses lateral osteotomy will not appropriately metalize the bony segments and medial osteotomy will result in passive movements of bony segments.

2. **When hump reduction is not performed** or has not resulted in an open roof of the bony vault; medial osteotomy will allow the osteotomy to be completed; otherwise excessive pressure if applied may lead to uncontrolled fractures.

3. **Deviated bony pyramid**: In this case complete reformation of the bony pyramid is necessary thus, total release of bony segments and repositioning may be necessary. [48-50]

7.4. Rocker deformity

Rocker deformity is a relatively common sequel of lateral osteotomy. In this complication a large bony spicule is seen and palpated after lateral osteotomy over nasal radix. Like many other complications the best is to avoid this deformity by limiting osteotomy line maximum up to lateral canthus and not to extend it in thicker bony compartments. In case rocker deformity is seen, sharp bony spicules may be gently trimmed and sometime crushed cartilages or fascia can be used to camouflage the deformity. [51]

7.5. Crooked bony vault

In some post-traumatic nasal deformities a conventional lateral osteotomy does not result in an ideal symmetric bony vault; a double layer osteotomy may solve the problem in most cases. In this technique a deep low or low lateral osteotomy is performed in the traditional way; the second line of osteotomy is started in a higher plane and then with light finger pressure the bony vault is molded. In case adequate results are not achieved a third line may be designed on one side or both sides of the nose. [52]

7.6. Important points

1. Internal continuous osteotomy may dislodge the fractured bony segments in two layer osteotomies, thus external perforating osteotomy is usually preferred in these deformities. As a predictable alternative, first deep osteotomy may be done by the internal method and the second line which is used to mold the segment may be added via the external approach.

2. Crushed cartilage may help the surgeon camouflage residual irregularities and asymmetries. In this technique a small part of crushed cartilage is gently placed on deficient parts, and then is molded until the ideal symmetric result is achieved.

Author details

Behnam Bohluli[1] and Payam Varedi[2*]

*Address all correspondence to: payam.varedi@yahoo.com

1 Department of Oral and Maxillofacial Surgery, Buali Hospital, Islamic Azad University of Medical Sciences, Tehran, Iran, and Craniomaxillofacial Research Center, Shariati Hospital, Tehran University of Medical Sciences, Tehran, Iran

2 Department of Oral and Maxillofacial Surgery, Qazvin University of Medical Sciences, Qazvin, Iran, and Researcher, Department of Oral and Maxillofacial Surgery, Craniomaxillofacial Research Center, Shariati Hospital, Tehran University of Medical Sciences, Tehran, Iran

References

[1] Tebbetts JB. Shaping and positioning the nasal tip without structural disruption: a new systematic approach. PlastReconstrSurg 94:61, 1994.

[2] McColloughEG,Mangat D. Systematic approach to correction of the nasal tip in rhinoplasty. Arch Otolaryngoll 07:12, 1981.

[3] Rich IS, Friedman WH, Pearlman SJ.The effects of lower lateral cartilage excision on nasal tip projection. Arch Otolaryngol Head Neck Surg 117:56, 1991.

[4] Gunter JP.The merits of the open approach in rhinoplasty. PlastReconstrSurg 99:863, 1997.

[5] TebbettsJB.The next dimension: rethinking the logic, sequence, and techniques of rhinoplasty. In Gunter JP, Rohrich RJ, Adams WP, eds. Dallas Rhinoplasty: Nasal Surgery by the Masters. St Louis: Quality Medical Publishing, 2002, p 219.

[6] TardyME Jr, Cheng E.Transdomal suture refinement of the nasal tip. Facial PlastSurg 4:317,1987.

[7] Daniel RK. Rhinoplasty: creating an aesthetic tip. PlastReconstrSurg 80:775, 1987.

[8] Daniel RK.Rhinoplasty: a simplified, three-stitch, open tip suture technique. Part I: primary rhinoplasty. PlastReconstrSurg 103:1491, 1999.

[9] Petroff MA, McCollough EG, Horn D, et al. Nasal tip projection: quantitative changes following rhinoplasty. Arch Otolaryngol Head Neck Surg 117:783, 1991.

[10] JanekelB,Wright WK. Studies on the support of the nasal tip. Arch Otolaryngol 94:458, 1971.

[11] Johnson CM Jr,Godin MS. The tension nose: open structure rhinoplasty approach. PlastReconstrSurg 95:43, 1995.

[12] Tardy ME Jr,Walter MA, PattBS.Theoverprojecting nose: anatomic component analysis and repair. Facial PlastSurg 9:306, 1993.

[13] Wise JB, Becker SS, Sparano A, et al. Intermediate crural overlay in rhinoplasty: a deprojection technique that shortens the medial leg of the tripod without lengthening the nose. Arch Facial PlastSurg 8:240, 2006.

[14] Sajjadian A, Guyuron B. An algorithm for treatment of the drooping nose. AesthetSurg J. 2009 May-Jun;29(3):199-206.

[15] Konior RJ. The droopy nasal tip. Facial PlastSurgClin North Am. 2006 Nov;14(4): 291-9, v. Review.

[16] Pedroza F. A 20-year review of the "new domes" technique for refining the drooping nasal tip. Arch Facial Plast Surg. 2002 Jul-Sep;4(3):157-63. Review.

[17] Bohluli B, Varedi P, Nazari S, Bagheri SC. Lateral crural suspension flap: a novel technique to modify and stabilize the nasolabial angle. J Oral Maxillofac Surg. 2013 Sep;71(9):1572-6.

[18] Tasman AJ, Lohuis PJ. Control of tip rotation. Facial Plast Surg. 2012 Apr;28(2): 243-50.

[19] Ponsky DC, Harvey DJ, Khan SW, Guyuron B.Nose elongation: a review and description of the septal extension tongue-and-groove technique.

[20] Chua DY, Park SS. Alar batten grafts. JAMA Facial Plast Surg. 2014 Sep 1;16(5):377-8.

[21] Bewick JC, Buchanan MA, Frosh AC. Internal nasal valve incompetence is effectively treated using batten graft functional rhinoplasty. Int J Otolaryngol. 2013;2013:734795.

[22] Sufyan AS, Hrisomalos E, Kokoska MS, Shipchandler TZ. The effects of alar batten grafts on nasal airway obstruction and nasal steroid use in patients with nasal valve collapse and nasal allergic symptoms: a prospective study. JAMA Facial Plast Surg. 2013 May;15(3):182-6.

[23] Kuran I, Oreroğlu AR. The sandwiched lateral crural reinforcement graft: a novel technique for lateral crus reinforcement in rhinoplasty.AesthetSurg J. 2014 Mar;34(3): 383-93.

[24] Gunter JP, Friedman RM. Lateral crural strut graft: technique and clinical applications in rhinoplasty. PlastReconstr Surg. 1997 Apr;99(4):943-52; discussion 953-5.

[25] Toriumi DM, Checcone MA. New concepts in nasal tip contouring. Facial PlastSurg-Clin North Am. 2009 Feb;17(1):55-90, vi. doi: 10.1016/j.fsc.2008.10.001. Review.

[26] Ashtiani AK, Bohluli B, Bateni H, Fatemi MJ, Sadr-Eshkevari P, Rashad A. Lateral crural transposition flap in tip correction: Tehran retrospective rhinoplasty experience.Ann Plast Surg. 2013 Jul;71(1):50-3. doi: 10.1097/SAP.0b013e318248b7f1. Erratum in: Ann Plast Surg. 2013 Aug;71(2):246

[27] Cohen JC, Pearlman SJ. Radix grafts in cosmetic rhinoplasty: lessons from an 8-year review. Arch Facial Plast Surg. 2012 Nov;14(6):456-61

[28] Besharatizadeh R, Ozkan BT, Tabrizi R. Complete or a partial sheet of deep temporal fascial graft as a radix graft for radix augmentation. Eur Arch Otorhinolaryngol. 2011 Oct;268(10):1449-53

[29] Baser B, Kothari S, Thakur M.Diced cartilage: an effective graft for post-traumatic and revision rhinoplasty. Indian J Otolaryngol Head Neck Surg. 2013 Aug;65(Suppl 2):356-9. doi: 10.1007/s12070-012-0525-6. Epub 2012 Feb 25.

[30] Moretti A, Sciuto S Rib grafts in septorhinoplasty.. ActaOtorhinolaryngol Ital. 2013 Jun;33(3):190-5.

[31] Christophel JJ, Hilger PA. Osseocartilaginous rib graft rhinoplasty: a stable, predictable technique for major dorsal reconstruction. Arch Facial Plast Surg. 2011 Mar-Apr; 13(2):78-83.

[32] Bussi M, Palonta F, Toma S. Grafting in revision rhinoplasty, ActaOtorhinolaryngol Ital. 2013 Jun; 33(3):183-9.

[33] Baker TM, Courtiss EH. Temporalis fascia grafts in open secondary rhinoplasty. PlastReconstr Surg. 1994 Apr;93(4):802-10.

[34] Cho JM, Jeong JH, Woo KV, Lee YH. Versatility of retroauricular mastoid donor site: a convenient valuable warehouse of various free graft tissues in cosmetic and reconstructive surgery. J Craniofac Surg. 2013; 24(5):e486-90.

[35] Nazari S, Bohluli B, Besharatizadeh R, Sadr-Eshkevari P, Rashad A. Neck hairline incision for simultaneous harvesting of temporal and mastoid fasciae: a technical note..J Oral Maxillofac Surg. 2013 Sep;71(9):1598-600.

[36] Erol OO. The Turkish delight: a pliable graft for rhinoplasty. PlastReconstr Surg. 2000 May;105(6):2229-41; discussion 2242-3.

[37] Gerbault O, Aiach G. Diced cartilage wrapped in deep temporal aponeurosis (DC-F): A new technique in augmentation rhinoplasty. Ann ChirPlastEsthet. 2009 Oct; 54(5): 477-85.

[38] Antohi N, Isac C, Stan V, Ionescu R.Dorsal nasal augmentation with "open sandwich" graft consisting of conchal cartilage and retroauricular fascia. AesthetSurg J. 2012 Sep;32(7):833-45.

[39] Varedi P, Bohluli B, Bayat M, Mohammadi F. Spreader graft placement: A simplified technique for young surgeons. Int J Oral Maxillofac Surg. 2014 Oct;43(10):1216-7.

[40] Hussein WK, Elwany S, Montaser M. Modified autospreader flap for nasal valve support: utilizing the spring effect of the upper lateral cartilage. Eur Arch Otorhinolaryngol. 2014 Sep 30

[41] Pepper JP, Baker SR. The autospreader flap in reduction rhinoplasty.Arch Facial Plast Surg. 2011 May-Jun;13(3):172.

[42] Moharamnejad N, Bohluli B. Docile splay graft for middle vault reconstruction. Br J Oral Maxillofac Surg. 2013 Dec;51(8):e307-9.

[43] Aaronson NL, Vining EM. Correction of the deviated septum: from ancient Egypt to the endoscopic era. Int Forum Allergy Rhinol. 2014 Aug 18

[44] Bohluli B, Motamedi MH, Varedi P, Malekzadeh M, Ghassemi A, Bagheri SC. Management of perforations of the nasal septum: can extracorporeal septoplasty be an effective option?J Oral Maxillofac Surg. 2014 Feb;72(2):391-5.

[45] Nazari S, Bohluli B, Varedi P, Besharatizade R. Carpentering in septorhinoplasty: a novel technique to straighten the deviated nasal septum.J Oral Maxillofac Surg. 2014 Jan;72(1):157-63.

[46] Karameşe M, Akdağ O, Akatekin A, Koplay TG, Koplay M, Tosun Z. Extracorporeal Septoplasty Combined With Valve Surgery in Rhinoplasty Patients.Ann Plast Surg. 2014 Oct 2.

[47] Ghassemi A, Ayoub A, Modabber A, Bohluli B, Prescher A. Lateral nasal osteotomy: a comparative study between the use of osteotome and a diamond surgical burr - a cadaver study. Head Face Med. 2013 Dec 19;9:41.

[48] Varedi P, Shirani G, Bohluli B, Besharati R, Keyhan SO. A simplified approach to the external lateral nasal osteotomy: a technical note.J Oral Maxillofac Surg. 2013 Aug; 71(8):1435-8.

[49] Bohluli B, Moharamnejad N, Bayat M. Dorsal hump surgery and lateral osteotomy.Oral MaxillofacSurgClin North Am. 2012 Feb;24(1):75-86.

[50] Harshbarger RJ, Sullivan PK. The optimal medial osteotomy: a study of nasal bone thickness and fracture patterns. PlastReconstr Surg. 2001 Dec;108(7):2114-9; discussion 2120-1.

[51] Cerkes N. The crooked nose: principles of treatment. AesthetSurg J. 2011Feb;31(2): 241-57.

[52] Levie P, Horoi M, Claes J, Monnoye JP, Verheyden PJ, Monnoye V, Lefebvre J, Millet B, Dartevelle D, Lemaire FX, Hatert AS, de Burbure C. External or internal lateral osteotomy: why I choose the external percutaneous approach.B-ENT. 2010;6Suppl 15:49-50.

[53] Helal MZ, El-Tarabishi M, MagdySabry S, Yassin A, Rabie A, Lin SJ. Effects of rhinoplasty on the internal nasal valve: a comparison between internal continuous and external perforating osteotomy. Ann Plast Surg. 2010 May;64(5):649-57.

[54] Sinha V, Gupta D, More Y, Prajapati B, Kedia BK, Singh SN. External vs. internal osteotomy in rhinoplasty. Indian J Otolaryngol Head Neck Surg. 2007 Mar;59(1):9-12.

[55] Rohrich RJ, Janis JE, Adams WP, Krueger JK.An update on the lateral nasal osteotomy in rhinoplasty: an anatomic endoscopic comparison of the external versus the internal approach. Plast Reconstr Surg. 2003 Jun; 111(7):2461-2; discussion 2463.

Chapter 33

Rhinoplasty in Adult Patients with Cleft — Lip Nasal Deformities

Fereydoun Pourdanesh and Behnam Bohluli

Additional information is available at the end of the chapter

http://dx.doi.org/10.5772/59237

1. Introduction

Among facial esthetic surgeons, secondary rhinoplasty in adult cleft –nose deformities is considered to be one of the most challenging surgical interventions due to the congenital distortion of the cartilaginous and bony nasal pyramid, which compromises both nasal esthetics and function. It is generally accepted that the cleft-lip nasal deformity (CLND) is challenging; It is attempted to do this either at the time of primary rhinoplasty in the early of age with repair of lip or by secondary rhinoplasty later on in life. CLND may vary from minor to severe deformity. Several techniques have been suggested and plenty of articles have discussed this issue but still there is no consensus on an optimal technique to manage all of the problems. The common techniques that we use in routine rhinoplasty may not yield good results in patients with CLND, and the reasons for that are:

1. The complexity of anatomical pathology which involves all layers, including skin, cartilage, vestibular lining and skeletal base platform.
2. Numerous former surgical interventions leading to significant scar tissue in the operating site
3. The inevitable effect of growth over time.

The clinical presentation of cleft nose deformities varies widely, requiring a full knowledge of surgical techniques; if deformity is severely asymmetric surgical correction is much more difficult. The clinical features of deformity in a unilateral cleft nose differ from that usually seen in bilateral CLND. The scenario of rhinoplasty in surgical techniques in bilateral CLND is entirely different from unilateral CLND. It seems complete correction of all deficiencies of some noses remain an intangible goal for many, and this is the reason why revision rhinoplasty is commonly needed in these patients. Furthermore, it should be noted that each patient with

CLND presents a unique challenge due to complexity and combination of aspects and certain techniques that may be more suitable than others in individual cases [1, 2].

2. Primary or secondary rhinoplasty

Primary rhinoplasty means performing rhinoplasty simultaneously with repair of cleft lip and secondary rhinoplasty means performing rhinoplasty at an early age i.e. during school going age(5-6 years), early adolescence (10-12 years) or later on in life (above 16 yrs. in women and age 18 yrs. in men). But as a working diagnosis, primary rhinoplasty in adults with CLND means the first attempt of surgical intervention on the nose and secondary rhinoplasty means revision rhinoplasty or second operation on the nose.

The best time to attempt correction of CLND is still controversial. With improvement in cleft lip surgery, there is an increasing interest for correction of the nose at the time of lip repair. Some authors strongly recommend a primary rhinoplasty and believe if the procedure is performed correctly it does not adversely affect the growth of the paranasal region. Primary rhinoplasty improves nasal symmetry in patients with unilateral cleft lip deformity. This does not exclude the possibility of later revisional surgery although there is tendency to doing an appropriate primary repair of cleft lip deformity but the fact is, small defects that are left after primary repair are amplified with the growth process and affect adjacent structures. It is become clear that primary and secondary rhinoplasty at the same time of lip repair or at age 7-8 can lead to some kind of deformities in adulthood. The adult deformity is related not only to the original embryological mesodermal deficiency and diminished growth potential, but also to the pattern of primary surgery, the degree of interceptive surgery during growth and the level of orthodontic skill practiced within a particular treatment. In our center most cases are referred for primary rhinoplasty in adulthood [3-9].

3. Clinical signs and symptoms

A variety of clinical signs may be seen in an operated cleft lip and palate patient as well as in unoperated cases. We are usually faced with a wide variety of signs and symptoms in a repaired cleft lip case with or without primary rhinoplasty. In this section the clinical signs of cleft nose deformity will be discussed.

3.1. Unilateral cleft lip nose deformity

Clinical features of cleft nose deformity from a cosmetic point of view have varied from minor to severe (Figure 1).

It is not easy to accurately describe the anatomic pathology of secondary CLND. Components of the nasal deformity include defects of all layers of skin, cartilages, septum, entire nasal pyramid as well as hypoplasia and mal positioning of the maxillary segments and the anatomic

http://dx.doi.org/10.5772/59237

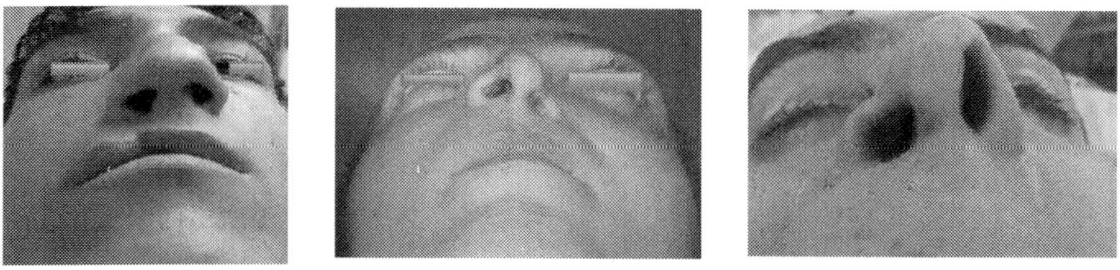

Figure 1. Basal view of minor and two difficult cases of unilateral cleft nose.

and functional deformity of the orbicularis muscle. It is accepted that patients who undergo appropriate primary repair for cleft lip will have secondary deformities [8]. Recently many three dimensional studies have been performed on cleft lip nose deformity patients; thanks to advances in technology we can define the details of the anatomic and functional deformity of each component [10]. The cleft deformity is not restricted to the skin and cartilage. Hogan represented the unilateral cleft nasal deformity as a tilted tripod (Figure 2).

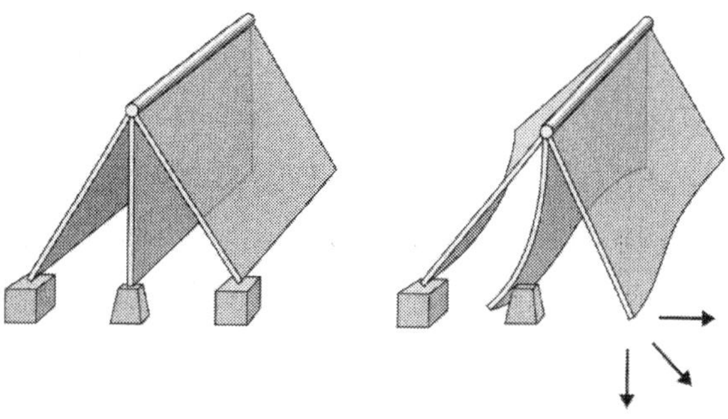

Figure 2. Tilted nasal tripod in CLND

Because of the lack of skeletal support, the alar base on the cleft side can, in some cases, become retro positioned with growth, even following an appropriate primary correction [9]. In most cases however good the primary correction, the patient is left with asymmetry of the nasal base and nares [11].

The ala on the cleft side is lengthened vertically and lies below the alae on the non- cleft side. The lower lateral cartilage is depressed and spread across the cleft. The nasal tip is deviated toward the left side. The columella on the left side is shortened significantly, as compared with the non-cleft side. The columella is obliquely oriented. With its base deviated to and located in the non-cleft side away from the midline. Bilateral alar bases are asymmetric, with the cleft side alar base inferiorly and posteriorly displaced. [12]

The deformities such as a deficient tubercle, vermilion deficiency, irregularities, the short upper lip, long upper lip, tight upper lip, and unfavorable scars may be common seen in the repaired lip [9]. Also the severity of septal deformity is variable. Typically, the septum is dislocated from the maxillary crest towards the non-cleft side resulting in a septal deflection towards the cleft side commonly causing nasal obstruction on that side. In addition, the inferior turbinate on the cleft side is also frequently hypertrophic, further adding to nasal obstruction on that side. [13] Lee [8] described seven cardinal deformities in unilateral cleft lip nose deformity include:

- Caudal deflection of the nasal septum to the non-cleft side
- Deviation of the nasal dorsum
- Low setting of the medial crus
- Tethering deformity of the lateral crus
- Discontinuity of the orbicularis oris muscle
- Long or short lip deformity
- Absence of the philtral column

Although Huffman and Lierle in 1949 published the most detailed descriptions of the cleft lip nasal deformity, over time it has changed; the typical clinical features of the unilateral cleft nasal deformity (Figure 3) is characterized as follow:

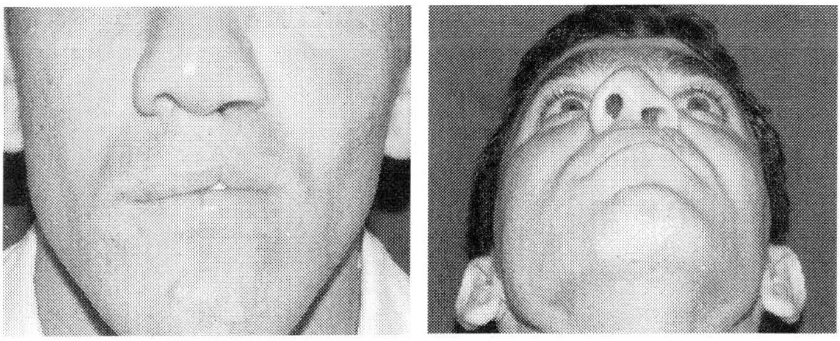

Figure 3. Typical deformity in unilateral cleft nose deformity

1. The tip of the nose and caudal septum are deviated towards the non-cleft side.
2. The base of the columella also deviates towards the non-cleft side.
3. The convexity of the septum on the side of the cleft impinges on the airway.
4. The angle between the medial and lateral crura on the cleft side is excessively obtuse.
5. The dome of the alar cartilage on the cleft side is depressed.
6. The interior of the cleft-side nostril, from its apex down the cephalic margin of the alar cartilage to the pyriform aperture, is bowed by a linear contracture—the vestibular web.
7. The lateral crus is caudally displaced on the cleft side.

8. The cleft side ala buckles inwardly (M configuration)
9. The cartilage on the cleft side smaller than the normal side
10. Absent alar-facial groove on the cleft side
11. Hypoplastic maxilla on cleft side
12. Ill-proportioned nares
13. Widened nostril floor on cleft side
14. Retrodisplaced medial crus on the cleft-side
15. Oblique slant of the columella [8-14]

3.2. Bilateral cleft nose deformities

Adult patients with bilateral cleft lip nose deformity (BLCND) show some asymmetry. Typical characteristics of BLCND include: a short columella, a short, depressed, thick nasal tip, flat–appearing nasal tip, sometimes notched in the midline, large diverging nostrils, wide nostril floors, an obtuse columella-labial angle, wide alae, a short nasal bridge, and a wide nasal root, lateral displacement of both alar domes with bilateral dislocation of the lateral crura from the septum, hooding of the alar rims and flaring alar bases.The short columella is the most common problem in bilateral cleft nose deformity. Although the residual deformity in bilateral cleft is symmetrical correction of nasal tip widening, the retro- positioning of the alar cartilage and shortening of the columella are all encountered and difficult to treat. The secondary deformity involves the nose and the lip as well as the facial profile (Figure 4) [12, 15, and 16].

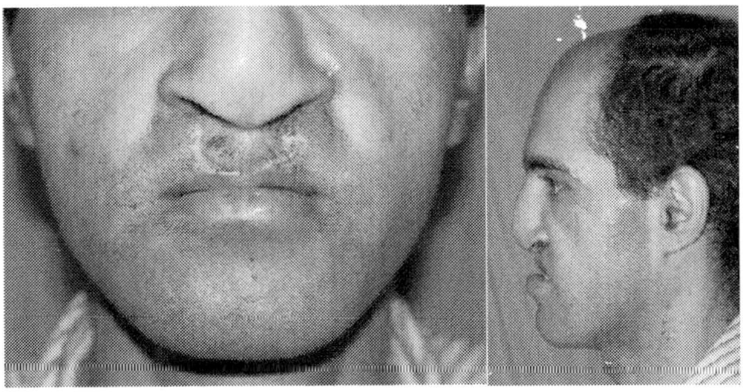

Figure 4. Preoperative views A: Frontal view B: lateral view

4. Diagnosis

In order to treat CLND, clinical diagnosis and complete knowledge of anatomy, pathology and physiology of the nasal pyramid, maxilla, and lip is imperative. Clinical examination consists of a careful examination of the bony and cartilaginous skeleton, anterior rhinoscopy evaluating the appearance of the nasal mucosa and the position of the anterior part of the septum is necessary. The problems present in a patient with a cleft lip nasal deformity must be recognized just as any other rhinoplasty patient and clearly defined in order to formulate a successful treatment plan. In fully grown adult we need to evaluate:

1. The nose and lip
2. Midface deficiency
3. Oro- nasal fistula
4. Occlusion and
5. Speech.

Significant improvement in growth, function and esthetics has been achieved by almost normal reconstruction of alveolar clefts.To establish the nasal skeletal base, three dimensional reconstruction of alveolar defects with bone grafting has been advocated by clinicians; different approaches at the different stages of life have been suggested (Figure 4).

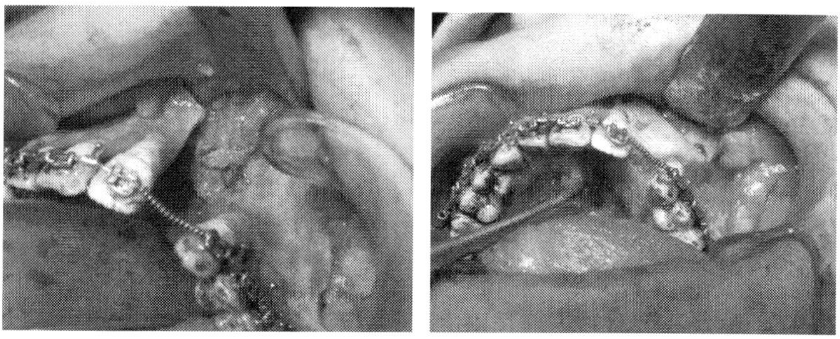

Figure 5. Intraoperative view of 3D reconstruction of alveolar cleft

Proper jaw relationship plays an important role in the skeletal base of the nose; obviously, final rhinoplasty must be postponed until completion of orthognathic surgeries. Although some authors suggested performing orthognathic surgery on growing cleft patients when mandated by psychological and / or functional concerns; but, because of postsurgical outcome the consensus of most clinicians is to delay orthognathic surgery until growth is completed. Different kinds of distraction procedures such as intraoral and extraoral devices may be used as an alternative to the orthognathic approaches in cleft patients; a proper position of the maxilla is mandatory before performing rhinoplasty in adults with cleft lip and nose deformity. Supposedly, the skeletal support enhances the projection of the lip and nose on the cleft side.

CT scan of paranasal sinuses in axial and coronal views may be helpful to define the deformation of the septum as well as other intranasal structures. It is important to identify both aesthetic and functional problems associated with the cleft nose deformity. Each component of the deformity must be addressed in an orderly manner including the skeletal base, nasal dorsal bone and cartilage, nasal tip cartilage, and, finally, the skin envelope [1, 8, 11, 17-21].

5. Non-surgical treatment

Before correction of the soft tissues, it is important to make sure if there are any dental problems that needs to be corrected first. Soft tissue correction before dental treatment can result in very embarrassing situation that may not be correctable later [22].

6. Surgical treatment

No single procedure has given sufficiently satisfactory results to provide a surgical standard for CLND correction. Despite considerable progress in the treatment of patients with cleft lip and palate, there is still no agreement about the optimal treatment method. Secondary deformity after the primary operation is a significant problem encountered in cleft-lip repair [23]. The knowledge and experience of the surgeon in rhinoplasty is the keystone for correcting deformity. Use of four basic techniques in rhinoplasty such as onlay grafting, suturing methods, cartilage transection, reorientation and cartilage repositioning can help the cosmetic surgeon to overcome many of the problems inherent to these patients. Familiarity with the numerous techniques in this regard and selection of the proper one to treat the existing deformity is essential. No matter which technique is used it is important to address all parts of the deformity and set all parts in anatomic position. Nostril asymmetry is one of the main complaints of adult patient with unilateral cleft nose deformities. In 1977, Tajima and Maruyama introduced an operation in which the deformed alar cartilage was fixed to the upper lateral cartilage through a reverse-U incision, and the insufficient area within the nostril was filled with the overhanging alar web tissues. We use this method for the correction of severe asymmetric nostrils. To obtain ideal treatment outcomes in unilateral cleft nose deformity the below list of procedures are used.

1. Using open rhinoplasty approach
2. Doing septoplasty and harvesting graft from the septum via open approach incision.
3. Release septum to upper lateral cartilage on the non-cleft side.
4. Release upper lateral cartilage from the skin and nasal pyriform
5. Correcting deformed caudal and dorsal part of the septum which is fixed to the non-cleft side.
6. Release and splitting of lower lateral cartilage on the cleft side.
7. Medial and lateral crus elevation
8. Using reverse U incision for correcting web.

9. Using Z- plasty incision in vestibular pica for vertical lengthening.
10. Reshaping and repositioning of lower lateral cartilage is essential for correcting nostril deformity.
11. Using multiple sutures to stabilize the final shape of lower and upper lateral cartilages.
12. Using autogenous graft for augmentation
13. Augmentation approach is better than reduction
14. Strut, tip, sheen and batten grafts are help to restore the nasal tip.
15. Unequal alar base resection
16. Release depressor septi muscles

Internal or external osteotomy can be used (Figure 5) [8, 24].

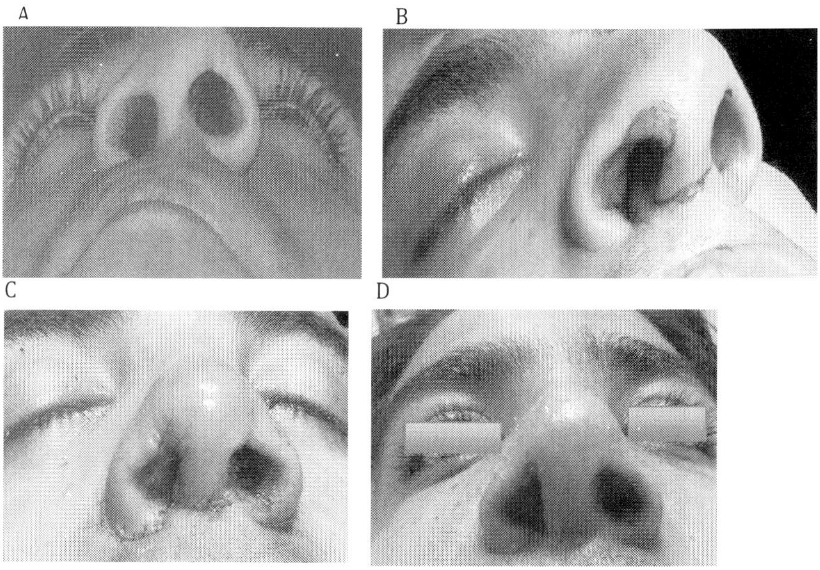

Figure 6. A, Before surgery: B, Intraoperative: C, Immediately after surgery: D, one week post surgery

In bilateral cleft nose deformity although confronted with almost symmetric deformities the lengthening of the columella, correction of the depressed nasal tip, bilateral dislocation of alar cartilage and eversion of the alar bases are on the top of the clinician's concern. There are many ways to elongate the shortness of the columella such as forked flap, v-y advancement, prolabium advancement flap combined with an Abbe flap, composite graft and skin rim rotation flap [26]. Using strong and proper struts, repositioning and reshaping lower lateral cartilages, supraperiosteal dissection of the pyriform area to allow the reposition of nasal

correcting alar component, use of different suturing methods and augmentation with autogenous grafts can help to achieve almost ideal results (Figure 6).

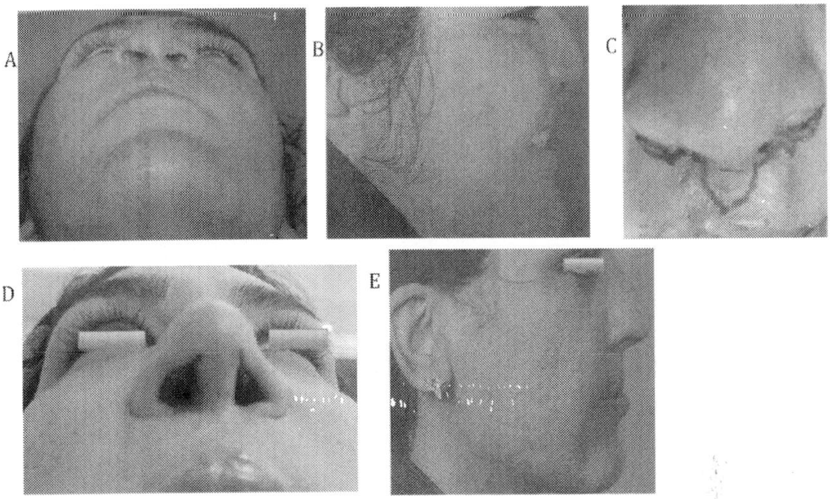

Figure 7. A and B, before surgery basal and lateral view, C: intraoperative D and E: 6 months after surgery

7. Outcomes

Normalized esthetics of the lip and nose is on the top of the specific goals of surgical care for children born with cleft lip and palate followed by nasal airway patency and normal speech [25]. The focus of secondary correction of unilateral cleft-lip nose deformity has been nasal symmetry. Importance has been placed on correction of the cleft-lip nasal deformity by translocation of the alar cartilage with its attached vestibular lining into a normal position, thereby establishing the normal vault and shape of the cartilage.[23] There is no doubt that definitive rhinoplasty should logically only be undertaken after reconstruction of skeletal base and correction of the jaws relationship. The key point is overcorrecting the cleft-side nostril and its alar cartilage is believed to produce better symmetry compensating for possible relapse during the postoperative period [12]

8. Complications

There is no difference between the complications associated with cleft lip rhinoplasty and traditional open rhinoplasty in non-cleft patients. Theoretically the risk of infection is more likely particularly when cartilage grafts are used. The risk of bleeding is similar to that of traditional rhinoplasty. Patients should be warned of possible need for secondary rhinoplasty, need for minor or even major revision, existence of nostril asymmetry, visible scars, skin necrosis, dysfunction of nasal system and anomalies associated with the donor site. Clinical failures using different kinds of grafts consisting of autograft, allograft and alloplastic materials may be seen in the future. Failure to achieve the desired nasal contour and normal looking appearance is a common finding in cleft lip nasal rhinoplasty.

Author details

Fereydoun Pourdanesh[1*] and Behnam Bohluli[2]

*Address all correspondence to: drpourdanesh@gmail.com

1 Associate Professor, Department of Oral and Maxillofacial Surgery, School of Dentistry, Shahid Beheshti University of Medical Sciences, Tehran, Iran

2 Associate Professor, Department of Oral and Maxillofacial Surgery, School of Dentistry, Azad University, Tehran, Iran

References

[1] Hellings P et al, Unique approach to secondary cleft lip rhinoplasty in facial plastic surgery, B-ENT, 2010,6:97-101

[2] Monasterio, O,F Ruas J,E, Cleft Lip Rhinoplasty: The Role of Bone and Cartilage grafts clinics in Plastic Surgery-Vol. 16, No. 1, January 1989,177-187

[3] Anastassov E.G,Joos U., Comprehensive management of cleft lip and palate deformities, Joms, Volume 59, Issue 9, 2001, Pages 1062–1075

[4] Thomas C, Primary Rhinoplasty for the Cleft Nasal Deformity. J Def Manag 2013 S3: 005. Doi:10.4172/2167-0374.S3-005

[5] Penfold C,Douminguez – gonzalez S Bilateral cleft lip and nose repair,bjomfs. Volume 49, Issue 3, 2011, Pages 165–17

[6] Nakajima T, Ogata H, Sakuma H, Long-term outcome of simultaneous repair of bilateral cleft lip and nose (a 15 year experience),brithis journal of plastic surgry,2003,(56),205-217

[7] El bestar M, Mansour O: Cleft lip nasal deformity : primary repair,Egypt.J,plast. Reconstr.surg.vol 28 No, 1 2004, pages 15-21

[8] Lee DW, Choi B-K, Park Be-Y.Y, Seven Fundamental Procedures for Definitive Correction of Unilateral Secondary Cleft Lip Nasal Deformity in Soft Tissue Aspects, J Oral Maxillofac Surg,2011 :69:e420-e430,

[9] BANKS P, the surgical anatomy of secondary cleft lip and palate deformity and its significance in reconstruction, british journal of oral surgery (1983) 21, 78-93

[10] Nakamura N, Okawachi, T, Nozoe E,, Nishihara K, and Matsunaga K, Three-Dimensional Analyses of Nasal Forms After Secondary Treatment of Bilateral cleftlip–Nose Deformity in Comparison to Those of Healthy Young Adults, J Oral Maxillofac Surg 69:e469-e481, 2011

[11] Hopper A.R, Cutting C, Grason B, chapter 23, cleft lip and palate,Grabb and smith's plastic surgery,6th edition by Charles H Thorne,2007,pages 201-225

[12] Banks p, the surgical anatomy of secondary cleft lip and palate deformity and its significance in reconstruction, British Journal of Oral Surgery (1983) 21, 78-93

[13] Lun-Jou Lo, Primary Correction of the Unilateral Cleft Lip Nasal Deformity: Achieving the Excellence, Chang Gung Med J 2006;29:262-7)

[14] Huffman WC,Leirle DM,studies on the pathologic anatomy of the unilateral harelip nose,plast reconstr surg,1949,4:225

[15] Yonehara, Y, Mori Y, Chikazu D, Saijo H, Tsuyoshi Takato T, Secondary Correction of Bilateral Cleft Lip and Nasal Deformity by Simultaneous Placement of an Abbe Flap, Septal Cartilage Graft, and Cantilevered Iliac Bone Graft, J Oral Maxillofac Surg 66:581-588, 2008

[16] Ahmed SA, Ramadan M.M, Correction of Secondary Deformities of the Cleft Lip Nose,Suez Canal Univ Med J Vol. 11, No. 1, March, 2008 1 -7

[17] Precious S.D, A New Reliable Method for Alveolar Bone Grafting at About 6 Years of Age, J Oral Maxillofac Surg 67:2045-2053, 2009

[18] Epker N.B, Correction of the Skeletal Nasal Base in Rhinoplasty, J Oral Maxillofac Surg 49:939-946, 1991

[19] Pourdanesh f.Behnia H, Using l-shaped bone graft to restore alar base region in patients with alveolar cleft, International Journal of Oral & Maxillofacial Surgery Volume 42, Issue 10, Page 1202, October 2013

[20] Wolford M.L, Cassano S.D, Cottrell A.D, El Deeb M, Karras, Goncalves R.J, Orthognathic Surgery in the Young Cleft Patient: Preliminary Study on Subsequent Facial Growth, J Oral Maxillofac Surg 66:2524-2536, 2008

[21] Showkatbakhsh R, Pourdanesh F, Jamilian A, Ghorbani A, Behnaz M. Hyrax application as a tooth-borne distractor for maxillary advancement., J Craniofac Surg. 2011 Jul;22(4):1361-6.

[22] Tung K.M, Management of Post Cleft Deformities of the Lip & Nose,medical bulletin,vol.12,no 11,November 2007

[23] Fujimoto T, Imai K, Hatano T, Makoto Takahashi, Tamai M, Follow-up of unilateral cleft-lip nose deformity after secondary repair with a modified reverse-U method, Journal of Plastic, Reconstructive & Aesthetic Surgery (2011) 64, 747e753

[24] Tajima S, Maruyama M: Reverse-U incision for secondary repair of cleft lip nose. Plast Reconstr Surg 60:256, 1977

[25] Taheri Talesh K, Kalantar Motamedi MH, cleft lip and palate surgery, A text book of advanced oral and maxillofacial surgery p 560- 569

[26] Nakamura N, Sasaguri M, Okawachi T, Nishihara K, Nozoe E, Secondary correction of bilateral cleft lip nose deformity e Clinical and three-dimensional observations on pre- and postoperative outcome, Journal of Cranio-Maxillo-Facial Surgery 39 (2011) 305e312

Section 13

Advanced Laser Applications

Chapter 34

Advanced Applications of the Er:YAG Laser in Oral and Maxillofacial Surgery

Dragana Gabrić, Anja Baraba, Goran Batinjan, Marko Blašković, Vanja Vučićević Boras, Irina Filipović Zore, Ivana Miletić and Elizabeta Gjorgievska

Additional information is available at the end of the chapter

http://dx.doi.org/10.5772/59273

1. Introduction

Lasers are becoming widely used in medicine and dentistry due to their beneficial effects such as: coagulation properties (less postoperative bleeding), less pain and edema. Lasers also allow good and rapid healing, a very low level of discomfort both during and after intervention and a rapid disappearance of symptoms.

Four responses within tissues are described when the laser beam hits the target tissue namely reflection, absorption, transmission and scattering. The main mechanisms of interaction between the lasers and biological tissues are: photothermic, photoacoustic and photochemical. The effect of lasers on the soft tissues is based on the transformation of light energy into heat. Operator-dependent factors affecting the effect of lasers are: power density, energy density, pulse repetition rate, pulse duration and the mode of energy transferred. Operator non-dependent factors which affect laser treated areas are specific laser wavelengths and optical properties of the target tissues [1].

Effects on the tissues when lasers are applied include the increase in the temperature, coagulation, hemostasis, tissue sterilization, tissue welding, incision, excision, ablation and vaporization [1]. When laser energy is absorbed in the water of the hard tissues, a rapid volume expansion of the evaporating water occurs as a result of a substantial temperature elevation at the interaction site. Micro-explosions are produced causing hard tissue disintegration. If pulp temperatures are raised beyond 5 degrees, pulp damage is irreversible. If heat is intensive and lasts for an extended period of time the consistency of the intracellular ground substance may not be preserved [1].

Erbium-yttrium-aluminum-garnet (Er: YAG) lasers produce invisible infrared light at a wavelength of 2.940 nm which is ideal for absorption by hydroxylapatite and water [2]. Therefore, they can be used for treatment of both soft and hard tissues (unlike for example diode lasers). As the Er: YAG wavelength corresponds to the absorption coefficient of water, Er: YAG laser irradiation transforms water within tissue into steam leading to the development of micro-explosions [3].

2. Advantages of Er: YAG laser treatment

Laser technology has certain advantages such as accuracy of the incision, absence of vibration and manual pressure during use; this is also true for Er: YAG laser application. Due to laser positive coagulation effects during surgical procedure, better sight of the work field is obtained. Komori [4] and Gouw-Soares [5] have reported that Er: YAG lasers are appropriate for the treatment of hard dental tissues without inducing discomfort, vibration or noise. Furthermore, risk of surgical field contamination and damage to the surrounding tissues is decreased when compared to the other similar techniques. Additionally Er: YAG lasers are characterized by low intraoperative and postoperative pain levels. Decreased pain levels by use of Er:YAG as well as other lasers may be explained by the fact that laser application leads to the formation of protein coagulum on the surface of the wound which acts as a dressing [6]. Furthermore, lasers have the ability to seal sensory nerve endings which results in decreased pain perception. Last but not least, Er: YAG lasers produce rapid wound healing [7].

3. Possible hazards of laser use

It is very important to acknowledge possible thermal damage induced by Er: YAG lasers in the clinical setting. Kreisler [8] suggested that temperature elevation did not exceed 47°C after 120 seconds of Er:YAG laser irradiation with pulse energy between 60 and 120 mJ and frequency of 10 Hz. Geminiani [9] reported that application of Er:YAG lasers in continuous mode for 10 seconds generated a high temperature which was above critical threshold. Monzavi [10] reported that use of Er: YAG was safe without cooling and that, an increase of 4.30°C was observed. Use of air and air water cooling eliminated the risk of possible thermal damage. Mitsunaga [11] retrieved literature data from the year 2001 to 2012 with regard to complications after laser irradiation such as cervicofacial subcutaneous emphysema. They [11] reported 13 such cases, of which eight had undergone CO2 laser treatment and two had undergone Er: YAG laser treatment. Nine patients had emphysema following laser irradiation for soft tissue incision [11].

4. Application of ER: YAG laser in soft tissue surgery

Lasers have played an integral part in the evolution of oral and maxillofacial surgery (OMS); and rapidly became the standard of care for many procedures performed by oral surgeons.

The reason for this transition is simple: many procedures can be executed more efficiently and with less morbidity using lasers when compared with scalpel, electrocautery or high frequency devices. Onisor [12] performed an *in vitro* study using Er: YAG and CO_2 laser for crown lengthening, gingivoplasty and maxillary labial frenectomy. The same authors [12] concluded that Er: YAG is able to provide good cutting and coagulation effects on soft tissues. Specific parameters have to be defined for each laser in order to obtain the desired effect. Reduced or absent water spray, defocused light beam, local anesthesia and use of long pulses are important in order to obtain optimal coagulation and bleeding control. Kaya [13] described a case of pyogenic granuloma around an implant seven years after its insertion which they treated by use of Er: YAG laser. Türer [14] compared Er: YAG laser to the scalpel in the preparation of the recipient site for free gingival grafts. The same authors [14] stated that Er: YAG laser may be used with similar effectiveness as the scalpel for this purpose.

Laser surgery has emerged as an established method in advanced medicine. Laser-induced remote tissue treatment provides a number of advantages: controllable coagulation and cutting of surgical tissues with wavelength tissue-specific cutting efficiency [15]. At the Department of Oral Surgery, School of Dental Medicine, University of Zagreb, two clinical studies of Er: YAG laser use for soft tissue surgery was performed.

4.1. Er: YAG laser-assisted surgery of benign oral tumors

The aim of first study was to evaluate the efficacy of a high power diode laser, Er:YAG and Nd:YAG laser in surgical therapy of benign oral lesions in comparison to the conventional methods on the basis of following temperature difference in surrounding tissue during the laser operation procedure.

Infrared thermography is a diagnostic method with ability to record infrared radiation emitted by the skin and convert it into electronic video signals. Infrared thermography is unique in its capability to show physiological and/or pathological temperature changes [16]. One hundred and twenty patients who had indication for surgical removal of benign oral lesions were randomly divided into four groups dependent on the type of therapy. First group (Diode group) received diode laser therapy with Laser (Hager & Werken GmbH & Co., Germany). Depending on the indications settings specified by the manufacturer for removal of fibroma a "Fibroma removal mode" was used (wavelength of 975 nm, power of 5W, CW). Second (Er: YAG) and third (Nd: YAG) groups received Er: YAG and Nd: YAG therapy modules. All settings of the Er: YAG and Nd: YAG laser were according to manufacturer specifications. Light Walker AT (Fotona, Slovenia) was used for Er: YAG and Nd: YAG treatments. The laser settings were 150 mJ for fibroma removal in pulse mode QSP and 15 Hz frequency. Non-contact X-Runner digitally controlled handpiece was used for treatments. The shape with the X-Runner handpiece was selected according to the required treatment area. The handpiece was held at the distance 15 mm from the treatment tissue, without water spray (Figures 1-3). In the fourth group (scalpel group) procedure was performed using the conventional methods using the cold knife for fibroma removal and afterwards the wounds were sutured.

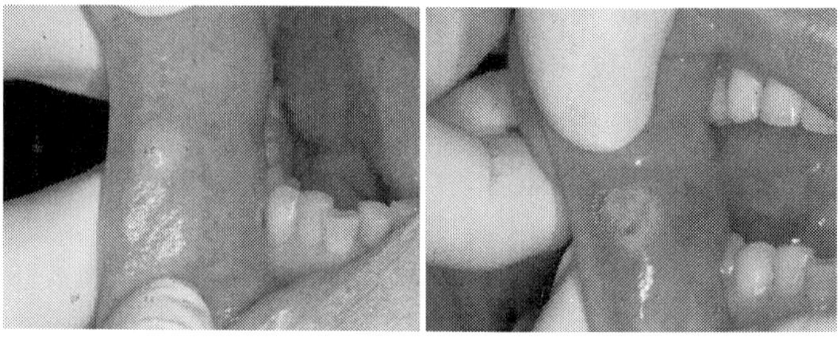

Figure 1. Fibroma of the right cheek (left) and removal of the lesion using Er: YAG laser with X-Runner handpiece (right)

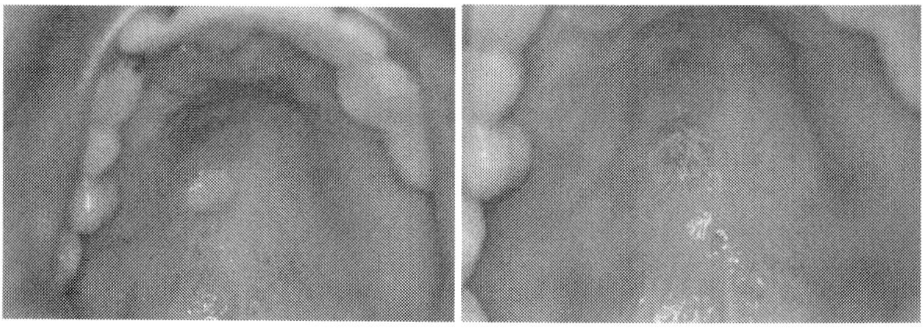

Figure 2. Fibroma of the hard palate (left) and removal of the lesion using Er: YAG laser with X-Runner handpiece (right)

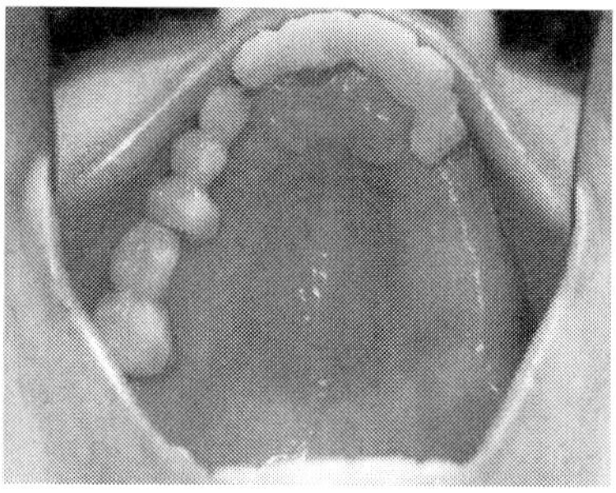

Figure 3. Follow-up (case from Figure 2), 3 weeks after surgery

4.2. Thermographic measurement and thermogram processing

Prior to the start of the procedure each patient spent 15 minutes in operating anteroom in which the temperature and humidity are the same as the operating room since both areas have controlled environment (air conditioned). Camera was set on a tripod at fixed, predetermined distance (30 cm from the head of the patient), thus camera settings were always the same. Infrared (IR) camera in general records temperature distribution in a given area. In this case it recorded temperature distribution in the oral cavity prior to, during and after laser treatment and during postoperative check-up. Taking thermographic images (thermograms) allowed us to monitor the effects of laser treatment on tissues, i.e. the changes in temperature of tissue treated with the laser (and surrounding tissue in close proximity) caused by the effects of laser on the tissues, i.e. the effects during the procedure. Thermographic images taken using FLIR T335 camera (Flir systems, USA) during laser procedure were stored on the computer for later processing. Images had to be spatially calibrated firstly during image interpretation in order to obtain data regarding spatial temperature distribution in the image. Spatial market, metal equilateral triangle of known dimensions, was used for that purpose. Metal triangle was easily visible on thermographic images since its temperature was a few degrees lower. Since the triangle dimensions were known and well defined, triangle outlines on the image were used for spatial measurement. In this procedure metal triangle was used as spatial marker in the same way as a ruler (as a "standard" spatial marker) is used (Figure 4, in the middle).

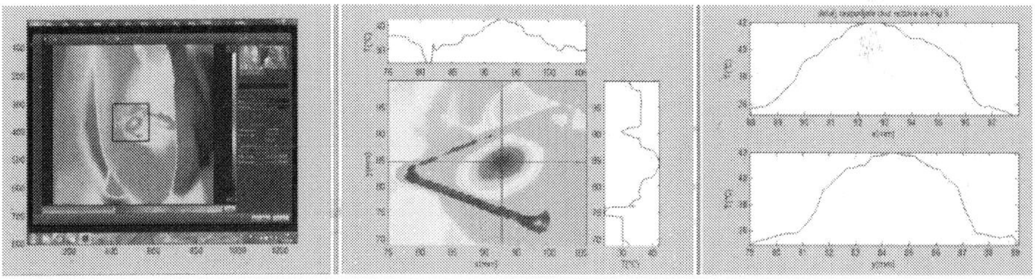

Figure 4. Thermographic image processing

In all the surgical procedures performed, thermal increase was evaluated until the end of the procedure; thermal decrease was evaluated in the few seconds after surgery. Matlab program (MathWorks, USA) was used for processing thermograms in the RGB format. The oral health related quality of life (OHRQoL) was assessed in all four groups after the surgical procedure. All participants filled-out the Oral Health Impact (OHIP) 14-CRO Questionnaire. The questions were related to the period during and after the surgical procedure. Patients answered each question using the 0-4 Likert scale (0=absence of problems; 4=the most severe problems). The OHIP Summary Score was calculated for statistical analysis. Results of this study showed no significant temperature differences between diode and Nd: YAG group during the surgical procedure. They had almost the same temperature in the region ($p=0.76$). Er: YAG group had significantly lower temperature increase in the operative areas when compared to the other two laser groups ($p<0.001$). The highest superficial thermal increase was recorded for diode laser, the lowest one for Er: YAG laser (Table 1). Participants in all three laser groups had significantly lower OHIP14-CRO summary scores ($p<0.001$, Table 2).

LASER	THERMAL EFFECT Mean (μm) ± SD
Er:YAG	38,92 ± 19,92
Nd:YAG	81,23 ± 3,53
Diode laser	82,76 ± 5,38

Table 1. Thermal effect of the operated area during the surgical procedure, mean value and standard deviation (SD)

	Group	mean (OHIP score)	SD	t	P
OHIP Summary score	Laser groups	12.65	3.84	-6.776	<0.001 *
	Scalpel group	26.50	8.29		

Degree of freedom = 38, * significant at 99% probability, p<0.01

Table 2. Difference in the OHIP 14 scores as well as in the OHIP 14 Summary Scores between the laser groups and the scalpel group together with significance of the differences

Most laser excisional or incisional procedures are accomplished at 100°C, where vaporization of intracellular and extracellular water causes ablation or removes biological tissues. Clinicians must be aware of the heat generated within tissues during a procedure. If the tissue temperature exceeds 200°C during a laser procedure, carbonization and irreversible tissue necrosis will occur. This adverse consequence can be avoided completely by using the lowest power setting necessary to achieve the desired treatment goal [17].

Er: YAG lasers operate at a higher wavelength on the principle of ablation in non-contact mode at a 2940 nm wavelength, while the diode and Nd: YAG laser work at smaller wavelength on the principle of excision in contact mode which denotes a more aggressive approach. That is probably the reason why the diode and Nd:YAG lasers cause higher heating of the surrounding tissues and a higher dispersion of energy which damages more surrounding structures within targeted therapeutic areas and result in slower healing. However, they result in better hemostasis and less swelling due to the effects of diode laser on tissue targets (melanin and hemoglobin). When considering use of diode laser for soft tissue surgery, the clinician must consider several factors. Diode lasers are attracted to pigment, and frena are typically thicker fibrous tissue and have very little pigment. The lack of pigment and more fibrous nature of the tissue mean that higher energies and patience are required to ablate this tissue. Other lasers, such as Er: YAG lasers may ablate frena faster, and can be used in non-contact mode, but the drawback compared to diode lasers is an increased risk of bleeding. Er: YAG lasers are not well absorbed in hemoglobin as the soft tissue diode lasers are, so hemostasis can be an issue with these wavelengths. Some studies [18-23] compared the efficacy of diode and Er: YAG lasers in soft tissue oral surgery. Some studies showed that the Er:YAG laser induced deeper gingival tissue injury than diode laser, as judged by bleeding at surgery, delayed healing and deformed specimen for histopathological analysis [23]. In some studies the use of diode laser showed additional advantages over Er: YAG in terms of less postoperative discomfort and pain, but some studies show no difference between these two lasers [3]. Some studies indicate that only the Er: YAG laser can be used for lingual frenectomy without local anesthesia, and there was no difference between the two groups regarding the degree of the postsurgical discomfort except in the first 3 hours [19]. Results indicate that the Er: YAG laser is more advantageous than the diode laser in minor soft-tissue surgery because it can be performed without local anesthesia and with only topical anesthesia.

Since the introduction of the lasers in clinical practice, different wavelengths have been used for oral surgery on the basis of the different characteristics and affinities of each. One study compared different laser wavelengths in relation to both thermal increase and "histological quality" in a model of soft tissue surgery procedures. Thermal evaluation was noticed, during laser-assisted surgery excision performed on a bovine tongue, by a thermal camera device to evaluate thermal increase on the surface of the sample and with four thermocouples to evaluate thermal increase on the depth of the specimen. Temperature was recorded before start of the surgical procedure and at the peak of every excision. The results of this study are similar to ours because the highest in depth thermal increase was recorded for the 5 W diode lasers, the lowest one for Er: YAG laser [21].

4.3. Evaluation of Er:YAG laser for surgical treatment of precancerous lesion (leukoplakia)

Leukoplakia is a white precancerous lesion of the oral cavity with a recognizable risk of malignant transformation. According to the World Health Organization, the name leukoplakia can be used to describe the clinical finding of white patches on the oral mucosa that cannot be removed or classified as other oral diseases. Histologically, leukoplakia consists of epithelial hyperplasia, with or without hyperkeratosis, minimal inflammation, and different degrees of dysplasia. Oral leukoplakia is the most common potentially malignant lesion of the oral cavity, and the incidence of malignant transformation increases during the years. Treatment options are: scalpel excision, electrocoagulation, cryotherapy and CO_2 laser therapy. Extremely extensive lesions are the biggest challenge. Pharmacological treatments include vitamin A and retinoids, topical antioxidants and bleomycin [24-26]. Out of all available ablative lasers in the treatment of leukoplakia Er: YAG laser is emphasized due to the highest degree of absorption in water. The latest laser technology allows extremely precise ablation or excision of these lesions using computerizing, automatic guided laser beams with precise and individually determined limits by use of QSP mode (X-Runner, LightWalker, Fotona, Slovenia, 2013). Besides complete visibility during ablation due to its coagulation effect, speed, precision of the procedure and rapid healing without postoperative complications or healing without scar are its main advantages [27].

We evaluated the effectiveness of ablative Er: YAG laser in the treatment of leukoplakia and frequency of recurrence after ablative laser therapy. By regular monitoring of postoperative pain via visual analogue scale of pain scores (VAS), the impact of leukoplakia at the quality of life (QoL) using OHIP-14 questionnaire was also assessed. The study was conducted at the School of Dentistry, University of Zagreb, Croatia. Ablative Er: YAG laser was used on 28 lesions with histologically confirmed diagnosis of oral leukoplakia. Lesions were measured (in millimeters), which was necessary for monitoring results and the potential recurrence, as well as for the choice of laser parameters. During surgery, after applying a local anesthetic (Ubistesin 2%, 3M ESPE), depending on the size of the lesion, the size of the working field of the laser was selected. All hyperkeratotic lesions were removed by ablation. Their degree was recorded as was the number of sessions required for ablation. Patients were seen at follow-up a week, two weeks, four weeks and eight weeks after the irradiation. At the follow-up, lesions were re-measured for each patient when applicable and the results were compared with the initial data. Postoperative pain was assessed by VAS where the patient rated the degree of pain after the procedure on the scale from 1-10. Also, each patient filled-out the OHIP - 14 questionnaire of the impact of lesions on the quality of their life (Figures 5-15). All data were used for statistical analysis.

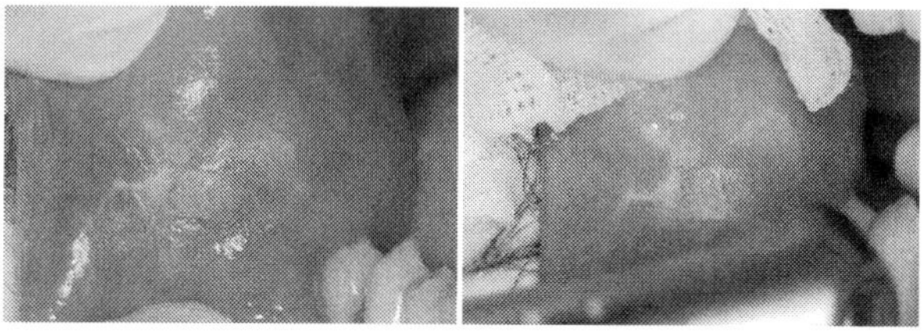

Figure 5. Leukoplakia of the right cheek (left) and removal using Er: YAG laser with X-Runner handpiece (right)

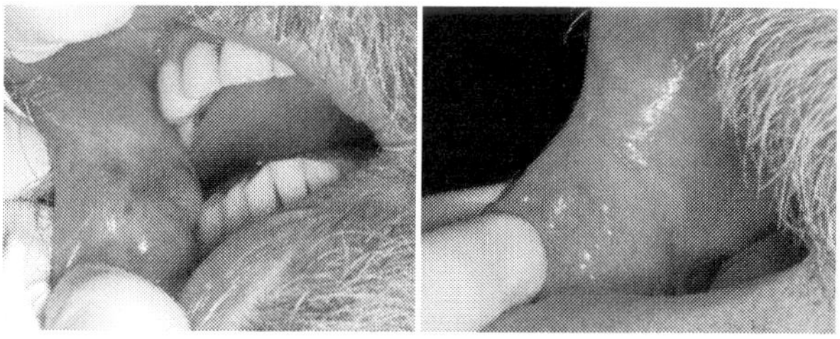

Figure 6. Immediate postoperative view (left) and follow-up 3 weeks after surgery (right)

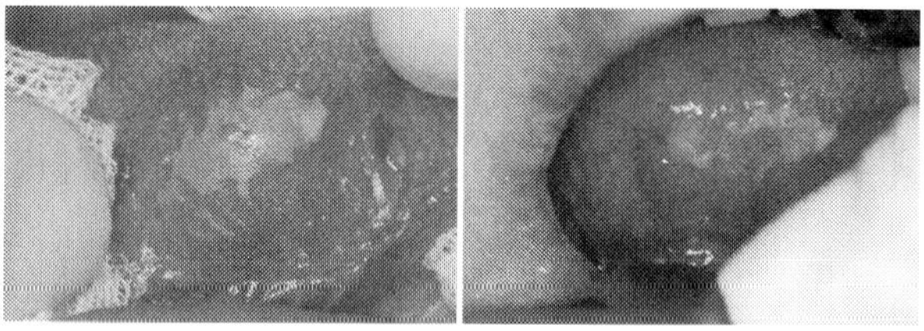

Figure 7. Leukoplakia of the right lateral tongue (left) and removal using Er: YAG laser with X-Runner handpiece (right)

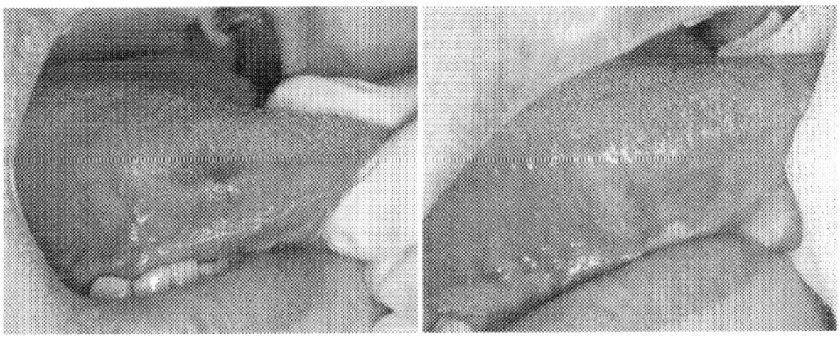

Figure 8. Immediate postoperative view (left) and follow-up 3 weeks after surgery (right)

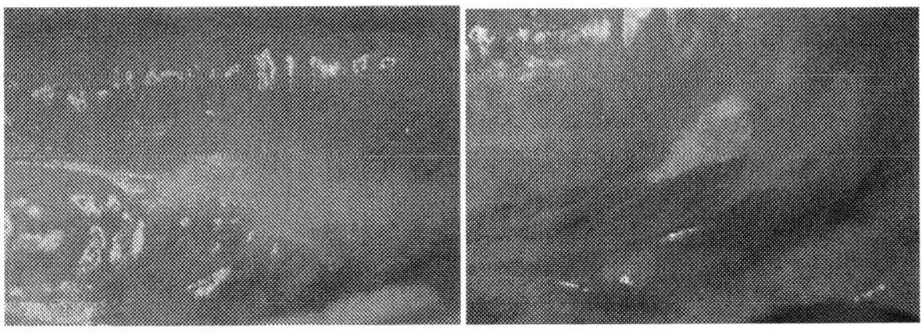

Figure 9. Leukoplakia of the left lateral tongue (left) and removal using Er: YAG laser with X-Runner handpiece (right)

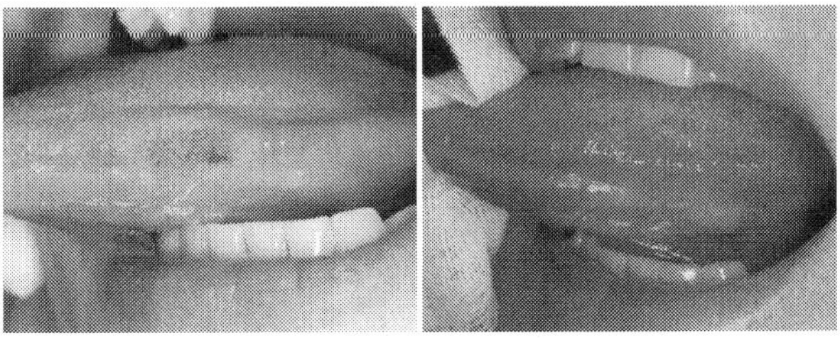

Figure 10. Immediate postoperative view (left) and follow-up 3 weeks after surgery (right)

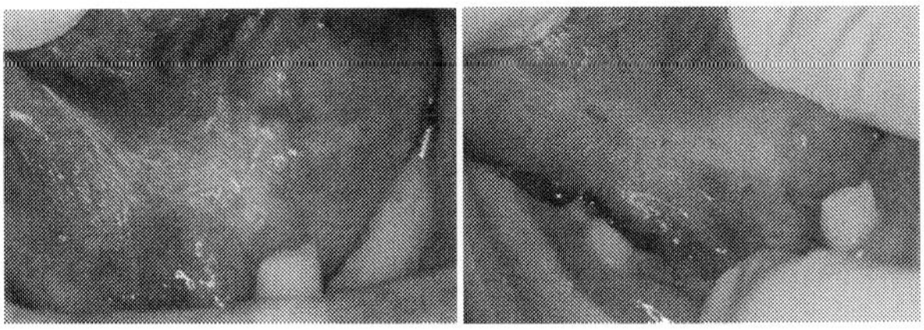

Figure 11. Sublingual leukoplakia (left) and immediate postsurgical view after removal using Er: YAG laser with X-Runner handpiece (right)

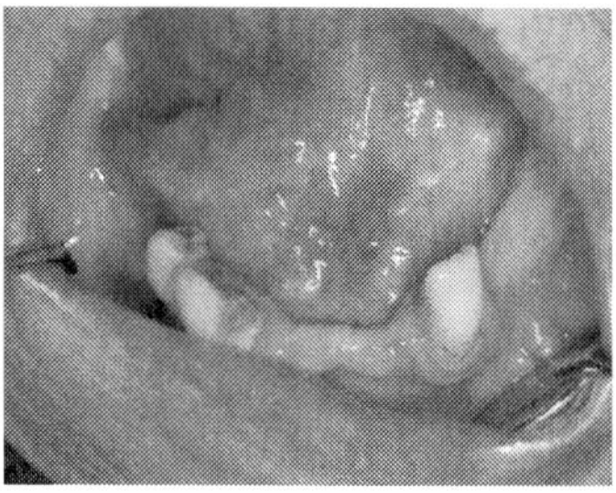

Figure 12. Follow-up 3 weeks after surgery

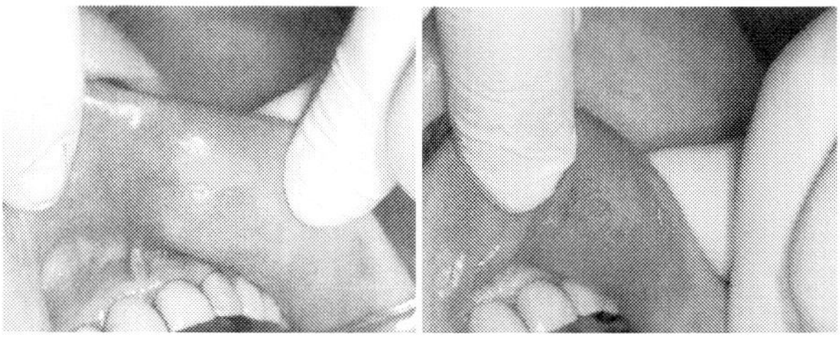

Figure 13. Leukoplakia of the upper lip (left) and removal using Er: YAG laser with X-Runner handpiece (right)

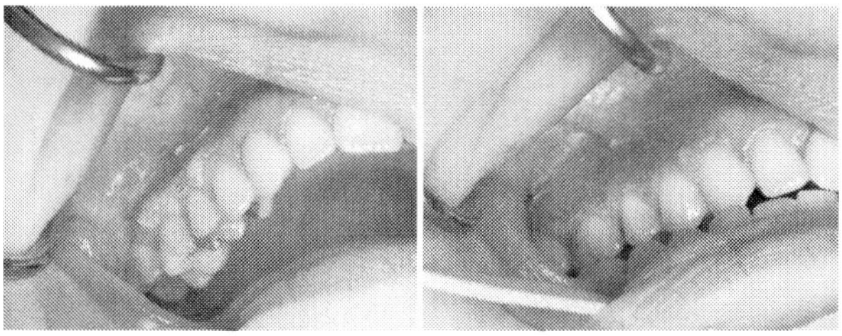

Figure 14. Leukoplakia of the alveolar ridge (left) and removal using Er: YAG laser with X-Runner handpiece (right)

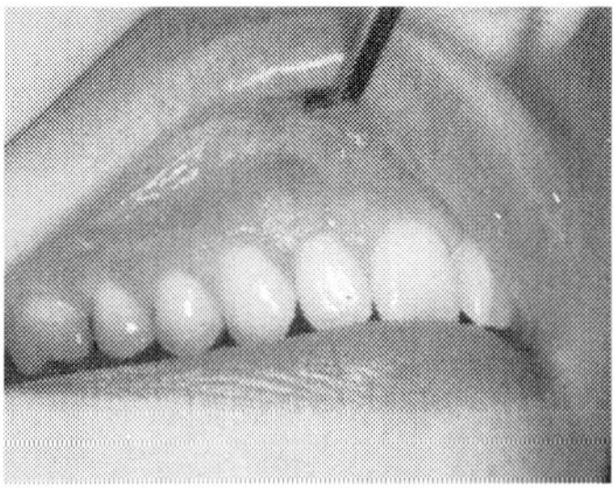

Figure 15. Follow-up 6 weeks after surgery

The results of our study confirmed that treatment of leukoplakia by Er: YAG laser had less edema, post-operative bleeding and pain, in comparison to the conventional surgical methods of treatment such as scalpel. The procedure was easily tolerated and postoperative pain was low or absent. Significant differences between men and women regarding the location of the lesions, number of laser sessions and VAS were found (Tables 3 and 4).

Gender N (%)		Differences in gender	Differences compared to the recurrence
Male	10 (37)		0.148
Female	17 (63)		
Age (mean ± SD)	53.3. ± 13.3	0.459	0.643
Smoking Yes	9 (33.3)	0.260	0.121
Smoking No	18 (66.7)		
Cigarettes per day (mean ± SD)	18.3 ± 10	0.809	0.471
Lesion in mm^2 (mean ± SD)	74.8 ± 90.4	0.166	0.381
Buccal mucosa	11 (40.7)	**<0.001***	**0.004***
Tongue	6 (22.2)		
Sublingual mucosa	3 (11.1)		
Other	7 (26)		

Table 3. Demographic data regarding participants and location of the leukoplakia lesions.

Laser parameters – shape N (%)		Differences in gender	Differences compared to the recurrence
Circle	10 (37)	0.456	0.926
Rectangle	8 (29.6)		
Combination	9 (33.3)		
Number of ablations ≤10	7 (25.9)	0.05	0.694
11-20	16 (59.3)		
>20	4 (14.8)		
Number of laser sessions (mean ± SD)	2.1 ± 0.8	**0.036***	**<0.001***
Recurrence Yes	20 (74.1)	0.148	
Recurrence No	7 (25.9)		
VAS (mean ± SD)	2.68 ± 3.28	**0.008***	0.200
OHIP	9.6 ± 9.8	0.493	0.283

Table 4. Data regarding laser parameters, number of ablations, recurrence rate as well as VAS scores and OHIP results.

The results indicate that sublingual leukoplakia lesions tend to recur less frequently in comparison to the ones situated on the buccal mucosa, tongue and on other parts of the oral mucosa. All leukoplakia lesions found sublingually were seen in women. Women tended to have higher VAS scores in comparison to the men. Men had less laser sessions compared to the women due to the fact that lesions in men were mostly located on the buccal mucosa.

In the published literature there are few papers on treatment of leukoplakia which is refractory to conventional therapy. In the recent years, lasers are having shown to be highly effective in the soft tissue surgery due to the properties of coagulation during surgery and post-operative swelling and pain reduction [28-31]. It was found that laser-assisted removal of the precancerous lesion with the non-contact, digitally controlled X-Runner handpiece was very safe and pleasant for the patient and very effective and comfortable for the operator. The operational field is very clear, especially because there is no bleeding during the operation with the QSP mode. The interventions were performed very quickly because of the automatic coverage of the area with the X-Runner handpiece [27].

4.4. Gingival melanin depigmentation

So far, there are not many published studies regarding the use of Er: YAG lasers in the treatment of gingival melanin pigmentations (Figures 16 and 17). The results of the study of Simsek Kaya. [3] have showed that both diode and Er:YAG laser applied at 1 W can perform gingival depigmentation. However, it seems that treatment duration is longer when Er: YAG lasers are applied compared to the diode lasers. This difference may be explained by the fact that diode lasers penetrate deeper in comparison to the Er: YAG lasers. Furthermore, wavelength of diode lasers lies within the spectrum absorbed by melatonin. Overall, it seems that Er: YAG lasers limit the thermal damage of the surrounding tissues due to the lower penetration force [3]. Ergun [32] reported a case of refractory pigmentations on the lips and oral mucosa in a female patient with Laugier-Hunziker syndrome, successfully treated with Er: YAG laser. Similar skin lesions (hyperkeratosis, nevus, spots and patches) can also be removed using Er: YAG laser with X-Runner handpiece (Figures 18 and 19).

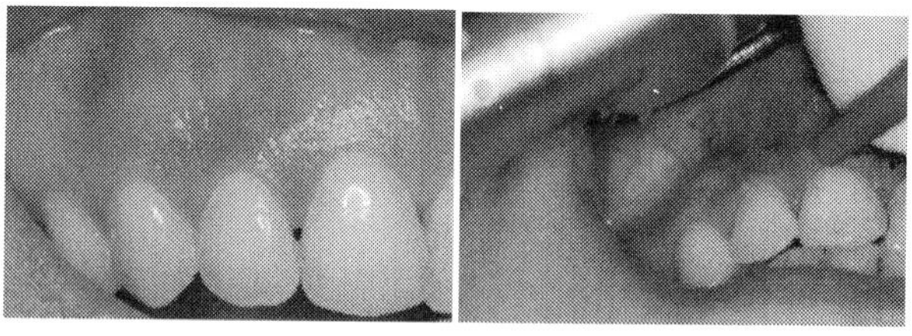

Figure 16. Gingival melanin pigmentation (left) and removal using Er: YAG laser with X-Runner handpiece (right); QSP mode, 120 mJ, 20 Hz, 10 ml/min

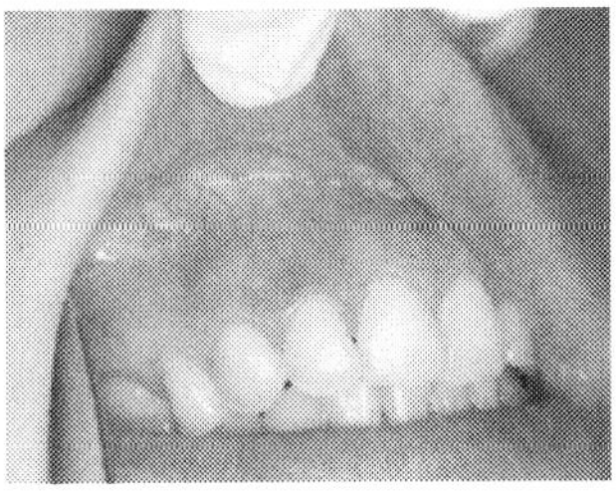

Figure 17. Follow-up 6 weeks after surgery

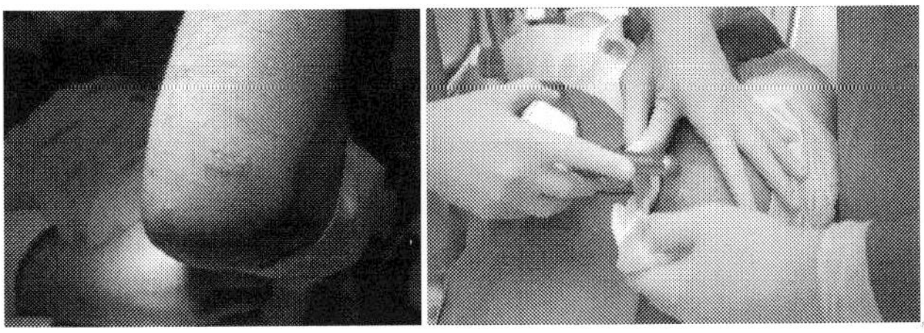

Figure 18. Isolated keratosis of the left elbow (left) and removal using Er: YAG laser with X-Runner handpiece (right); QSP mode, 120 mJ, 20 Hz, 10 ml/min

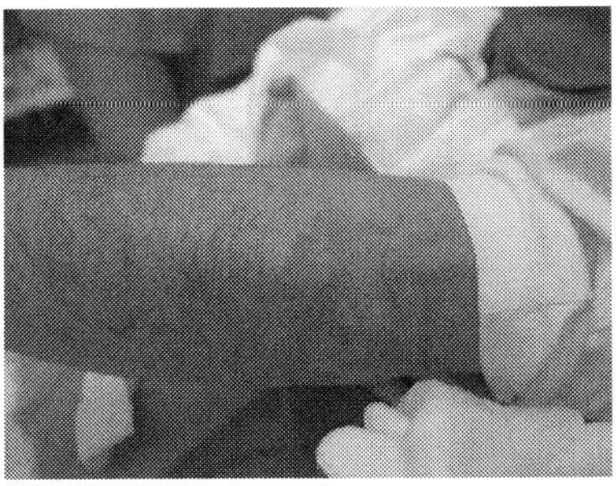

Figure 19. Immediate postoperative view

5. Application of ER: YAG laser in endodontic surgery

The main goal of endodontic treatment is to remove necrotic tissue and microorganisms from root canals by means of mechanical preparation and disinfection in order to seal the root canal space and to prevent subsequent recontamination. According to the literature, the success of primary endodontic treatment reaches values from 47-97% [33]. Failures of orthograde root canal fillings occur in cases with pre-operative presence of periapical radiolucency, root canal filling with voids or root canal fillings more than 2 mm short of the radiographic apex and inadequate coronal restoration [34]. If microorganisms remain present in the root canal system or invade the periradicular tissues or periradicular tissues become contaminated with root canal filling materials, inflammatory and immune response or foreign body reaction may occur, causing local bone destruction and impairment of tissue healing. Failures in endodontic treatment can be managed by retreatment or endodontic surgery although certain clinical situations can only be resolved by means of surgical endodontics. Endodontic surgery has been reported to have a success rate from 44-95% [35] while modern techniques and materials used in endodontic surgery nowadays yield even more consistent success rates, from 88-96% [36-8].

5.1. Endodontic surgery indications

- periradicular disease due to iatrogenic or developmental anomalies which prevent orthograde root canal treatment;
- periradicular disease in root canal of filled teeth in which conventional retreatment cannot be performed or has failed or if the orthograde access to root canal may be detrimental to the retention of the tooth;
- when biopsy of periradicular tissue is required;
- when visualization of the periradicular tissues and tooth root is required, i.e. when perforation or root fracture is suspected [39].

Although there are only few absolute contraindications for endodontic surgery, some factors should be considered. Regarding patients, it is important to assess medical history and the presence of any systemic diseases as well as psychological conditions (uncooperative patient) [40]. Factors which may also preclude surgical approach are local anatomical factors (e.g., inaccessible root end), unusual bony or root configurations, possible involvement of neurovascular structures, tooth with inadequate periodontal support and nonrestorable tooth or tooth without function [40]. Skills, training and experience of the operator as well as available facilities should also be considered.

Endodontic surgical treatment or apicectomy is a procedure performed through a transosseous approach with resection of the root apex, removal of inflammatory periapical tissue and retrograde obturation of root apex in order to prevent microbes or their byproducts from reaching the periapical tissues.

Conventional techniques for apicectomy may include the use of scalpels, curettes, burs and ultrasound tips. This surgical procedure starts with soft tissue flap design depending on a number of factors such as: access to and size of the periradicular lesion, periodontal status, state of coronal tooth structure, the nature and extent of coronal restorations, aesthetics and adjacent anatomical structures. After flap reflection, hard tissue management or osteotomy is performed and the bone should be removed accurately in order to have an access to the root. Bone can be removed using diamond, steel or tungsten carbide burs with continuous cooling with saline sterile water. In cases of missing or very thin cortical bone plate even curettes may be used for osteotomy. Although osteotomy should provide clear visibility and adequate access to root apex, microsurgical approach is recommended [41]. Soft tissue in the periradicular inflammatory region should be removed, usually using curettes, ensuring good visualization of the operating field. When resecting the root, the angle of the resection should be 90 degrees to the long axis of the tooth in order to reduce the number of exposed dentinal tubules [42]. Regarding the length of the resected part of the root, at least 3 mm of root end should be resected to eliminate the majority of anomalies in the apical third. Traditionally, root end resection is done using rotating burs. It is important to examine the resected root surface for presence of any cracks or canal irregularities [43, 44]. The traditional way for root-end preparation is using small round or inverted cone steel burs. The goal of root-end preparation is to surgically remove root canal ramifications, enhance access to the apex, create a working surface for retrograde preparation, facilitate debridement of periapical tissues and to remove irritants from root canal space [45]. Root end preparation should ensure space for root end obturation providing adequate seal apically and optimizing conditions for pariapical tissue healing [45]. This preparation should be 3 mm deep, following the long axis of the tooth. This became easier to achieve in the early 1990s, when sonically or ultrasonically driven microsurgical retrotips were commercially available. When compared to burs, the advantages of ultrasonic tips are: easier access to root ends, smaller osteotomy needed due to angulation and small size of the retrotips, preparation of deeper cavities following more closely the original path of the root canal which also lessens the risk of lateral perforations [45, 46]. The use of retrotips does not require a beveled root end resection decreasing the possible leakage through dentinal tubules. Furthermore, ultrasonic preparations demonstrated less smear layer when compared to the bur preparation, however, bur preparations showed less superficial debris and better canal debridement of gutta-percha [45]. More cracks and microfractures were found after sonic or ultrasonic root-end preparation but it is still unknown if these influence the healing success [45]. Apical leakage studies did not show any difference between the bur and retrotip cavity preparation, although when coronal leakage was investigated using polymicrobial marker, a better seal was established with ultrasonically prepared cavities [45].

Lasers can also be used in periapical surgery for apex resection or for improving the apical sealing following apicectomy and retrograde filling. Different authors have evaluated ruby, CO_2, Nd: YAG, Er: YAG, excimer and argon laser or combinations of different lasers and their effects upon soft and hard tissues, as well as on dental materials and instruments [47-50]. The main advantages of laser use in endodontic surgery in comparison to the conventional techniques are reduction in tissue trauma and lower risk of contamination [47].

Among all other lasers, Er: YAG laser has shown the greatest potential in periapical surgery application. This laser can be used in almost all steps of periradicular surgery: incision for flap lifting, bone removal, removal of granulation tissues, apex resection and retrograde cavity preparation because of its efficacy in soft tissue, bone and hard dental tissues removal.

Er: YAG laser was approved by the FDA (Food and Drug Administration) in 1997 and has been since used in dentistry. This laser has a wavelength of 2.940 nm which coincides with the peak of water absorption. The main principle of Er: YAG laser operation is that during laser irradiation, the energy delivered causes vaporization of water within a mineral substrate giving volume expansion and disruption of dental tissues by micro-explosions, with ejection of both organic and inorganic particles [51, 52]. There is also a small absorption at around 2.800 nm by the hydroxyl group of the hydroxyapatite, although water is the main absorber of laser energy. Regarding mineralized tissues, water is present among the crystals in enamel, dentin, bone and cementum in ascending quantity [53, 54].

Oral soft tissues also contain water and when healthy or minimally pigmented, wavelengths which are highly absorbed in water, like the wavelength of Er: YAG laser, will provide efficient ablation [55]. Er: YAG laser affects 10 to 50 microns thick layers in soft tissues which are important to avoid thermal damage to underlying periosteum and hard dental tissues which are vulnerable to excessive heat, especially in sites with thin oral mucosa [56, 57]. Er: YAG laser use for management of soft oral tissues is advantageous in comparison to scalpel as it provides better hemostasis [58, 59]. Hemostasis occurs due to tissue absorption of laser energy and controlled heating of the tissues, resulting in blood proteins coagulation and sealing of small blood vessels [60-62]. After surgical treatment, bacteria can cause infection and subsequent reduction of bacteria by using Er: YAG laser is also important. Several different mechanisms are responsible for bactericidal effect of the Er: YAG laser. High temperatures during laser irradiation cause changes in the cell wall and membrane of bacteria, denaturization of proteins and damage of nucleic acid which result in bacterial death via photothermal effects [63].

Photothermal effect after absorption of a laser beam in water also causes microexplosions and breakup of bacteria [64]. Yamaguchi [65] found that lipopolysaccharides in the cell membrane of Gram negative bacteria have peak value of absorption of 2.92 μm, which is close to the wavelength of the Er:YAG laser. Furthermore, it was also found that amines and amine groups which are present in bacteria also absorb the wavelength of the Er: YAG laser leading to bacterial death due to photochemical effects [66]. One study performed on the animals compared nociceptive response during Er: YAG laser oral tissue incision and scalpel incision and found less pain when the laser was used [67], which is promising. All these beneficial effects make Er: YAG laser a desirable tool for incision of soft oral tissues for endodontic surgery procedures. Besides the incision, Er: YAG laser may also be used for vaporization of granulation tissue.

Removal of bone by conventional drills in order to perform apicectomy increases the chance of thermal bone damage, causes bacterial decontamination and produces vibrations which are uncomfortable for the patient. Er: YAG laser enables bone ablation to be carried out with minimal thermal damage and the whole procedure is more convenient for the patient due to reduced vibration. In a study by Gabric Panduric [68] Er:YAG laser showed shorter preparation time, a lower heat generation, sharp edges of the preparation sites without bone fragments and minimal thermal alterations of the bone tissues in comparison to the surgical drill. Studies investigating healing of laser-ablated bone showed that the reduction of physical trauma, tissue heating and bacterial contamination may lead to uncomplicated healing processes when compared to conventional surgical methods [69-71]. When compared to the mechanical bur and CO_2 laser groups, Er:YAG irradiated bone tissue showed a more pronounced inflammatory cell infiltration, fibroblastic reaction and a faster revascularization adjacent to the irradiated bone surface with a significantly greater and more rapid bone neo-formation [70], all being desirable after surgical treatments.

Er: YAG laser is also efficient in hard dental tissue removal, namely enamel, dentin and cement. However, the lower ablation rates of the early Er: YAG lasers in comparison to the mechanical bur presented a limitation of their use in dental practice [72-74]. With development of new technology incorporated into Er: YAG laser system with high energies and low pulse durations, the speed of ablation is faster than the diffusion of heat into the tissue, enabling a cold and efficient ablation. Therefore, ablation rates even higher than those obtained with a mechanical handpiece can be achieved [75, 76]. After using different pulses of Er: YAG laser, dentin surface is irregular and clean, with open dentin tubules and no smear layer [76] which may enhance apical seal with modern retrograde filling materials. This makes Er: YAG laser suitable for both root-end resection and preparation.

Different studies have investigated the performance of Er: YAG laser in endodontic surgery. In comparison to Ho: YAG laser, Er: YAG laser produced smoother and cleaner surfaces in the resection area without any thermal damages [77]. Er: YAG laser was also superior in reduction of postoperative complaints and showed better wound healing in comparison to the ultrasound and diamond drills [78]. Another study also confirmed better postoperative healing with Er: YAG laser when compared to the traditional surgical techniques [79]. Cavities prepared with Er: YAG laser had significantly lower microleakage of different retrograde filling materials in comparison to the cavities prepared with ultrasonic [80]. In a study by Grgurevic [81], optimal settings for apicectomy with Er: YAG laser were 380 mJ/100 at microseconds/20 Hz and there was no difference in time needed for root resection in comparison to mechanical handpiece.

Beneficial effects of Er: YAG laser in periradicular surgery are attributed to biostimulatory effect and disinfection of the operating field which promote early healing [82], as well as stimulation of platelet-derived growth factor which enhances the healing of osteotomy sites [83]. Furthermore, Er:YAG laser enhances osteoblast proliferation through activation of the mitogen-activated protein kinase which helps promote healing in periodontal or implant sites [84].

Therefore, Er: YAG laser can be considered as a suitable method for periapical surgery (Figures 20 and 21) as it is an efficient and safe surgical method which ensures good post-operative healing.

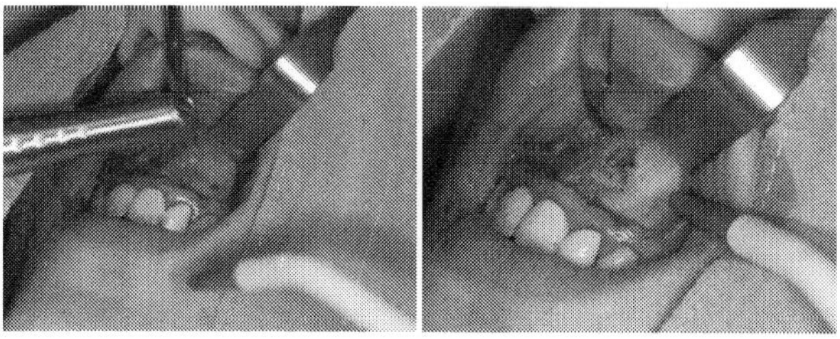

Figure 20. Use of Er: YAG laser for bone removal prior to apicectomy (X-Runner, QSP mode, 750 mJ, 10 Hz, 10 ml/min)

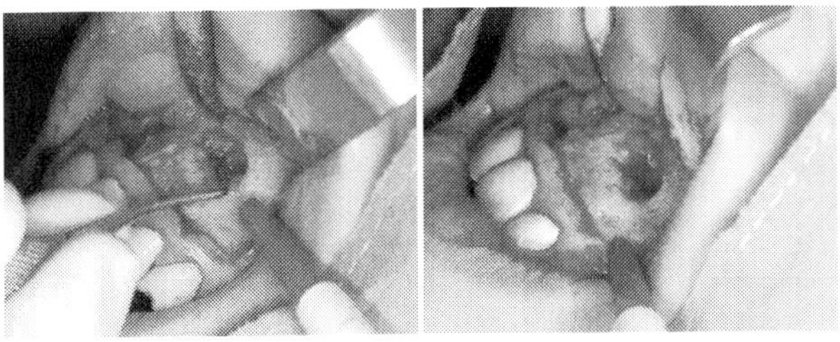

Figure 21. Laser-assisted apicectomy of the upper left central and lateral incisors (X-Runner, QSP mode, 750 mJ, 10 Hz, 10 ml/min)

6. Application of ER: YAG laser in bone surgery

Common instruments used for osteotomies in oral surgery are diamond or steel burrs, oscillating saws, chisels or mills [85, 86]. Despite the fact that they are considered a gold standard for bone osteotomies, these instruments have some disadvantages; they are used in contact with the bone tissue with some extent of grinding pressure causing increase of focal temperature, deposition of metal shavings, biomechanical stress, microfractures and dispersal of bony particles and debris into surrounding tissue and osteotomy walls. Bone fragments and fibrin like debris can be found which cover the osteotomy walls after drill instrumentation and can be contributing factor in the infection. The debris can interfere with the wound healing process thus impairing the adhesion of blood elements to the osteotomy walls [68, 86-89]. Hence, alternative methods have been developed for hard tissue surgery [90]. Continuous wave (CW) carbon dioxide (CO_2) laser was the first laser in oral surgery for soft tissue treatment which was introduced in the year 1964 [91]. Shortly after, the development and research of hard tissue laser assisted ablation began [92, 93]. Different types of high energy laser have been investigated, among which the Erbium: Yttrium-Aluminum-garnet (Er: YAG) laser demonstrated the most promising results [94-99]. Er: YAG emits at a wavelength 2.94 μm which has a high absorption in water and hydroxyl ions of hydroxyapatite [100- 102]. The water absorption coefficient of Er: YAG laser is 10 higher than the CO_2 lasers, and 15,000- 20,000 times higher than Nd: YAG lasers [103]. This high absorption rate enables bone ablation with minimal adjacent thermal damage, making Er: YAG lasers safe for use in oral surgical procedures [68, 104, 105, 106]. Erbium laser was the first dental laser cleared by the US Food and Drug Administration for use in cutting human teeth *in vivo* [107].

6.1. Removal of partially erupted third molars

The Er: YAG laser can be used successfully for third molar removal. Histological analyses found no signs of carbonization or charred surfaces which might lead to undisturbed bone healing. Another advantage of laser ablation was no bone particle or other kind of debris deposits found within the surgery site, absence of mechanical pressure and accurate cut geometry [68, 98, 105-121]. Higher percentage of patients found that the laser assisted surgery was more acceptable compared to the standard drill osteotomy which was explained by the absence of friction sound and vibration. On the other side, the laser osteotomy is more time consuming. Inadequate suction of operative field may lead to prolonged ablation time because increase in volume of irrigation fluid and blood slow down the laser ablation [121]. When a contact free handpiece was used, the ablation process was faster but the intraoral maneuverability of the articulated arm was more difficult, requiring additional care to ensure only ablation of the target tissues [121]. Prolonged treatment may be responsible for an elevated incidence of trismus and swelling in the patients treated with laser in comparison to the surgical bur [122]. Er: YAG lasers lack the feedback of depth control. Hence, in cases of tooth apex proximity to the inferior alveolar nerve, it is recommendable to finish the osteotomy using the surgical bur in order to prevent nerve damage [121].

6.2. Bone graft harvesting

The osteotomy for harvesting bone blocks plays an important role in the success of the bone grafting technique. Incorrect harvesting technique may cause mechanical and thermal damage with reduced or loss of bone vitality. When performed with classical surgical bur or oscillating saw, clinicians are faced with some limitations during bone block grafting due to the mechanical pressure and vibrations, accumulation of debris within the osteotomy lines and in the adjacent soft tissue as well as possible injury of adjacent vital structures. When Er:YAG contact free handpiece with variable squared pulse (VPS) was employed for bone block harvesting excellent results were obtained resulting in reasonable time necessary to finish the osteotomies (2 minutes for the chin bone block harvesting) [105, 114, 123]. The histological results obtained from the bone blocks specimens, showed sharp cutting edges (Figures 22 and 23) and vital bone containing osteocyte lacunae occupied with cells thus presenting normal osteocyte structural characteristics [124]. The anatomical situation in the distal part of the lower jaw limited the access of the laser handpiece preventing the maintenance of predetermined distance between bone surface and the handpiece. Furthermore, deficient aspiration led to water and blood accumulation which inhibited laser ablation because the accumulated fluid formed a protective layer against the laser beam. Afore mentioned reasons make the Er: YAG block osteotomy difficult or impossible in the ramus region [123]. On the other hand, the osteotomy in the symphysis area is straightforward, allowing control of the direction of laser beam and maintenance of predetermined distance. The procedure was much more comfortable for the patients owing to the absence of mechanical stress or vibrations. Lasers are less traumatic when ablating bone compared to surgical burs, hence less bleeding tendency can be observed (Figures 25-27). One major disadvantage of lasers is the lack of depth control which is time consuming and difficult in the ramus region. Periodontal probes can be used for controlling the osteotomy depth [123].

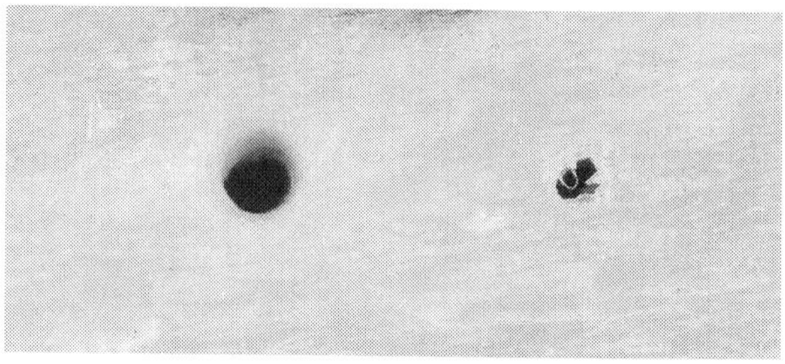

Figure 22. Macroscopic comparison of laser (left) and surgical drill (right) osteotomy (106)

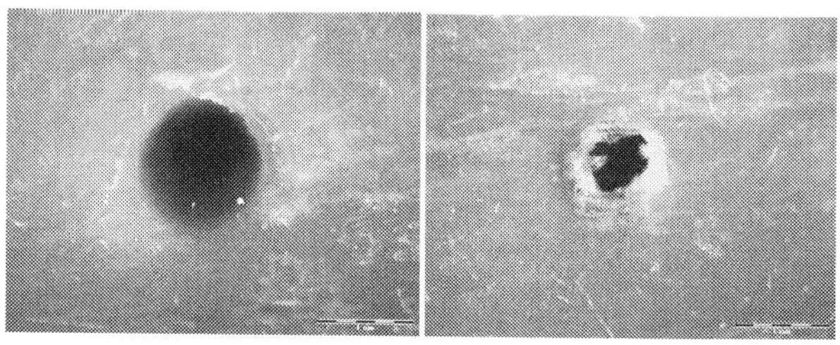

Figure 23. Light microscopy comparison of laser (left) and surgical drill (right) osteotomy (106)

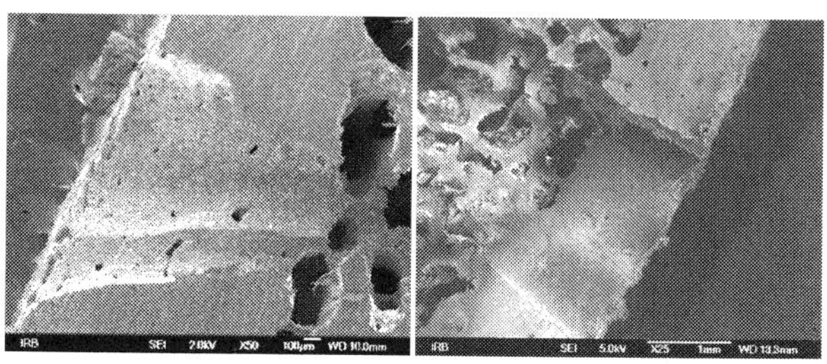

Figure 24. SEM (scanning electron microscopy) comparison of laser (left) and surgical drill (right) osteotomy (106)

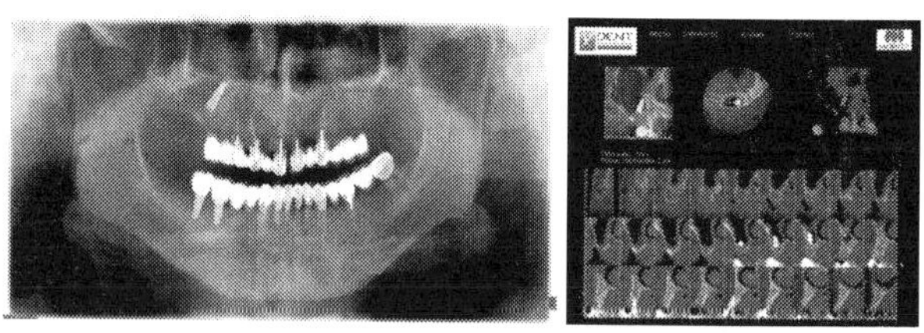

Figure 25. OPG and CBCT of the patient with dislocated dental implant in the right maxillary sinus, after transcrestal sinus floor elevation procedure

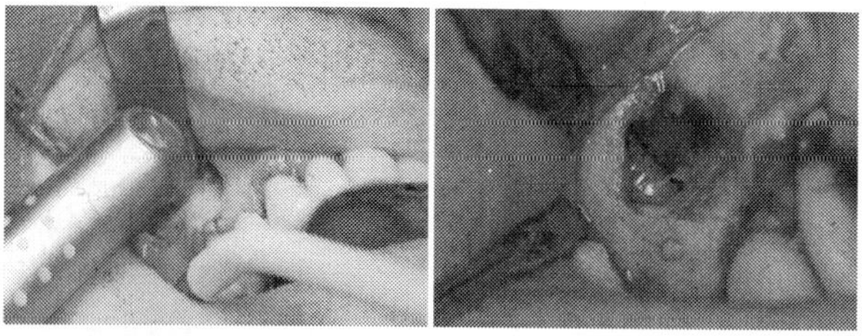

Figure 26. Removal of the cortical plate of the maxilla using Er: YAG laser (X-Runner, QSP mode, 750 mJ, 10 Hz, 10 ml/min) to show the implant within the sinus and to allow implant removal

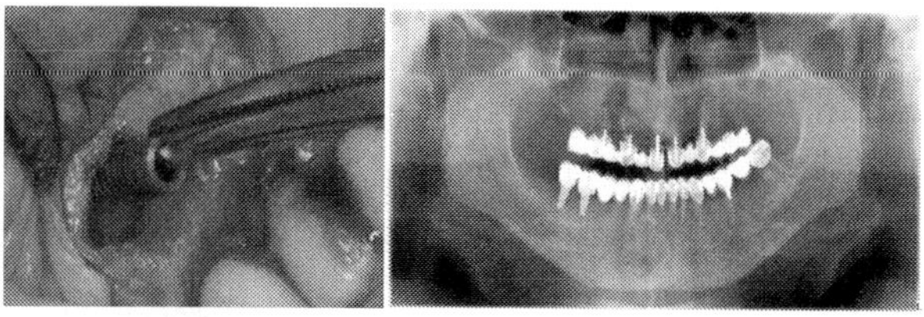

Figure 27. Removal of the implant after laser-assisted sinus surgery (left) and follow-up OPG 3 months after surgery (right)

6.3. Use of Er: YAG laser in the treatment of bisphosphonate-related osteonecrosis of the jaws

In the last decade, there has been an exponentially increasing number of bisphosphonate-related osteonecrosis of the jaws (BRONJ) reports; however its treatment still remains a dilemma. Promising results were accomplished using lasers in the therapy for BRONJ. Er: YAG laser therapy was used for ablation of necrotic bone [105, 83, 125, 126]. When the laser ablation was used in combination with low level laser therapy (LLLT) additional benefits were observed in terms of mucosal healing [83, 125]. Surgical sites treated with Er: YAG showed superior results when compared with traditional surgical treatment and remained stable for a mean follow-up period of 13 months [83]. Atalay [127] evaluated the use of Er:YAG laser (200 mJ, 20 Hz) using a fiber tip 1.3 mm in diameter and 12 mm in length in order to remove necrotic and granulation tissue from the area of avascular necrosis in 10 patients with BRONJ. Their findings [127] suggest that Er: YAG laser surgery is a beneficial alternative in the treatment of patients with BRONJ.

Laser ablation of oral hard tissues has progressively improved. Initial drawbacks, extensive thermal damage of the adjacent tissue, impaired haling and prolonged time necessary for laser osteotomy, were gradually resolved by development of Er: YAG laser with the pulse mode and water spray cooling. Numerous advantages associated with laser bone ablation lead to the fast and safe procedure resulting in the less trauma to the surrounding tissues. Some of these advantages are: minimal thermal damage to the bone, rapid osseous healing, precise cut geometry with regular shaped borders, absence of organic debris or metal shavings, reduced hard tissue bleeding, the possibility of operating with non contact handpiece, elimination of pressure and vibration from the procedure and decreased risk of injury to the adjacent tissues. Despite these advantages, routine use of Er: a YAG laser has not been established in clinical practice. Some factors which limit the everyday clinical application of lasers in bone ablation are: difficult access in the distal part of the lower jaw, inhibited laser ablation because the fluid accumulation in the deep parts of the surgical field and the lack of depth control. These issues are to be improved in the future. The main disadvantage of laser osteotomies is the inability to control the depth of the cut which my complicate the procedure.

7. Application of ER: YAG laser in dental implantology

7.1. Implant site preparation and second stage surgery

The bone preparation for implant site determines the beginning and the progression of bone healing and the subsequent success of osseointegration of the implant. Direct bone to implant contact (BIC) established without the interposition of non-bone or connective tissue is mandatory for successful osseointegration. Atraumatic bone ostetomy leads to less bone injury, less bone remodeling, better implant to bone contact and hence better implant stability in the early stage of healing [105, 115, 116] (Figures 28 and 29).

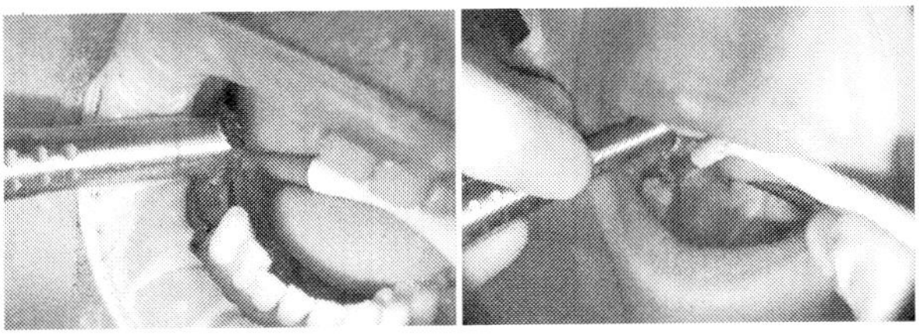

Figure 28. Er:YAG laser (LightWalker, Fotona, Slovenia) usage for preparation of the dental implant site in the lateral part of the right mandible; cortical bone – H02, SP mode, 1000 mJ, 20 Hz, 20 W, water 6, air 4; spongious bone – H14, SP mode, 600 mJ, 20 Hz, 12 W, water 6, air 2 (Courtesy of Dr. Jean Jacques Paverani)

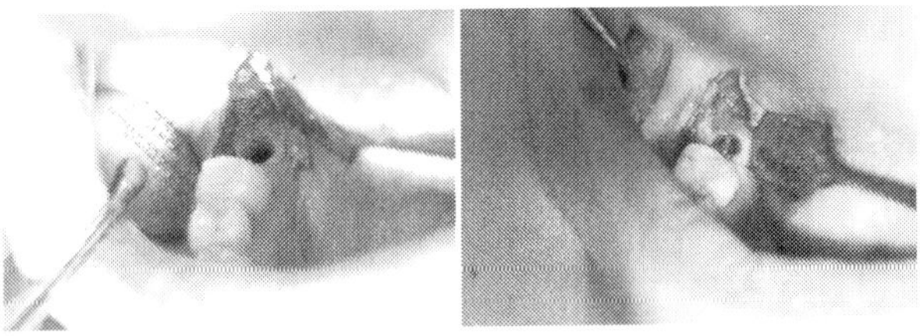

Figure 29. Implant site prepared using laser-assisted surgery (left) and dental implant inserted after laser preparation (right) (Courtesy of Dr. Jean Jacques Paverani)

Since the late 1990 different Er: YAG lasers were tested for implant bed preparation in numerous animal studies. The primary concern was how the thermally changed layer of bone tissue would affect the bone healing and osseointegration. All the authors demonstrated that osseointegration could be successfully achieved after Er: YAG implant bad bone preparation [117-120]. The carbonized amorphous tissue layer produced no irreversible damage and was progressively substituted with new bone in the first 2-12 weeks [118]. Significantly better bone-to-implant contact (BIC) was seen in the surgical drili group compared to the Er: YAG group within first two weeks. Afterwards the differences gradually disappeared and after 12 weeks they were not evident [119]. Some authors found even better results for Er: YAG group compared to the surgical drill group. Histological evaluation revealed higher BIC percentages in the laser prepared bone compared to the drill prepared bone after 3 weeks and 3 months of healing [120].

It can be concluded that Er:YAG laser ablation presents a promising tool for implant bed preparation and second stage surgery for dental implants exposure (Figures 30-32), but some major disadvantages limit the everyday clinical application: manual guided laser osteotomy resulted in a more imprecise osteotomy with a wide gap around implant. Prolonged time required for Er: YAG ablation compared to the surgical drill preparation caused by bleeding at the bottom of the osteotomy cavity can be a potential risk of accidental tissue damage [105].

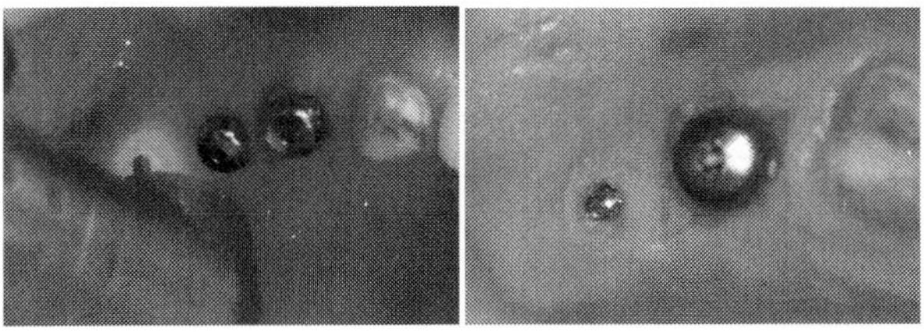

Figure 30. Second stage surgery using Er: YAG laser (X-Runner, QSP mode, 120 mJ, 20 Hz, 10 ml/min)

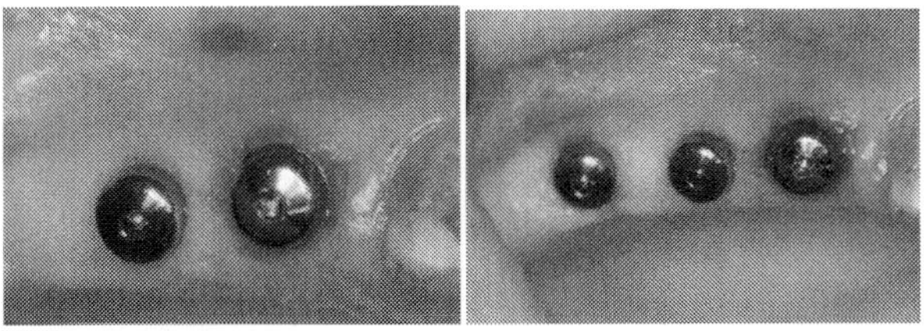

Figure 31. Comparison between Er: YAG laser (lateral implants) and scalpel for second stage surgery (first/mesial implant)

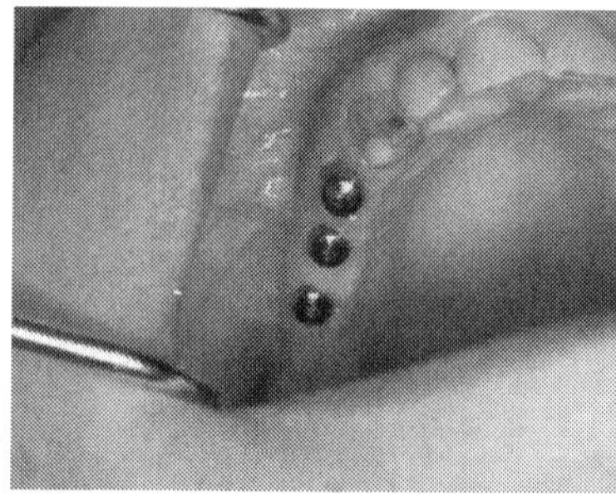

Figure 32. Follow-up healing evaluation 3 days after surgery, same patient.

7.2. Implant surface temperature changes during Er: YAG laser irradiation

It is known that Er: YAG lasers do not induce damage to the titanium implant surfaces when used within appropriate energies. The results of studies have showed that Er: YAG irradiation at 100 mJ/pulse and 10 pps for 60 seconds was safe for use on hydroxylapatite implant surfaces without any microscopic changes noticed. Furthermore, bacterial load on implant surfaces decreased up to 98%. It has been reported that energies exceeding 140-180 mJ/pulse result in implant surface alterations. Monzavi [10] used Er:YAG laser with a wavelength of 2.94 on the sheep model, energy output of 100 mJ/pulse, repetition rates of 10 pps and pulse duration of 230 μs delivered with a non-contact handpiece (4 mm above surface) for 60 seconds. However, Leja [128] reported that irradiation of Er: YAG laser on dental implants for 18 seconds increased the temperature up to 10°C. Fornaini [129] studied in an animal model thermal elevation induced by four different laser wavelengths (diode, Nd: YAG, Er: YAG, KTP) during implant uncovering. The same authors [129] reported that thermocouples recorded a lower increase in temperature for Er: YAG and KTP laser; Nd: YAG and diode lasers produced similar increase in temperature characterized by higher values. The thermo-camera pointed out lower increase for Er: YAG and higher for diode laser. KTP laser resulted in faster uncovering of the implants and diode laser was the one with which more time was needed for the same procedure. This *in vitro* study showed that laser utilization with the recommended parameters is without risk of dangerous thermal elevation to the tissues and implants [129]. Geminiani [9] concluded that irradiation of implant surfaces with CO_2 and Er: YAG lasers may produce a temperature increase above the critical threshold 10ºC after ten seconds of continuous irradiation. Galli [130] reported that Er:YAG laser at energy levels at 150 and 200 mJ/pulse at 10 Hz can alter the surface profile of titanium implants and that these changes may negatively affect the viability and the activity of osteoblastic cells. Therefore, the same authors [130] concluded that Er: YAG lasers should be used with caution on titanium surfaces. Shin [131] evaluated surface roughness and microscopic changes of irradiated dental implant surfaces *in vitro* after use of Er: YAG laser. Irradiation with Er: YAG laser led to the decrease in implant surface roughness that was not significant. The melting and fusion phenomenon of implant surfaces were observed with at all application times (1, 1.5 or 2 minutes) with 180 mJ/pulse irradiation. The sand-blasted, large-grit and acid-etched (SLA) surface implants are stable with laser intensities of less than

140 mJ/pulse and irradiation times less than 2 minutes. With SLA surfaces no significant change in surface texture could be found on any implant surface in the 100 and 140 mJ/pulse subgroups. The anodic oxidized surfaces were not stable with laser intensities of 100 mJ/pulse when Er: YAG laser was used to detoxify implant surfaces [131].

7.3. Implant surface microbial changes during Er: YAG laser irradiation

Tosun [132] examined CO_2, diode and Er:YAG laser irradiation on *Staphylococcus aureus* contaminated, sandblasted, large-grit, acid-etched surface titanium discs and concluded that complete or near complete elimination of surface bacteria on titanium surfaces can be accomplished *in vitro* by use of CO_2, diode and Er:YAG laser as long as appropriate parameters are used [132].

7.4. Treatment of peri-implantitis

In the published literature, there are several reports upon use of Er: YAG lasers for debridement which results in decontamination of implant surface in patients suffering from peri-implantitis [133-137]. As lasers use unidirectional light beams they gain better access to all implant surfaces in comparison to the manual curettes and ultrasonic tips. Furthermore, Er: YAG does not cause alterations of the implant surface. Also Er: YAG lasers are suitable for calculus elimination. Badran [138] used Er: YAG laser (energy 120 mJ; frequency 10 Hz) and sterile water irrigation for the treatment of severe peri-implantitis. Each site was irradiated with Er: YAG laser for 60 seconds, with a 10-15 degree working angulation during six weeks. The results of their study [138] showed that severe cases of peri-implantitis may be cured by use of Er: YAG laser. Fast healing, ease of use, bactericidal effect, effective ablation, hemostasis and adaptation with irregular implant surface are the main advantages of laser beam for treatment of peri-implantitis. Major side effects of laser application on metal objects inserted in the vital bone is thermal increase. Eriksson [139] demonstrated that increase of 10°C during 60 seconds leads to the permanent damage of bone tissues. Renvert [140] compared treatment of severe peri-implantitis either by use of air-abrasive or Er: YAG monotherapy. The same authors concluded that there were no differences between the bleeding on probing (BOP), periodontal pocket depth (PPD) and bone gain regarding the type of the aforementioned treatments [140]. Schwarz [141] reported that 4-year clinical outcomes obtained following combined surgical resective-regenerative therapy of advanced peri-implantitis were not influenced by the method of surface decontamination, i.e. Er: YAG laser or with plastic curettes/cotton pellets/ sterile saline. Taniguchi [137] concluded that optimized irradiation parameters effectively removed calcified deposits from contaminated titanium microstructures without causing substantial thermal damage. It seems that Er:YAG laser irradiation at pulse energies below 30 mJ/pulse (10.6 J/cm^2/pulse) and 30 Hz with water spray in near contact mode did not cause damage and resulted in effective debriding of the microstructure surfaces (except for anodized microstructures). Nevins [142] investigated use of Er:YAG laser in order to decontaminate complex rough surface of the implant by stripping the contaminated oxide laser for induction of hard and soft tissue adaptation to a compromised or failing implant. The results have shown that new bone-implant contact was established along the whole defect area without any evidence of inflammation.

8. Conclusion

Laser technology has made rapid progress over the past decades, and lasers have found a niche in many surgical specialties. Because of their many advantages, lasers have become indispensable in OMS as a additional modality for soft and hard tissue surgery. There are many uses for lasers in OMS, and the advent of new wavelengths will undoubtedly lead to new procedures that can be performed with laser technology. Practitioners should seek novel clinical approaches with a sound scientific basis. Despite the enthusiastic acceptance of this technology by professionals and the public, further research, including controlled clinical studies, to investigate the higher efficacy, as well as side effects of laser therapy, are still needed.

> *"The medical application of the laser is fascinating for two reasons. It is an optimistic mission, on the one hand, while on the other it counteracts the original impression of the laser being a death ray."*

Dr. Theodore Maiman, the inventor of the first laser

Acknowledgements

The authors are grateful to Fotona D.D. for technical support. We would like to thank our clinical photographers Mirjana Krajačić and Darije Petolas, and especially all employees of the Department of Oral Surgery and Department of Oral Medicine, School of Dental Medicine, University of Zagreb.

Author details

Dragana Gabrić[1*], Anja Baraba[2], Goran Batinjan[1], Marko Blašković[1], Vanja Vučićević Boras[3], Irina Filipović Zore[1], Ivana Miletić[2] and Elizabeta Gjorgievska[4]

*Address all correspondence to: dgabric@sfzg.hr

1 Department of Oral Surgery, School of Dental Medicine, University of Zagreb; University Dental Clinic, Clinical Hospital Center Zagreb, Zagreb, Croatia

2 Department of Endodontics and Restorative Dentistry, School of Dental Medicine, University of Zagreb; University Dental Clinic, Clinical Hospital Center Zagreb, Zagreb, Croatia

3 Department of Oral Medicine, School of Dental Medicine, University of Zagreb; University Dental Clinic, Clinical Hospital Center Zagreb, Zagreb, Croatia

4 Department of Pediatric and Preventive Dentistry, Faculty of Dentistry, University of Skopje, Macedonia

References

[1] Moshonov J, Stabholz A, Leopold Y, Rosenberg I, Stabholz A. Lasers in dentistry. Part B-Interaction with biological tissues and the effect on the soft tissues of the oral cavity, the hard tissues of the tooth and the dental pulp. Refuat Hapeh Vehashinayim 2001;18(3-4): 107-108.

[2] Fujii T, Bachni PC, Kawai O, Kwawkomi T, Matsuda K, Kowashi Y. Scanning electron microscopic study of the Er:YAG laser on root cementum. Journal of Periodontology 1998;69(11): 1283-1290.

[3] Simşek Kaya G, Yapici Yavuz G, Sümbüllü MA, Dayi E. A comparison of diode laser and Er:YAG lasers in the treatment of gingival melanin pigmentation. Oral Surgery Oral Medicine Oral Pathology Oral Radiology and Endodontology 2012; 113(3): 293-9.

[4] Komori T, Yokoyama K, Matsumoto Y, Matsumoto K. Erbium:YAG and holmium: YAG laser root resection of extracted human teeth. Journal of Clinical Laser Medicine Surgery 1997; 15(1): 9-13.

[5] Gouw-Soares S, Tanji E, Haypek P, Cardoso W, Eduardo CP. The use of Er:YAG, Nd:YAG and Ga-Al-As lasers in periapical surgery: a 3-year clinical study. Journal of Clinical Laser Medicine Surgery 2001;19(4): 193-198.

[6] Fisher SE, Frame JW, Browne RM, Tranter RM. A comparative histological study of wound healing following CO_2 laser and conventional surgical excision of canine buccal mucosa. Archives of Oral Biology 1983;28(4): 287-291.

[7] Schuller DE. Use of laser in the oral cavity. Otorhinolaryngology Clinics of North America 1990;23(1): 31-42.

[8] Kreisler M, Al Haj H, d'Hoedt B. Temperature changes at the implant-bone interface during simulated surface decontamination with an Er:YAG laser. International Journal of Prosthodontics 2002;15(6): 582-7.

[9] Geminiani A, Caton JG, Romanos GE. Temperature increase during CO_2 and Er:YAG irradiation on implant surfaces. Implant Dentistry 2011;20(5): 379-382.

[10] Monzavi A, Shahabi S, Fekrazad R, Behruzi R, Chiniforush N. Implant surface temperature changes during Er:YAG laser irradiation with different cooling systems. Journal of Dentistry 2014;11(2): 210-215.

[11] Mitsunaga S, Iwai T, Kitajima H, Yajima Y, Ohya T, Hirota M Cervicofacial subcutaneous emphysema associated with dental laser treatment. Australian Dental Journal 2013;58(4): 424-427.

[12] Onisor I, Pecie R, Cheskelis I, Krejci I. Cutting and coagulation during intraoral soft tissue surgery using Er:YAG laser. European Journal of Paediatric Dentistry 2013;14(2): 140-145.

[13] Kaya A, Ugurlu F, Basel B, Sener CB. Oral pyogenic granuloma associated with a dental implant treated with an Er:YAG laser: a case report. Journal of Oral Implantology 2013; doi: 10.1563/AAID-JOI-D-13-00251

[14] Türer CC, Ipek H, Kirtiloglu T, Acikgoz G. Dimensional changes in free gingival grafts: scalpel versus Er:YAG laser: a preliminary study. Lasers in Medical Science 2013; doi: 10.1007/s10103-013-1349-7

[15] Stelzle F, Terwey I, Knipfer C, Adler W, Tangermann-Gerk K, Nkenke E The impact of laser ablation on optical soft tissue differentiation for tissue specific laser surgery-an experimental ex vivo study. Journal of Translational Medicine 2012; doi: 10.1186/1479-5876-10-123

[16] Fikáčková H, Navrátilová B, Dylevský I, Navrátil L, Jirman R. Assessment of the effect of non invasive laser on the process of healing of an extraction wound by infrared thermography: preliminary study. Journal of Applied Biomedicine 2003; 1: 175–180.

[17] Lomke MA. Clinical applications of dental lasers. General Dentistry 2009; 57(1): 47-59.

[18] Namour, S. Atlas of current oral laser surgery. Florida, USA: Universal-Publishers Boca Raton;2011.

[19] Aras MH, Göregen M, Güngörmüş M, Akgül HM. Comparison of diode laser and Er:YAG lasers in the treatment of ankyloglossia. Photomedicine and Laser Surgery 2010; 2: 173-177.

[20] Koort HJ, Hopp M, Gabrić Pandurić D. A combined device for optimal soft tissue applicaions in laser dentistry. Laser 2013;5(4) 24-29.

[21] Merigo E, Clini F, Fornaini C, Oppici A, Paties C, Zangrandi A, Laser-assisted surgery with different wavelengths: a preliminary ex vivo study on thermal increase and histological evaluation. Lasers in Medical Science 2013; 28(2): 497-504.

[22] Fornaini C, Rocca JP, Bertrand MF, Merigo E, Nammour S, Vescovi P. Nd:YAG and diode laser in the surgical management of soft tissues related to orthodontic treatment and laser surgery. Photomedicine and Laser Surgery 2007; 25(5): 381-392.

[23] Tomov GT, Bachurska SY, Tashkova DA, Ivanov GP. Pathomorphological distinction between Er:YAG and diode lasers on the excisional biopsy of the oral mucosa. Russian Open Medical Journal 2013; 2(1): 107-111.

[24] van der Waal I. Potentially malignant disorders of the oral and oropharyngeal mucosa; present concepts of management. Oral Oncology 2010;46(6): 423-425.

[25] Lodi G, Porter S. Management of potentially malignant disorders: evidence and critique. Journal of Oral Pathology and Medicine 2008;37(2): 63-69.

[26] van der Waal I, Schepman KP, van der Meij EH, Smeele LE. Oral leukoplakia: a clinicopathological review. Oral Oncology 1997;33(5): 291–301.

[27] Gabrić Pandurić D, Katanec D, Filipović Zore I. Clinical cases of soft-tissue surgery with X-Runner in QSP mode. Journal of Laser and Health Academy 2013;2(2) 34-37.

[28] Brouns E, Baart J, Karagozoglu K, Aartman I, Bloemena E, van der Waal I. Treatment results of CO(2) laser vaporisation in a cohort of 35 patients with oral leukoplakia. Oral Diseases 2013;19(2): 212-216.

[29] Jerjes W, Upile T, Hamdoon Z, Al-Khawalde M, Morcos M, Mosse CA, Hopper C.CO2 laser of oral dysplasia: clinicopathological features of recurrence and malignant transformation. Lasers in Medical Science 2012;27(1): 169-179.

[30] Deppe H, Mücke T, Hohlweg-Majert B, Hauck W, Wagenpfeil S, Hölzle F. Different CO2 laser vaporization protocols for the therapy of oral precancerous lesions and precancerous conditions: a 10-year follow-up. Lasers in Medical Science 2012;27(1): 59-63.

[31] Roodenburg JL. Dissertations 25 years after date 29. CO2 laser surgery of leukoplakia of the oral mucosa. Nederlands Tijdschrift voor Tandheelkunde 2011;118(10): 496-500.

[32] Ergun S, Saruhanoglu A, Migliari DA, Maden I, Tanyeri H. Refractory pigmentation associated with Laugier-Hunziker syndrome following Er:YAG laser treatment. Case Reports in Dentistry 2013; doi: 10.1155/2013/561040.

[33] Friedman S. Treatment outcome and prognosis of endodontic therapy. In: Ørstavik D, Pitt Ford TR, eds. Essential endodontology: Prevention and treatment of apical periodontitis. Oxford: Blackwell Science; 1998.

[34] Ng YL, Mann V, Rahbaran S, Lewsey J, Gulabivala K. Outcome of primary root canal treatment: systematic review of the literature– Part 2: Influence of clinical factors. International Endodontic Journal 2008;41(1) 6–31.

[35] Rahbaran S, Gilthorpe MS, Harrison SD, Gulabivala K Comparison of clinical outcome of periapical surgery in endodontic and oral surgery units of a teaching hospi-

tal: A retrospective study. Oral Surgery Oral Medicine Oral Pathology Oral Radiology and Endodontology 2001;91(6) 700–709.

[36] Saunders WP. A prospective clinical study of periradicular surgery using mineral trioxide aggregate as a root-end filling. Journal of Endodontics 2008;34(6) 660–665.

[37] Tsesis I, Faivishevsky, Kfir A, Rosen E. Outcome of surgical endodontic treatment performed by a modern technique: a meta-analysis of the literature. Journal of Endodontics 2009;35(11) 1505–1511.

[38] Setzer FC, Shah SB, Kohli MR, Karabucak B, Kim S. Outcome of endodontic surgery: A meta-analysis of the literature –Part 1: Comparison of traditional root-end surgery and endodontic microsurgery. Journal of Endodontics 2010;36(11) 1757–1765.

[39] el-Swiah JM, Walker RT. Reasons for apicectomies. A retrospective study. Endodontics & Dental Traumatology 1996;12(4) 185–191.

[40] ESE/European Society of Endodontology: Consensus report of the European Society of Endodontology on quality guidelines for endodontic treatment. International Endodontic Journal 1994;27(3) 115-124.

[41] Tsesis I, Faivishevsky, Kfir A, Rosen E. Outcome of surgical endodontic treatment performed by a modern technique: a meta-analysis of the literature. Journal of Endodontics 2009;35(11) 1505–1511.

[42] Gilheany PA, Figdor D, Tyas MJ. Apical dentin permeability and microleakage associated with root end resection and retrograde filling. Journal of Endodontics 1994;20(1) 22–26.

[43] Hsu YY, Kim S. The resected root surface. The issue of canal isthmuses. Dental Clinics of North America 1997;41(3) 529–540.

[44] Wada M, Takase T, Nakanuma K, Arisue K, Nagahama F, Yamazaki M. Clinical study of refractory apical periodontitis treated by apicectomy – Part 1: Root canal morphology of resected apex. International Endodontic Journal 1998;31(1) 53–56.

[45] von Arx T, Walker WA. Microsurgical instruments for root-end cavity preparation following apicectomy: a literature review. Endodontics & Dental Traumatology 2000;16(2) 47–62.

[46] von Arx T, Kurt B, Ilgenstein B, Hardt N Preliminary results and analysis of a new set of sonic instruments for root-end cavity preparation. International Endodontic Journal 1998;31(1) 32-38.

[47] Bader G, Lejeune S. Prospective study of two retrograde endodontic apical preparations with and without the use of CO_2 laser. Endodontics & Dental Traumatology 1998;14(2) 75-78.

[48] Moritz A, Gutknecht N, Goharkhay K, Schoop U, Wemish J, Sperr W. The carbon dioxide laser as an aid in apicectomy: an in vitro study. Journal of Clinical Laser Medicine & Surgery 1997;15(4) 185-188.

[49] Kimura Y, Wilder-Smith P, Matsumoto K. Lasers in endodontics. A review. International Endodontic Journal 2000;33(3) 173-185.

[50] Gouw-Soares S, Tanji E, Haypek P, Cardoso W, Eduardo CP. The use of Er:YAG, Nd:YAG and Ga-Al-As lasers in periapical surgery: a 3-year clinical study. Journal of Clinical Laser Medicine & Surgery 2001;19(4) 193-198.

[51] Gurgan S, Kiremitci A, Cakir FY, Yazici E, Gorucu J, Gutknecht N. Shear bond strength of composite bonded to erbium:yttrium-aluminum-garnet laser-prepared dentin. Lasers in Medical Science 2009;24(1) 117-122.

[52] Hossain M, Nakamura Y, Yamada Y, Kimura Y, Nakamura G, Matsumoto K. Ablation depths and morphological changes in human enamel and entin after Er:YAG laser irradiation with or without water mist. Journal of Clinical Laser Medicine & Surgery 1999;17(3) 105-109.

[53] Meister J, Franzen R, Forner K, Grebe H, Stanzel S, Lampert F, Apel C. Influence of water content in dental on ablation with erbium YAG and erbium YSGG lasers. Journal of Biomedical Optics 2006;11(3) 34030.

[54] Wigdor H, Abt E, Ashrafi S, Walash JT Jr. The effect of lasers on dental hard tissues. Journal of American Dental Association 1993;124(2) 65-70.

[55] Coluzzi D. Fundamentals of dental lasers: Science and instruments. Dental Clinics of North America 2004;48(4) 751-770.

[56] Walsh JT Jr, Flotte TJ, Deutsch TF. Er:YAG laser ablation of tissue: Effect of pulse duration and tissue type on thermal damage. Lasers in Surgery and Medicine 1989;9(4) 314-326.

[57] Cobb C, Low SB, Coluzzi DJ. Lasers and the treatment of chronic periodontitis. Dental Clinics of North America 2010;54(1) 35-53.

[58] Ishikawa I, Aoki A, Takasaki AA. Potential applications of erbium:YAG laser in periodontics. Journal of Periodontal Research 2004;39(4) 275-285.

[59] Coluzzi DJ. Fundamentals of lasers in dentistry: Basic science, tissue interaction, and instrumentation. Journal of Laser Dentistry 2008;16(Spec. Issue) 4-10.

[60] Black JF, Barton JK. Chemical and structural changes in blood undergoing laser photocoagulation. Photochemistry and Photobiology 2004;80 89-97.

[61] Zhu D, Luo Q, Zhu G, Liu W. Kinetic thermal response and damage in laser coagulation of tissue. Lasers in Surgery and Medicine 2002;31(5) 313-321.

[62] Mordon S, Rochon P, Dhelin G, Lesage JC. Dynamics of temperature dependent modifications of blood in the near-infrared. Lasers in Surgery and Medicine 2005;37(4) 301-307.

[63] Wilson M. Photolysis of oral bacteria and its potential use in the treatment of caries and periodontal disease. The Journal of Applied Bacteriology 1993;75(4) 299-306.

[64] Ando Y, Aoki A, Watanabe H, Ishikawa I. Bactericidal effect of Erbium YAG laser on periodontopathic bacteria. Lasers in Surgery and Medicine. 1996;19(2) 190-200.

[65] Yamaguchi H, Kobayashi K, Osada R, Sakurabe E, Nomura T, Arai T, Nakamura J. Effects of irradiation of an erbium:YAG laser on root surfaces. Journal of Periodontology 1997;68(12) 1151-1155.

[66] Socrates G. Infrared and Raman Characteristics group frequencies: tables and charts, Chichester: John Wiley & Sons; 2001.

[67] Zeredo JL, Sasaki Km, Yozgatian JH, Okada Y, Toda K. Comparison of jaw-opening reflexes evoked by Er:YAG laser versus scalpel incisions in rats. Oral Surgery Oral Medicine Oral Pathol Oral Radiology and Endododontology 2005;100(1) 31-35.

[68] Gabrić Pandurić D, Bago I, Katanec D, Zabkar J, Miletić I, Anić I. Comparison of Er:YAG laser and surgical drill for osteotomy in oral surgery: an experimental study. Journal of Oral and Maxillofacial Surgery 2012;70(11) 2515-2521.

[69] Wang X, Ishizaki NT, Suzuki N, Kimura Y, Matsumoto K. Morphological changes of bovine mandibular bone irradiated by Er:YSSG laser: An in vitro study. Journal of Clinical Laser Medicine and Surgery 2002;20(5) 245-250.

[70] Pourzarandian A, Watanabe H, Aoki A, Ichinose S, Sasaki KM, Nitta H, Ishikawa I. Histological and TEM examination of early stages of bone healing after Er:YAG laser irradiation. Photomedicine and Laser Surgery 2004;22(4) 342-350.

[71] Donnell RJ, Deutsch RJ, Flotte RJ, Lorente CA, Tomford WW, Mankin HJ, Schomacker KT. Effect of Er:YAG laser on osteoinduction in demineralized rat calvarial allografts. Journal of Orthopaedic Research 1996;14(1) 108-113.

[72] Jelínková H, Dostálová T, Doležalová L, Krejsa O, Hamal K, Kubelka J, Prochazka S. Comparison of preparation speed of Er:YAG laser and conventional drilling machine. Lasers in Dentistry III. 1997; doi:10.1117/12.273573.

[73] Yamada Y, Hossin M, Nakamura Y, Suzuki N, Matsumoto K. Comparison between the removal effect of mechanical, Nd: YAG, and Er: YAG laser systems in carious dentin. Journal of Clinical Laser Medicine & Surgery 2001; 19(5) 239-243.

[74] Furtado Messias DC, de Souza-Gabriel AE, Palma-Dibb RG, Rodriguez AL, Campos Serra M. Efficiency and effectivness of Er: YAG laser on carious tissue renoval. Journal of Oral Laser Applications 2006; 6 181-186.

[75] Lukac M, Marincek M, Grad L, Bozic Z. Dental laser drilling: State of art with the latest of the Variable Square Pulse Erbium dental laser systems. Journal of the Laser and Health Academy 2007;6(1) 1-4.

[76] Baraba A, Miletić I, Jukić Krmek S, Perhavec T, Božić Ž, Anić I. Ablative potential of the Er:YAG laser and conventional handpieces: A comparative study. Photomedicine and Laser Surgery 2009;27(6) 921-927.

[77] Komori T, Yokoyama K, Matsumoto Y, Matsumoto K. Erbium:YAG and holmium:YAG laser root resection of extracted human teeth. Journal of Clinical Laser Medicine & Surgery 1997;15(1) 9–13.

[78] Zhao XY, Wang SM, Zhang CF. Root resection by Er:YAG laser: a scanning electron microscope study. Hua Xi Kou Qiang Yi Xue Za Zhi 2010;28(5) 526–528.

[79] Lietzau M, Smeets R, Hanken H, Heiland M, Apel C. Apicectomy using Er:YAG laser in association with microscope: a comparative retrospective investigation. Photomedicine and Laser Surgery. 2013;31(3) 110-115.

[80] Karlovic Z, Pezelj-Ribaric S, Miletic I, Jukic S, Grgurevic J, Anic I. Erbium:YAG laser versus ultrasonic in preparation of root-end cavities. Journal of Endodontics 2005;31(11) 821-823.

[81] Grgurević J, Grgurević L, Miletić I, Karlović Z, Jukić Krmek S, Anić I. In vitro study of the variable square pulse Er:YAG laser cutting efficacy for apicectomy. Lasers in Surgery and Medicine 2005;36(5) 347–350.

[82] Vescovi P, Manfredi M, Mergio E, Meleti M, Fornaini C, Rocca JP, Nammour S. Surgical approach with Er:YAG laser on osteonecrosis of the jaws (ONJ) in patients under bisphosphonate therapy (BPT). Lasers in Medical Science 2010;25(1) 101–113.

[83] Kesler G, Shvero DK, Tov YS, Romanos G. Platelet derived growth factor secretion and bone healing after Er:YAG laser bone irradiation. Journal of Oral Implantology 2011;37(Spec No) 195–204.

[84] Aleksic V, Aoki A, Iwasaki K, Takasaki AA, Wang CY, Abiko Y, Ishikawa I, Izumi Y. Low-level Er:YAG laser irradiation enhances osteoblast proliferation through activation of MAPK/ERK. Lasers in Medical Science 2012;25(4) 559–569.

[85] Stopp S, Deppe H, Lueth T. A new concept for navigated laser surgery. Lasers in Medical Science 2008;23(3) 261-6.

[86] Rupprecht S, Tangermann K, Kessler P, Neukam FW, Wiltfang J. Er:YAG laser osteotomy directed by sensor controlled systems. Journal of Craniomaxillofacial Surgery 2003;31(6) 337-42.

[87] Barone CM, Jimenez DF, Yule GJ, Strauch B. Analysis of bone formation after cranial osteotomies with a high-speed drill. Journal of Craniomaxillofacial Surgery 1997;8(6): 466-70.

[88] Kerawala CJ, Martin IC, Allan W, Williams ED. The effects of operator technique and bur design on temperature during osseous preparation for osteosynthesis self-tapping screws. Oral Surgery Oral Medicine Oral Pathology Oral Radiology and Endodontology 1999;88(2) 145-50.

[89] Kondo S, Okada Y, Iseki H, Hori T, Takakura K, Kobayashi A, Nagata H. Thermological study of drilling bone tissue with a high-speed drill. Neurosurgery 2000;46(5) 1162-8.

[90] Sulewski JG. Historical survey of laser dentistry. Dental Clinics of North America 2000;44(4) 717-752.

[91] Wlodawsky RN, Strauss RA. Intraoral laser surgery. Oral Maxillofacial Surgery Clinics of North America 2004;16(2) 149-163.

[92] Horch HH. Current status of laser osteotomy. Der Orthopade 1984;13(2):125-132.

[93] Clayman L, Fuller T, Beckman H. Healing of continuous-wave and rapid superpulsed, carbon dioxide, laser-induced bone defects. Journal of Oral Surgery 1978;36(12) 932-937.

[94] Peavy GM, Reinisch L, Payne JT, Venugopalan V. Comparison of cortical bone ablations by using infrared laser wavelengths 2.9 to 9.2 microm. Lasers in Medical Science 1999;25(5) 421-434.

[95] Bader C, Krejci I. Indications and limitations of Er:YAG laser applications in dentistry. American Journal of Dentistry 2006;19(3) 178-186.

[96] Bornstein ES, Lomke MA. The safety and effectiveness of dental Er:YAG lasers. A literature review with specific reference to bone. Dentistry Today 2003;22(10) 129-133.

[97] Buchelt M, Kutschera HP, Katterschafka T, Kiss H, Lang S, Beer R, Losert U. Er:YAG and Hol:YAG laser osteotomy: the effect of laser ablation on bone healing. Lasers in Surgery and Medicine 1994;15(4) 373-381.

[98] Sasaki KM, Aoki A, Ichinose S, Ishikawa I. Ultrastructural analysis of bone tissue irradiated by Er:YAG. Lasers in Surgery and Medicine 2002;31(5) 322-332

[99] Sasaki KM, Aoki A, Ichinose S, Yoshino T, Yamada S, Ishikawa I. Scanning electron microscopy and Fourier transformed infrared spectroscopy analysis of bone removal using Er:YAG and CO2 lasers. Journal of Periodontology 2002;73(6) 643-652.

[100] Iaria G. Clinical, morphological, and ultrastructural aspects with the use of Er:YAG and Er,Cr:YSGG lasers in restorative dentistry. General Dentistry 2008;56(7) 636-639.

[101] Convissar RA. The biologic rationale for the use of lasers in dentistry. Dental Clinics North America 2004;48(4) 771-794.

[102] Kang HW, Oh J, Welch AJ. Investigations on laser hard tissue ablation under various environments. Physics in Medicine and Biology 2008 ;53(12) 3381-3390.

[103] Schwarz F, Aoki A, Sculean A, Becker J. The impact of laser application on periodontal and peri-implant wound healing. Periodontology 2000. 2009; doi: 10.1111/j.1600-0757.2009.00301.x..

[104] Pandurić DG, Jurić IB, Musić S, Molčanov K, Sušić M, Anić I. Morphological and ultrastructural comparative analysis of bone tissue after Er:YAG laser and surgical drill osteotomy. Photomedicine and Laser Surgery 2014;32(7) 401-408.

[105] Stübinger S. Advances in bone surgery: the Er:YAG laser in oral surgery and implant dentistry. Clinical, Cosmetic and Investigational Dentistry 2010;2(1) 47-62.

[106] Gabrić Pandurić D. Physical and ultrastructural bone effect comparison between laser and surgical drill. PhD thesis. University of Zagreb; 2010.

[107] Cozean C, Arcoria CJ, Pelagalli J, Powell GL. Dentistry for the 21st century? Erbium:YAG laser for teeth. Journal of the American Dental Association 1997;128(8) 1080-1087.

[108] Nuss RC, Fabian RL, Sarkar R, Puliafito CA. Infrared laser bone ablation. Lasers in Surgery and Medicine. 1988;8(4) 381-391.

[109] Nanni C. Complications of laser surgery. Dermatology Clinics. 1997;15(3) 521-534.

[110] Walsh JT Jr, Deutsch TF. Er:YAG laser ablation of tissue: measurement of ablation rates. Lasers in Surgery and Medicine 1989;9(4) 327-337.

[111] de Mello ED, Pagnoncelli RM, Munin E, Filho MS, de Mello GP, Arisawa EA, de Oliveira MG. Comparative histological analysis of bone healing of standardized bone defects performed with the Er:YAG laser and steel burs. Lasers in Medical Science 2008;23(3) 253-260.

[112] Choi B, Welch AJ. Analysis of thermal relaxation during laser irradiation of tissue. Lasers in Surgery and Medicine 2001;29(4) 351-359.

[113] Yoshino T, Aoki A, Oda S, Takasaki AA, Mizutani K, Sasaki KM, Kinoshita A, Watanabe H, Ishikawa I, Izumi Y. Long-term histologic analysis of bone tissue alteration and healing following Er:YAG laser irradiation compared to electrosurgery. Journal of Periodontology 2009;80(1) 82-92.

[114] Stübinger S, Landes C, Seitz O, Sader R. Er:YAG laser osteotomy for intraoral bone grafting procedures: a case series with a fiber-optic delivery system. Journal of Periodontology 2007;78(12) 2389-2394.

[115] Sharawy M, Misch CE, Weller N, Tehemar S. Heat generation during implant drilling: the significance of motor speed. Journal of Oral and Maxillofacial Surgery 2002;60(10) 1160-1169.

[116] Wu X, Deng F, Wang Z, Zhao Z, Wang J. Biomechanical and histomorphometric analysis of the osseointegration of microscrews with different surgical techniques in

beagle dogs. Oral Surgery Oral Medicine Oral Pathology Oral Radiology and Endodontology 2008;106(5) 644-650.

[117] el-Montaser M, Devlin H, Dickinson MR, Sloan P, Lloyd RE. Osseointegration of titanium metal implants in erbium-YAG laser-prepared bone. Implant Dentistry 1999;8(1) 79-85.

[118] Salina S, Maiorana C, Iezzi G, Colombo A, Fontana F, Piattelli A. Histological evaluation, in rabbit tibiae, of osseointegration of mini-implants in sites prepared with Er:YAG laser versus sites prepared with traditional burs. Journal of long-term effects of medical implants 2006;16(2) 145-156.

[119] Schwarz F, Olivier W, Herten M, Sager M, Chaker A, Becker J. Influence of implant bed preparation using an Er:YAG laser on the osseointegration of titanium implants: a histomorphometrical study in dogs. Journal of Oral Rehabilitation. 2007;34(4) 273-281.

[120] Kesler G, Romanos G, Koren R. Use of Er:YAG laser to improve osseointegration of titanium alloy implants--a comparison of bone healing. International Journal of Oral & Maxillofacial Implants. 2006;21(3) 375-379.

[121] Stübinger S, von Rechenberg vB, Zeilhofer HF, Sader R, Landes C. Er:YAG laser osteotomy for removal of impacted teeth: clinical comparison of two techniques. Lasers in Surgery and Medicine 2007;39(7) 583-588.

[122] Abu-Serriah M, Critchlow H, Whitters CJ, Ayoub A. Removal of partially erupted third molars using an Erbium (Er):YAG laser: a randomised controlled clinical trial. British Journal of Oral & Maxillofacial Surgery. 2004;42(3) 203-208.

[123] Stübinger S, Nuss K, Landes C, von Rechenberg B, Sader R. Harvesting of intraoral autogenous block grafts from the chin and ramus region: preliminary results with a variablesquare pulse Er:YAG laser. Lasers in Surgery and Medicine. 2008;40(5) 312-318.

[124] Stübinger S, Ghanaati S, Saldamli B, Kirkpatrick CJ, Sader R Er:YAG laser osteotomy: preliminary clinical and histological results of a new technique for contact-free bone-surgery. European Surgical Research 2009;42(3) 150-156.

[125] Vescovi P, Merigo E, Meleti M, Manfredi M, Fornaini C, Nammour S. Surgical Approach and Laser Applications in BRONJ Osteoporotic and Cancer Patients. Journal of Osteoporosis 2012;doi:10.1155/2012/585434.

[126] Angiero F, Sannino C, Borloni R, Crippa R, Benedicenti S, Romanos GE. Osteonecrosis of the jaws caused by bisphosphonates: evaluation of a new therapeuticapproach using the Er:YAG laser. Lasers in Medical Science 2009;24(6) 849-856.

[127] Atalay B, Yalcin S, Emes Y, Aktas I, Aybar B, Issever H, Mandel NM, Cetin O, Oncu B. Bisphosphonate-related osteonecrosis: laser-assisted surgical treatment or conventional surgery? Lasers in Medical Science 2011; 26(6) 815-823.

[128] Leja C, Geminiani A, Caton J, Romanos GE. Thermodynamic effects of laser irradiation of implants placed in bone: an in vitro study. Lasers in Medical Science 2013;28(6) 1435-1440.

[129] Fornaini C, Merigo E, Vescovi P, Bonanini M, Antonietti W, Leoci L, Lagori G, Meleti M. Different laser wavelengths comparison in the second-stage implant surgery: an ex vivo study. Lasers in Medical Science 2014; doi: 10.1007/s10103-014-1623-3.

[130] Galli C, Macaluso GM, Elezi E, Ravanetti F, Cacchioli A, Gualini G, Passeri G. The effects of Er:YAG laser treatment on titanium surfce profile and osteoblastic cell activity: an in vitro study. Journal of Periodontology 2011; 82(8) 1169-1177.

[131] Shin Sl, Min HK, Park BH, Kwon YH, Park JB, Herr Y, Heo SJ, Chung JH. The effect of Er:YAG laser irradiation on the scanning electron microscopic structure and surface roughness of various implant surfaces: an in vitro study. Lasers in Medical Science 2011; 26(6) 767-776.

[132] Tosun E, Tasar F, Strauss R, Kivanc DG, Ungor C. Comparative evaluation of antimicrobial effects of Er:YAG, diode and CO_2 lasers on titanium discs: an experimental study. Journal of Oral and Maxillofacial Surgery 2012; 70(5): 1064-1069.

[133] Stubinger S, Homann F, Etter C, Miskiewicz M, Wjeland M, Sader R. Effect of Er:YAG, CO_2 and diode laser irradiation on surface properties of zirconia endosseous dental implants. Lasers in Surgery and Medicine 2008; 40(3): 223-228.

[134] Takasaki AA, Aoki A, Mizutani K, Kikuchi S, Oda S, Ishikawa I. Er:YAG laser therapy for peri-implant infection: a histological study. Lasers in Medical Science 2007; 22(3): 143-157.

[135] Sculean A, Schwarz F, Becker J. Anti-infective therapy with an Er:YAG laser: influence on peri-implant healing. Expert Review of Medical Devices 2005; 2(3): 267-276.

[136] Schwarz F, Sculean A, Rothamel D, Schwenzer K, Georg T, Becker J. Clinical evaluation of an Er:YAG laser for non-surgical treatment of peri-implantitis: a pilot study. Clin Oral Implants Research 2005; 16(1): 44-52.

[137] Taniguchi Y, Aoki A, Mizutani K, Takeuchi Y, Ichinose S, Takasaki AA, Schwarz F, Izumi Y. Optimal Er:YAG laser irradiation parameters for debridement of microstructured fixture surfaces of titanium dental implants. Lasers in Medical Science 2013; 28(4): 1057-1068.

[138] Badran Z, Bories C, Struillou X, Saffarzadeh A, Verner C, Soueidan A. Er:YAG laser in the clinical management of severe peri-implantitis: a case report. Journal of Oral Implantology 2013; 37:212-217.

[139] Eriksson AR, Albrektsson T. Temperature threshold levels for heat-induced bone tissue injury: a vital microscopic study in the rabbit. Journal of Prosthetic Dentistry 1983; 50(1):101-107.

[140] Renvert S, Lindahl C, Roos Jansaker AM, Persson GR. Treatment of peri-implantitis using an Er:YAG laser or an air-abrasive device: a randomized clinical trial. Journal of Clinical Periodontology 2011; 38(1) 65-73.

[141] Schwarz F, Hegewald A, John G, Sahm N, Becker J. Four-year follow-up of combined surgical therapy of advanced peri-implantitis evaluating two methods of surface decontamination. Journal of Clinical Periodontology 2013; 40(10) 962-967.

[142] Nevins M, Nevins ML, Yamamoto A, Yoshino T, Ono Y, Wang CW, Kim DM. Use of Er:YAG laser to decontaminate infected implant surface in preparation for reestablishment of bone to implant contact. International Journal of Periodontics and Restorative Dentistry 2014; 34(4) 461-466.

Section 14

Basics of Craniofacial Surgery

Chapter 35

Basics of Craniofacial Surgery

Hamid Mahmood Hashemi, Farnoush Mohammadi, Iman Tavakoli and Amirsalar Sayedyahossein

Additional information is available at the end of the chapter

http://dx.doi.org/10.5772/59966

1. Introduction

1.1. History

Craniofacial surgery includes a wide range of procedures in the face and cranium from congenital malformations such as orofacial clefts to traumatic deformities. Many scientists contributed to develop this field of surgery. Rene Le Fort was a French surgeon who discovered the lines of weakness in the facial skeleton. He classified the pattern of fractures through these lines into three categories known as LeFort 1, 2 and 3.[1] Gillies was the first surgeon who performed Le Fort 3 osteotomy for a patient with Crouzon or Pfeiffer syndrome, but the result was not satisfactory.[2] Tessier accomplished LeFort 3 osteotomy in a different and of course a more accurate way for a child with Crouzon's syndrome.[3] The presentation of this surgery had a great influence on this remarkable field and become a turning point in craniofacial surgery. Tessier introduced different approaches to the craniofacial skeleton such as transcranial approach to the orbital hypertelorism, transconjunctival approach to the orbital floor or development of subperiosteal facelift technique.[1]-[3] He is named the father of craniofacial surgery. During the years much progress has been made in this field. Refined surgical techniques and instruments, new imaging techniques like 3D computed tomography(CT) scan has had a great impact on craniofacial surgery, not only in diagnosis of craniofacial anomalies but also in treatment planning of surgery. Stereolithic models are 3D printing models which can replicate the actual shape of the defect. These models facilitate reconstruction of prosthesis; they can help in determining the site of insertion of prosthesis or the correct position of the plates or devices like distraction osteogenesis.

2. Craniofacial anomalies

Craniofacial anomalies (CFA) include different dysmorphogenic conditions in this region of the body. People with these anomalies generally have problems not only in function but also with their ordinary life in the society. These people, especially children with CFA have less social competence and lack of self-esteem. The aim of craniofacial surgery is to give a normal appearance to the patients. Specialized centers would be a great help in treating patients with CFA. Accurate data of epidemiology of CFA is of utmost importance for managing and treatment of patients.

Cleft lip and palate are the most common congenital anomalies which affect the orofacial region. The incidence of oral clefts in United States is 1 in 700 births.[4] Orofacial clefts are more common in boys but cleft palate without cleft lip have a slight tendency to involve girls. One fourth of oral clefts are bilateral and the rest are unilateral. In unilateral cases the left side is affected more frequently.

Craniosynostosis means premature fusion of cranial vault sutures. There are six major cranial vault sutures. Any of these sutures can be affected in craniosynostosis, alone or in combination with other sutures. In this section we discuss the prevalence of nonsyndromic single suture synostosis.

Sagittal suture synostosis or scaphocephaly is the most common single suture synostosis with the prevalence of 1 in 5000 live births. [5] Boys are affected three times more frequently than girls.

Coronal suture synostosis or anterior plagiocephaly is the second most common single suture synostosis. The prevalence is approximately 1 in 10000 births. [6]

Metopic suture craniosynostosis or trigoncephaly is an unusual type of synostosis with an approximate prevalence of 1 in 15000. [7]

Lambdoid suture synostosis or posterior plagiocephaly is a rare entity with a prevalence of 1 in 150000 live births. [8]

Bilateral coronal suture craniosynostosis or brachycephaly is also rare.

3. Craniofacial pathology

Pathology includes any deviations from normal function and structure. The pathologic conditions show themselves as aplastic, hypoplastic, hyperplastic, neoplastic, traumatic or developmental entities. In craniofacial pathology a good access to the lesion and preservation of vital structures are important factors in a successful operation. Most operations in this field should be carried out in a team work manner engaging both the maxillofacial surgeon and the neurosurgeon.

http://dx.doi.org/10.5772/59966

3.1. Fibrous dysplasia

Fibrous dysplasia is a benign fibro-osseous lesion. Fibro-osseous lesions are a category of entities in which normal bone tissue is replaced with fibrous and mineralized tissue. In fibrous dysplasia normal bone is substituted with cellular fibrous tissue and immature bone.[9]

In most of cases it is monostotic involving a single bone.[10] The rate of growth is very slow. The maxilla and frontal bone are the most affected sites.[11] The most common feature is painless swelling. Radiographic feature of ground glass is of significant importance for diagnosis. This pattern is due to superimposition of disorganized poorly calcified bone trabecular.

Polyostotic Fibrous dysplasia is uncommon. In syndromic conditions like Jaffe-Lichtenstein, McCune-Albright and Mazabraud syndromes, polyostotic fibrous dysplasia forms an important part of these syndromes.

Treatment of fibrous dysplasia depends on the degree of functional or cosmetic impairment from shaving of involved area to resection. The aim is not to remove the entire lesion but to have an acceptable appearance. Regrowth after surgical reduction is unpredictable.

3.2. Sarcoma

One of the most important issues in morbidity and mortality of children is malignant neoplasms.[12] One third of malignant solid tissue tumors during infancy and childhood are caused by sarcomas.[13] The most common sarcoma in children is rhabdomyosarcoma and after that fibrosarcoma.[14] For management of rhabdomyosarcoma, radiotherapy and chemotherapy in combination with surgery are recommended in accessible tumors by many authors.

3.3. Lymphoma

Malignant lymphoid tissue tumors are common in head and neck region. There are different types of classification for lymphoma but separation to Hodgkin and non- Hodgkin types is the most common. Both have manifestations in the head and neck area. In Africa, another type of this condition known as Burkitt's lymphoma is common in children. Surgery is usually not indicated and chemotherapy should be done by an oncologist.

3.4. Melanoma

Approximately 20% of melanomas occur in head and neck regions.[15] An important etiologic factor is excessive exposure to ultraviolet light but many risk factors have been proposed in development of this lethal entity. Most of them arise from pigmented lesions. Melanoma can be categorized to superficial spreading, nodular, lentigo maligna, acral lentigenous and desmoplastic type according to clinical and histological evaluations. Excision of the lesion is the treatment of choice. Elective lymph node dissection is a controversial matter.

4. Nonsyndromic craniosynostosis

The pathophysiology of malformed skulls was described in the 18th century. It was reported that "bony expansion ceases in a direction perpendicular to the synostosed suture with compensatory expansion in the opposite direction." This is called the Virchow's law. Early closure of cranial sutures is termed as craniosynostosis which can be categorized to syndromic and non-syndromic synostosis. The latter is the main point of concern of this chapter.

4.1. Anterior plagiocephaly

Plagiocephaly is simply the Greek synonym for slanted head. It is reported in 5% to 25 % of deliveries. It can be associated with external forces or synostosis. Those associated with external forces are deformational and are commonly the result of compressive forces applied by the maternal pelvis to the head of the fetus which is more common on the left side. Anterior plagiocephaly can be due to unilateral coronal synostosis (UCS). This is almost nonsyndromic but can be seen in a familial feature relating to a mutation in fibroblast growth factor receptor gene. A surgical approach to treat this condition is basically to decompress the intracranial pressure which can itself cause brain damage and ophthalmic consequences due to optic atrophy. The superior forehead and superior orbital region is the main affected site. The ipsilateral superior orbital rim is displaced superiorly and nasal root is displaced to the problematic side. Presurgical radiological evaluation of the patient is best carried out by 3D CT scans which are available now and a multidisciplinary approach involving pediatric craniofacial surgeon, pediatric neurosurgeon, ophthalmologist and radiologist is necessary.

The surgical technique presented by Posnick is based on removing, reshaping and reassembling the cranial vault and bilateral three-quarter orbital osteotomies. The procedure is started by a postauricular coronal incision with wide subperiosteal dissection anteriorly to bilateral infraorbital rim regions and superior of the zygomatic bone and maxilla and posteriorly half way from the coronal to lambdoid suture. Bilateral lateral canthotomy is carried out. Frontal bone is removed from the preferred marked lines then the osteotomy is carried out including orbital roof, superior aspect of orbital medial wall, lateral orbital wall and lateral side of inferior orbital floor to the inferior orbital fissure.

4.2. Trigonocephaly

The prevalence of this type of craniosynostosis is 1 in every 15000 newborns. This results from early closure of the metopic suture which makes a triangular shape deformity of anterior cranial vault and anterior cranial base and orbits presents with orbital dystopia. Correction of the position of the superior and lateral orbital rims is the main concern in trigonocephalic patients. Beside the esthetic considerations, preventing the increase in intracranial pressure in growth is an important indication for surgical intervention.

If there is no sign of deficits due to increased intracranial pressure then it is recommended to postpone the surgical intervention 9 to 11 months of infant age. This supports the fact that at

http://dx.doi.org/10.5772/59966

that age most of the brain growth is done and the outcome is less dependent on brain growth. Also better bony reshaping can be performed and hemodynamic concerns at the time of surgery are more controllable.

It is obvious that every surgical treatment plan should be programmed based on the individual characteristics of the deformity but a general surgical approach involves releasing of the metopic suture and also osteotomies of the anterior cranial vault, temporal and three-quarter orbital osteotomies. A postauricular coronal incision with subperiosteal dissection is carried out. Bilateral lateral canthotomy is performed. Frontal craniotomies are performed by the neurosurgeon considering the retraction of frontal and temporal lobes and remaining anterior to the olfactory bulbs. Orbital osteotomies are done including orbital roof and lateral aspect of orbital floor to the inferior orbital fissure. For better correction of the orbital segment a vertical split osteotomy can be done in the midline to separate sides from each other. Temporal osteotomy can then be performed and reshaping, repositioning and reassembling of frontal bone in strip figures are done.

Bony gaps can be filled with autogenous grafts and segments are fixed by means of screws and microplates.

4.3. Scaphocephaly

Early closure of the sagittal suture which makes the calvarium grow more in the anteroposterior direction is called scaphocephalia. This leads to a more prominent frontal and occipital region. This condition is seen in 1 in every 5000 births. Like other synostotic conditions increased intracranial pressure and hydrocephalus are points of concern. It is accepted that craniotomies can at least release the external pressure on the brain. Papilledema and optic atrophy are other possible situations related to synostotic conditions that can lead to blindness.

There can be 3 types of scaphocephalia depending on the location of synostosis along the sagittal suture. If the anterior portion is involved in synostosis then posterior projection and prominence of the skull occurs. If posterior parts of the suture gets involve then anterior skull projection is seen and there is a condition when the whole suture is synostotic that leads to a more significant growth of the skull in the anteroposterior direction. Again it is recommended that surgical intervention occurs at 9 to 11 months of age supporting the concept that it is the age that most of brain tissue growth has occurred and bony tissue can be reshaped easier and estimated blood loss during the operation is a lesser challenge.

The general concept in the surgical approach which is done again by a post auricular coronal approach is to remove the sagittal suture and portions of temporal bone then reshaping the segments in a manner to decrease the anteroposterior projection while increasing the biparietal length. Dissections are carried out anteriorly to the periorbital regions and posteriorly to the occipital prominence of the skull. Craniotomies are done and brain tissue is retracted gently to allow the surgeon to have access for orbital osteotomies. Strip portions of bone are reshaped in an individualized manner to correct the deformity.

4.4. Brachycephaly

Brachycephaly is the Greek synonym for short headedness, occurs in bilateral coronal synostosis. This condition can be seen in some syndromes like Crouzon, Apert and Pfeiffer. In syndromic conditions other synostoses can be seen like in cranial base and upper face that leads to concave facial profile, proptosis and midface deficiency. In non-syndromic conditions no midface deficiency is present. Forehead height is apparently increased and the orbits are retruded and widened. The general concept in surgical approach is to increase the cranial capacity and therefore decrease the intracranial pressure preventing brain damage and conditions like hydrocephalus. Beside the esthetic concerns these conditions if left untreated may lead to ophthalmic deterioration and even blindness.

Again like other synostotic conditions the forehead and upper parts of the orbit are the center of concern for reconstruction. In these patients the forehead has a retruded position. In a normal condition the eyebrows are slightly more projected anteriorly comparing to the globes in contrast to brachiocephalic patients whose forehead and upper orbital rims have a retruded position. Here an anterior coronal flap is preferred because the malformed bony parts are located in the anterior skull region. Subperiosteal dissection anteriorly to periorbital region and posteriorly halfway between coronal and lambdoid sutures is carried out. As was said before the aim is to remove the synostotic and bad shaped bony parts and reshaping and reassembling them in a new position to correct the deformity. Osteotomies of the frontal and temporal bone are done as well as osteotomies of the orbital roofs. A vertical osteotomy should be carried out in the midline to help reduce the width of the superior orbital parts. In all the dissections in any form of cranial synostosis where lateral canthotomy is performed, at the end of operation lateral canthopexies are done using wire sutures.

5. Distraction osteogenesis

This method increases the length of bone by means of gradual distraction. Distraction techniques provide circumstances to achieve large advancements in craniofacial anomalies. Not only lengthening of the skeleton but also distracting the overlying soft tissue occurs with this technique. Because of this fact, some prefer to use the term "distraction histogenesis" than distraction osteogenesis. Ilizarov a Russian orthopedic surgeon published the first case series of DO for limb lengthening.[16] The first reports of mandibular lengthening by DO were reported by Molina and McCarthy.[17],[18] Since that time DO has been used for patients with various craniofacial deformities. Advantages of DO include achieving large advancements, obviating bone grafting and lesser risk of relapse than conventional osteotomies. We may however, encounter some problems. Higher rates of postoperation infection than conventional osteotomy, difficulty in control of vector direction, nonunion or malunion of the surgical site are disadvantages of this method.

The procedure of DO entails a corticotomy at the site where the device would be placed. During the procedure special consideration should be given to protection of periosteum. Minimal disturbance of the periosteum is an important matter in success of DO.[4] The aim of this step

http://dx.doi.org/10.5772/59966

is to provide an environment for remodeling and growth of the bone without significant tissue damage or vascular supply insufficiency. Corticotomy and device placement cause tissue damage like other surgical procedures. A latency period is needed for inflammatory mediators and subsequent inflammation to subside. This period ranges from 0 to 10 days depending on the age of the patient and conditions of the surgical site. After this period, distraction phase begins. Distraction rate is approximately 1mm per day. Soft tissue matrix covering the bone is distracted with this rate of traction. The term distraction histogenesis can describe this phenomenon better than distraction osteogenesis. Distraction at a higher rate may result in malunion or nonunion of involved bone and distraction at a lower rate will cause bone healing without any changes in length of the bone. After distraction, consolidation begins. Time lapse for this phase ranges from 3 months to 6 months depending on the amount of advancement, age of the patient and the type of deformity. Consolidation phase can be confirmed with radiography.[19]

5.1. Mandibular distraction osteogenesis

In severe mandibular retrognathia DO is indicated. This condition can be acquired or congenital. Congenital mandibular retrognathia includes craniofacial anomalies such as Treacher-Collin's syndrome, Pierre Robin sequence and hemifacial microsomia. Acquired anomalies include traumatic events to the mandible such as condylar fractures in young children in which ankylosis of the temporomandibular joint and subsequently, retardation of mandibular growth occur.[19], [20]

5.2. Maxillary distraction osteogenesis

Midface deficiency can occur in a variety of syndromic and nonsyndromic patients. In cleft patients, post-surgical scar tissue causes retardation in maxillary growth. Because of scar tissue formation, Le Fort advancement with conventional osteotomy and rigid fixation are not appropriate for these patients. Difficulty in mobilization of the maxilla and a tendency to relapse are the major concerns in these cases with conventional osteotomy.[21], [22] Craniofacial syndromes like Apert, Crouzon or Pfeiffer's syndromes show different degrees of paranasal hypoplasia. Midface advancement at the Le Fort 1 or 3 levels with DO technique is a good method for large advancements. Lower rate of relapse is another advantage of this technique.

5.3. Cranial vault distraction osteogenesis

Conventional treatment for patients with craniosynostosis is an aggressive dismantling of the cranial vault. A high rate of morbidity and even mortality in some cases is of major concern in these patients. Recently, corticotomy of the cranial vault and slow distraction with DO has shown new horizons in correction of calvarial deformities. Although some advantages like decreasing morbidity or reducing scar formation are mentioned for distraction techniques, its disadvantages cannot be ignored.[23], [24] A 3D deformity cannot be corrected with a unidirectional force. However, accurate selection of position of the appliance and prebending it as much as possible may be helpful.

Author details

Hamid Mahmood Hashemi*, Farnoush Mohammadi, Iman Tavakoli and Amirsalar Sayedyahossein

*Address all correspondence to: hamid5212@yahoo.com

Tehran University of medical sciences Tehran, Iran

References

[1] Le Fort R. Etude expérimentalsur les fractures de la machoiresupérieure 1901

[2] Gillies HD, Millard DR. The principles and art of plastic surgery. Boston, little, brown, 1995.

[3] Tessier P. The definitive plastic surgical treatment of the severe facial deformities of craniofacial dysostosis. Crozoun's and Apert's diseases. PlastReconst Surg. 1971;48: 419-442

[4] Jones C: The genetics of cleft lip and palate: information for families, Chapel Hill, NC, 2000, Cleft Palate Foundation.

[5] Lajeunie E, Le Merrer M, Bonaïti-Pellie C, Marchac D, Renier D. Genetic study of scaphocephaly.Am J Med Genet. 1996;62(3):282-5

[6] Cohen MM Jr.An etiologic and nosologic overview of craniosynostosis syndromes.Birth Defects Orig Artic Ser. 1975;11(2):137-89.

[7] Lajeunie E, Le Merrer M, Marchac D, Renier D.Syndromal and nonsyndromal primary trigonocephaly: analysis of a series of 237 patients. Am J Med Genet. 1998;75(2): 211-5.

[8] Cohen MM Jr.Craniosynostosis update 1987.Am J Med Genet Suppl. 1988;4:99-148.

[9] Daves MI, Yurdley JH. Fibrous dysplasia of bone. Am J Med Sci. 1957 Nov;234(5): 590-606.

[10] Fries JW. The roentgen features of fibrous dysplasia of the skull and facial bones; a critical analysis of thirty-nine pathologically proved cases. Am J Roentgenol Radium TherNucl Med. 1957; 77(1):71-88.

[11] Firat D, Stutzman L. Fibrous dysplasia of the bone. Review of twenty-four cases. Am J Med. 1968 Mar;44(3):421-9.

[12] Anderson GJ, Tom LW, Womer RB, et al. Rhabdomyosarcoma of the head and neck in children. Arch Otolaryngol Head Neck Surg. 1990;116:428-31

[13] Enneking WF: Reticuloendothelial lesions. In musculoskeletal tumor surgery. New York, Churchill-Livingstone, 1983, p1345.

[14] Schuller DE, Lawrence TL, Newton WA Jr. Childhood rhabdomyosarcomas of the head and neck. Arch Otolaryngol.1979 ;105:689-94.

[15] Rigel DS. Epidemiology and prognostic factors in malignant melanoma. Ann Plast Surg. 1992 ;28:7-8.

[16] Ilizarov GA.The principles of the Ilizarov method. 1988. Bull HospJt Dis. 1997;56(1): 49-53

[17] McCarthy JG, Schreiber J, Karp N, et al. Lengthening the human mandible by gradual distraction.PlastReconstr Surg. 1992;89(1):1-8

[18] Molina F, Ortiz Monasterio F. Mandibular elongation and remodeling by distraction: a farewell to major osteotomies.PlastReconstr Surg. 1995;96(4):825-40

[19] Choi IH, Shim JS, Seong SC, et al. Effect of the distraction rate on the activity of the osteoblast lineage in distraction osteogenesis of rat's tibia. Immunostaining study of the proliferating cell nuclear antigen, osteocalcin, and transglutaminase C. Bull HospJt Dis. 1997;56(1):34-40

[20] Walker D. Management of severe mandibular retrognathia in the adult patient using distraction osteogenesis. J Oral Maxillofac Surg. 2002;60(11):1341-6

[21] Yadav R, Bhutia O, Shukla G, et al. Distraction osteogenesis for management of obstructive sleep apnoea in temporomandibular joint ankylosis patients before the release of joint. J Craniomaxillofac Surg. 2014 Jul;42(5):588-94.

[22] Gateno J, Engel ER, Teichgraeber JF, et al. A new Le Fort I internal distraction device in the treatment of severe maxillary hypoplasia. J Oral Maxillofac Surg. 2005;63(1): 148-54.

[23] Houston WJ[1], James DR, Jones E, et al. Le Fort I maxillary osteotomies in cleft palate cases. Surgical changes and stability. J Craniomaxillofac Surg. 1989;17(1):9-15.

[24] Yonehara Y, Hirabayashi S, Sugawara Y, et al. Complications associated with gradual cranial vault distraction osteogenesis for the treatment of craniofacial synostosis. J Craniofac Surg. 2003;14(4):526-8.